Diagnosis and Management of the Hospitalized Child

Diagnosis and Management of the Hospitalized Child

Howard B. Levy, M.D.
Chairman, Department of Pediatrics
Mt. Sinai Hospital Medical Center, and
Chairperson, Joint Program in
Pediatric Nephrology
Mt. Sinai Hospital and Rush Presbyterian
St. Lukes Hospital, and
Associate Professor of Pediatrics
Rush Medical College
Chicago, Illinois

Stephen H. Sheldon, D.O.
Director, Division of Educational
Development and Systems Research, and
Assistant Professor of Pediatrics
and Preventive Medicine
Rush Medical College
Chicago, Illinois

Rabi F. Sulayman, M.D.
Program Director, Department of Pediatrics
Christ Hospital; and
Associate Professor of Pediatrics
Rush Medical College
Chicago, Illinois

Raven Press ■ New York

Raven Press, 1140 Avenue of the Americas, New York, New York 10036

Made in the United States of America

Library of Congress Cataloging in Publication Data

Levy, Howard B.
   Diagnosis and management of the hospitalized child.

   Bibliography: p.
   Includes index.
   1. Pediatrics—Handbooks, manuals, etc.   2. Children—
Hospital care—Handbooks, manuals, etc.   I. Sheldon, Stephen H.
II. Sulayman, Rabi F.   III. Title.   [DNLM:
1. Diagnosis—In infancy and childhood—Handbooks.
2. Pediatrics—Handbooks.   WS 39 S544d]
RJ48.S576   1984   618.92   84-6829
ISBN 0-89004-913-0

To the infants, children and adolescents
who have taught us the art of medicine

Preface

This volume is designed for the house officer and practicing physician as a guide to the management of hospitalized children. There are many pocket handbooks that cover all aspects of practical patient care. They usually focus on the description, evaluation, and management of various diseases and disease processes, though not necessarily under the same cover. Existing manuals utilize either long narratives or complicated outline formats, making the extraction of practical information difficult. The result is the "bulging white coat syndrome," pockets stuffed with a variety of quick reference volumes. The more inclusive the manual, however, the more it usually approaches textbook size, rendering it impossible to fit into the already overflowing pocket library.

Diagnosis and Management of the Hospitalized Child fills the gap and provides complete, up-to-date information organized by subject in a minimal amount of space. It includes a brief discussion of the disease entity or clinical syndrome, a review of the signs and symptoms, a differential diagnosis, pathophysiology (in modular easily understandable flowchart form), comprehensive stepwise diagnostic plans and various sequential treatment protocols. Appendixes include handy, rapidly accessible reference material, drugs and their dosages, laboratory tests and their interpretation along with other material required for comprehensive management of children and adolescents. A bibliography is also included which provides access to in-depth information. This handbook is all that is required in the white coat pocket of pediatricians and other physicians who treat hospitalized children.

Acknowledgments

To our parents, spouses, children, and friends who provided us wih the energy and support we needed to write this book , Aida, Fuad, Karim, Jeannie, David, Susan, Marian, and Ralph.

We would also like to acknowledge two staff members who typed, corrected and made this book otherwise readable, Ms. Sherrie Lynn Gorney and Ms. Kathy Sims, along with the editorial staff at Raven Press, without whose tireless efforts this book would not have come to pass, Dr. Diana Schneider and Ms. Anne Friedman.

We would like our readers to note that the sequence of the authors does not necessarily reflect or detract from the importance of their respective contributions.

Contents

Appendixes

Diagnosis and Management of the Hospitalized Child

Learning from Problem Solving

The transition of a physician from an unskilled student to a masterful problem solver is long and difficult. It is not a mystical road where junctions are reached and the traveler is anointed with powers to diagnose and treat. It is a pathway of modification of behavior, habit development, and thought processing. It is also a pathway leading to the development of new learning behavior. The rapidly expanding knowledge base of medicine requires life-long, continuing education and the practitioner must develop learning styles that will permit him or her to keep up-to-date on changing content and practices. It is for this reason that a chapter on learning by problem solving is included in a manual on diagnostic and therapeutic protocols. It is also included because a physician's learning behavior, which begins in the clinical clerkships of medical school, is drastically different from the traditional educational model that pervades primary and secondary schools, colleges, and preclinical medical education.

It is assumed that the successful preclinical student will easily make the transition from the traditional teacher-centered, content-based learning of earlier educational experiences to the problem-based, self-directed study required during clerkships, residency programs, fellowships, and continuing education. In fact, many students have difficulty in making the transition. It is not easy to break old learning habits that have been successful and rewarding. It is not easy for the student instantaneously to develop the internal rewards that are required for learning after the clinical clerkships have begun (i.e., successful problem solving through the resolution of learning issues). No longer are the external rewards of grades significant in the learning process. A major difficulty is that students of medicine, previously having used grades to measure successful learning and thus having gained comfort from the fact that they had learned what the teacher thought necessary, no longer have grades to go by. Success and comfort in the educational process now need to be obtained in other unfamiliar ways. This new learning process requires maturity on the part of medical students.

This chapter is intended, therefore, to assist the student, resident, fellow, and practitioner in adopting new learning techniques. For the first time in his or her formal education, learning occurs during the solution of particular patient-related problems when the student begins a clerkship. Limits of learning are no longer set for the student. What is learned is what is needed to diagnose and treat human diseases effectively.

One of the most important aspects of learning from problem solving is the establishment of specific learning objectives. Students will be guided by the objectives set by the clerkship director and also by internal objectives set by what the students want to learn and need to learn to pass examinations. The residents' objectives are set by the residency program director and requirements for passing certification examinations. Also important are objectives set by the patient's problem for accurate and complete diagnosis and management. Attending physicians' objectives are usually guided by what they need to know to manage their patients accurately and comprehensively and also by what is necessary to keep currently informed.

It has been shown that knowledge gained from lectures and conferences (teacher-centered, content-based) is rapidly forgotten. Learning coupled to problem solving is retained longer and reinforced whenever a similar problem presents itself. The successful clinician is always referring to patients managed in the past for stimulation of retrieval of knowledge gained during the previous encounter. It is common to hear the experienced clinician saying, "I once had a patient who had similar findings." Effective development of learning issues and utilizing resources will result in greater retention of information.

Table 1 shows the steps in the clinical reasoning process and describes how this process may be used to develop learning issues. Specific learning issues can be generated at each step of the process. The issues that are developed are guided by the objectives set prior to the encounter. The following examples may aid the student and practitioner in developing learning skills required in medical education.

Example 1: The Student

Every patient encounter is a learning experience for the student. Regardless of the problem or the frequency of presentation, something can be learned from any patient

TABLE 1. *Clinical reasoning process and development of learning issues*

Clinical Reasoning Process	
Patient situation Cue perception Hypothesis generation	These steps occur instantaneously and often unconsciously. They guide the direction of the line of questioning and make the medical history-taking and physical examination purposeful diagnostically
Problem formulation	

Inquiry design
  History of present illness
  Systems review
  Family history
  Social history
  Patient's past medical history
	This step consists of two types of inquiries: (1) Searching questions guided by the generated hypotheses, questions asked to test the particular hypotheses and (2) scanning questions asked for the completeness of inquiry and to give the practitioner time to think

Clinical skills
  Including the physical examination and
   other diagnostic modalities	

Development of Learning Issues	
Closure Diagnostic plans Therapeutic plans	After the learning issues are resolved, the new knowledge is related to the patient situation and the cascade is continued through problem formulation, inquiry design, and clinical skills until adequate closure is achieved

Modified from Barrows (1980).

situation. The successful clinical student should first establish learning goals prior to the encounter (i.e., determine what it is that he or she will learn from the patient-student interaction). The objectives may be broad and relate to either a basic or a clinical science issue. Diagnosis and /or management issues may also be considered. During the encounter, the student should attempt to follow the steps in the clinical reasoning process. During the progression, specific learning issues should be generated. The student should take notes on the learning issues for later reference (perhaps in a small loose-leaf note book carried in the clinic coat pocket) so that appropriate resources can be sought for resolution. After the initial encounter reaches a point where more knowledge is needed and learning issues need resolution appropriate resources should be sought. The new knowledge should then be applied to the original patient problem that generated the issue in order to reach closure.

A child admitted to the hospital for tonsillectomy and adenoidectomy might generate the following learning issues:

1. Position of the tonsils and adenoids in the posterior pharynx and their adjacent structures.

2. Function of lymphoid tissues.

3. Mechanisms of action of preoperative drugs.

4. Indications and contraindications of tonsillectomy and adenoidectomy.

Example 2: The Resident

The learning principles that apply to the student are equally important for the house officer to master. Application of basic and clinical sciences is essential for effective diagnosis and management of patients' problems. Hypotheses generation is an important step. A complete set of hypotheses will guide the house officer through the medical history-taking and physical examination (data collection mechanism) and guide appropriate laboratory diagnostic tests. Alternate hypotheses should also be generated and tested in parallel. The generation of hypotheses will help to avoid ritualistic history-taking and physical examination, and ordering inappropriate laboratory tests. Hypothesis generation will also assist in generating learning issues related to the clinical sciences, diagnosis, and management.

A 3-year-old child is admitted to the hospital with the chief complaint of wheezing. The differential diagnosis might include asthma, pneumonia, foreign-body aspiration, congestive heart failure. Possible learning issues might be:

1. The pathophysiological mechanisms of wheezing in asthma and how the treatment regimen might be designed according to these mechanisms.

2. The most common organisms causing pneumonia in a 3-year-old child.

3. The most common mechanism for aspiration of a foreign body.

4. Cardiovascular diseases which present with an acute onset of wheezing.

Example 3: The Attending

Learning from problem solving is the major mechanism for acquisition of new knowledge and continuing education for the attending physician. Knowledge is acquired for two basic reasons: (1) to better diagnose and treat particular diseases and

(2) to keep up with rapidly expanding body of medical knowledge. (A third reason, collecting the necessary credits for relicensure, will not be considered here.)

An 11-year-old boy is admitted to the hospital in diabetic ketoacidosis. Possible learning issues might include:

1. Current thoughts on continuous insulin infusions.

2. Split dosage schedules for long-acting insulin.

A bdominal Pain

Abdominal pain is one of the most common symptoms in children. Recurrent pain is defined as at least three episodes of pain, severe enough to interfere with the normal activity of the child, occurring over a period of 3 months or more. The pain is usually vague, difficult to describe, frequently periumbilical, and bears no constant relationship to meals, time of day, or any particular activity. The frequency and duration of the pain are variable. There are usually similar complaints in other family members, but the patient's past medical history is usually unremarkable.

Recurrent abdominal pain occurs in 10% of all children. A definite etiology is found in only 10% of these patients: 15% to 25% may have associated symptoms such as diarrhea, vomiting, headache, fever, pallor, sleepiness after the episode, and asymmetry of pupillary size. The pain is usually real to the child regardless of its etiology.

Acute abdominal pain is also a common complaint in childhood. There is an abrupt onset of abdominal complaints, which may or may not be localized and may or may not be associated in the clinical findings. All episodes of acute abdominal complaints should be investigated for the possibility of intra-abdominal disease (many patients may require a complete medical history and physical examination).

PATHOPHYSIOLOGY

The abdominal pain may be visceral, parietal, or referred. Visceral pain is dull or crampy and tends to be midline. Parietal pain is deeper, more lateralized, and arises from irritation of the parietal peritoneum. The farther away the pain is from the midline, the more likely there is an organic etiology (Apley's law) (Fig. 1).

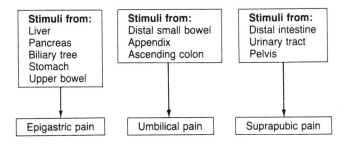

FIG. 1. Pathophysiology of abdominal pain.

5

SIGNS AND SYMPTOMS

The signs and symptoms in patients with acute or recurrent abdominal pain are extremely variable. Localization may be present or the pain may be diffuse and nonspecific. The character of the pain ranges from a dull ache to incapacitating colicky paroxysms. An accurate description of the pain is extremely important in making the correct diagnosis.

DIFFERENTIAL DIAGNOSIS

Acute Abdominal Pain

1. **Newborn**
   a. Necrotizing enterocolitis
   b. Malrotation
   c. Volvulus
   d. Congenital bands
   e. Intestinal atresias
   f. Meconium ileus
   g. Aganglionic megacolon
   h. Sepsis

2. **1 month to 2 years of age**
   a. Intussusception
   b. Incarcerated hernia

3. **>2 years of age**
   a. Appendicitis

4. **Possible causes**
   a. Mesenteric lymphadenitis
   b. Basilar pneumonias

   c. Pyelonephritis
   d. Pericarditis
   e. Rheumatic fever
   f. Sickle-cell anemia
   g. Henoch-Schönlein purpura
   h. Food poisoning
   i. Hyperlipidemia
   j. Hypoglycemia
   k. Porphyria
   l. Diabetic ketoacidosis
   m. Torsion of ovary or testes
   n. Pelvic inflammatory disease
   o. Inflammatory bowel disease
   p. Streptococcal pharyngitis
   q. Inflammed Meckel's diverticulum
   r. Peritonitis
   s. Parasitic infection (e.g., giardiasis and entamebiasis)

Recurrent Abdominal Pain

I. *Functional (90% of Total)*
II. *Organic (10% of Total)*
A. **Gastrointestional system**
   1. Hiatus hernia
   2. Peptic ulcer

3. Malrotation or volvulus
4. Polyps
5. Duplications
6. Meckel's diverticulum
7. Crohn's disease

8. Ulcerative colitis
9. Hernia
10. Hirschsprung's disease
11. Constipation
12. Bacterial or parasitic infections
13. Trauma
14. Superior mesenteric artery syndrome
15. Annular pancreas
16. Food intolerance
17. Irritable colon syndrome
18. Foreign body
19. Malabsorption syndromes
20. Hepatitis
21. Gallbladder disease
22. Pancreatitis

B. Genitourinary system
1. Ureteral obstruction and hydronephrosis
2. Ectopic kidney
3. Pyelonephritis
4. Dysmenorrhea
5. Torsion of ovary or testes
6. Renal stones
7. Endometriosis
8. Ruptured ovarian follicle

C. Metabolic causes
1. Lead poisoning
2. Porphyria
3. Hereditary angioedema
4. Diabetic ketoacidosis
5. Hyperlipemia
6. Henoch-Schönlein purpura
7. Collagen disease
8. Congestive heart failure
9. Rheumatic fever

D. Respiratory system
1. Tonsillitis
2. Asthma
3. Cystic fibrosis
4. Pneumonia

E. Other causes
1. Brain tumors
2. Epilepsy
3. Migraine
4. Sickle-cell anemia
5. Leukemia, lymphoma, neuroblastoma
6. Syphilis
7. Trauma and injury

F. Unlikely causes
1. Pinworms
2. Lordosis
3. Milk ingestion

DIAGNOSTIC PROTOCOL

Acute Pain

1. A problem for which immediate intervention is required should be ruled out first and as soon as possible.
2. Obtain a detailed medical history. Symptoms suggestive of acute and/or surgical

problems include trauma, sudden onset of pain, constant and continuous pain, weight loss, and other associated symptoms such as anorexia, fever, vomiting, diarrhea, or constipation. Symptoms suggestive of nonacute problems include absence of trauma, recurrent pain, weight maintenance, and no associated symptoms.

3. Perform a careful physical examination of the abdomen, including a rectal and/ or vaginal examination. Vital signs should be closely monitored if an acute process is suspected. Signs suggestive of an acute and/or surgical problem include abdominal distention or rigidity, no bowel sounds, localized tenderness, no other focus of disease, and a positive rectal and/or vaginal examination. Signs suggestive of a benign process include absence of abdominal distention or rigidity, normal bowel sounds, diffuse or no abdominal tenderness, other focus of disease, and a negative rectal and/or vaginal examination.

4. If the medical history and physical examination are not helpful in determining the correct diagnosis, the following procedures should be performed:

   a. Complete blood cell count: Repeat every 6 hr; examine white blood cells and left shifts to rule out appendicitis; examine hematocrit to rule out gastrointestinal bleeding.

   b. Urinalysis.

   c. Chest radiograph: Examine for absent air in right lower quandrant, scoliosis, sentinel loop, ileus, free air and/or fecalith.

   d. Blood glucose, blood urea nitrogen, electrolytes, and amylase.

   e. Repeat physical examination every 6 hr, including monitoring of vital signs.

Recurrent Pain

After an acute abdominal problem has been ruled out, the following diagnostic steps should be taken if the pain persists or recurs.

1. **First-stage orders:**

   a. Sickle-cell preparation

   b. Erythrocyte sedimentation rate

   c. Urine culture

   d. Multiple stool examinations for occult blood, ova, or parasites

   e. Stool pH and reducing sustances

   f. Biochemical screening, including SMA-12 and lipid profile

   g. Purified protein derivative (PPD) test

2. **Second-stage orders** (performed if any of the above tests is positive or if the pain is persistent and no cause is found):

   a. Intravenous pyelogram (IVP)

   b. Voiding cystourethrogram

c. Barium enema

d. Upper gastrointestinal (UGI) series

e. Abdominal ultrasound

f. Isotope scan for Meckel's diverticulum

g. Endoscopy: Done after the UGI series if the child has hematemesis, melena, and midepigastric pain; done before the UGI series if the child has UGI hemorrhage

h. Psychological interview with family and child: Emotional markers include modeling, separation, anxiety, gain, high-strung personality

3. If an **organic** etiology is still highly suspected, the following tests should be considered:

a. Cholecystography

b. CT scan

c. Electroencephalogram

d. Urine test for porphobilinogen

e. Serum lead level

f. Immunoglobulins

g. Antinuclear antibodies (ANA) test, including anti-DNA

h. Abdominal angiography

i. Laparotomy

4. If a **nonorganic** etiology is highly suspected, the following procedures should be considered:

a. Psychological testing

b. Meeting with family to explain results of tests (pain is real)

c. Send child to school or to resume normal activities

d. Trial of milk-free diet (medications are not indicated)

e. Psychotherapy

TREATMENT PROTOCOL

---

1. If the patient is in shock or bleeding, resuscitate and stabilize.

2. Allow nothing by mouth.

3. Insert a nasogastric tube.

4. Begin intravenous fluids to hydrate and correct electrolytes and/or acid-base balance.

5. Consider liver-spleen scan, emergency IVP, and/or surgical consultation.

Abnormal Facies

This chapter describes the currently accepted definitions and terminology applied to patients with syndromes associated with dysmorphic facies and describes a logical method for appropriate diagnosis and management of these syndromes. Other malformation syndromes are discussed in the Bibliography. Appropriate diagnosis of craniofacial anomalies is crucial, since it has prognostic implications and is the cornerstone of genetic counseling.

DEFINITIONS

1. **Dysmorphology:** The study of abnormalities in morphogenesis regardless of etiology, timing, or severity.

2. **Malformation:** A primary structural defect resulting from a localized error of morphogenesis (e.g., cleft lip).

3. **Deformation:** An alteration in shape and/or structure of a previously normally formed part (e.g., torticollis)

4. **Anomalad:** A malformation together with its subsequently derived structural changes.

5. **Malformation syndromes:** Recognized patterns of malformation presumably having the same etiology and currently not interpreted as the consequence of a single localized error in morphogenesis (e.g., Down's syndrome).

6. **Association:** A recognized pattern of malformations that currently is not considered to constitute a syndrome or an anomalad.

7. **Prenatal onset defects:** Structural abnormalities observed at birth.

8. **Postnatal onset defects:** Abnormalities not observed at birth but developing secondary to deterioration of structures that have developed normally.

PATHOPHYSIOLOGY

Facial elements begin to appear during the fourth embryonic week, and the definitive fetal face is apparent by the eighth week. Deformed and displaced features result from interruption in morphogenesis of any of the following:

1. Lateral-to-mesial migration of the optic vesicles.

2. The lateral and superior migration of the ears.

3. The mesial and inferior migration of the nose.

4. The bipartite origins of the nose, maxilla, and mandible.

Genetic, multifactorial, environmental, chromosomal (rare cause of facial anomalies), and teratogenic (e.g., maternal ingestion of hydantoin, warfarin, alcohol, or trimethadione) factors are all known to induce facial anomalies.

SIGNS AND SYMPTOMS

The morphogenic craniofacial alterations appear to result from either suture fusion or clefting. This postulated mechanism of deformity combined with the affected region forms the basis of the classification of these anomalies.

I. Suture Stenosis

A. Cranium

  1. Craniosynostosis: Premature suture fusion. The brain may grow normally, in which case the skull will be deformed. May be associated with agenesis of the corpus callosum or hydrocephalus

  2. Plagiocephaly: Unilateral coronal suture stenosis

  3. Trigonocephaly: Metopic synostosis, causing a "triangular head"

B. Midface

  1. Craniofacial dysostoses (Crouzon, Apert, Pfeiffer, Carpenter, and Saethre-Chotzen syndromes)

  2. Isolated maxillary retrusions

  3. Maxillary proganthism

II. Clefting

A. Orbit

  1. Hyper- and hypotelorism: Increased or decreased width between the pupils and the medial orbital walls

  2. Dystopias: Displaced bony orbits

  3. Microphthalmia, anophthalmia, cyclopia

  4. Lid ptosis

B. Asymmetric deformities

  1. Craniofacial microsomia

  2. Unilateral (non-midline) clefts

C. Symmetrical deformities

  1. Mandibulofacial dysostosis (Treacher-Collins syndrome)

  2. Midline clefts (bifid nose, arrhinocephaly, holopros-encephaly)

  3. Bilateral clefts

D. The ear

   1. Low-set ears

   2. Protruding ears

   3. Constricted ears

   4. Microtia with or without aplasia of the external auditory canal, tympanic membrane, and middle ear ossicles

E. The mandible

   1. Micrognathia

   2. Retrognathia (mostly with symmetrical facial deformities)

   3. Proganthism (mandibular hyperplasia)

F. The nose

   1. Bifidity and bridge hypoplasia (with midline and paramedian clefts)

   2. Cleft lip/nasal deformities

   3. Aplasia

G. Cleft lip and cleft palate (most frequent craniofacial anomalies)

DIAGNOSTIC PROTOCOL

This approach may be used whenever structural defects are observed, whether they are craniofacial or not.

A complete medical history and physical examination must be performed to determine if the defect is of prenatal or postnatal onset. Prenatal onset defects (e.g., chromosomal abnormalities) are usually characterized by decreased intensity of fetal activity, polyhydramnios or oligohydramnios, breech presentation, small for gestational age, problems with respiratory and neonatal adaptation, and positive physical examination at birth. Postnatal onset defects (e.g., mucopolysaccharidosis) are usually characterized by a full-term newborn, normal fetal activity, no abnormalities of the amniotic fluid, vertex presentation, normal weight, normal respiratory adaptation, and usually no abnormalities noted at birth.

Prenatal Onset Deformities

   1. List the abnormalities and note whether they are deformities or malformations.

   2. Determine if the abnormalities are secondary to a **single defect** (e.g., mandibular hypoplasia causing glossoptosis and cleft palate) or secondary to a **multiple malformation syndrome.** (There are some multiple malformation syndromes that have concomitant single defect abnormalities.)

   3. If the infant has a malformation syndrome, obtain the following information:

      a. **Maternal age:** Consider Down's syndrome if over 45 years old.

      b. **Paternal age:** Consider achondroplasia, Apert's or Marfan's syndrome if over 36 years old.

c. **Consanguinity:** Consider autosomal recessive disorders.

d. History of **frequent abortion:** Consider X-linked dominant disorders or chromosomal abnormalities in which either parent is a balanced translocation carrier.

4. Consider chromosomal studies if the infant has multiple organ involvement, abnormal growth parameters, and psychomotor retardation, or any of the criteria in Table 1.

5. Evaluate the phenotype of patient and family members and consult the atlas of the face in Goodman and Gorlin's *Genetic Disorders* (see Bibliography).

TABLE 1. *Craniofacial features of some common malformation syndromes*

Facial features	Syndrome	Associations
Flat occiput, oblique palpebral fissures, epicanthic folds, speckled iris, protruding tongue, malformed ears, flat nasal bridge	Trisomy 21	Mental retardation, hypotonia, simian crease, short and/or broad hands, congenital heart disease (CHD), undescended testes, imperforate anus
Prominent occiput, small features, micrognathia, low-set malformed ears	Trisomy 18	Mental retardation, hypertonia, failure-to-thrive (FTT), low birth weight, CHD
Microcephaly, cleft lip and/or cleft palate, microphthalmia, colobomas, low-set ears	Trisomy 13	Mental retardation, FTT, seizures, polydactyly; CHD
Short palpebral fissures, midfacial hypoplasia, epicanthic folds	Fetal alcohol syndrome	Microcephaly, abnormal prenatal and postnatal growth, developmental delay, fine motor dysfunction, CHD
Microcephaly, round face, hypertelorism, epicanthic folds, downward slant of palpebral fissures, strabismus, low-set ears, facial asymmetry	Cri-du-chat syndrome (partial deletion of short arm of chromosome 5)	Low birth weight, hypotonia, cat-like cry in infancy, and mental deficiency
Narrow maxilla (palate), small mandible, inner canthal folds	Turner's syndrome (XO)	Short stature, widely spaced nipples, low hairline, learning impairment
Microbradycephaly, bushy eyebrows, small nose, anteverted nares, thin lips with midline beak of the upper lip, high-arched palate, micrognathia, downward curving of the angle of the mouth	De Lange syndrome	Hirsutism, mental retardation, micromelia
Macrocephaly, narrow forehead, coarse facial features, full lips, macroglossia, low nasal bridge, bushy eyebrows	Mucopolysaccharidosis (Hunter-Hurler, Maroteaux, Morquio, Sanfilippo, and Scheie syndromes)	Hirsutism, hepatosplenomegaly

6. Rule out teratogenic infections and chemical agents; consult Shepard's *A Catalog of Teratogenic Agents* (see Bibliography); common agents include toxoplasmosis, rubella, cytomegalovirus, herpes, syphilis, hydantoins, and alcohol.

7. Unknown (sporadic) etiology (e.g., Cornelia DeLange and Prader-Willi syndromes).

Postnatal Onset Deformities

1. List the time of onset and the observed abnormalities.

2. Determine if the abnormalities are accompanied by evidence of any of the following disorders:

   a. Metabolic.

   b. Neurological.

   c. Combined (e.g., cataracts, sparse hair, coarse facies, unusual skin pigmentation, hepatosplenomegaly).

   d. Environmental insult (e.g., trauma, infection, hypoxia).

3. Identify minor malformations that may or may not be of any significance early in life, but could be later on.

   a. Aberrant scalp hair pattern (unruly scalp hair) may be associated with defects in CNS development.

   b. Prominent lateral palatine ridges may be associated with neuromuscular dysfunction.

   c. Joint contractures suggesting decreased fetal movements, which suggests neuromuscular dysfunction.

   d. Hypoplasia of the thenar eminence may be associated with tracheoesophageal fistula and esophageal atresia.

   e. Hemihypertrophy may be associated with Wilm's tumor, hepatoma, or renal carcinoma.

   f. Asymmetrical crying facies may be associated with cardiac defects.

TREATMENT PROTOCOL

1. Life support if the abnormalities are life-threatening.

2. Treatment of the associated complications (metabolic function, cardiac, neurological, renal).

3. Reconstructive surgery.

4. Support services, especially if the abnormalities are associated with psychomotor retardation.

5. Every attempt should be made to achieve a diagnosis because of the important prognostic and genetic implications.

6. Genetic counseling.

Accidents and Accidental Trauma

Accidents are the leading cause of death in childhood. The goal of outpatient care is prevention of accidents (Table 1). In many cases, accidents cannot be prevented, but injury can. When injury cannot be prevented, the goal is to minimize the degree of injury and provide adequate treatment to avoid sequelae of the trauma (Table 2).

A complete medical history should be taken and a physical examination should be performed on all injured patients. If the history is inconsistent with the degree or type of injury encountered, child abuse should be suspected.

The following procedures should be performed at the site of an accident.

1. Immediately stop any obvious external bleeding with pressure.

2. Do not move the patient, unless further trauma is risked.

3. Check pulse and respiration. If absent, begin cardiopulmonary resuscitation.

4. If the patient's condition is stable, arrange for transportation to a hospital. Stabilize any area of the body that may be injured (e.g., arm, leg, neck) to prevent further injury during transport.

In the emergency department, treat the accident victim as follows.

1. Identify and stop any external bleeding.

2. Assure and maintain an adequate airway.

3. Treat shock.

4. Obtain pertinent medical history and rapidly perform a complete physical examination.

5. Further evaluation and treatment should be guided by the medical history and physical examination. It is important to remember, however, that in many accidents, multiple trauma may occur and evaluation and treatment must not be based only on the obvious gross trauma.

TABLE 1. *Causes and prevention of accidents*

Major etiological factors	Preventive measures
Automobile Accidents	
Carrying children unrestrained while riding in an automobile	All passengers in a moving vehicle should be appropriately restrained
Riding on an adult's lap in the right front seat of the car (especially dangerous)	Children from birth to approximately 20 lb should ride in an approved rear-facing

TABLE 1. *(continued)*

Major etiological factors	Preventive measures
Young drivers; adolescent drivers are responsible for many fatal automobile accidents and should be considered high risks Alcohol; drunk drivers are responsible for many fatal auto accidents	infant's car seat Children weighing 20 to 40 lb should ride in an approved front-facing child's car seat; it should be secured in the back seat by the car's seat belt and a back tether, if required Children weighing >40 lb should ride in the back seat, using the car's lap belt; the shoulder harness should not be used until the child is tall enough for the strap to fit over the shoulder and not the neck All drivers should drive defensively and obey the speed limit and other rules of the road

Fire and Smoke Accidents

Lack of an early warning system (i.e., smoke detectors) Lack of knowledge of multiple escape routes Lack of knowledge of how to act during a fire emergency Playing on or near stoves and ovens Smoking Wearing flammable night clothes Hot water temperature set too high, causing accidental scalds	Installation of smoke alarms in multiple areas of the home Planned and rehearsed fire drills Keep matches out of children's reach Take care when smoking cigarettes; do not smoke in bed Purchase night clothes made of flame retardant fabric Keep children from playing in the kitchen Boil water on the back burner and keep hot liquids out of children's reach Keep thermostat of hot water heater between 120 and 140° F

Drowning Accidents

Lack of proper respect for bodies of water, no matter how small or shallow Lack of adequate adult supervision. This is the most common cause of drowning accidents Insufficient knowledge of water survival techniques and inability to swim Lack of obstructive barriers, permitting easy access to the water	Never leave an infant or a child unattended in a tub of water, even for a short time Never allow children access to areas containing accumulated water without adequate adult supervision (infants have been known to drown in a pail of water) Never swim alone Swim within endurance capabilities Swimming should be taught to all children when they can hold their breath on command All children should be taught a healthy respect for water

Falling Accidents

Leaving infants unattended on an elevated surface Failure to raise the side rail of a crib Normal developmental landmarks (rolling over, cruising, walking, and climbing) predispose children to accidental falls A child's normal insatiable curiosity Open unobstructed windows with easy access	Never leave an infant or child unattended on an elevated surface, even for a short time Always raise the side rail of a crib when an infant is left unattended Infants and small children should sleep in a crib until the side rail is two-thirds of the child's height; slats should be no wider than 2⅜ inches (or no less than 12 slats per side); if no crib is available, a padded

Major etiological factors	Preventive measures

drawer or box placed on the floor will usually suffice
Doors should be kept locked
All interior and exterior staircases should be barricaded with a gate or door
Windows should not be opened wide enough to allow a child to fit through; bars and other permanent obstructions should be avoided (they prevent access and escape in fire emergencies); screens should not be considered childproof

Ingestion Accidents

Major etiological factors	Preventive measures
Children's curiosity along with their normal oral sensory stimulation behavior predisposes them to ingestion accidents Lack of anticipated attainment of normal developmental landmarks Leaving poisonous or ingestible objects within the reach of a child Toys with easily removable parts that may fit into a child's mouth	Store medications under lock and key out of children's reach Keep all medications, household cleaning fluids, and pesticides out of children's reach Store all detergents, pesticides, medications, and cleaning agents in their original containers; assure that cabinets, especially under a sink, cannot be opened by a child Have immediate access to the telephone number of the nearest poison control center

Aspiration Accidents

Major etiological factors	Preventive measures
Small, hard foods (e.g., peanuts, popcorn) given to small children who cannot adequately chew Holding small, hard foods or objects in the mouth while running or playing	Small children should not be given foods such as peanuts, popcorn, or small hard candies until they are old enough to chew them adequately Toys that are small enough to swallow should be kept away from small children Avoid running, jumping, playing, or laughing while eating or holding something in the mouth

Bicycle and Pedestrian Accidents

Major etiological factors	Preventive measures

Pedestrian
  Disobeying traffic safety rules
  Walking on the roadway at night wearing dark clothing
  Failure to take adequate precautions crossing the street (e.g., running from between parked cars)
Bicycle
  Horseplay
  Riding tandem on a bicycle not designed for two
  Amateur modification of the bicycle
  Riding a bike of the wrong size
  Failure to obey traffic rules
	All persons riding a bicycle must learn the rules of the road and follow them
	Pedestrians should not walk on the roadway; if there is no sidewalk, walk facing the oncoming traffic
	Bright clothing or reflective strips should be worn when walking or riding a bicycle at night
	Bicycles should be kept in good repair and amateur modifications should be avoided
	Bicycles should be ridden with the flow of automobile traffic, and all rules of the road should be followed
	Riding a bicycle in areas with a heavy flow of automobile traffic should be avoided
	Tandem riding should be avoided, unless the bicycle was designed for tandem use

TABLE 2. *Accidental trauma: Diagnostic and treatment protocols*

Diagnosis	Treatment

Closed Head Trauma

Diagnosis	Treatment
The diagnosis of accidental trauma rests primarily on the medical history and physical examination The history should focus on the type of trauma incurred and on assessment of the forces involved, loss of consciousness, and retrograde or anterograde amnesia Physical examination should focus on the identification of external injuries and on a complete neurological evaluation, including mental status, cranial nerve evaluation, motor and sensory system evaluation, and reflexes Skull radiographs may be indicated if the trauma is significant and linear or depressed fractures are suspected CT scan may be indicated if intracranial disease or increased intracranial pressure is suspected Evaluate the patient for cervical spine injuries	Observe patient for evidence of developing intracranial disturbance Establish an airway and intravenous line; closely monitor vital signs and neurological status Elevated intracranial pressure may be controlled temporarily with fluid restriction, hyperventilation, and mannitol (1-2 g/kg, i.v. push) Subdural tap Definitive treatment is surgical if a subdural or epidural hematoma is present; evacuation of an expanding intracranial/extracerebral lesion is required; surgical elevation of a depressed skull fracture is also required

Closed Chest Trauma

Diagnosis	Treatment
A rapid and complete medical history and physical examination are essential, with special emphasis on the chest and its contents Obtain chest radiograph to evaluate the heart, lungs, mediastinum, musculoskeletal system, pleural space, and diaphragm A barium swallow should be considered if esophageal injury is suspected Angiography is indicated if there is injury to the great vessels Electrocardiogram (ECG) is indicated if there is suspected injury to the heart or if a pericardial effusion is suspected Complete blood cell count, urinalysis, abdominal radiographs, and coagulation profile should be ordered and blood typed and crossmatched for 40 cc/kg of whole blood	Assure and maintain an adequate airway Establish an intravenous line and treat shock If pneumothorax is present, insert a chest tube to evacuate pleural air Perform pericardiocentesis if a pericardial effusion is present and tamponade is imminent The chest wall should be stabilized if a flail chest is present (sandbags or strapping may be used) Treat hemothorax with tube thoracotomy Surgical intervention may be required for definitive treatment

Closed Abdominal Trauma

Diagnosis	Treatment
Rapid and complete medical history and physical examination are essential Vital signs should be closely monitored; hypotension strongly suggests intra-abdominal bleeding. Abdominal pain, guarding, tenderness, and rebound strongly suggest hemoperitoneum or rupture of a hollow viscus (e.g., intestine, bladder)	Assure and maintain an adequate airway Establish an intravenous line and treat shock Insert a nasogastric tube and an indwelling urinary catheter Admit patient to the hospital for observation or in preparation for surgical intervention

Diagnosis	Treatment

Intravenous pyelogram (IVP) may be indicated if renal trauma is suspected (hematuria is usually present)

A nucleotide scan of the liver and spleen may be indicated if trauma to these organs is suspected

Venography

Complete blood cell count, urinalysis, abdominal radiograph, coagulation profile, and type and crossmatch whole blood

Paracentesis may be indicated if intra-abdominal bleeding is suspected

Dental Trauma

Obtain the medical history and perform a complete physical examination	Definitive treatment should be performed by a dentist or oral surgeon
Dental radiographs should be taken to rule out fractures of the root of the tooth or alveolar process of the mandible and/or the maxilla	Avulsed teeth should be preserved in moist saline (or carried in the parent's mouth) and transported with the patient; reimplantation can occur and is frequently successful if the avulsion occurred <30 min before the reimplantation
Obtain radiographs of facial bones if there is significant trauma to other areas of the face, or if there is significant lateral malocclusion of the teeth after the injury	
A chest radiograph should be obtained if aspiration of a tooth or its fragment is suspected	

Drowning Trauma

Obtain the medical history and rapidly perform a physical examination to rule out other associated injuries (e.g., head and neck)	Establish and maintain an airway (intubation or tracheostomy; laryngospasm is common)
Monitor blood gases and pH	Establish an intravenous line and treat shock
Complete blood cell count, electrolytes, blood urea nitrogen, and creatinine	Assure adequate ventilation with 100% oxygen
Specific radiographs may be indicated, depending on the presence of associated trauma	Acidosis should be appropriately treated
Obtain a base-line chest radiograph	Further management should be dictated by the clinical evaluation and laboratory findings
	Aminophylline, 5 mg/kg, may be given if bronchospasm is present
	Note: Cardiopulmonary resuscitation (CPR) should be attempted in almost all drowning accidents; the survival rate is generally good, especially if cold water is involved

Fractures

Obtain the medical history and perform a complete physical examination	Appropriate stabilization proximal and distal to the fracture
Obtain appropriate radiographs to determine the presence, type, and extent of a fracture and to guide the treatment	Appropriate physiological immobilization

Ocular Trauma

Obtain the medical history and perform a complete physical examination	Minor traumatic injuries may be treated conservatively with observation,

TABLE 2. *(continued)*

Diagnosis	Treatment
Most trauma to the eye results from foreign bodies, penetrating trauma, or blunt trauma The eye must be examined with adequate light and magnification Fluorescein staining may show corneal ulceration or disruption Examine the anterior chamber for blood (hyphema), the pupil for symmetry and reactivity, and examine the fundus; be sure a red reflex can be obtained The visual acuity should be checked Radiographs of the orbits and facial bones are indicated if a fracture is suspected	especially subconjunctival hemorrhage; other trauma, especially if the cornea is involved, should be managed with the help of an ophthalmologist The eye should be patched before patient is transported Corneal foreign bodies should be removed by an ophthalmologist Patients with hyphema, evidence of intraocular injury, or orbital fractures should be admitted to the hospital

Urogenital Trauma

Obtain the medical history and rapidly perform a complete physical examination; injury may occur anywhere along the urinary tract (e.g., kidney, ureter, bladder, or urethra) Complete blood cell count and urinalysis Obtain chest and abdominal radiographs IVP and cystoscopy may be indicated Urethrography	Appropriate stabilization of the patient is indicated, and definitive treatment is usually surgical; it should be conducted in consultation with a urologist and nephrologist Assure and maintain an adequate airway Treat shock Prepare the patient for operation, if necessary

Wringer Injury

Obtain the medical history and perform a physical examination Determine the duration of entrapment Obtain radiographs of the involved limb **Note: The degree of soft-tissue injury is usually more significant than it initially appears on physical examination**	The patient should be hospitalized and evaluated with the help of an orthopedic surgeon and a plastic surgeon Special wrapping and immobilization is not necessary, unless a fracture is present

A cetaminophen Intoxication

Accidental ingestion of medication occurs most commonly in children younger than 5 years of age. Drug overdoses in patients in middle childhood, adolescents, and adults are usually intentional (i.e., suicide gestures and attempts). Safety caps on over-the-counter and prescription medication have significantly reduced the incidence of accidental intoxication with aspirin, but the problem still exists. Because of the increasing use of acetaminophen as an alternative for aspirin, toxic ingestions of this drug are being seen more frequently. Although acetaminophen is a potentially lethal drug, it is more benign than aspirin in children younger than 5 years of age. Nevertheless, fatalities occur in any age group. Also, unlike aspirin, an antidote is available that will block the toxic effects of the drug until excretion occurs.

PATHOPHYSIOLOGY

The toxic effects of acetaminophen are directed toward the liver. **It is hepatotoxic and may cause severe hepatic necrosis** manifested by elevated liver enzymes, bilirubin, and prothrombin time. For adults, ingestion of more than 10 g may be associated with hepatic toxicity, and more than 15 g may be lethal.

SIGNS AND SYMPTOMS

There is a **triphasic clinical course** associated with acetaminophen intoxication. First, symptoms of gastrointestinal irritability occur shortly after the ingestion (nausea, vomiting, diaphoresis). Twelve to 24 hr after the first symptoms appear, a latent phase begins. This usually lasts 24 to 48 hr, but may be as long as 4 days. Symptoms of liver involvement appear with hepatomegaly, abdominal pain and tenderness (usually right upper quadrant), and abnormal liver function tests. In the last phase, significant hepatic necrosis occurs. Symptoms depend on the severity of the intoxication and are those of liver necrosis and failure.

Many patients progress only to the first phase and no farther. Most rarely progress past the second phase, and recovery is the rule. Therapy should begin as soon after the ingestion as possible and should be guided by acetaminophen levels. Resolution of the hepatic damage is usually complete if the patient is adequately treated and survives the insult.

DIAGNOSTIC PROTOCOL

1. Serum electrolytes, carbon dioxide, blood urea nitrogen, and creatinine.

2. SGOT, SGPT.[1]

3. Bilirubin.[1]

4. Prothrombin time.[1]

5. Blood glucose.

6. Drug screen: If there is suspicion of the ingestion of other drugs in addition to acetaminophen, and in patients who ingest acetaminophen compounds; depressed central nervous system function initially suggests ingestion of drugs other than acetaminophen.

7. Estimate the amount of acetaminophen ingested.

8. Acetaminophen level: Monitor at least 4 hr after the ingestion (repeat if obtained prior to 4 hr); if the acetaminophen level falls more than 25% below the level of probable toxicity, the N-acetylcysteine may be discontinued (see nomogram in Appendixes).

9. Lead level: The accidental ingestion of a medication may be a manifestation of pica.

TREATMENT PROTOCOL

1. Empty the patient's stomach. Induction of emesis is the preferred method. Syrup of ipecac (15–30 ml for children; 30–60 ml for adults), followed by a large amount of fluids, is usually sufficient to cause emesis in most patients; the dose may be repeated if emesis does not occur in 20 min; gastric lavage is recommended if ipecac fails to induce vomiting.

2. **Activated charcoal should not be given; it may interfere with the absorption of N-acetylcysteine.**

3. Loading dose of N-acetylcysteine, 140 mg/kg p.o.

4. The loading dose should be followed in 4 hr by a maintenance dose of 70 mg/kg for 17 doses (the loading dose and maintenance doses may be repeated if vomiting occurs within 1 hr of the dose).

5. Maintain and monitor fluid and electrolyte balance, but avoid forced diuresis and diuretics.

6. Treat hypoglycemia and coagulation abnormalities if they occur.

[1]Repeat every 4 days until acetaminophen level falls below toxic level.

A cidosis and Alkalosis

The physician who treats children probably encounters acid-base problems long before he or she becomes cognizant of the frequency with which they occur. Most abnormalities of the acid-base system are mild and well tolerated by the body's buffer systems. These buffering systems maintain the blood pH within narrow limits (7.35–7.45) by an interactive system of chemical and physiological regulation of hydrogen ions.

A growing child produces 2 to 3 mEq/kg of H^+ each day due to the release of hydrogen ions when the calcium ion is cleaved from its base (carbonate) and to the catabolism of ingested foodstuffs. As hydrogen ions are released into circulation, they are almost immediately neutralized by chemical buffers in the cells and extracellular fluids. As a consequence, with any increase in the concentration of hydrogen ions, a concomitant decrease in the blood pH is minimized. This neutralization of hydrogen ions occurs on a one-for-one exchange (i.e., for every hydrogen ion buffered, a bicarbonate ion is consumed). To prevent depletion of the bicarbonate system, the kidney generates a quantity of new bicarbonate in an amount exactly equal to that utilized. This mechanism of bicarbonate reclamation and regeneration occurs in a complex fashion within the renal tubules. The kidney's partner in the physiological buffering process is the respiratory system, which is responsible for excreting carbon dioxide (produced by the metabolism of fat and carbohydrates). **It is important to recognize that the physiological systems (respiratory and renal) do not function independently.** They are interactive through the carbonic acid-bicarbonate buffer system. When a change occurs in P_{CO_2} (pulmonary), the renal system compensates and thus, a constant ratio of $HCO_3^-:H_2CO_3$ is maintained at 20:1.

This finely tuned system may be disrupted when the body is acutely and massively insulted, thereby becoming alkalemic or acidemic. The chemical buffering system reacts instantaneously, the pulmonary system providing help within a matter of 10–12 min. The renal system, the metabolic component of pH regulation, requires several hours to effect any change (between 10–12 hr to have any significant effect on rectifying acid-base disturbance).

Children tend to tolerate not only significant variations in the quality and quantity of their diet but also significant stresses to the acid-base buffer system (multiple viral infections of the upper respiratory tract). They infrequently require exogenous medication or other support. Only when the systems are overwhelmed is the body unable to compensate. After a primary insult (e.g., respiratory alkalosis with pneumonia, or metabolic acidosis following severe diarrhea), a compensating mechanism occurs, usually of the uninvolved physiological system. In the case of alkalosis with pneumonia, the renal system aggressively attempts to compensate for what it perceives as an excess of bicarbonate. It ceases to reabsorb quantities of bicarbonate ion and thus partially conpensates for the alkalosis. The compensation mechanism rarely overshoots (i.e., it will compensate very closely to the normal blood gas values, but will not overcompensate).

A complicating factor in understanding acid-base balance is the situation in which there is more than one primary etiological factor, resulting in a mixed acid-base disorder. A classic example is in the child who ingests toxic levels of salicylates and subsequently develops a respiratory alkalosis and severe metabolic acidosis.

A thorough medical history and physical examination are important in dealing effectively with acid-base disturbances; the information from them will very often provide a diagnosis. Nonetheless, there are four important laboratory tests that must be obtained to evaluate acid-base status adequately:

1. Arterial pH (or hydrogen ion concentration): Calculated from the equation

$$H^+ = (80) - 100(pH_{actual} - 7.00)$$

2. Plasma bicarbonate level (essentially equal to the CO_2 content)

3. Arterial partial pressure of carbon dioxide (obtained in a normal state, i.e., the child should not have undergone protracted crying or breath holding).

4. Measurement of the anion gap (defined as the difference between the serum cations and anions); there is normally a small anion gap due to circulating organic acids and proteins; normal values, $\leq$ 22 in children up to 3 years old and $\leq$ 16 in children above 3 years old; if significant acidemia is present, a quick calculation may provide an answer to a very complex mixed acid-base disturbance, especially when the 95% confidence band shows that hydrogen ion values are greater than expected (see Fig. 1).

DIFFERENTIAL DIAGNOSIS

Acidosis

Respiratory (alveolar hypoventilation) (Fig. 2)

1. Airway obstruction (laryngospasm, bronchospasm)

2. Respiratory center depression (anesthesia, trauma)

3. Disorders restricting ventilation (fibrosis, pneumothorax)

4. Neuromuscular disorders (Guillain-Barré, severe hypokalemia, myopathies)

FIG. 1. Acid-base relationships can be interpreted by use of confidence bands, representing the ranges of H^+ or pH and of HCO_3^-, each in relationship to P_{CO_2}. The bands encompass values prevalent in 95% of cases of uncomplicated primary respiratory acidosis or alkalosis; values that fall outside the bands suggest a mixed disturbance. Confidence bands have been calculated for acute, but not chronic, disturbances in humans; however, acid-base data from dogs are close enough to human data to be clinically useful. *Hatched lines*, acute acidosis; *dots*, acute alkalosis; *horizontal bars*, chronic acidosis; *open circles*, chronic alkalosis. (From Kassirer, J.P., and Madias, N.E. (1980): *Hosp. Pract.*, 15:68, with permission.)

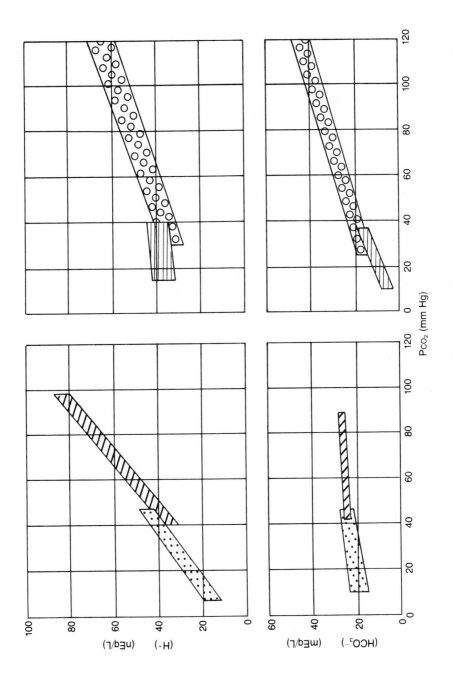

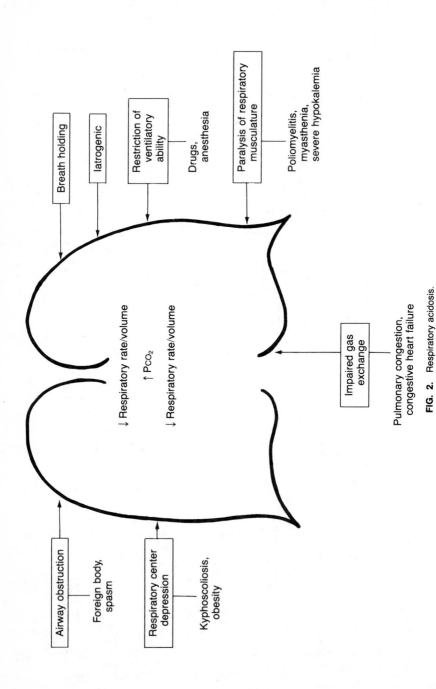

FIG. 2. Respiratory acidosis.

Breath holding

Iatrogenic

Restriction of ventilatory ability

Drugs, anesthesia

Paralysis of respiratory musculature

Poliomyelitis, myasthenia, severe hypokalemia

↓ Respiratory rate/volume

↑ P_{CO_2}

↓ Respiratory rate/volume

Impaired gas exchange

Pulmonary congestion, congestive heart failure

Airway obstruction

Foreign body, spasm

Respiratory center depression

Kyphoscoliosis, obesity

5. Smoke inhalation

6. Iatrogenic (mechanical ventilation)

7. Obesity

8. Pickwickian syndrome

9. Cardiac arrest

10. Toxins or medications (curare, aminoglycosides)

Metabolic (Fig. 3)

1. Lactic acidosis (primary, secondary)

2. Renal failure or insufficiency, tubular acidosis

3. Gastrointestinal disorder (diarrhea)

4. Genetic or inborn errors of metabolism

5. Toxins or medications (acetazolamide, ethanol ingestion)

6. Cardiac arrest

7. Endocrine disorders (adrenal insufficiency)

8. Phosphate depletion

9. Hyperparathyroid states (primary, secondary)

Alkalosis

Respiratory (Fig. 4)

1. Pneumonias

2. CNS irritation (infection, bleeding)

3. Reye's syndrome

4. Hepatic failure

5. Medications or toxins

6. Mechanical ventilation

7. Fever

8. Protracted crying

Metabolic (Fig. 5)

1. Mineralocorticoid excess

2. Bartter's syndrome

3. Glucocorticoid excess

4. Hypercalcemia

5. Hypokalemia

6. Diuretic excess

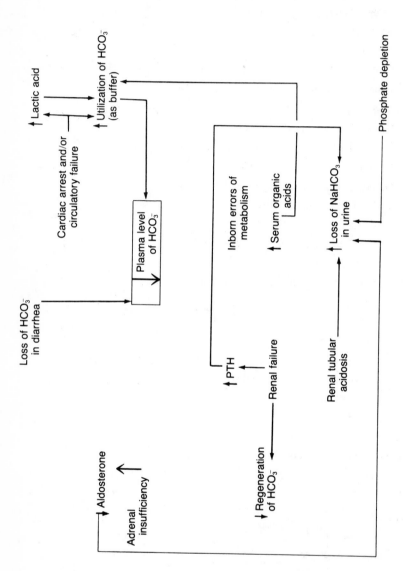

FIG. 3. Metabolic acidosis.

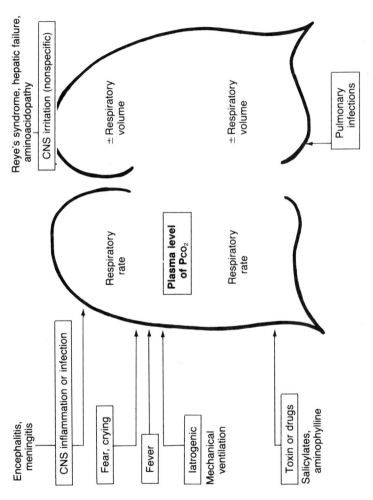

FIG. 4. Respiratory alkalosis.

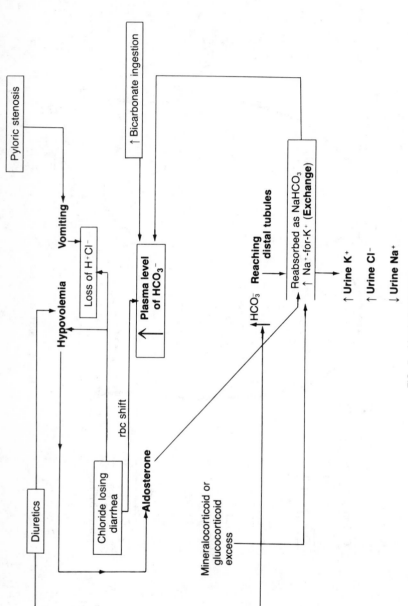

FIG. 5. Metabolic alkalosis.

7. Cystic fibrosis

8. Excess exogenous bicarbonate in renal failure

9. Loss of stomach contents

10. Chloride-losing diarrhea

11. Ingestion of low chloride foods

DIAGNOSTIC AND TREATMENT PROTOCOLS

Table 1 gives diagnostic and treatment protocols for acidosis and Table 2 gives diagnostic and treatment protocols for alkalosis.

TABLE 1. *Acidosis: Diagnostic and treatment protocols*

Diagnosis[a]	Treatment
Respiratory Acidosis (Alveolar Hypoventilation)	

Medical history:
  Airway obstruction
  CNS (respiratory center) depression
  Smoke inhalation
  Paralyzed respiratory muscles
  Limited excursions of thorax
  Impaired gas exchange
Clinical findings:
  Respiratory embarrassment and
    concomitant hypoxia
  Dyspnea, breathlessness
  Cyanosis
  Interference with myocardial contractility,
    producing potential arrythmias, including
    ventricular fibrillation (K^+ depletion is
    additive to this feature)
  Asterixis
  Signs and symptoms of increased
    intracranial pressure
  Papilledema
  Confusion, stupor
Laboratory findings:
  Increased Pco_2 (primary)
  HCO_3^- (compensatory)
  pH < 7.35 (uncompensated)
  pH ≤ 7.35 (partially compensated)
  Normal base excess
  Acid urine pH (increased chloride excretion)
	Spontaneous compensatory attempts and
	  changes by the body:
	  Increased reabsorption of HCO_3^-
	  Increased excretion of H^+ and NH_3^+
	  Increased chloride excretion
	Pulmonary stimulation of respiratory center by
	  high Pco_2 and low pH
	In acute (emergent) situation, regardless of
	  the cause, attention must be directed at
	  restoring adequate ventilation
	Because of severe acidosis, HCO_3^- may be
	  required but is a temporizing measure, at
	  best
	If less acute in origin, then acidosis will
	  probably not be so severe and treatment
	  should maximize alveolar ventilation with
	  bronchodilators, physiotherapy, and
	  diuretics for congestive heart failure, or
	  assisted ventilation

Metabolic Acidosis	

Medical history:
  Cardiac arrest
  Renal failure (acute or chronic)
  Genetic or inborn error of metabolism
  Gastroenteritis
  Recurrent renal stones
  Nonspecific symptoms (anorexia, fatigue,
    dyspnea on exertion)
	Spontaneous compensatory changes by the
	  body:
	  Hyperventilation
	  Decreased excretion of HCO_3^-
	Correct underlying medical defect.
	If acidosis is severe, administer buffer
	Rehydrate or restore fluid volume as
	  needed; dehydration is both a cause and

TABLE 1. *(continued)*

Diagnosis[a]	Treatment

Signs of hypercatabolism (fever, trauma)
Clinical findings:
  Weakness
  Headache
  Nausea and vomiting
  Hyperpnea
  Abdominal pain
  Symptomatology related to the underlying
   disease
Laboratory findings:
  Decreased HCO_3^-
  Decreased PCO_2 (compensatory)
  pH < 7.35 (uncompensated)
  pH ≤ 7.35 (partially compensated)[b]
  Negative base excess
  Acid urine pH (chloride < 10 mEq/L except
   with severe K^+ depletion and/or
   hypercalcemia)
	result of metabolic acidosis
	Chemical buffers (see Respiratory Acidosis)

[a]Individual causes of respiratory or metabolic acidosis are discussed in the pertinent chapters.
[b]As body compensates, pH should approach 7.35 but never exceed it unless secondary to iatrogenic manipulations.

TABLE 2. *Alkalosis: Diagnostic and treatment protocols*

Diagnosis[a]	Treatment
Respiratory Alkalosis	

Medical history:
  Stimulation of respiratory center
  CNS disease
  Toxin
  Hypoxia
  Fever
  Hepatic coma or hepatic insufficiency
  Secondary to metabolic acidosis; diabetic
   ketoacidosis (DKA)
Clinical findings:
  Hyperventilation
  Dizziness
  Paresthesias
  Diaphoresis
  Tinnitus
  Possible tetany
  Pyrexia
  Nuchal rigidity
  Possible cardiac arrythmias, signs and
   symptoms of the underlying dysfunction
   (secondary)
Laboratory findings:
  Decreased PCO_2 (primary)
  Decreased $[HCO_3^-]$s (compensatory)
  pH > 7.45 (uncompensated)
  pH ≤ 7.45 (partially compensated)
	Spontaneous primary and secondary
	  compensation:
	  Spontaneous endogenous compensatory
	   efforts by the body (chemical buffer
	   system, i.e., red blood cells, protein, acts
	   to take excess HCO_3^-
	  Secondary compensation:
	  Kidney attempts to excrete increased HCO_3
	   and retain H^+ and Cl^-
	If hypocapnia is secondary, i.e., due to a
	  metabolic acidosis, diabetic ketoacidosis
	  therapy must be directed at the primary
	  metabolic insult

Diagnosis[a]	Treatment

Normal base excess (partially
compensated)
Alkaline urine pH (not in severe potassium
depletion)

Metabolic Alkalosis

Medical history:
  Diuretics
  Chloride-losing diarrhea
  Intestinal obstruction
  Endogenous or exogenous steroids
  Hypovolemia
  Hyperparathyroidism
Clinical findings may reflect the disease state
  and symptoms due to electrolyte imbalance:
  Dehydration or hypovolemia
  Cushing's syndrome (fat distribution and
    hypertension)
Laboratory findings:
  Increased bicarbonate (primary)
  Increased P_{CO_2} (compensatory)
  pH > 7.45 (uncompensated)
  pH ≤ 7.45 (partially compensated)
  Positive base excess
  Basic urine pH (decreased chloride
    excretion)

Spontaneous compensatory changes by the
  body:
  Increased P_{CO_2}
  Increased excretion of $HCO_3{}^-$
  Decreased excretion of Cl^-
Therapy should be directed at correcting the
  primary underlying defect
If hypokalemia is severe and/or chronic, the
  metabolic alkalosis will be difficult to
  correct unless the K^+ is corrected
If volume depletion is present, then
  expansion of the plasma volume is of
  prime importance
Chemical buffers (see Respiratory Alkalosis)

---

[a]Individual causes of respiratory or metabolic alkalosis are discussed in the pertinent chapters.

Acute Renal Failure

Acute renal failure is a relatively common and invariably serious clinical syndrome with multiple causes. From a functional viewpoint, regardless of the etiology, the kidneys are unable to maintain homeostasis. This dysfunction is manifested by an accumulation of waste products in the blood.

Oliguric renal failure, which is the usual presentation, is arbitrarily defined as urine output of <0.5 ml/kg/hr over a 4-hr period in infants or <300 ml/m²/24 hr in older children. These values relate to the lower limit of glomerular filtration necessary to excrete an average daily solute load if the kidneys were able to maximally concentrate urine. Along with this reduction in the volume of urine output, there is a commensurate increase in the nitrogenous metabolic by-products.

Acute renal failure (vasospastic nephropathy) is classified pathophysiologically as prerenal, parenchymal, and postrenal failure. Prerenal failure connotes functional renal failure resulting from an extrarenal hemodynamic alteration. It is usually readily reversible if the primary insult (e.g., hypovolemia, low cardiac output) is corrected expeditiously. Parenchymal renal failure results from primary renal disease of immunological, nephrotoxic, infectious, or hereditary origin. This type of failure may or may not be reversible, depending on the specific etiology and severity. Postrenal failure (obstructive uropathy) is secondary to complete or incomplete obstruction of the renal outflow tract.

The anatomical (functional) approach to categorizing renal failure (Fig. 1) represents the early or initiating events of the process. Prerenal or postrenal failure may convert to parenchymal failure if the process is not reversed early in its course.

SIGNS AND SYMPTOMS

The clinical findings in renal failure may be those of the primary precipitating event, or they may be a result of the accumulation of metabolic by-products. The presentation of renal failure may be subtle (e.g., an infant who, within 3 days of birth, has not voided urine, but is otherwise asymptomatic) or explosive (e.g., an adolescent who sustains a severe crush injury and, within a matter of 1 or 2 days, requires dialysis because of hypertension, hypervolemia, hyperkalemia, and other electrolyte imbalances) (Figs. 2 and 3).

DIFFERENTIAL DIAGNOSIS

Prerenal (see Table 1)

1. Hypovolemia (gastroenteritis, cardiac surgery, abdominal surgery, burns)

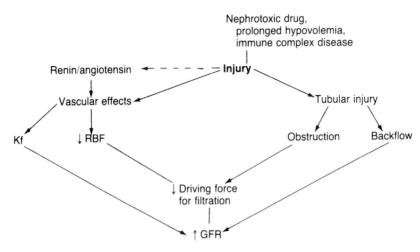

FIG. 1. Kf (glomerular capillary ultrafiltration coefficient) = glomerular permeability × effective filtering surface area. Backflow: filtrate leaks across injured tubular membrane and is reabsorbed. Vascular effects: prolonged or transient vasospasm. Renin/angiotensin: intrarenal activation.

  2. Hypotension (septic shock, hypothermia)

Renal (see Table 1)

  1. Collagen-vascular disease

  2. Large kidney hematuria syndrome in neonates (renal vein thrombosis, polycystic kidney disease, medullary necrosis, cortical necrosis, idiosyncratic vasodilatory effect)

  3. Hemolytic uremic syndrome

  4. Congenital parenchymal maldevelopment

  5. Congenital glomerular and tubular disease

  6. Immune complex disease

Postrenal

  1. Posterior urethral valves

  2. Uric acid obstruction

  3. Ureteropelvic junction (UPJ) obstruction

DIAGNOSTIC PROTOCOL

Medical History

  1. Birth and perinatal history (asphyxia and urine stream); adequate amniotic fluid

  2. Trauma

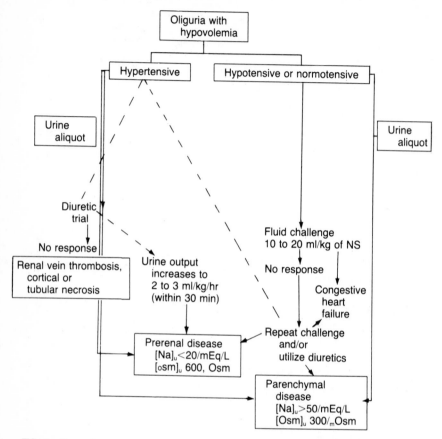

FIG. 2. Prerenal versus renal disease. [Na]u, urine sodium concentration; [Osm]u, urine osmolality; NS, normal saline.

3. Drugs

4. Hobbies

5. Travels

6. Recent illness

7. Recent exposure to illness

8. Family history

    a. Hearing or ophthalmological abnormalities

    b. Platelet abnormalities (qualitative and quantitative)

    c. Neurological disorders

    d. Renal disease (hypertension, edema)

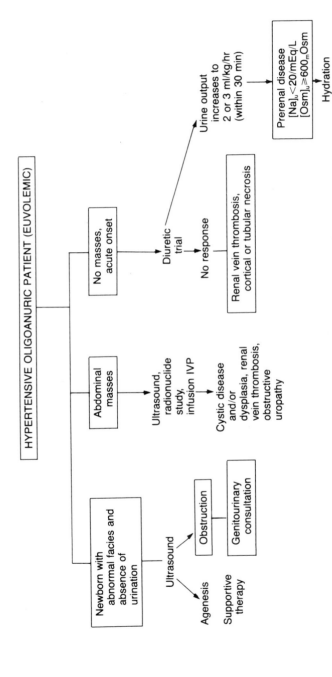

FIG. 3. Postrenal versus renal versus prerenal failure. [Na]$_u$, urine sodium concentration; [Osm]$_u$, urine osmolality.

TABLE 1. *Laboratory tests to aid in differential diagnosis of prerenal and renal failure*

Test	Prerenal failure	Renal failure
Urine specific gravity	>1.016	1.010
$[Osm]_u$	>600 mOsm	<400 mOsm
$[Na]_u$	<20 mEq/L	>50 mEq/L
FE_{Na} $\dfrac{[Na]_u \times [Cr]_s}{[Cr]_u \times [Na]_s}$	<1%	>2%
$[Osm]_u/[Osm]_s$ ratio	>1.5	≤0.8–1.2
Fluid challenge: normal saline 10 to 20 ml/ kg i.v. over a period of 30 to 45 min	Output increases within 30 to 45 min[a]	(±) No effect
Diuretic challenge: mannitol, 0.5 mg/kg i.v. *and/or* furosemide (Lasix®), 2 to 5 mg/kg i.v.	Output increases within 30 to 45 min[a]	(±) No effect

[a]Urine volume increases to 2 to 3 ml/kg/hr or urine output occurs in place of prior anuria; always palpate the abdomen to detect a palpable or possibly obstructed bladder.
$[Osm]_u$: Urine osmolality; $[Na]_u$: urine sodium concentration; FE_{Na}: fractional excretion of sodium; $[Cr]_s$: serum creatinine concentration; $[Cr]_u$: urine creatinine concentration; $[Na]_s$: serum sodium concentration; $[Osm]_s$: serum osmolality.

  e. Heredity traits

  f. Stillborn children

  g. Collagen diseases

  h. Blood disorders

Physical Examination

1. Growth and developmental state
2. Vital signs
3. State of hydration
4. Pallor, flushing
5. Skin lesions
6. Dysmorphic features
7. Abdominal masses
8. Genitals
9. Edema
10. Mental status

Laboratory Investigations

1. Complete blood cell count, platelets, reticulocyte count, peripheral smear, SS prep
2. Urinalysis and urine culture
3. Serum and urine electrolytes
4. Creatinine, blood urea nitrogen

5. Creatinine clearance and urine protein excretion

6. Collagen evaluation (complement, antinuclear antibodies, LE preparation)

7. Uric acid, calcium, phosphorus

8. Urine and serum osmolality

9. Radiographic evaluation and/or renal biopsy (individually determined)

TREATMENT PROTOCOL

Survival depends on the cause and is more likely (80% to 90%) if the renal failure is secondary to primary renal disease (without multisystem involvement) than if it is secondary to a major operative procedure.

Prophylaxis and Early Intervention

1. Early diagnosis of the major category (prerenal, renal, postrenal)

2. Volume repletion

3. Diuretics

4. Delineation of the anatomical involvement, if applicable (e.g., obstruction, congenital or other malformations) by ultrasound, radionuclide studies, intravenous pyelogram (IVP), and/or cystoscopy with retrograde pyelography (rarely indicated in children)

5. Surgical diversion, if necessary (e.g., obstructive uropathy)

Infections

Polymorphonuclear cell function is often abnormal, and elevated urea may suppress a febrile response.

1. Avoid the use of catheters

2. Avoid prophylactic antibiotics

3. Aggressive diagnosis and treatment of infections (alter dose of antibiotics based on degree of renal failure)

Nutrition

1. **Fluids:** D_5, D_{10}, i.e., 5% or 10% dextrose in water, etc. (insensible loss of fluids):

    a. 300 ml/m²/day plus urine output (urine replacement is ml/ml quantity and quality)

    b. Electrolytes: Free except for urine replacement

    c. Daily weight loss of 0.5% to 1.0% of body weight/day is expected over first few days

2. **Calories:** Approximately 400 cal/m²/24 hr are required to minimize protein breakdown.

3. **Salt (NaCl) requirement:** Be wary of any restriction in medullary disease.

   a. Depends on urinary excretion under usual conditions

   b. Tolerance ranges widely from a minimum of 2 mEq/day to a maximum of 1,000 mEq/day

4. **Potassium:** Intake must be markedly restricted because of the limitation in excretion but not so severe that minimal protein ingestion (0.5 to 1.0/g/kg/day) is obviated.

   Consider less intake of essential amino acids, which allows reutilization of nonessential amino acids and promotes recovery.

Complications and Intercurrent Problems (Figs. 4, 5, and 6)

1. Fluid overload or dehydration

2. Hyponatremia or hypernatremia

3. Hypertension

4. Congestive heart failure

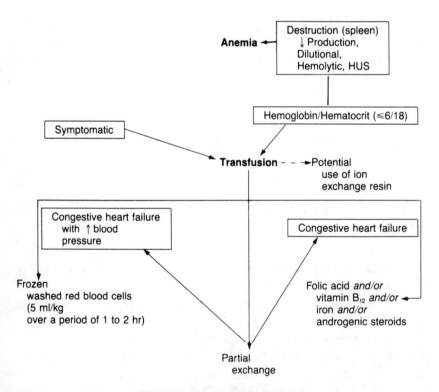

FIG. 4. Anemia in acute renal failure.

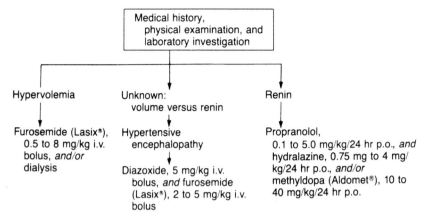

FIG. 5.   Hypertension in acute renal failure.

5. Hyperkalemia
6. Acidosis
7. Anemia
8. Seizures or coma
9. Hypocalcemia
10. Bleeding diathesis

Indications for Dialysis

1. Hyperkalemia (unresponsive to exchange resin and/or excessive level)
2. Refractory congestive heart failure
3. Refractory hypertension (volume related)
4. Refractory acidosis
5. Dialyzable drug (toxic ingestions)
6. Uremia
7. Signs of hypercatabolism
8. Severe hyperphosphatemia or hypernatremia
9. Preoperative dialysis to improve surgical outcome
10. In children there is a tendency not to dialyze at a specific creatinine and/or blood urea nitrogen level, but more in relation to the clinical state

Contraindications for Peritoneal Dialysis

1. **Absolute:**
   a. Absence of the diaphragm
   b. Inadequate nursing or supervisory care

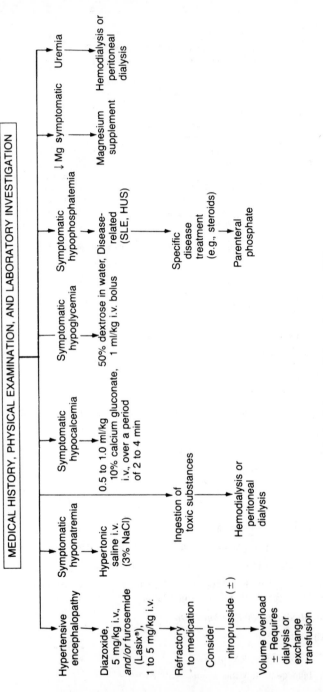

FIG. 6. Seizures and/or coma in acute renal failure.

2. **Relative:**

   a. Bleeding diathesis

   b. Bowel obstruction

   c. Recent abdominal surgery with use of prosthetic material

   d. Extensive adhesions

   e. Renal agenesis

   f. Trisomy or other genetic abnormality

   g. Focal peritonitis

   h. Fecal fistula or colostomy

   i. Major vascular anastomosis

   j. Undiagnosed abdominal illness

Contraindications for Percutaneous Renal Biopsy

1. **Absolute:**

   a. Unilateral kidney

   b. Coagulation abnormality

   c. Malignant disease or perinephritis

   d. Polycystic disease

   e. Uncontrolled hypertension

   f. Small kidneys

2. **Relative:**

   a. Atypical renal position (high, low, rotated)

   b. Pregnancy

   c. Severe hydronephrosis

   d. Suspected renal vein thrombosis

   e. Renal artery aneurysm

   f. Uremia (if chronic, kidneys may also be small and the associated bleeding diathesis may cause severe bleeding)

APPENDIX 1
RENAL FUNCTION TESTS

Urine Collection

1. Accurate urine collections are possible at all ages, although slightly more difficult in an infant.

2. A plastic bag (i.e., Hollister urine collection bag) should be applied to the infant's perineum.

3. Supervisory personnel must watch the infant carefully so that the bag is emptied as soon as the child voids.

4. It is also imperative that the perineal area be thoroughly cleansed to minimize the possibility of contamination.

5. If the child has not voided in approximately 30 min, the bag must be replaced.

6. It is often helpful to feed the child with tempting fluids at the time of, or just after, applying the urine collection device.

Suprapubic Tap

1. Suprapubic fluid examination is a valid way of determining urinary tract infection in a child in whom there has been some difficulty with previously contaminated samples.

2. The infant is fed 30 to 40 min prior to performance of the test.

3. At the time of the test, the infant is cleansed thoroughly, just after the bladder is palpated.

4. The needle is then inserted in the midline, just above the symphysis pubis, and urine is collected through the needle into the attached syringe.

5. Any organism grown from this sample, regardless of quantity, is indicative of a urinary tract infection.

Urine Volume

1. The quantity of urine passed by a child is a reflection of the concentrating ability, the osmotic load that must be excreted.

2. The solute load depends on dietary intake and metabolic state.

3. For every 100 calories ingested, a urine volume of 20 to 30 ml is required to excrete the concomitant solids.

4. Oliguria is defined as urinary excretion of <0.5 ml/kg/hr in a 4-hr period, or <240 ml/m^2/day.

Urinalysis

1. The accuracy of the urinalysis will, in large part, depend on the lack of contamination of the urine, as well as its timely analysis.

2. If urine is not promptly analyzed after collection (within 20 to 30 min) there is a change in the bacterial content, as well as early breakdown of the sediment.

3. If the urine cannot be promptly analyzed, it should be refrigerated.

4. Clean, first voided, morning urine is a good random screening test for urine concentrating ability.

5. Turbid urine does not necessarily reflect infection and, in fact, more often reflects the presence of amorphous phosphates and/or urates, particularly if the urine is concentrated. If there is some concern about a urinary tract infection, several

drops of alkaline substance placed in the urine will dissolve the amorphous materials and remove some of the turbidity.

Concentration of the Urine

1. See water deprivation test (see Appendix 2).
2. Healthy children, from their toddler years through adolescence, are able to achieve maximal osmolality of close to 1,200 mOsm.
3. A reasonable screening test for urine concentration is to analyze the first voided morning urine for osmolality.
4. Urine specific gravities may range from 1.001 to slightly beyond 1.030, with respective osmolalities of 40 to 1,200 mOsm/kg.
5. Specific gravity will be significantly affected by any exogenous substances imparting increased density to the urine (e.g., IVP dye).
6. Osmolality is a more valid test, in the presence of exogenous substances, because it measures osmotically active particles rather than urine density.
7. Protein and glucose will increase the osmolality and specific gravity of the urine.

Protein

1. See Proteinuria chapter.
2. Screening methods such as dip stick tests, do not detect all proteins in the urine.
3. Albumin, under normal conditions, is the main urinary protein, and is detected by the dip stick test at $\simeq$150 mg/L of urine.

Glucose

Glucose oxidase is the catalytic enzyme utilized in this test and may give false negative results if vitamin C, tetracycline, and/or certain other agents are present in the urine or the urine container. Hydrogen peroxide, bleach, and several antibiotics may give false positive tests.

pH

The kidneys are able to vary the urine pH between 4.5 and 8.5, but routine screening methods detect urine pH as low as 5.5 and as high as 7.5. Under circumstances where it is desirable to have more exact measurements, collection under oil and analysis with a pH meter are necessary.

Microscopic Analysis

1. The urine is collected as previously described.
2. The urine must be promptly analyzed (optimal, $\simeq$30 min; tolerable lapse, 1 hr).

3. The urine specimen is centrifuged at about 2,000 rpm for approximately 5 min. The supernatant is then discarded and several drops of a staining substance, such as Sedistain®, may be added to help delineate red and white blood cells.

4. Pyuria does not necessarily indicate urinary tract infection; it is also seen in dehydration, inflammatory diseases of the kidneys, and glomerulonephritis.

5. Fine granular or hyalin casts may be seen in the urine under normal circumstances, but red and white blood cell casts are distinctly unusual and should lead to further evaluation of the child.

6. Urine samples continuously showing more than five red blood cells per high power field are abnormal.

7. The number of acceptable white blood cells differs for males and females, and the normal number for females is still controversial; males should have no more than 10 white blood cells per high power field.

Glomerular Filtration Rate

1. Creatinine clearance is an estimate of glomerular filtration rate (GFR).

2. Creatinine must be freely filterable at the glomerularis and have minimal secretory or reabsorbed activities to avoid falsely increasing or decreasing the clearance.

3. Although creatinine is secreted to a small degree by the renal tubules, thus falsely elevating its clearance rate slightly, it is still thought to be a valid test.

4. Creatinine is a normal metabolic product of muscle creatine and is excreted daily in the urine proportional to individual muscle mass (relatively constant for each age group); its amount in the blood is usually constant with normal renal and thyroid functioning.

5. A rule of thumb for normal serum creatinine is to add 0.1 mg/year of age after 1 year.

6. There is a diurnal variation of creatinine, with its highest levels occurring late in the day.

7. Male muscle mass is greater than that of comparable females by about 12 years of age; therefore, at that time, creatinine in pubescent males tends to be slightly higher than in females.

8. Creatinine clearance (CrCl) must be corrected for surface area to be applicable to a child.

   a. CrCl (real) = (CrCl measured) $\times$ (1.73 m^2 patient's surface area)

   b. $$CrCl \text{ (in ml/min)} = \frac{Cr_u \blacktriangle V_u}{Cr_s} \div 1{,}440 \text{ min/day}$$

   where Cr_u is urine creatinine concentration, V_u is urine volume, and Cr_s is serum creatinine concentration.

   c. GFR = 0.55 $\times$ length of patient (cm)/Cr_s

d. In a chronic or stable state of renal failure, a gross measure of CrCl may be derived from Cr_s:

$$Cr_s \ 2 \ mg/dl = 40 \ ml/min \tag{1}$$

$$Cr_s \ 3 \ mg/dl = 20 \ to \ 30 \ ml/min \tag{2}$$

$$Cr_s \ 4 \ mg/dl = 10 \ ml/min \tag{3}$$

Selectivity of Proteinuria

Minimal lesions of the glomeruli will allow passage of small proteins, while glomeruli with more frequent lesions will allow the passage of larger proteins, and therefore, be less selective (see Proteinuria and Nephrotic Syndrome chapters).

APPENDIX 2
WATER DEPRIVATION TEST

Objective

To determine the intactness of the concentrating mechanism of the kidney and the antidiuretic hormone (ADH) secretory ability.

Methods

1. General: Initial fluid deprivation followed by the administration of ADH.

2. Specific:

a. Obtain base-line weight and urine sample (specific gravity and osmolality) and monitor electrolyte levels just prior to initiating the test and every 2 to 4 hr during the test, if possible. In infants, the test, by necessity, will be shorter and the sampling more frequent.

b. Restrict fluid for 12 to 16 hr or until patient loses 3% to 5% of his body weight.

c. Normal urine osmolality or adequate response to this test is 800 mOsm. If this concentration is not achieved, 3 to 5 units of aqueous vasopressin should be given subcutaneously and the urine osmolality monitored over the next 1 to 2 hr.

d. An increase in urine osmolality of more than 10% suggests central diabetes insipidus; no change in osmolality suggests a renal defect.

APPENDIX 3. *Commonly used antimicrobials that require dose-modification in renal failure*

Drugs	Carbenicillin (i.v.)	Celazolin (i.m., i.v.)	Cephalexin (oral)	Cephalothin (i.v.)	Gentamycin (i.m., i.v.)	Kanamycin (i.m.)	Streptomycin (i.m.)	Tetracycline (oral)	Tobramycin (i.m., i.v.)	Vancomycin (i.v.)
Therapeutic serum levels	25–100 µg/ml	—	—		4–8 µg/ml	10 µg/ml	—	—	6–12 µg/ml	5–10 µg/ml
Loading dose	4–6 g	0.5 g	0.5 g	1–3 g	1–2 mg/kg	7 mg/kg	1.0 g	0.5–1.0 g	1.0 mg/kg	1.0 g
Ccr 80		Usual dose								
70										
60	4–5 g/4 hr									
50			500 mg/4–6 hr	1–2 g/4–6 hr	1–5 mg/kg/8 hr	7 mg/kg/every third T½				
40		250 mg/6 hr	500 mg/8–12 hr		0.5 mg/kg/(Cr × 4) hr	($T½ = Cr × 3$)			$kg/Cr = mg$ of tobramycin/8 hr or 1.0–1.5 mg/kg/(Cr × 6) hr	
30					0.5–0.8 mg/8 hr		0.5–1.0 g/2–3 days			
20	2–4 g/6–12 hr	250 mg/6–12 hr	250 mg/12 hr	1–2 g/6–8hr	0.3 mg/kg/8 hr	0.25 g/24 hr		0.5 g/day		
10			250 mg/12 hr			0.25 g/48 hr				
5	2 g/12 hr	250 mg/48 hr	250 mg/12–24 hr	1–2 g/8–12 hr	0.2 mg/kg/8 hr	7 mg/kg/5–7 days	0.5 g/3–4 days	0.25 g/day	0.1 mg/kg/8 hr	1.0 g/10–14 days
Hemodialysis	2 g/12–24 hr and 2 g/PHD	250 mg/48 hr and 250 mg PHD	250 mg/12–24 hr and 500 mg PHD	1–2 g/8–12 hr and 1–2 g PHD	0.25 mg/kg/12 hr or 1.0–1.5 mg/kg PHD	7 mg/kg/every other HD	0.5 g/3–4 days and 250 mg PHD	0.25 g/day and 0.25 g PHD	1 mg/kg PHD	1.0 g/7–10 days
Peritoneal dialysis	2 g/6–12 hr			1 mg/kg/12 hr	1 mg/kg/12 hr	3.5 mg/kg 24 hr or 0.25 g/24 hr				
Cautions	1 g contains 4.7 mEq Na⁺	—	—	Nephrotoxic probably dose related (ARF)	Nephrotoxic dose related (ARF, rarely tubular dysfunction)	Nephrotoxic dose related (ARF, rarely tubular dysfunction)	Nephrotoxic dose related (ARF)	Nephrotoxic dose related (ARF), increases catabolism	Nephrotoxic dose related (ARF)	Nephrotoxic dose related (ARF)

Note: hr = hours, ARF = acute renal failure, Cr = serum creatinine (mg/100 ml), Ccr = creatinine clearance (ml/min). $T½$ = half-life (hr), P = post, HD = hemodialysis. i.v. = intravenously; i.m. = intramuscularly; Na⁺ = sodium ion, kg = body weight in kg.
From Cheigh, J. S. (1977): Commonly used antimicrobials that require dose-modification in renal failure. *Am. J. Med.*, 62 (4) 557, with permission.

Adrenal Hyperfunction

Excess secretion of adrenal hormones may be caused by a variety of factors, such as adrenal hyperplasia, adrenal tumors, or direct stimulation from the pituitary gland. The clinical manifestations depend on which hormone has been excessively secreted. Generally, the manifestations are those of excess glucocorticoid, mineralocorticoids, androgenic hormones, aldosterone, and catecholamines. In congenital adrenal hyperplasia (adrenogenital syndrome), the presence of enzyme defects prevents the formation of some of these adrenal hormones and, hence, the clinical manifestations are those of deficiency of the hormones and an excess of their precursors or the hormones not affected by the enzyme deficiency, which are stimulated by excessive pituitary adrenocorticotropic hormone (ACTH) secretion.

Adrenal hyperfunction is manifested by four distinct, but closely related, clinical syndromes:

Glucocorticoid excess (Cushing's Syndrome)

May be associated with excess adrenal androgens and to a lesser degree with increased mineralocorticoids.

Cortisol Precursors' Excess (Adrenogenital Syndrome)

Depending on the enzyme defect, androgens and mineralocorticoids may be decreased or increased in 18-hydroxylase deficiency; only mineralocorticoids are decreased and cortisol and sexual development are normal.

Aldosterone Excess (Primary Hyperaldosteronism)

Other steroids are variable.

Catecholamine Excess (Pheochromocytoma)

The excess catecholamines may be secreted from tumors of the adrenal medulla or extramedullary tissue.

Adrenal hyperfunction should be suspected in any infant or child with the following characteristics:

1. Family history of unexplained deaths in infancy.

2. Family history of tall children with sexual precocity but short adults.

3. Signs of virilization, such as hirsutism, acne, hypertrophied genitalia.

4. Overweight and obesity.

5. Hypertension.

6. Ambiguous genitalia.

7. Vague symptoms, such as fatigue, weakness, tachycardia, failure to gain weight, polydipsia, and polyuria.

8. Abnormal carbohydrate or fat metabolism (abnormal glucose tolerance test).

9. Abnormal electrolytes, such as hyponatremia with hyperkalemia or hypernatremia with hypokalemia or hyperkalemia.

10. Unexplained metabolic acidosis or alkalosis.

11. Menstrual irregularities.

DIAGNOSTIC PROTOCOL

Cushing's Syndrome

1. **Etiology:** Iatrogenic (secondary to steroid therapy), adrenal tumor, adenoma of pituitary, adrenal hyperplasia, extrapituitary ACTH-producing tumor.

2. **Clinical manifestations:** "Buffalo" adiposity with moon facies, fatigue and weakness, diabetes mellitus, hypertension and edema, osteoporosis, growth retardation, menstrual irregularities.

3. **Blood:** Elevated serum cortisol; ACTH decreased in patients with tumors slightly increased in hyperplasia, and greatly increased in pituitary tumors; serum androgens may be increased; hypokalemic, hypochloremic, hypernatremic, alkalosis; hyperglycemia.

4. **Urine:** Elevated free cortisol, elevated 17-hydroxycorticosteroids, normal 17-ketosteroids (elevated in tumors only), glycosuria.

5. **ACTH stimulation:** Excessive response in cases of adrenal hyperplasia, poor response in cases of adrenal tumor.

6. **Dexamethasone suppression:** Causes suppression in cases of hyperplasia; no effect in cases of tumors, even in large doses.

7. **Bone age:** Decreased osteoporosis.

8. **Other procedures:** Intravenous pyelogram (IVP) and adrenal arteriogram.

Adrenogenital Syndrome

1. **Etiology:** Inherited deficiency of an enzyme required for adrenocortical hormone production, with pituitary excretion of an excess of ACTH in compensation, resulting in adrenal hyperplasia and accumulation of corticol precursors; virilizing maternal tumors or androgen administration in the first trimester; tumors of adrenal gland, testes, or ovary; idiopathic adrenal hyperplasia later in life.

2. **Clinical manifestations:** Depends on the specific enzyme deficiency (see Table 1).

3. **Blood:** See Table 1.

TABLE 1. *Adrenogenital syndrome*

| Enzyme deficiency | Genitalia | | Symptoms | Diagnostic abnormalities | |
	Females	Males		Urine	Serum
17-Hydroxylase	Virilized with enlarged clitoris, labial fusion, or both (pseudohermaphrodite); phallus formation	Virilized	Salt losing crisis in 30% with vomiting, circulatory collapse, and death	Increased 17-ketosteroids and pregnanetriol	Increased 17-hydroxy-progesterone, decreased sodium, elevated potassium, increased renin
11β-Hydroxylase	Virilized	Virilized	Hypertension	Increased 17-ketosteroids, pregnanetriol, deoxy-corticosterone, 11-deoxycortisol, and testosterone	Increased 11-deoxycortisol
3β-Hydroxysteroid dehydrogenase	Mild virilization	Incomplete masculinization, cryptorchidism, hypospadius	Salt losing crisis	Moderately increased 17-ketosteroids	Increased dehydroepiandosterone
20,20-Desmolase	Normal	Incomplete masculinization	Salt losing crisis	Normal or decreased 17-ketosteroids	
17-Hydroxylase	Normal	Incomplete masculinization	Hypertension	Increased pregnanetriol, decreased 17-ketosteroids and aldosterone	
18-Hydroxylase	Normal	Normal	Mineralocorticoid deficiency	Normal cortisol	Normal cortisol synthesis

4. **Urine:** See Table 1.

5. **Dexamethasone suppression:** Causes 17-ketosteroids to return to normal in cases of hyperplasia, but not in cases of adenoma.

6. **Bone age:** Advanced after 1 year of age.

7. **Other procedures:** Vaginogram, IVP, buccal smear.

Primary Hyperaldosteronism

1. **Etiology:** Adrenal tumor, adrenal hyperplasia.

2. **Clinical manifestations:** Paresthesias and tetany, weakness and fatigue, hypertension, edema.

3. **Blood:** Elevated serum aldosterone, abnormal glucose tolerance test, decreased plasma renin (increased in secondary aldosteronism), hypernatremic, hypokalemic, metabolic alkalosis.

4. **Urine:** Alkaline with low fixed specific gravity, proteinuria, elevated aldosterone.

5. **ACTH stimulation:** Further increases aldosterone excretion.

Pheochromocytoma

1. **Etiology:** Tumors of the adrenal medulla, extramedullary tumors.

2. **Clinical manifestations:** Intermittent hypertension, headache, tachycardia, palpitations, weight loss, anxiety and nervousness, hyperhydrosis, visual changes, polydipsia and polyuria, tremors.

3. **Blood:** Elevated serum epinephrine, norepinephrine, and metanephrine.

4. **Urine:** Increased urinary epinephrine, norepinephrine, and metanephrine; increased urinary vanillylmandelic acid.

5. **Dexamethasone suppression:** Spironolactone may be used to antagonize aldosterone and cause a decrease in alkalosis, hypokalemia, and hypernatremia.

6. **Other procedures:** Laparotomy to localize the tumor.

TREATMENT PROTOCOL

Cushing's Syndrome

1. Surgical resection of adrenal tumor.

2. Surgical resection and/or radiation or electrocoagulation of pituitary tumors.

3. Metyrapone (which blocks cortisol) or mitotane (adrenolytic) may be given before surgical resection or to cause a medical adrenalectomy.

4. Total resection in cases of hyperplasia.

5. ACTH and supplemental therapy are necessary pre- and postoperatively; watch for hypertension and poor wound healing.

Adrenogenital Syndrome

1. Vigorous fluid volume and salt replacement with 5% dextrose in normal saline solution, 150 mg/kg/day, in salt losing crisis.

2. Cortisone acetate, 10 to 25 mg/day p.o. for infants and 25 to 100 mg/day p.o. for older children (give 50% of the dose in the evening).

3. After stabilization, use maintenance doses as in Addison's disease.

4. Clitororesection and/or vaginoplasty.

5. Adjust medications by following growth, 17-ketosteroids, bone age, and blood pressure; dosage needed in newborn infants appears to be 2.5 mg of hydrocortisone every 8 hr for 1 year and then 10 to 20 mg/m^2/day in three divided doses; desoxycorticosterone acetate (DOCA) appears to be needed also.

Primary Hyperaldosteronism

1. Glucocorticoid administration.

2. Surgical resection of the tumor.

3. Total or subtotal adrenalectomy for hyperplasia.

Pheochromocytoma

1. Control blood pressure with dibenzamine before diagnostic procedures and surgical intervention.

2. Surgical resection of the tumor.

Airway Obstruction

Airway obstruction results from abnormalities and diseases that affect the conducting airways (nose, pharynx, larynx, trachea, bronchi, and bronchioles) (Fig. 1).

SIGNS AND SYMPTOMS

The signs and symptoms of airway obstruction depend on the anatomical area involved and the age of the patient. In general, patients with upper airway obstruction have stridor, dyspnea, and prolongation of inspiration, whereas those with lower airway obstruction show rhonchi, wheezes, tachypnea, and prolongation of expiration. However, infants with an upper airway lesion may show signs and symptoms of lower airway obstruction.

DIFFERENTIAL DIAGNOSIS

Upper Airway Obstruction

1. Choanal atresia
2. Laryngotracheomalacia
3. Laryngeal web
4. Laryngeal cyst
5. Laryngotracheoesophageal cleft
6. Vocal cord paralysis
7. Glottic or subglottic tumor
8. Hypoplasia of the mandible
9. Mediastinal masses:

    a. Anterior mediastinum: Thymoma, lymphoma

    b. Posterior mediastinum: Neurogenic tumors, gastrointestinal duplications, aortic aneurysms

    c. Middle mediastinum: Pericardial cysts, anomalies of the great vessels

10. Vascular rings: Right aortic arch and left ligamentum arteriosum, double aortic arch, anomalous innominate artery, anomalous right carotid artery, aberrant left subclavian artery.
11. Mucous plug
12. Macroglossia
13. Epiglottic malformation
14. Laryngeal injury and fracture
15. Tracheoesophageal fistula
16. Laryngotracheal bronchitis
17. Subglottic stenosis
18. Epiglottis
19. Mucous retention cyst
20. Thyroglossal duct remnants
21. Bronchial cleft cyst

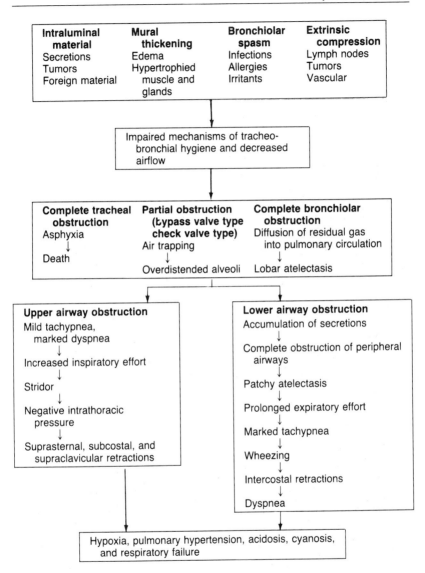

FIG. 1. Pathophysiology of airway obstruction.

22. Lemangioma

23. Lymphangioma

24. Pierre Robin syndrome

25. Congenital goiter

26. Phrenic nerve paralysis

27. Allergic reactions and angioneurotic edema

28. Foreign body

29. Hypertrophied tonsils and adenoids

Lower Airway Obstruction

1. Respiratory distress syndrome
2. Bronchopulmonary dysplasia
3. Wilson-Mikity syndrome
4. Aspiration
5. Esophageal chalasia and gastroesophageal reflux
6. Cystic fibrosis
7. α_1-Antitrypsin deficiency
8. Congenital heart disease
9. Congestive heart failure
10. Lung edema
11. Pneumonia: *Pneumocystis carinii, Chlamydia*
12. Lobar emphysema
13. Pulmonary hypoplasia
14. Diaphragmatic hernia
15. Pulmonary lymphangiectasis
16. Intracranial lesion
17. Metabolic disturbance
18. Immune deficiency
19. Bronchial adenoma
20. Allergy
21. Pertussis
22. Asthma
23. Organophosphorus poisoning
24. Tropical eosinophilia
25. Bronchiectasis
26. Bronchiolitis obliterans
27. Microlithiasis
28. Alveolar proteinosis

DIAGNOSTIC PROTOCOL

1. Patient must be attended during the procedures.

2. Immediate intervention (intubation or tracheostomy, positive pressure breathing, oxygen, suction) may be necessary before any procedure is done if patient is in respiratory failure with impending asphyxia, respiratory and/or cardiac arrest.

3. Measurement of arterial blood gases and pH allows immediate evaluation of the respiratory status.

4. Chest radiographs (posterior/anterior, and lateral) with fluoroscopy allow recognition of mediastinal masses, infiltrates, and pneumonias, cardiomegaly and heart failure, lung edema, emphysema, hyperinflation, diaphragmatic problems, bronchiectasis, atelectasis, or foreign body.

5. Posterior/anterior, and lateral radiographs of the neck yield diagnostic information about the retropharyngeal space, subglottic area, epiglottis, and subglottic space.

6. Other diagnostic tests: Complete blood cell count, circulating eosinophils, blood glucose, blood urea nitrogen, electrolytes, urinalysis, nasal smear for eosinophils, electrocardiogram.

7. Asthma. (See Diagnostic Protocol in Asthma chapter.)

8. Infection: Nasotracheal cultures, blood cultures, cultures and smears for pertussis, *Chlamydia*, and *Pneumocystis carinii*, epiglottitis, laryngotracheal bronchitis, bronchiolitis.

9. Foreign body: Immediate surgical consultation for bronchoscopy.

10. Congenital heart disease: See chapter on congestive heart failure.

11. If above procedures show no abnormalities, fluoroscopy with barium swallow is indicated.

   a. Give only 0.5 ml of barium if esophageal atresia is suspected.

   b. Inject barium through a catheter if H-type tracheoesophageal fistula is suspected.

   c. Evaluate vascular rings and swallowing because gastroesophageal reflux can give symptoms of airway disease.

12. If fluoroscopic examination shows no abnormalities, the following procedures are indicated.

   a. Tomograms to evaluate masses in upper airway obstruction (do not use routinely because of high doses of radiation).

   b. Serum levels of immunoglobulins (including IgE), α_1-antitrypsin, calcium, and magnesium, and sweat chloride level in lower airway obstruction.

13. If above studies show no abnormalities, consider the following procedures:

   a. Laryngoscopy (with a small fiber optic bronchoscope) or bronchoscopy in upper airway obstruction.

   b. Esophageal mobility and pH studies.

   c. Lung perfusion scan.

   d. Bronchography.

   e. Brain scan.

14. If findings are negative, consider the following procedures:

   a. Cardiac catheterization.

   b. Pulmonary and aortic angiograms.

   c. Epinephrine (bronchodilators dose for infants is indicated, although it is said that infants do not have enough muscle strength to react).

TREATMENT PROTOCOL [1]

Treatment depends on the etiology of the airway obstruction.

[1] If obstruction is complete: laryngoscopy (do not push the F.B.); Heimlich emergency maneuver; if these measures unsuccessful: emergency cricothyroidotomy incision or needle between the cricoid and thyroid cartilages, emergency bronchoscopy (experienced), tracheostomy.
Do not slap, shake, or give vigorous physiotherapy.
Do not attempt intubation if obstruction is complete.

1. Suction, oxygen, emergency radiographs, arterial blood gases (ABG), intravenous fluids, allow nothing by mouth.

2. Respiratory failure

   a. P_{CO_2}: 60 mm Hg

   b. P_{O_2}: 60 mm Hg

   c. pH: 7.3

2. Epiglottitis

   a. Intubation, antibiotics

3. Foreign body

   a. Surgical consultation for bronchoscopy

4. Croup (Consider each modality separately depending on the patient's condition.)

   a. Symptomatic treatment in mist tent

   b. Racemic epinephrine

   c. Cool mist with 25% to 30% oxygen

   d. Dexamethasone, 0.5 mg/kg/day in four doses for 1 to 3 days

   e. Tracheostomy

   f. Gastrostomy

   g. Pulmonary function testing

5. Infection: Ampicillin, 300 mg/kg/day in six divided doses, and chloramphenicol, 100 mg/kg/day in four divided doses if *H. influenzae* is considered

6. Tonsillectomy and adenoidectomy (if indicated)

7. Dilatation of airway (if indicated)

8. Pulmonary physiotherapy

9. Surgical evaluation

10. Bronchodilators

A llergic Reactions

Allergies represent an altered clinical state in the host following a challenge with an allergen. The resulting manifestation to this challenge may represent a hypersensitivity reaction, an immune reaction, or both. Unfortunately, the body's immune system, which normally defends against foreign elements, may precipitate an abnormal allergic reaction. Antithetically, if the immune system is not functioning adequately, an immunodeficient disease state may result. Therefore, allergies are examples of the body's active, but inappropriate, immune responses.

An individual's allergic constitution is dictated, in part, by his or her genetic background. The clinical syndromes that develop depend on which surface (e.g., bronchi, gut) the antibody-forming target resides. One of the more dramatic examples is that in which the target cell is a mast cell, and the antibody produced by the body's immune system is fixed or attached to this target cell. Following significant antigenic stimulation or challenge, the mast cell releases histamine, slow reacting substance of anaphylaxis (SRS-A), bradykinin, and/or eosinophilic chemotactic factor of anaphylaxis (ECF-A).

The clinical reaction to this mast cell degranulation will depend on where the target organ is located. Food allergies, urticaria, and allergic rhinitis are, therefore, merely reflections of the specific "surface lining" which is attacked (Fig. 1).

DIFFERENTIAL DIAGNOSIS

1. **Type I:** Immediate
   a. Anaphylaxis (drugs, insect stings, antitoxins)
   b. Allergy (hay fever, asthma)
2. **Type II:** Cytotoxic
   a. Complement-fixing (transfusion reaction)
   b. Immunoprotein recognition (granulocytopenia)
3. **Type III:** Soluble antigen-antibody complexes (immune complexes)
   a. Arthus' reaction
   b. Serum sickness
   c. Massive complement activation (Waterhouse-Friderichsen syndrome)

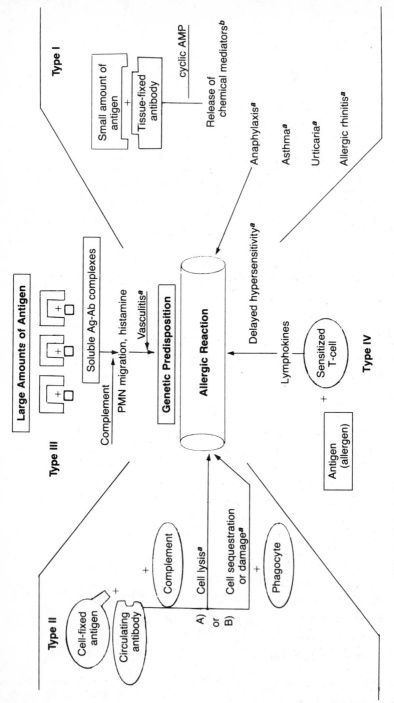

FIG. 1. Pathophysiology of allergic reactions in children. [a]Anticipated reaction. [b]Histamine, SRS-A, kinins.

4. Type IV: Delayed hypersensitivity (cell-mediated)

  a. Contact dermatitis

  b. Tuberculosis

DIAGNOSTIC AND TREATMENT PROTOCOLS

Table 1 gives diagnostic and treatment protocols for the four types of allergic reactions.

TABLE 1. *Allergic reactions: Diagnostic and treatment protocols*

Diagnosis	Treatment
Type I: Immediate	
Requires prior exposure to an antigen; dependent upon fixation of IgE to the mast cell	Immediate recognition and concomitant therapy are essential; death may occur very rapidly
Begins within seconds to minutes after exposure to the antigen	Discontinue the provoking medication immediately
Collapse, hypotension, upper and lower airway obstruction urticarial rash, vomiting, and diahrrea, in any combination, are common symptoms	Epinephrine 1:1,000, 0.01 ml/kg i.v. or s.c. 0.3–0.5 ml maximum dose; repeated every 3 min as needed
Heterologous serum, human gamma gobulin, pollen extracts, insect venom, foods, and drugs have all been implicated	Apply a tourniquet to the extremity in which antigenic material was injected
Diagnosis depends on a history of prior exposure to the antigen (not necessarily known by the patient and not needed if clinical diagnosis is apparent) and recognition of the characteristic signs and symptoms	Inject epinephrine 1:1,000, 0.2 ml/kg s.c., into the antigenic site
	Remove insect stinger, if this was the source of the insult
	Initiate intravenous infusion to provide for the administration of diluted epinephrine in the event of vascular collapse (volume expanders and vasopressors may be mandatory)
	Oxygen, endotracheal intubation, and/or tracheotomy may be life-saving measures
	Diphenhydramine (Benadryl®) may be used for prolonged reaction and/or urticaria and angioedema (1–2 mg/kg slow i.v.) or i.m.
	Aminophylline boluses (4 mg/kg) infused intermittently to decrease broncho spasm
	Corticosteroids are not helpful during the acute reaction, but may be used in persistent bronchospasm or hypotension
	Once the patient's condition is stabilized, and further medical history obtained, including characterization of the antigen, an attempt should be made at desensitization, in conjunction with the allergist; desensitization is important for *Hymenoptera*-induced anaphylaxis

TABLE 1. *(continued)*

Diagnosis	Treatment

Asthma

See Asthma chapter

Urticaria and Angioedema

Classify, for example, as idiopathic, infective, secondary to food or drugs, physical factors, collagen diseases

Differentiate from urticaria pigmentosa (a diffuse mast-cell disease), papular urticaria (insect bites), and hereditary angioedema (a specific complement deficiency)

Dietary history (3% to 5% of cases are caused by food and its additives)

Physical examination, including tests of dermographism, ice cube and heat tests

Laboratory investigation:
Complete blood cell count with an eosinophil count, erythrocyte sedimentation rate; urinalysis, complement levels (THC, C3, C4); cryoglobulins; screening test for syphilis; other serological investigations as needed

Stool examination for ova and parasites; vaginal smears for *Candida* and *Trichomonas*

Skin tests, for yeast-containing foods, for example, may be indicated based on the patient's history

Eliminate the defined etiological or aggravating factors

Antihistamines such as diphenhydramine (Benadryl®), 5 mg/kg/ 24 hr, i.v., i.m., p.o. for acute urticaria, Chlortimeton® 2 mg every 6 hr for chronic urticaria; Periactin®, Atarax®, and Vistaril® may be used in various combinations as needed

Epinephrine 1:1000, 0.01 ml/kg, during the acute symptomatic stage, especially in edema of the pharyngeal area

Dietary manipulations need to be considered (a diary on the diet is helpful)

Use of steroids in acute is questionable; may be used in urticaria; for chronic urticaria (by five years, <1% of patients with chronic urticaria are still plagued; most have ceased to have urticaria by the end of the first year)

Allergic Rhinitis

History of sneezing, nasal itching, conjunctivitis, cough and varying degrees of nasal obstruction

Affects approximately 15% of children; one of the most common problems for pediatricians and family practitioners

Hereditary predisposition;

Onset is usually at young age

May be perennial (intermittent or continuous symptoms without seasonal variation), seasonal (pollinosis, hay fever), or both

Mucous membranes are often swollen and red with clear mucus discharge early in the course, becoming pale and boggy with chronic rhinitis

Adenoids and tonsils are often enlarged; child <3 years of age with enlarged tonsils probably has an allergic diathesis or a positive family history of allergy

Sinus radiographs may show cloudiness and be accompanied by tenderness over the maxillary sinuses

Differential diagnosis: vasomotor rhinitis, infectious rhinitis, nasal polyps, aspirin sensitivity

Avoid the offending agent, which may involve environmental controls (dustproofing, electrostatic filters, and airconditioning)

Hyposensitization may or may not be helpful; oral medication, including antihistamines, especially HI receptor antihistamines (e.g., Optimine® or Azactidin®) may be used

Intranasal medication, such as cromolyn, and the use of decongestants may be worthwhile, as may corticosteroids

Diagnosis	Treatment

Laboratory investigation: Complete blood cell count, eosinophil count, nasal eosinophils, RAST testing

Skin testing (scratch and intradermal) is important; the test for seasonal rhinitis will be markedly positive, thus differentiating it from perennial rhinitis

House dust, molds, animal dander, and various occupational products may give positive skin or other provocation tests

The main confusion is attempting to distinguish allergic rhinitis from vasomotor rhinitis (other than skin tests, positive nasal eosinophils may be helpful); a purulent nasal discharge suggests infectious or vasomotor rhinitis and mitigates against allergic rhinitis

Atopic Dermatitis

A common skin disorder of children

Atopic dermatitis, hay fever, or asthma is often found among the families of patients with atopic dermatitis

More prevalent during certain seasons, especially during the winter; exacerbated by the cold

Scratching plays a major role in worsening; summing up the idea of atopic dermatitis as genetically abnormal or predisposed skin, subject to many different irritants that involve it in an itch-scratch cycle, with pruritus possibly being the primary event; the itch-scratch cycle allows the dermatitis to fluctuate between eczematization and lichenification; the flare factor an exacerbating variable, makes "the itch the problem" (different in each person) and must be identified so that specific treatment can be instituted

Young infants may have marked vesicular lesions, as opposed to xerosis (dry skin) in older children

Instruct the parents about the concept of dry skin inheritance and the coexistence of an allergic constitution

Treat skin infections aggressively with erythromycin or, alternatively, ampicillin

Remove basic irritants from the environment (e.g., wool clothing); control home temperature (sweating tends to exacerbate the phenomena by increasing itching); cut fingernails and file daily to remove rough edges

Relieve the itching with Benadryl® Periactin® and/or Atarax®.

Bathing in soap and water should be limited, in time and frequency of baths

Cetaphil® lotion creates a monomolecular film, which retains moisture

Type II: Cytotoxic

Antibodies are formed against cell-surface antigens; antibody-coated cell is then destroyed by complement-dependent lysis, phagocytosis and lysis of the cell, or K-cell lysis

ABO or RH incompatability

History of potential prior exposure to a similar antigen

History of any ongoing disease process that predisposes to complement or other mediated hemolytic reactions (i.e., Addison's or Goodpasture's disease, in which preformed antibodies may exist)

TABLE 1. *(continued)*

Diagnosis	Treatment

History of neonatal hemolytic episodes in the newborn period

Clinical manifestations and laboratory confirmation

Type III: Immune Complex

Mediated hypersensitivity reaction: Arthus-type reaction; serum-sickness type reaction (immune complex glomerulonephritis, immune complex arteritis, and immune complex associated with connective tissue disease, such as rheumatoid arthritis)

Involves soluble antigen-antibody complexes, with antibody or antigen excess

Systemic lupus erythemotosus, with serological confirmation

Type IV: Cell-Mediated

Antigen interacts with specific receptors on surface of a responsive T lymphocyte, which in turn triggers effector functions, including lymphokines, cytotoxicity, suppressor-cell or helper-cell activity

History of exposure to tuberculosis and/or a positive skin test

Ambiguous Genitalia

The birth of a child with ambiguous genitalia is an emergency for the parents even though the infant may be in no immediate danger. Rapid evaluation of the child before gender assignment is essential. Four major factors (genetic, gonadal, hormonal, and genitalia) interdependently determine the sex of the individual. Any alteration of these factors can lead to a child with ambiguous external genitalia (Fig. 1).

SIGNS AND SYMPTOMS

Manifestations of ambiguous genitalia are directly related to the time of development and the specific factors affected. Regardless of pathogenesis, the ambiguous external genitalia are remarkably similar along a continuum with an appearance somewhere between normal male and female phenotype. The external anatomy of these children may vary from clitoral enlargement (with congenital adrenal hyperplasia) to complete absence of the penis and lack of fusion of the median raphe.

A classic example of ambiguous external genitalia and one of the more common clinical variants is congenital adrenal hyperplasia. In this entity, a normal female neonate, although born with a slightly prominent clitoris, does well clinically until the end of the first week of life. At that time, the baby begins vomiting, develops hyperkalemia, and progresses rapidly into a shocklike state. Although these manifestations are extreme, the example is provided to convey the principle that a child with ambiguous genitalia may have not only anatomical defects but also a combination of defects accompanied by clinical manifestations of concomitant hormonal imbalance.

DIFFERENTIAL DIAGNOSIS (Fig. 2)

---

1. Congenital adrenal hyperplasia
2. Mixed gonadal dysgenesis
3. Maternal androgen ingestion
4. Male dysgenesis
5. True hermaphrodite
6. Testosterone subresponsiveness
7. Testicular feminizing syndrome
8. Third-degree hypospadias
9. Bilateral cryptorchidism
10. Ovarian tumor

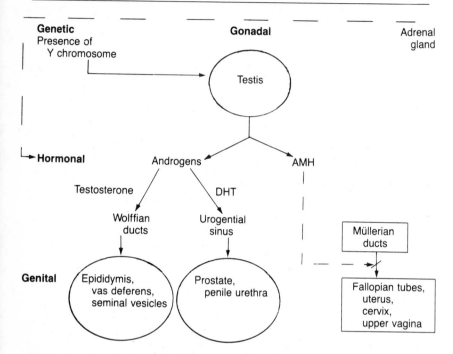

FIG. 1. Formation of male genitalia in the presence of the Y chromosome. AMH, Antimullerian hormone; DHT, Dihydrotestosterone.

TREATMENT PROTOCOL

1. Sexual behavior and gender assignment: The gender should be determined as soon as possible, and the parents should be informed of this decision immediately. In the face of difficulties in determining the gender, it is helpful to convene a gender board or committee composed of the primary care physician along with an endocrinologist, urologist, gynecologist, and psychiatrist, each of whom actively shares in evaluating the case and in reaching a decision regarding the ultimate gender assignment.

2. Surgical therapy: Following a thorough diagnostic evaluation, it is possible that the infant may require surgical anatomical alteration. The four areas that require the technical skill and patience of a surgical consultant often involve:

   a. Penile reconstruction (size, formation of urethral tube)

   b. Vaginal construction

FIG. 2. Diagnostic protocol. In screening with buccal smear for Barr bodies, neonates may have falsely negative test in the first 2 weeks of life. 17-P, plasma 17--hydroxyprogesterone; 17-KS, urinary 17-ketosteroids; CAH, congenital adrenal hyperplasia. Modified and reproduced with permission from Rosenfield, R. L., et al. (1980): The diagnosis and management of intersex. In: L. Gluck, et al. (eds.), *Current Problems in Pediatrics.* Year Book Medical Publishers Inc., Chicago.

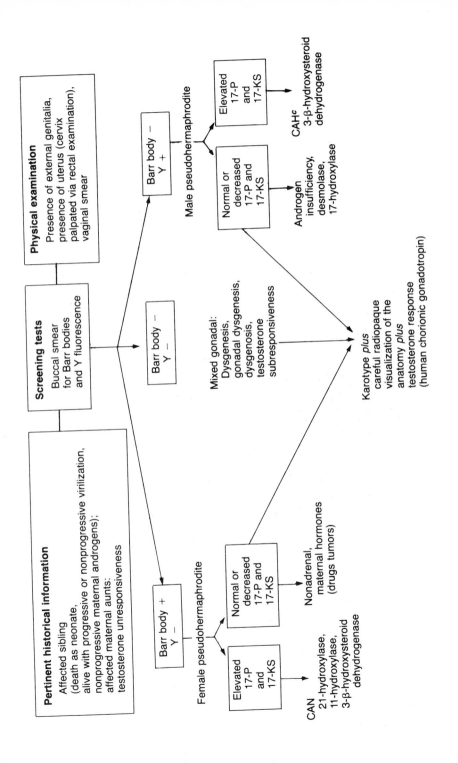

Pertinent historical information

Affected sibling (death as neonate, alive with progressive or nonprogressive virilization, nonprogressive maternal androgens); affected maternal aunts: testosterone unresponsiveness

Screening tests

Buccal smear for Barr bodies and Y fluorescence

Physical examination

Presence of external genitalia, presence of uterus (cervix palpated via rectal examination), vaginal smear

Barr body +
Y –

Female pseudohermaphrodite

Elevated 17-P and 17-KS

CAN
21-hydroxylase, 11-hydroxylase, 3-β-hydroxysteroid dehydrogenase

Normal or decreased 17-P and 17-KS

Nonadrenal, maternal hormones (drugs tumors)

Barr body –
Y –

Mixed gonadal: Dysgenesis, gonadal dysgenesis, dysgenosis, testosterone subresponsiveness

Barr body –
Y +

Male pseudohermaphrodite

Normal or decreased 17-P and 17-KS

Androgen insufficiency, desmolase, 17-hydroxylase

Elevated 17-P and 17-KS

CAHc
3-β-hydroxysteroid dehydrogenase

Karotype *plus* careful radiopaque visualization of the anatomy *plus* testosterone response (human chorionic gonadotropin)

   c. Clitoral reconstruction (clitoridectomy, clitoral reduction, clitoroplasty)

   d. Removal of gonadal elements (in an intersex patient with a Y chromosome).

3. Pharmacological and fluid therapy: Salt-losing crisis of congenital adrenal hyperplasia is used as an example.

   a. Acute therapy

   (1) Immediate fluid therapy may be required to restore volume and/or blood pressure; 0.75 normal saline infused at 200 ml/kg over the first 24-hr period will usually stabilize the infant (plasma or plasma substitutes may be substituted initially if shock is imminent).

   (2) Mineralocorticoid therapy: Deoxycorticosterone acetate (DOC), 1 mg/day i.m., should be administered as part of the neonate's resuscitative phase.

   (3) Glucocorticoid therapy: Often administered in the form of hydrocortisone, 50 mg/m^2 i.v. every 6 hr (10 mg in neonates), and cortisone acetate, 125 mg/m^2/day i.m. (25 mg in neonates)

   b. Postcrisis therapy

   (1) Oral feedings should be initiated as soon as the baby's condition is stable and should include at least 1 g of sodium chloride daily (about 15 ml of normal saline with the first or second ounce of each of the infant's six feedings).

   (2) Hydrocortisone may be discontinued at this time, but parenteral cortisone acetate (DOC) should be continued until the baby is considered clinically well.

   c. Stabilization

   (1) The maintenance dose of sodium chloride should average approximately 0.5 g daily, and toward the end of the first week of therapy, the infant should be expected to have normal electrolytes and appear well.

   (2) At this time, a long-acting form of DOC should be initiated (start with 25 mg i.m. every month).

   (3) Glucocorticoid therapy may be required, with 3.3 mg of hydrocortisone every 8 hr in neonates (average maintenance dose, 25 mg/m^2/day, p.o.)

   d. Long-term therapy should be monitored by a consultant and will often include maintenance glucocorticoid therapy as well as mineralocorticoid therapy in the form of a fluorinated steroid after the first year.

   These patients require the active supervision and consultative skills of a pediatric endocrinologist, who monitors their medications and its potential side effects and works closely with the primary care physician.

4. Sex hormone therapy: Patients who require hormone therapy for feminization because of their gonadal status require careful choice of an estrogen and close observation to avoid stunting of their growth.

   Male children may require hormone therapy as treatment for microphallus or pubertal masculinization (depot testosterone enanthate, 100 mg/m^2/month).

Amino Acid Disorders

Amino acid disorders result from inborn errors of metabolism, usually absent activity of a specific enzyme. Aberrations in the metabolic pathways affect the development and function of almost every organ system. The manifestations of amino acid disorders and other inborn errors of metabolism are, therefore, usually systemic, reflecting multisystem involvement (Fig.1). Almost all of these disorders are inherited.

This chapter summarizes some of the more common amino acid abnormalities (Table 1). Complete discussions and specific details of these and other inborn errors of metabolism are given in standard textbooks of pediatrics.

SIGNS AND SYMPTOMS

The various amino acid disorders often have similar clinical manifestations usually since they reflect multisystem dysfunction. Amino acid disorders should be suspected in any infant (especially a neonate) who presents with

1. Vomiting
2. Failure to thrive
3. CNS manifestations (e.g., seizures, lethargy, coma)
4. Unexplained metabolic acidosis
5. Unusual odor to the urine

Amino acid disorders should be ruled out in infants or children who present with any developmental disorder associated with mental retardation and/or speech defects.

DIFFERENTIAL DIAGNOSIS

1. Intestinal atresia
2. Anoxic brain damage
3. Intracranial hemorrhage
4. Other metabolic disorders
5. Chromosomal abnormalities
6. Congenital and acquired infections

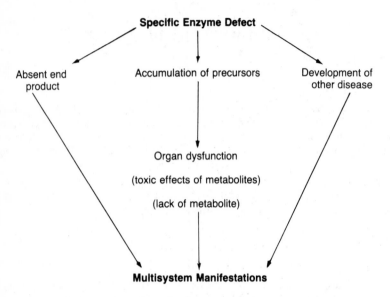

FIG. 1.   Pathophysiology of amino acid disorders.

TABLE 1. *Amino acid abnormalities*

Phenylalanine	Proline and hydroxyproline
Phenylketonuria	Prolinemia
Phenylalaninemia	Hydroxyprolinemia
Dihydropteridine reductase defect	Prolinuria
Methylmandelic aciduria	Valine, leucine, and isoleucine
Parahydroxyphenylacetic aciduria	Maple syrup urine disease
Tyrosine	Valinemia
Transient neonatal tyrosinemia	Isovaleric acidemia
Richner-Hanhart syndrome	Propionic acidemia
Albinism	Methylmalonic acidemia
Parkinsonism	Cystine
Alcaptonuria	Cystinuria
Tryptophan	Cystinosis
Hartnup disease	Methionine
Kynureninase defects	Methioninemia
Xanthurenic aciduria	Homocystinemia
Glycine	Histidine
Glycinemia	Histidinemia
Oxaluria and oxalosis	Urea cycle
	Ornithinemia and citrullinemia

DIAGNOSTIC PROTOCOL

Many disorders of amino acid metabolism result in myelinization defects and mental retardation. If diagnosis and treatment occur soon after birth, this sequela is often preventable. Diagnosis by amniotic fluid assay during the prenatal period may be indicated if the family history is suggestive of metabolic abnormalities.

1. The diagnosis almost always starts with a high index of suspicion.

2. Physical examination is usually nonspecific, except for the odor of the urine in certain disorders (e.g., maple syrup urine disease).

3. Other causes of presenting symptomatology must be ruled out.

    a. If infection is suspected, a septic evaluation should be done.

    b. If a noninfectious CNS disorder is suspected, ultrasound scan and/or CT scan may be obtained.

    c. If obstructive gastrointestinal disease pathology is suspected, an upper gastrointestinal series and barium swallow may be indicated.

4. Ferric chloride test on a wet diaper may give clues to the presence or absence of an amino acidopathy.

5. Monitor blood glucose, blood urea nitrogen, ammonia, electrolytes, calcium, and magnesium levels and arterial blood gas and pH.

6. If all of the aforementioned evaluations are normal or if the ferric chloride test is suggestive, and symptoms of acidosis are evident, serum and urinary levels of amino acids should be obtained.

7. The specific diagnosis is made by assaying the activity of the specific enzyme suspected.

GENERAL TREATMENT PROTOCOL

1. Prevention of mental retardation and attainment of normal growth and development are the primary goals of treatment.

2. Treat the patient for life-threatening complications (e.g., seizures, severe metabolic acidosis); dialysis and/or an exchange transfusion may be required.

3. A geneticist should be consulted.

4. Eliminate the specific offending dietary substrate.

5. Ensure the intake of adequate, but specifically limited, dietary proteins and amino acids to allow for normal growth and development.

6. Supportive and symptomatic treatment.

More specific diagnostic and treatment protocols are given in Table 2 for several amino acid disorders.

TABLE 2. *Diagnostic and treatment protocols*

Diagnosis	Treatment

Phenylketonuria

Clinical manifestations: Mousy urine odor, mental retardation, seizures, light complexion, eczema, and/or autistic behavior
Serum phenylalanine: >20 mg/ml after one week of age
Low serum tyrosine
Urinary excretion of phenylpyruvic acid and hydroxyphenylacetic acid
Positive urine ferric chloride test

Low phenylalanine diet (LOFENALAC®)
Monitor growth, hematocrit, and hemoglobin; serial phenylalanine determinations
Diet therapy may be discontinued after 6 years of age in some patients

Tyrosinemia

Clinical manifestations: Vomiting, hyperkeratosis, jaundice, and possible CNS impairment
High serum tyrosine (6 to 35 mg/ml)
Phenylpyruvic acid and phenylacetic acid are excreted in the urine in large concentrations

Limit protein intake to 2 g/kg/day
Provide adequate intake of vitamin C (50 to 100 mg/day)
If there is evidence of liver damage, use a low phenylalanine and low tyrosine diet

Methylmalonic Acidemia

Clinical manifestations: Vomiting, failure to thrive, severe acidosis, hyper ammonemia, and/or possible mental retardation
Hyperglycinemia and hyperglycinuria

Restrict protein intake
Vitamin B_{12}, 1 mg/day should be provided in infants with blocks in vitamin B_{12} metabolism

Maple Syrup Urine Disease

Clinical manifestations: Lethargy, poor feeding, and seizures
Ketoacidosis
No ketoacid decarboxylase activity in cultured cells

Limit dietary intake of protein
Diet therapy should be continued throughout life

Orotic Aciduria

Clinical manifestations include failure to thrive and vomiting
Increased urinary excretion of orotic acid
Megaloblastic anemias occur

Uridine

Lesch-Nyhan Syndrome

Clinical manifestations: Severe retardation, choreoathetosis, spasticity, self-mutilation behavior, and/or ureterolithiasis
Hyperuricemia and hyperuricosuria
No hypoxanthine-guanine phosphoribosyl transferase activity

Allopurinol and probenecid

Histinemia

Clinical manifestations: Impaired speech, retarded growth, and possible mental retardation
Positive urine ferric chloride test
Elevated plasma histidine level

Nonspecific, supportive, and symptomatic

Anemia

Anemia is a common disease of children and is frequently related to nutrition. Rarely does it become severe enough to warrant inpatient diagnosis and management. Congenital anemia and acquired anemias that are other than nutritional in origin may require long-term management in conjunction with a specialist in hematological disorders. Occasionally, a nutritional deficiency will be significant and require management in the hospital.

The medical history and physical examination are extremely important in the evaluation of a patient with anemia and will guide the diagnostic evaluation (and ultimately the treatment). The medical history may point to the diagnosis of anemia (e.g., poor or unusual diet, lethargy, malaise) or may give clues to the type of anemia present (e.g., parents with sickle-cell trait). Pallor, jaundice, petechiae, and failure to thrive are physical findings that may point to a specific diagnosis. Symptoms of anemia vary from simple pallor to severe congestive heart failure (Fig. 1).

INITIAL DIAGNOSTIC PROTOCOL

---

1. Complete blood cell count with examination of the peripheral smear.

    a. Microcytic and/or hypochromic red blood cells: Iron deficiency, thalassemia, lead poisoning, chronic blood loss, spherocytosis.

    b. Macrocytic: Vitamin B_{12} deficiency, folic acid deficiency, intestinal parasitosis.

    c. Normocytic: Acute blood loss.

2. Elevated reticulocyte count (may occur with iron deficiency after treatment with iron, or after acute blood loss; if medical history and physical examination suggest neither, hemolytic anemia may be present).

    a. Congenital: Sickle-cell disease, thalassemia, glucose 6-phosphatase deficiency, hereditary spherocytosis.

    b. Immunological: Erythroblastosis, autoimmune hemolytic anemia.

    c. Other: Hemolytic-uremic syndrome, drugs, poisons, hypersplenism, infection, nonautoimmune hemolytic anemia.

3. Decreased platelet count and pancytopenia (if bone marrow suppression is suspected from absence of obvious causes of pancytopenia, bone marrow examination is indicated).

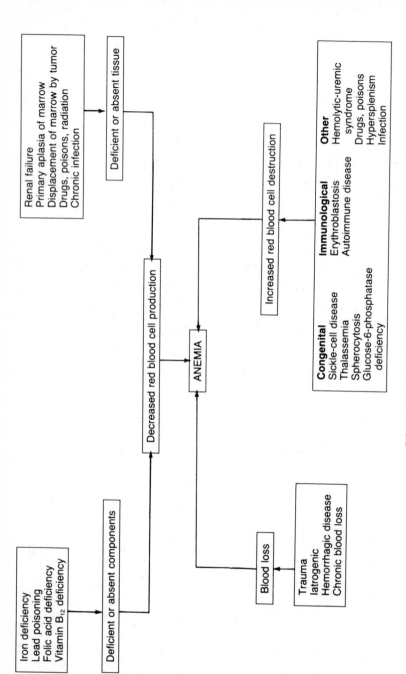

FIG. 1. Pathophysiology of anemia.

a. Congenital: Congenital aplastic anemia.

b. Acquired: Drugs, poisons, radiation, displacement of bone marrow by tumor.

DIAGNOSTIC AND TREATMENT PROTOCOLS

Table 1 gives the diagnostic and treatment protocols for a variety of anemia disorders.

TABLE 1. *Anemia: Diagnostic and treatment protocols*

Diagnosis	Treatment
Aplastic Anemia, Constitutional	
Bone marrow: Hypocellularity Chromosome evaluation Skeletal studies, as indicated	Supportive transfusions Androgens: Oxymetholone, 5 mg/kg/day Steroids: Prednisone, 1 mg/kg/day Taper the above medications and monitor the CBC. Attempt to achieve the lowest dose of medications required to maintain a hemoglobin concentration of 12 g/100 ml
Blood Loss, Acute	
Medical history and physical examination to help determine site of blood loss Diagnostic protocol is guided by medical history and physical examination	Acute blood loss may cause shock; immediate treatment is indicated; whole blood transfusion is best, but usually is not immediately available; other fluids and volume expanders may be used Blood transfusion if the patient is symptomatic secondary to the anemia or if the hemoglobin level falls below 7 g/100 ml
Blood Loss, Chronic	
Medical history and physical examination of blood loss to help determine site Stool guaiac testing Stool examination for ova and parasites Urinalysis Further diagnostic protocol is guided by the medical history and physical examination	Treatment depends on the etiology of the blood loss Patients are usually well compensated despite extremely low hemoglobin levels; transfusion is usually not necessary unless the patient is symptomatic secondary to the anemia (10 cc of packed red blood cells per kg of body weight slowly transfused is usually sufficient) Treatment of the iron deficiency is indicated in absence of blood transfusion
Drugs, Poisons	
Complete medical history and physical examination are important Drug screening of blood and urine	Discontinue offending medication or avoid the poison Supportive treatment until the marrow recovers (red blood cell and platelet transfusions) Androgens and steroids: Marrow shows a very poor response as compared with constitutional aplastic anemia

TABLE 1. *(Continued)*

Diagnosis	Treatment
	Bone marrow transplantation (if a transplant is anticipated, red blood cell transfusions should be avoided)

Erythroblastosis

Diagnosis	Treatment
Blood type Coombs' test (direct and indirect) Peripheral smear Rh_oD antibody titer Autoantibody titers Minor blood group crossmatch Serum bilirubin (and cord blood bilirubin)	Therapy is directed at the etiology of the erythroblastosis and the severity of rise in bilirubin Phototherapy for treatment of hyperbilirubinemia Exchange transfusion **Note: Exchange transfusion is obligatory when cord blood bilirubin is >4 mg/100 ml and/or cord blood hemoglobin is <13 g/100 ml, and/or the rate of rise of bilirubin is >1 mg/100 ml/hr**

Folic Acid Deficiency

Diagnosis	Treatment
Peripheral smear Folic acid level: Low Vitamin B_{12} level: Normal Schilling test: Normal A history of feeding goat's milk is often elicited	Folate, 20 to 200 μg i.m. or p.o. daily for 10 days If there is a therapeutic response, 1 to 5 mg of folate is given orally for 4 weeks; this dose will usually replenish folate stores

Glucose 6-Phosphatase Deficiency

Diagnosis	Treatment
Red blood cell glucose 6-phosophatase level	Avoid the drugs that result in hemolysis

Hemolytic Anemia, Autoimmune

Diagnosis	Treatment
Coombs' test: Positive Reticulocyte count: Elevated Warm and cold agglutination test	Prednisone, 2 to 4 mg/kg/day; several weeks may be required for a response Splenectomy: May be indicated if the steroids fail Patients with warm antibodies respond better to the above regimen

Hemolytic Anemia, Congenital Nonspherocytic

Diagnosis	Treatment
Coombs' test: Negative Evaluation of patient's cells for specific enzyme defect Peripheral smear: Burr cells, Heinz bodies	Splenectomy is usually recommended after the patient is 4 years old

Hemolytic-Uremic Syndrome

Diagnosis	Treatment
Medical history and physical examination usually show upper respiratory tract infection or gastroenteritis followed by pallor or jaundice Platelet count: Low Peripheral smear: Reflects microangiopathy Blood urea nitrogen and creatinine: Reflect acute renal failure Urinalysis: Reflects hemolysis and renal disease Diagnostic triad: Hemolytic anemia, thrombocytopenia, and acute renal failure	Manage renal failure, restrict fluids, and perform peritoneal dialysis when necessary Supportive care The use of heparin and corticosteroids is very controversial

Diagnosis	Treatment

Hypersplenism

Complete blood cell count: Reveals pancytopenia
Physical examination: Reveals spleen enlargement
Bone marrow: Normal or hypercellular
Absence of other causes for pancytopenia
Red blood cell survival time

Splenectomy: Improvement in the blood picture confirms the diagnosis

Infection

Appropriate cultures as guided by the medical history and physical examination
Iron stores: Normal, but impaired release of iron by the reticuloendothelial system

Treat the infection
Transfusions may be necessary (packed red blood cells), but usually not until the hemoglobin is <7g/100 ml

Iron Deficiency

Ferritin level: Low
Serum iron level: Low
Iron binding capacity: Elevated
Percent saturation (Fe/TIBC $\times$ 100) is <16%
Therapeutic trial of iron: Reticulocytosis should occur along with an elevation of the hemoglobin after 1 week of treatment
Bone marrow examination is not helpful in children <2 years of age; most of their iron is stored in their red cell mass, not in the marrow

Elemental iron, 4 to 6 mg/kg/day, equal to 30 mg/kg/day of ferrous sulfate, divided into three equal doses; treat for at least 2 to 3 months after the hemoglobin returns to normal to replenish iron stores
Each gram of hemoglobin contains approximately 3.4 mg of iron
Blood transfusions are rarely necessary unless the hemoglobin level falls below 3 g/100 ml or congestive heart failure is present; transfusion should be done slowly

Lead Poisoning

Peripheral smear: Basophilic stippling of red blood cells
Blood lead level
Free erythrocyte protoporphyrin level (>100 is elevated; >250 is severe intoxication)
Lead chips may be visible on a flat-plate abdominal radiograph
EDTA-lead excretion test. (EDTA challenge: EDTA 50 mg/kg/24 hr; positive result, >1 μg of lead per mg of EDTA
Urinary protoporphyrin level
Metaphyseal radiographs

For a complete discussion see Lead Poisoning chapter
Penicillamine, 20 to 40 mg/kg/day for 30 days; recheck the lead level and monitor the CBC and liver functions
EDTA, 50 mg/kg i.m. or i.v. for 5 days
Dimercaprol (BAL), 12 to 14 mg/kg/24 hrs
Supportive and symptomatic care

Parasitic Disease

Peripheral smear
Stool examination for ova and parasites
Vitamin B_{12} and folate levels
Further diagnostic protocol is guided by medical history and physical examination

The infection must be appropriately treated
Other therapy is guided by the diagnosis

Sickle-Cell Anemia

Peripheral smear
Sickle-cell preparation
Hemoglobin electrophoresis on the patient's, parents', and siblings' blood
Serum bilirubin
Reticulocyte count
Urinalysis

Treatment of sickle-cell anemia is directed toward the management of individual types of crises
Pain crisis: Hydrate with 5% dextrose in 0.45 normal saline at 1½ to 2 times maintenance; supplemental oxygen; transfusion therapy (or partial exchange):

TABLE 1. *(Continued)*

Diagnosis	Treatment
Serum electrolytes, blood urea nitrogen, and creatinine	Approximately 10 ml/kg of packed red blood cells are given to raise the hemoglobin level to approximately 12 g (or partial exchange, to raise the hemoglobin A to >50%) Aplastic crisis: Slow transfusion of 2 to 3 ml/kg of packed red blood cells to raise the hemoglobin level to >7 g; supplemental oxygen Sequestration crisis: Correct hypovolemia with volume expanders or whole blood Hemolytic crisis: Transfuse as necessary when indicated; supportive care with fluids and oxygen as needed; treat the cause (e.g., infection) Folic acid supplementation

Spherocytosis

Diagnosis	Treatment
Peripheral smear Osmotic fragility testing	Splenectomy after 4 years of age Prophylaxis for splenectomized patients

Thalassemia

Diagnosis	Treatment
Peripheral smear: Target cells Hemoglobin electrophoresis: thalassemia major, Elevated hemoglobin F; thalassemia minor, Elevated hemoglobin A_2	Thalassemia minor and thalassemia trait usually require no treatment Thalassemia major requires transfusion therapy; 10 to 20 ml/kg of packed red blood cells are given at frequent intervals to suppress the marrow; the hemoglobin is kept at 10 to 12 g/100 ml Splenectomy, if indicated Deferoxamine to chelate iron overload from frequent transfusions Folic acid, 1 mg/day

Vitamin B_{12} Deficiency

Diagnosis	Treatment
Peripheral smear: Macrocytosis Vitamin B_{12} level Folic acid level Schilling test Therapeutic trial of vitamin B_{12} Monitor potassium closely during therapy Watch for elevation of the uric acid level during therapy	Vitamin B_{12}, 1 to 3 μg i.m. for 10 days; a reticulocyte response occurs in 3 days and there is conversion of the marrow; the hemoglobin usually normalizes in 4 to 6 weeks Vitamin B_{12}, 100 μg/day i.m. for 2 weeks will usually replenish the depleted stores Vitamin B_{12}, 100 to 1,000 μg/month, should be given thereafter

Apnea

Apnea is defined as an episode of cessation of effective respiration for longer than 15 sec (more than 11 sec if the infant is 3 months or older). Apneic episodes are also considered significant if they are accompanied by bradycardia (heart rate less than 100 beats per min at birth) or cyanosis (hypoxia). Bradycardia and cyanosis may occur after 20 sec of apnea. After 40 sec, pallor and hypotonia may occur. Most premature infants of less than 30 weeks' gestation have occasional short apneic spells.

Apnea may be obstructive, nonobstructive (Fig. 1), or a combination of both. The causes of apnea are varied (Table 1), but if uninterrupted, apnea of all types may culminate in death. Apnea occurring during sleep has been correlated with the sudden infant death syndrome (SIDS). However, because many causes for the apnea of SIDS have been described, it is unlikely that SIDS represents a homogeneous group of children, or it may be that the apnea of SIDS may represent a primary sleep disorder of idiopathic nature. At present, it is safe to assume that SIDS is a specific disease entity and that apnea is a nonspecific symptom that may be caused by many factors. (For a detailed discussion of SIDS, see Sudden Infant Death Syndrome chapter.)

DIAGNOSTIC PROTOCOL

When an infant presents with the complaint of apnea (or cyanotic episodes), a pathological state should be considered even though the infant appears to be well developed and healthy and shows no abnormalities on the physical examination. It also should not be dismissed after a few days of observation in the hospital, even if no apneic or cyanotic episodes are observed.

The initial step is admission to the hospital, and a systematic search for the cause of the apnea should immediately commence. The following steps may be helpful in developing the diagnostic plan:

1. Admit the patient to the pediatric intensive care unit.

2. Monitor: Heart rate (electrocardiograph channel), respiratory rate (waveform channel), and percutanous Po_2, Pco_2 and pH (waveform channel).

3. Obtain a complete medical history; the following factors may be associated with apnea:

    a. Prenatal factors: Maternal health, smoking, alcohol intake, diet, age, hematocrit and hemoglobin levels.

    b. Natal factors: Gestational age, maternal anesthesia, length of labor and its complications, birth weight.

79

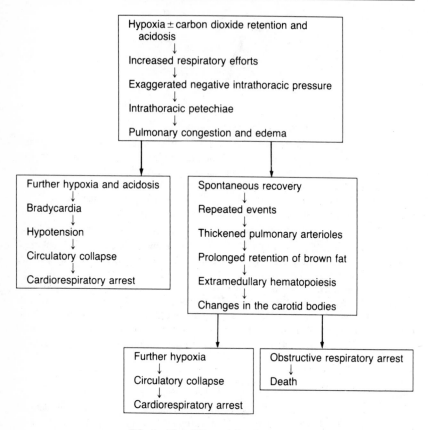

FIG. 1. Idiopathic nonobstructive apnea.

    c. Neonatal factors: Respiratory, cardiac, or CNS problems, feeding habits.

4. Perform a careful physical examination (most often, the physical examination is noncontributory).

5. Laboratory evaluations.

    a. First-stage orders

        (1) Complete blood cell count

        (2) Urinalysis

        (3) Nasopharyngeal, blood, and urine cultures

        (4) Blood glucose, blood urea nitrogen, electrolytes, calcium, and magnesium

        (5) Base-line arterial blood gases and pH

        (6) Electrocardiogram

        (7) Chest radiograph

TABLE 1. *Causes of apnea*

Nonobstructive apnea
  Hypoxemia due to any cause
  Respiratory distress syndrome
  Congenital heart disease
  PDA in premature infants
  Anemia or hypovolemia
  Respiratory center depression: CNS prematurity (neurogenic
    imbalance in the brainstem or autonomic nervous system);
    hpoglycemia, hypocalcemia, electrolyte disorders, sepsis, drugs,
    CNS hemorrhage, or seizures
  Viral infections
  Arrhythmias
  Hypothermia
  Idiopathic
Obstructive apnea
  Passive neck flexion
  Laryngospasm
  Muscle relaxation of the oropharynx
  Laryngeal chemoreceptor apnea (chalasia)
  Reflexive apnea during feeding or sucking
  Vascular rings (or other external pressures)
  Mucous plugs

b. Second-stage orders (if above tests show no abnormalities)

  (1) Barium swallow

  (2) Brain ultrasound scan and/or CT scan

  (3) Electroencephalogram

  (4) 24-hr Holter cardiac monitoring

  (5) Viral cultures and/or titers

  (6) Esophageal pH and motility studies

c. Third-stage orders (if second-stage tests show no abnormalities)

  (1) Carbon dioxide exhalation levels (to determine if there is retention).

  (2) Pneumogram (24-hr recording of heart rate and respiration).

  (3) If a polygraph is available, it may be possible to record several variables simultaneously for 6 to 24 hr, including EEG, heart rate, respiration, blood gases and eye movements to correlate with sleep stages (Table 2).

Respiration may be monitored by chest pick-up electrodes, which record actual chest movement, or by a nasal thermister, which records the actual respiratory effort. If obstructive apnea is suspected, the thermister must be used, since chest movements may continue. Direct laryngoscopy and/or cardiac catheterization and angiography may have to be performed (if the special procedures do not yield useful information).

TREATMENT PROTOCOL

1. Attempt to establish a cause for the apnea (e.g., to rule out seizures, the infant should have a normal EEG and a simultaneously normal respiratory pattern. To

TABLE 2. *Pneumogram or pneumocardiogram*

Definition: Continuous recording for 12 to 24 hr of infant's heartbeat and respiration (recording may be transformed into waveforms by use of an analyzer or computer and recorded on ECG paper at variable speeds for interpretation)

Technical aspects

Obtain recording at night when infant is asleep

Do not disturb infant to measure vital signs, feed, or change diapers during recording

Keep a record describing hourly condition of infant, whether apnea or bradycardia alarms sounded, whether infant was asleep or awake, and whether any form of resuscitation (e.g., stimulation, ventilation) was required

Record for at least 300 min of sleep for a meaningful interpretation

Respiratory and cardiac patterns

Shallow breathing: Normal all the time except if the Pco_2 [or Tco_2] becomes abnormal during apneic episodes, which may occur with or without bradycardia

Periodic breathing: Three episodes of apnea lasting not longer than 3 sec within periods of normal sleep, totaling 20 min. Percentage of periodic breathing as compared with normal breathing should not exceed 0.4%. Observed more commonly at home than in hospital, especially if infant is >2 months of age

Disorganized breathing: Apneic episodes of any duration within periods of irregular (short amplitude) breathing always associated with bradycardia. Usually associated with obstructive apnea. Occurs more often in premature infants

Bradycardia: At birth, heart rate of ≤100 beats per minute for >10 sec; at 1 to 3 months of age, <70 beats per minute; at 3 months of age, <60 beats per minute

Cardiac arrhythmia: Bradycardia, nodal and escape rhythm associated with supraventricular tachycardia (may or may not manifest during a recording)

Short apnea: Premature infants, <20 sec; full-term infants, <16 sec; >3 months of age, <11 sec

Prolonged apnea: Premature infants, >20 sec; full-term infants up to 3 months of age, 16 sec; >3 months of age, 11 sec

Irregular breathing: Occurs without apnea; considered abnormal if associated with bradycardia

Combination patterns: Apnea without bradycardia—abnormal if prolonged; apnea with bradycardia—always abnormal; bradycardia without apnea—associated with CNS lesions and hypoxia, often seen in near-miss SIDS infants

Heart rate variability: Variations in R-R interval may be abnormal even though heart rate per minute may be normal; also of prognostic importance

Calculated parameters

Percentage of periodic breathing: Normal, <0.4%; siblings of SIDS infants, 1.6% to 1.8%

Apnea index: Relationship between total seconds of short apnea (usually <6 sec) and total sleep time; normal, <0.5%

Total active sleep time

Total deep sleep time

Response to carbon dioxide inhalation: Normal response is to increase the minute ventilation by increasing the tidal volume (near-miss SIDS infants show no change in ventilation, i.e., central chemoreceptors show decreased responsiveness to carbon dioxide)

rule out gastroesophageal reflux, simultaneous esophageal pH determination and a pneumogram must be performed).

2. Treat first-degree cause, if identified (e.g., seizures, patent ductus arteriosus (POA), upper airway obstruction by mucous plugs, congenital abnormalities or vascular rings, metabolic problems, and infection).

Premature Infants

1. Place on apnea and cardiac monitors.

2. Tactile stimulation.

3. If no response, ventilate with bag and mask with FIO_2 of <0.40.

4. If apneic episodes are repeated frequently, decrease the environmental temperature to the low end of the neutral thermal environment (heat shield is needed to prevent temperature swings).

5. Small increases in FIO_2 (0.25–0.26) with continuous electrode oxygen monitoring.

6. Blood transfusions to keep the hematocrit above 45%.

7. Nasal continuous positive airway pressure (CPAP) at low pressures (3–4 cm H_2O).

8. Theophylline, 2 to 4 mg/kg every 8 hr, or a loading dose of 5.5 mg/kg i.v. over a 20 min-period followed by 1.1 mg/kg every 8 hr; monitor blood theophylline levels and maintain at 7 to 13 mg/ml.

9. Mechanical ventilation may be required.

10. Check theophylline level once a month.

11. Premature infants most probably will improve within 2 to 4 weeks; if they do not improve and continue to be symptomatic they should be monitored.

Healthy Full-Term Infants and Infants 1 to 6 Months of Age

These infants will probably continue to be symptomatic in the first year of life and will require specialized management programs that incorporate continuous electronic respiratory and cardiac monitoring at home[1] (see Table 3), medications[2], and/or periodic reevaluation.

All of these procedures should be used in healthy full-term infants with the following signs and symptoms:

1. Prolonged apnea

2. Short apnea and bradycardia

3. Apnea index $>0.5\%$

4. Periodic breathing index $>3.5\%$

5. Disorganized breathing

6. Irregular breathing and bradycardia

7. Shallow breathing and bradycardia

Home monitoring and periodic reevaluation should be used in the following children. Do not give medications, since the decreased heart rate may be secondary to hypoxia.

1. Infants with near-miss SIDS

---

[1]Home monitoring is also indicated if the parents request it.
[2]Maintain theophylline level at 5 to 8 mg/ml if pneumogram is mildly abnormal and at 11 to 15 mg/ml if pneumogram is severely abnormal.

TABLE 3. *Home monitoring of infants with apnea*

Plans and Procedures for Home Monitoring

Make available technical back-up to the parents

Teach the parents cardiopulmonary resuscitation (CPR) and have them certified by the Red Cross or other certifying agency

Teach parents of very sick infants how to suction, how and when to administer oxygen, chest physiotherapy, nasogastric feeding, nutrition, how to recognize complications (e.g., serious infection, gastrointestinal bleeding)

Make available, as necessary, visiting nurse support, psychosocial support, medical support, emergency support (e.g., ambulance, paramedics, emergency room), and financial support (private or government)

Services can best be provided through special parent training and outreach programs based in major hospitals

Discharge planner (specialized nurse)

Referral to public health nurse for home assessment

Gradual training of parents

Summary of plan to primary physician

Glossary of terms (i.e., description of apnea, bradycardia, monitor, pneumogram)

Detailed description of theophylline dosage schedule and side effects

Rooming-in at least one or two nights before hospital discharge (simulate home environment)

Keep infant's file in hospital with someone who can be reached by the parents at any time (e.g., chief resident, senior resident, emergency room)

Coordinate with home monitoring company

Advise parents to train their babysitters

Discontinuation of Monitoring

Asymptomatic infant with normal pneumogram: (near-miss SIDS or sibling of patient with SIDS): If pneumogram is persistently normal after 1 year of age, discontinue monitoring

Premature infant with problems at birth (e.g., hypoxia, did not gain weight, treated with drugs): Discontinue theophylline at 1 to 3 months of age for 48 hr and repeat the pneumogram; if normal, discontinue monitoring

Older infants: Reevaluate at age of 6 months or 1 year; discontinue aminophylline for 48 hr and repeat the pneumogram; if normal and if infant has had no apnea or bradycardia, discontinue monitoring

---

2. Siblings of SIDS infants

3. Infants with bradycardia but no apnea

DISCHARGE INSTRUCTIONS

To be accomplished before discharge:

1. Nurses' evaluation

    a. Medical aspects

    b. Parental interaction

    c. Identification of potential problem

2. Social service evaluation

    a. Home situation

    b. Financial situation

    c. Family relationships

3. Home assessment by public health nurse

4. Education of parents on how to deal with the problems, nurse, psych., Red Cross, home monitoring company, visiting nurse, etc.

5. Instruction sheet (care plan)

   a. Identifying problem(s) and how to deal with them

   b. Potential problems and how to deal with them

   c. Medications—dose—side effects, etc.

   d. Important phone numbers: Electric company; police; ambulance; physicians; chief resident

   e. Glossary of terms

6. Allow rooming-in for at least one night before discharge to simulate home environment

7. Helpful literature

   a. Red Cross manual for CPR

   b. SIDS Foundation literature

8. Parent support groups

   a. Monthly meetings

   b. Weekly visits

   c. Offer to babysit or provide babysitters who know CPR

9. Send summary of all of above to referring physician

10. Coordinate all above with home monitoring company

Asthma

Asthma is a diffuse obstructive disease of the lower pulmonary tract with hyper-irritability or hyperreactivity of the airways to a variety of stimuli, including allergic reactions, upper and lower respiratory tract infections, rapid changes in temperature, air pollutants, exercise, and emotional stress. The process is also characterized by a high degree of reversibility with or without treatment. Inheritance is compatible with polygenic or multifactorial determinants. Failure of response to drugs that are usually effective in relieving bronchoconstriction results in status asthmaticus and hypoxemia, which are life-threatening and necessitate immediate, intensive monitoring and therapy (Fig. 1).

SIGNS AND SYMPTOMS

Acute episodes of asthma manifest by tight nonproductive cough, wheezing, tachypnea, dyspnea, prolonged expiration, use of accessory muscles of respiration, cyanosis, hyperinflated chest, tachycardia, and abdominal pain. In very severe cases, wheezing might be absent, but there may be profuse sweating and even low-grade fever without evidence of infection. Dehydration may also be present.

DIFFERENTIAL DIAGNOSIS

1. Congenital malformation of respiratory tract, cardiovascular system, or gastrointestinal system
2. Foreign body
3. Bronchiolitis
4. Cystic fibrosis
5. Immune deficiencies
6. Hypersensitivity pneumonia
7. Endobronchial tuberculosis
8. Fungal disease
9. α_1-Antitrypsin deficiency
10. Bronchial adenoma

DIAGNOSTIC PROTOCOL

1. **Mild to moderate** respiratory distress
   a. No special laboratory tests are required.

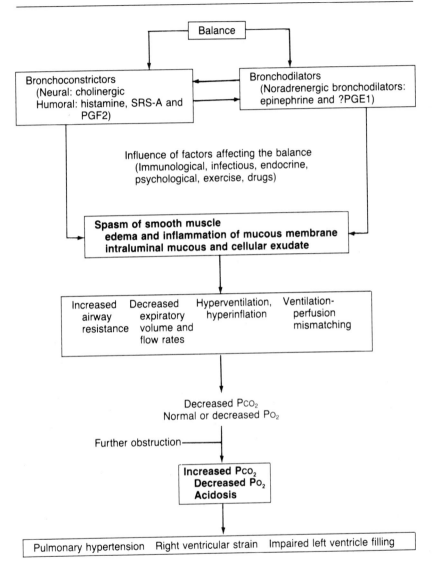

FIG. 1. Pathophysiology of asthma.

b. Epinephrine 1:1,000 aqueous solution, 0.01 cc/kg s.c. (maximum dose 0.2–0.3 cc).

c. Repeat epinephrine every 20 min (maximum of three doses) if there is no improvement.

d. If the patient improves, give epinephrine (Sus-Phrine®)1:200 solution, 0.005 cc/kg s.c.; patient may be discharged with close follow-up.

2. Moderate to severe respiratory distress

a. Epinephrine 1:1,000 aqueous solution, 0.01 cc/kg s.c. (maximum 0.2–0.3 cc).

b. Repeat epinephrine every 20 min (maximum of three doses) if there is no improvement.

c. Chest radiograph: To search for infection and/or atelectasis.

d. Arterial blood gases: To check for hypoxia, carbon dioxide retention, and acidosis.

e. Trial of intravenous aminophylline or aerosolized bronchodilator.

f. Intravenous fluid administration.

3. Nonresponsive severe respiratory distress

a. Chest radiograph with fluoroscopy: To rule out foreign body.

b. Sweat chloride test: To rule out cystic fibrosis.

c. Purified protein derivative (PPD) test (intermediate strength).

d. Serum immunoglobulin and IgE levels.

e. Serum α_1-antitrypsin level.

f. Absolute total eosinophil count.

g. Eosinophils in sputum and nasopharyngeal smear.

h. Pulmonary function tests before and after aerosol therapy.

i. Allergic skin testing.

j. Inhalation bronchial challenge.

k. Alveolar-arterial oxygen gradient with or without oxygen inhalation: To differentiate hypoxia secondary to ventilation/perfusion problem or diffusion defects secondary to anatomical shunts.

l. Blood urea nitrogen, blood glucose, and electrolytes.

m. Blood and sputum cultures for infection.

TREATMENT PROTOCOL

1. Epinephrine 1:1,000 aqueous solution, 0.01 cc/kg s.c. (maximum 0.2–0.3cc); may be repeated every 20 min (maximum of three doses) if patient does not improve.

2. Responds to epinephrine

a. Epinephrine (Sus-Phrine®)1:200 solution, 0.005 cc/kg s.c.

b. Aminophylline, 5 mg/kg p.o. every 6 hr.

c. Discharge patient with close follow-up.

d. Do not use narcotics, excessive epinephrine, excessive aerosols, mist or oxygen tents.

3. No response to epinephrine

a. Intravenous fluids (5% dextrose in 0.2 normal saline); set rate at 24-hr maintenance level.

b. Moisturized oxygen by mask or nasal prongs (3–4 liter/min).

c. Aminophylline, 4 to 6 mg/kg i.v. over a 20-min period; repeat every 6 hr; *or* 0.6 to 1.0 mg/kg/hr as continuous i.v. drip after a loading dose of 4 to 6 mg/kg i.v. (therapeutic blood level, 10 to 20 ug/dl).

d. Arterial blood gases: Normal or increased Pco_2 may indicate impending respiratory failure.

e. Sodium bicarbonate: If pH is <7.3.

f. Measure arterial blood gases and pH 10 min after sodium bicarbonate administration.

g. If condition is unchanged or worsens: Isoproterenol (Isuprel®)1:200 by inhalation, or other adrenergic aerosols (e.g., Bronchosol® 1:100, 10 drops in 2 cc saline).

h. Corticosteroids (e.g., Solu-cortef®, 4 mg/kg i.v. every 4 hr): May be used if patient has been on steroids or if there is no response to aforementioned treatments.

i. Add potassium to intravenous fluids after the patient has urinated and monitor fluid intake by output, weight, blood urea nitrogen, serum electrolytes, and serum and urine osmolality.

4. No response to aminophylline and steroids (respiratory failure is imminent)

a. Arterial blood gases: Measure frequently (every 15 min); $Pco_2 > 60$ and $Po_2 < 50$ indicates respiratory failure.

b. Isuprel® (0.1 mg/kg/min) by continuous infusion through a second intravenous line; may be increased by the same amount every 15 to 30 min until there is improvement or the heart rate is 180 beats per minute. Isuprel® administration should be administered under constant cardiac and vital sign monitoring.

c. If there is decreasing respiratory distress and improvement in blood gases, Isuprel® may be decreased slowly over the next 30 to 36 hr; other treatment should be continued and tapered as significant improvement occurs; patient should not be discharged until condition is stabilized with oral medications.

d. If the condition continues to worsen and blood gases indicate impending respiratory failure, patient should be intubated with controlled respiration.

e. Chloral hydrate (15 mg/kg rectally) may be used for anxiety.

f. Antibiotics may be used as indicated for susceptible precipitating infections.

Bites and Stings

Animal bites and stings are common problems presenting to the pediatric practitioner.

Most are minor and do not require inpatient management. Office or emergency department treatment usually will suffice. Occasionally, bite wounds are extensive and require surgical as well as medical management. Stings frequently involve local and/or systemic toxic or immunological reactions, and their management depends on the extent of the stinging injury. Treatment also depends on the severity and type of immunological reaction to the venom.

Initial diagnosis of bite and sting injuries usually rests in the medical history and physical examination. The biting animal or stinging insect may be easily identified or frustratingly obscure. Physical examination may reveal wounds characteristic of a bite or sting by a specific agent. Many wounds, however, may be simple puncture wounds or nonspecific lacerations or abrasions. The bite or sting may be obscured by the results or subsequent immunological reaction.

Cleansing and/or debridement of the wound is the most immediate treatment modality. Cleansing is best performed with soap and water. A quaternary ammonium compound is sometimes recommended.

Tetanus toxoid is usually indicated in most bite wounds. Clostridial organisms are common oral flora of many animals. Stings do not usually require tetanus prophylaxis. If the child's immunization status is up to date, no additional immunization is required.

Antibiotic treatment is usually indicated in severe bite wounds or deep puncture wounds, or when cellulitis (or other obvious infection) is present.

DIAGNOSTIC AND TREATMENT PROTOCOLS

Table 1 gives diagnostic and treatment protocols for a variety of bites and stings.

POSTEXPOSURE RABIES PROPHYLAXIS

Diagnosis

Medical History

The species of animal involved must be identified. It must be determined whether the animal is available for observation. The situation surrounding the attack must be

TABLE 1. *Bites and stings: diagnostic and treatment protocols*

Diagnosis	Treatment

Domestic Animals: Dogs and Cats

Rabies is unusual in the domestic dog and cat population (except for certain areas near the Mexican border)

The dog or cat should be captured and quarantined for 10 days

If the animal shows signs of rabies during the period of quarantine, it should be sacrificed and examined for the presence of Negri bodies in the brain tissue; rabies prophylaxis should begin at the first sign of illness in the animal

If the animal remains well for 10 days, no rabies prophylaxis is indicated

If the animal is lost, rabies prophylaxis is indicated

Thoroughly clean the wound with soap and water

Tetanus prophylaxis (0.5 cc of TT, Td, or DT) is indicated

Rabies prophylaxis should be given when indicated (see Postexposure Rabies Prophylaxis)

Antibiotic prophylaxis should be given when the bite is penetrating or severe (penicillin V, 300,000–600,000 units twice a day for 3 to 5 days)

If infection is present, it should be treated in accordance with the presenting type (e.g. osteomyelitis, cellulitis) and guided by the Gram stain, culture, and sensitivity tests

Domestic Animals: Gerbils, Hamsters, and Mice/Rats

Rabies is unusual in rodents other than bats, and rabies prophylaxis is usually not required

If possible, the animal should be quarantined and observed; if the animal is unobtainable, rabies prophylaxis is not usually indicated

The wound should be thoroughly cleaned

Tetanus prophylaxis should be given when indicated

The wound should be closely observed, and infection, if it occurs, should be appropriately treated; prophylaxis with antibiotics is usually not necessary since most bites from these animals are superficial and mild

Wild Animals: Fox, Skunk, Bat, Racoon, Coyote

Every attempt should be made to capture the animal; if the animal is available for **immediate** examination, prophylaxis may be deferred until the results are obtained

If the animal is lost, unknown, or not immediately available for examination, rabies prophylaxis is indicated

The wound should be thoroughly cleaned with soap, water, and a quaternary ammonium compound (Zephiran® 20%)

Tetanus prophylaxis should be given when indicated

Rabies prophylaxis is obligatory ·

Wild Animals: Squirrels, Chipmunks, Birds

These wild animals, rodents (except bats), and birds are rarely rabid, and rabies prophylaxis is usually not indicated

If infection is present, appropriate aerobic and anaerobic cultures should be taken

The wound should be thoroughly cleaned

Tetanus prophylaxis should be given when indicated

Antibiotic prophylaxis is usually not necessary unless the bite is severe

Infection should be treated with appropriate antibiotics as guided by the culture, Gram stain, and sensitivity

Human Bites

Appropriate history should include the exact time of infliction of the bite wound and how the wound was inflicted (punching inflictions during fights are usually severe)

Appropriate aerobic and anaerobic cultures should be obtained

Uninfected and superficially infected:
Thorough cleansing of the wound
Frequent soaks and elevation of the extremity
Do not suture
Tetanus prophylaxis

TABLE 1. *(Continued)*

Diagnosis	Treatment

Classification of the wound
  Uninfected and superficially infected
    (superficial laceration, local tenderness
    and pain, local inflammation, and serous
    drainage)
  Moderate and severe infection (stiffness,
    swelling, significant cellulitis/lymphangitis,
    purulent discharge, involvement of deep
    structures, osteomyelitis, septicemia)
Radiographs may be required
	Penicillin V. 300,000 to 600,000 units orally
	  twice a day for 3 to 5 days (alternate:
	  cephalexin, 50 mg/kg/day)
	Moderate to severe infection:
	  Immediate hospitalization
	  Thorough cleansing and local debridement
	  Frequent soaks or compresses
	  Elevation of the involved part
	  Tetanus prophylaxis
	Antibiotic use should be guided by culture,
	  sensitivity, and Gram stain (initial antibiotic
	  may be cephalexin, 100 mg/kg/day i.v. for
	  at least 10 days and longer if osteomyelitis
	  is present)

Common Insect Stings: Fire Ants, Harvester Ants, Bees, Hornets, Wasps, Yellow Jackets

Diagnosis	Treatment

The diagnosis is usually made historically
Stings may result in a gamut of reactions from
  mild local involvement to severe systemic
  collapse
Local reaction to ant stings (commonly
  multiple) are characterized by pain, wheal
  and flare reaction, vesiculation (within 6 hr),
  pustulization (lasting 1 week), and nodule
  formation
Local reaction to bee, hornet, wasp, and
  yellow jacket stings (commonly single) are
  characterized by pain, wheal and flare
  reaction, local pruritis, and swelling, which
  may be local or extensive
Systemic reactions are common and range
  from serum sickness to anaphylaxis and
  death
	Local reactions:
	  The stinger should be removed by scraping
	  Clean the lesion with soap and water
	  Cold compresses may be applied
	  A papain solution may be applied to the
	    sting site (made by combining 1/4
	    teaspoon of meat tenderizer to 1
	    teaspoon of water)
	  Diphenhydramine, 5 mg/kg/day p.o. in four
	    divided doses
	Systemic reactions:
	  Any patient with a history of generalized
	    reactions to a sting should receive
	    immediate systemic therapy
	  Cardiorespiratory support
	  Epinephrine 1:1000 aqueous solution, 0.01
	    cc/kg s.c.
	  Diphenhydramine, 5 mg/kg/day i.m. in four
	    divided doses
	Prophylaxis:
	  Avoid stings by avoiding flower beds,
	    wearing sweet-smelling perfume or after
	    shave lotion, and bright flowery clothing
	  An insect sting kit should be immediately
	    available and the patient and family
	    should be familiar with its use
	  Desensitization

Common Marine-Life Stings: Jelly Fish, Man-of-War

Diagnosis	Treatment

The diagnosis is made historically and by
  physical examination
Local reactions are characterized by severe
  pain and erythema (frequently linear or
  serpigenous)
Generalized reactions occur and range from
  myalgia to severe anaphylaxis
	The sting site should be washed with normal
	  saline or sea water
	The tentacles should be removed with gloves
	Alcohol should be poured over the sting site
	A papain preparation may be applied to the
	  lesions (see Common Stinging Insects)

Common Arachnid Bites: Black Widow

Diagnosis	Treatment
The diagnosis is usually based on historical information	Clean the bite with soap and water **Antivenin: Lyovac®**

Diagnosis	Treatment

Clinical diagnosis:
  Local erythema and "fang" marks
  Paresthesias, severe pain, and muscle
    spasm (usually lasts 2 days)
  Severe abdominal pain with rigidity
  Severe back pains
  Muscle fasciculation may occur
  Seizures, coma, and death occur, more
    commonly in children than adults (death
    occurs in 4% to 5% of affected patients)
	Test for equine serum sensitivity
	If negative, give 2.5 cc i.m. (dose is the
	  same for children and adults)
	Calcium gluconate (10% = 100 mg/ml): 5 ml/
	  kg/24 hr i.v. to control muscle spasms
	Supportive and symptomatic care

Common Arachnid Bites: Brown Recluse

Diagnosis	Treatment

Diagnosis is usually based on historical
  information
Clinical manifestations vary from mild local
  reactions to severe systemic reactions and
  death
Local reaction: Pain, erythema, and
  vesiculation; in 3 to 4 days, the lesion turns
  a violaceous color and ulcerates; eschar
  formation follows
Systemic reaction: Onset within 24 to 48 hr
  after the bite, with nonspecific symptoms of
  nausea, vomiting, chills, and fever;
  petechial rash may be seen; hemolysis,
  disseminated intravascular coagulation, and
  renal failure occur
	Treatment of the wound is mainly surgical
	  (excision of the area); antibiotics may be
	  required if infection is present
	Antihistamines may be useful to control
	  pruritis
	Parenteral steroids may be indicated if a
	  systemic reaction occurs
	Analgesics may be required
	Exchange transfusion may be required
	Complications (e.g., renal failure) should be
	  treated as they arise

explored. Unprovoked attacks are considered more likely of a rabid animal. Provocation takes many forms (e.g., taunting, teasing, petting, feeding, disturbing an animal who is eating, walking or running in the direction of an animal). Lastly, the immunization status of both the animal (rabies) and the patient (tetanus) must be determined.

Physical Examination

The extent and the severity of the wounds must be determined. Any bite or lick by a rabid animal on the neck or above is considered severe. Any bite or lick on the fingers or hands, any deep laceration, and any deep puncture wounds are also considered severe exposure. Superficial puncture wounds, lacerations, or abrasions (as well as licks by nonrabid animals) are considered mild exposures.

Indications for Prophylaxis

If the animal is wild, has been caught, and rabies is endemic in the species, prophylaxis must begin and the animal must be sacrificed for examination of the brain for Negri bodies. If the animal has escaped, whether wild (coyote, skunk, fox, bat, or unknown) or domestic (dog, cat), it should be considered rabid and prophylaxis must begin. There is no specific diagnostic test in the early stages of rabies exposure.

Corneal Scrapings

In patients infected with rabies virus, corneal scrapings may be diagnostic and yield the organism.

Treatment

Local Therapy

Local therapy is the single most important initial step in the prophylaxis of rabies.The wound should be washed well with soap and water, followed by thorough cleansing with a quaternary ammonium compound (Zepharin® 20%). Care must be taken to assure that all soap has been removed from the wound before the quaternary ammonium compound is applied.

Passive Immunization

Passive immunization with rabies immune globulin should be the second step. The recommended dose is 20 IU/kg. Half of the dose is infiltrated around the wound and the remainder is given deep intramuscularly. (The package insert should be consulted for proper dose, side effects, contraindications, and precautions.)

Active Immunization

Five doses (1 ml i.m.) of human diploid cell vaccine (HDCV) are required on days 0, 3, 7, 14, and 28 after initiation of treatment. Blood specimens for antirabies anitbody titers should be drawn on day 0 and day 28. If inadequate titers are present on day 28, a sixth booster dose may be given. HDCV is an inactivated virus vaccine that is superior to duck embryo vaccine (DEV) in immunogenicity and exhibits significantly fewer side effects and complications. If HDCV is unavailable, DEV should be given.

Twenty-one daily doses (1 ml s.c.) of duck embryo vaccine are given, followed by a booster dose 10 days after the final immunization (day 31 postexposure) and another booster dose 10 days after the first (day 41 postexposure). Blood samples for antirabies antibody titers should be drawn. If the titer is adequate, no further doses are required. If inadequate, a third booster dose is recommended.

$\mathbf{B}$leeding Disorders

Hemorrhagic diatheses take many forms and may be manifested clinically by gross bleeding (e.g., epistaxis, hematochezia, macroscopic hematuria), occult bleeding (e.g., hematoma, hemarthrosis), and bleeding into the skin (e.g., petechiae, ecchymosis, purpura). The diagnosis may be suspected by a history of easy bruising, prolonged nosebleeds, or a family history of a bleeding disorder. Physical examination may reveal the site of bleeding or give clues to the diagnosis, such as an enlarged spleen, toxic appearance, isolated swollen joint, or purpura. Although the medical history and physical examination may point to a specific disorder, the diagnosis most often rests in the laboratory evaluation of the patient (Fig. 1).

INITIAL DIAGNOSTIC PROTOCOL

1. Complete blood cell count, including platelet count and reticulocyte count
2. Prothrombin time
3. Activated partial thromboplastin time
4. Bleeding time
5. Coagulation factor assay
6. Fibrinogen level
7. Fibrin split products

DIAGNOSTIC FINDINGS

Table 1 gives diagnostic findings for a variety of bleeding disorders.

DIAGNOSTIC AND TREATMENT PROTOCOLS

Table 2 gives diagnostic and treatment protocols for those disorders given in Table 1.

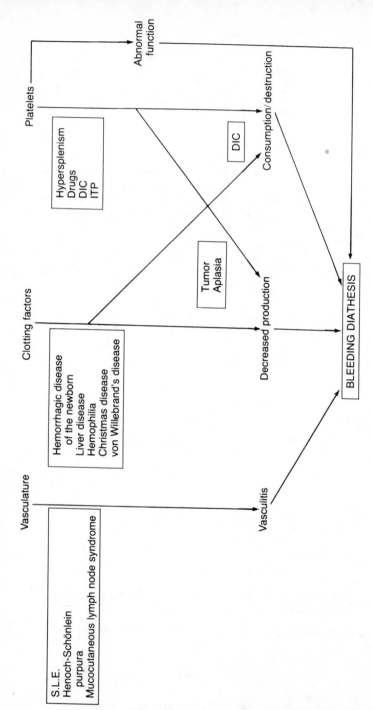

FIG. 1. Pathophysiology of bleeding disorders.

TABLE 1. *Diagnostic findings*

Disorder	Platelets	PT	PTT	BT	FSP	1	2	3	5	7	8	9	10	11	12	13
Christmas disease	—	—	P	—	—	—	—	—	—	—	—	L	—	—	—	—
Disseminated intravascular coagulation	L	P	P	P	I	L	—	—	—	—	L	—	—	—	—	—
Drug-induced thrombocytopenia	L	—	—	P	—	—	—	—	—	—	—	—	—	—	—	—
Hemophilia	—	—	P	—	—	—	—	—	—	—	L	—	—	—	—	—
Hemorrhagic disease of newborn	—	P	P	P	—	—	L	—	—	L	—	L	L	—	—	—
Henoch-Schönlein purpura	—	—	—	—	—	—	—	—	—	—	—	—	—	—	—	—
Hypersplenism	L	—	—	—	—	—	—	—	—	—	—	—	—	—	—	—
Idiopathic thrombocytopenic purpura	L	—	—	—	—	—	—	—	—	—	—	—	—	—	—	—
Liver disease	L or —	P	P	P	I	—	—	—	L	—	L	—	—	—	—	—
Von Willebrand's disease	—	—	P	P	—	—	—	—	—	—	L	—	—	—	—	—

PT, prothrombin time; PTT, partial thromboplastin time; BT, bleeding time; FSP, fibrin split products.
1, fibrinogen; 2, prothrombin; 3, thromboplastin; 5, labile factor, proaccerlerin; 7, stable factor, proconvertin; 8, antihemophilic factor; 9, plasma thromboplastin component; 10, Stuart-Prower factor; 11, plasma thromboplastin antecedent; 12, Hageman factor; 13, fibrin stabilizing factor; there were no findings for 4, calcium; or 6, activated labile factor, accelerin.
P, prolonged; L, low, I, increased; —, normal.

TABLE 2. *Hemorrhagic disorders: diagnostic and treatment protocols*

Diagnosis	Treatment

Christmas Disease: (Factor IX Deficiency; X-Linked Recessive)

Medical history and physical examination Platelet count: Normal PT: Normal PTT: Prolonged (monitor during treatment) Bleeding time: Normal Coagulation factors: factor IX decreased	Mild soft-tissue bleeding: Fresh frozen plasma, 15 cc/kg immediately, *then* 10 cc/kg every 12 hr b(approximately 1 unit/kg of factor IX will raise the plasma level 1%) Factor IX concentrate, 40 units/kg immediately, *then* 15 units/kg every 12 hr for the next 10 days; especially useful before surgery (There is a risk of hepatitis when the concentrate is used)

Disseminated Intravascular Coagulation (Consumptive Coagulopathy)

Medical history and physical examination Platelet count: Decreased PT: Prolonged PTT: Prolonged Bleeding time: Prolonged Coagulation factors: Factor VIII decreased Fibrinogen: Low Fibrin split products: Increased Peripheral smear: Schistocytes, fragmented red blood cells	Treat the cause (e.g., sepsis) Platelet concentrate: Frequently used to control bleeding Fresh frozen plasma, 10 to 15 cc/kg; also used to control bleeding The use of heparin in this disorder is controversial

Drug-Induced Thrombocytopenia

Medical history and physical examination Thrombocytopenia may be due to increased platelet destruction by cross-reacting antibody production or by decreased production of platelets secondary to marrow depression, diagnostic protocol is dictated by assessment of etiology Complete blood cell count	Discontinue the offending drug Platelet transfusions (if the count is less than 10,000 and/or if bleeding occurs, (especially CNS), and/or steroids (prednisone, 1 to 2 mg/kg/day for 14 days)

Hemophilia (Factor VIII Deficiency; X-Linked Recessive)

A complete medical history and physical examination should be performed; results may be variable since the presentation frequently depends on the severity. There may be a positive or negative family history and/or history of bleeding tendencies Platelet count: Normal PT: Normal PTT: Prolonged (when factor VIII is less than 40% of normal) Bleeding time: Normal Coagulation factors: Factor VIII decreased 1 to 30% of normal (less than 3% of normal is considered severe)	Mild soft-tissue bleeding: **Fresh frozen plasma,** 15 cc/kg immediately, *then* 10 cc/kg every 12 hr **Cryoprecipitate,** 20 units/kg, is used for most bleeding diatheses, including hemarthrosis; for every unit of cryoprecipitate transfused, the plasma level of factor VIII increases by approximately 2%; if hemarthrosis is present, 20 units/kg should be repeated every 12 hr for 2 to 3 days; splinting and aspiration of the joint may also be required; for surgical procedures: 50 units/kg is given immediately, *then* 30 units/kg every 12 hr for 10 days For dental procedures: Epsilon-aminocaproic acid (EACA) 3 g/M^2 p.o.; (should not be used if bleeding is from the urinary tract) If the patient has factor VIII antibodies no factor VIII should be given; use activated factors (bypass factor VIII)

Diagnosis	Treatment

Hemorrhagic Disease of the Newborn (Deficiency of Vitamin K-Dependent Factors in the First Few Days of Life)

Prenatal and maternal history, medical history, and physical examination; history frequently reveals that the newborn failed to receive vitamin K
The site(s) of bleeding may be obvious or occult
Platelet count: Normal
Fibrinogen: Normal
Coagulation factors: Factors II, VII, IX, and X are decreased
PT: Prolonged
PTT: Prolonged

Vitamin K$_1$: 0.5 to 1.0 mg i.m. is prophylactic
Vitamin K$_1$ (aqueous colloidal), 1 to 2 mg i.v. slowly, or **fresh frozen plasma,** 10 cc/kg
Packed red blood cells may be required if bleeding is severe and anemia is present

Henoch-Schönlein Purpura

A complete medical history and physical examination should be performed; typical urticarial (iris) lesions may be seen; joint and kidney involvement is common
Platelet count: Normal
Urinalysis: May show blood and/or protein
Complement level: Normal
IgA: May be elevated
ASO titer: Normal

Aspirin, 60 to 100 mg/kg/day, for joint symptoms
Supportive and symptomatic care
Treat concomitant processes (e.g., acute renal failure)
Use of steroids in the treatment of Henoch-Schönlein purpura is controversial

Hypersplenism

Medical history and physical examination; splenomegaly may be present
Complete blood cell count: Anemia and thrombocytopenia

Splenectomy: Not usually done for thrombocytopenia alone; bleeding and anemia are usually more significant

Idiopathic Thrombocytopenic Purpura

Medical history and physical examination; may reveal petechiae, purpura, ecchymosis, hematomas, or epistaxis
Hemoglobin is normal, white blood cells are normal, and the platelet count is usually less than 50,000/cu mm
Antiplatelet antibodies: Present in 60% of the patients
Coombs test: Negative
Bone marrow: Shows adequate megakaryocytes; it may also be done to rule out infiltration of the marrow by tumor prior to instituting steroid therapy

Usually no therapy is necessary. It is reserved for patients with acute bleeding (CNS and GI are the most common sites); mortality is less than 1%
Prednisone, 2 mg/kg/day for 2 weeks
Chronic ITP: Occurs in 20% of patients; splenectomy is curative in approximately 65%

Liver Disease

Medical history and physical examination
Platelet count: Usually normal but may be low if a consumptive coagulopathy is occurring
Fibrinogen: Decreased
Fibrin split products: Mild to markedly elevated
Coagulation factors: Factors V and VII are low
PT: Prolonged
PTT: Prolonged

Vitamin K$_1$: 1 to 5 mg by slow i.v. infusion, or fresh frozen plasma if the bleeding is severe and not corrected by vitamin K

TABLE 2. *(continued)*

Diagnosis	Treatment

Von Willebrand's Disease (Autosomal Dominant)

Diagnosis	Treatment
Medical history and physical examination; may reveal mild bleeding tendencies (e.g., gingival bleeding, epistaxis, menorrhagia) Platelet count: Normal PT: Normal PTT: Prolonged Bleeding time: Prolonged Coagulation factors: Factor VIII decreased	Cryoprecipitate, 10 units/kg in a single dose will usually correct the level of factor VIII for 1 to 2 days

Bronchiolitis

Bronchiolitis is an acute viral illness of children younger than 1 year of age. It involves primarily the lower respiratory tract. The symptoms may be preceded by upper respiratory tract symptoms of coryza and low-grade fever (Fig. 1).

The smaller the diameter of the airway, the less constriction required to significantly increase the airway resistance. Airway resistance is proportional to the radius of the airway raised to the fourth power. Therefore, a small change in the radius will significantly affect the resistance.

SIGNS AND SYMPTOMS

The prominent physical finding in bronchiolitis is wheezing. The degree of respiratory distress is variable and may be mild, moderate, or severe. The wheezing and distress are frequently progressive. Stridor is usually absent. Cyanosis and acute respiratory failure may occur.

DIFFERENTIAL DIAGNOSIS

1. Asthma (reversible bronchospastic lower airway disease)
2. Pneumonia
3. Bronchiolitis
4. Foreign body aspiration
5. Cystic fibrosis
6. Tumor
7. Tuberculosis

DIAGNOSTIC PROTOCOL

1. Complete blood cell count: Usually not impressive; it may show mild leukocytosis with a predominance of lymphocytes.
2. Chest radiograph: May show no abnormalities, but it usually shows some degree of air trapping; may be streaky infiltrates, but lobar consolidation is unusual; patchy atelectasis may occur; also used to rule out foreign body aspiration.

Respiratory syncitial virus
↓
Lower respiratory tract infection
↓
Inflammation of bronchiolar tissue
↓
Swelling of mucosa and secretions/exudation
↓

| INCREASED BRONCHIOLAR RESISTANCE |

FIG. 1.   Pathophysiology of bronchiolitis.

3. Urinalysis: To assess renal status and state of hydration.

4. Serum electrolytes, blood urea nitrogen and creatinine: To assess acid-base status, electrolyte balance, and renal function.

5. Blood cultures.

6. Blood gases: Dependent on the severity of the respiratory distress.

7. Respiratory syncitial virus titers (fluorescent antibody technique).

8. Bronchodilators: Response (or lack of response) is not considered to be a diagnostic test for bronchiolitis.

TREATMENT PROTOCOL

The intensity of therapy depends on the degree of distress and the progression of the disease process.

1. Adequate cardiorespiratory support should be provided if the baby is in severe distress or if respiratory failure is imminent.

2. Children with respiratory rates >60/min or those in moderate to severe respiratory distress should receive nothing by mouth.

3. Intravenous fluids of 5% dextrose in 0.2 normal saline should be given (modification may be required and is guided by the electrolyte status) at 24-hr maintenance levels plus any ongoing losses.

4. Humidified oxygen.

5. Chest physical therapy is employed to mobilize secretions.

6. Postural drainage is also employed to aid in the mobilization of secretions.

7. Antibiotics are not usually required. Secondary bacterial infections can occur and should be treated according to culture results.

8. Bronchodilators appear to be of little value in the management of patients with bronchiolitis. However, they may be indicated in patients with severe respiratory distress or hypoxia. A few patients with bronchiolitis will respond to theophylline, especially when steroids are used concurrently. It is virtually impossible to differentiate bronchiolitis from reversible bronchospastic disease in children younger than 1 year of age.

9. Cardiorespiratory monitoring is indicated in infants in moderate to severe distress and in those whose symptoms are becoming progressively more severe.

10. Assisted ventilation and intensive therapy may be required in patients with imminent respiratory failure and collapse. Steroids may be indicated in these situations.

Burns

Approximately 2,600 children younger than 15 years of age die each year from burns. Accidental burns rank second in the age group 1 to 4 years and third in the age group 5 to 14 years as a major cause of death. Automobile accidents and drownings are the only other types of accidents accounting for more deaths in these populations.

The majority of fatalities occur at night, in the home, and most frequently involve children 2 to 3 years of age. Epidemiological data on burns are similar in most industrialized countries.

Morbidity as well as mortality is high. The amount of skin surface involved is the most important factor in determining outcome, with the depth of the burn affecting the incidence of infectious complications. Life is endangered when more than 10% of the total body surface area is involved. The risk of death is great when 30% of the body surface area is involved, and there is virtually no chance of survival if more than 80% of the body is burned.

CLASSIFICATION

Burns are classified according to the depth of involvement and the severity of the burn (minor, moderate, or severe). Partial-thickness burns involving only the epithelial surface are first degree burns. They are clinically manifested by erythema and pain. Second degree burns involve both the epithelium and part of the corium. The major portion of the dermis is spared and re-epithelization can occur. Bullae formation is characteristic. The underlying epidermal surface is vascular, blanches on pressure, and is generally tender to touch. A full-thickness burn, destroying all layers of skin (third degree) is avascular. Generally, the surface does not blanch with pressure, is frequently painless, and is nontender. Epithelialization can only occur from the edges of the lesion, and infection is not uncommon.

The severity of the burn is assessed by both the depth of the lesion and the extent. Minor burns are first or second degree involving less than 5% of the body or a third degree burn involving an area less than 3 cm in diameter. Moderate burns are second degree burns of 5 to 10% surface area or those involving the hands, face, feet, or genitalia. Third degree burns greater than 3 cm but less than 10% surface area are also considered moderate. Severe burns are characterized by second or third degree involvement of greater than 10% of the body's surface area (Fig. 1).

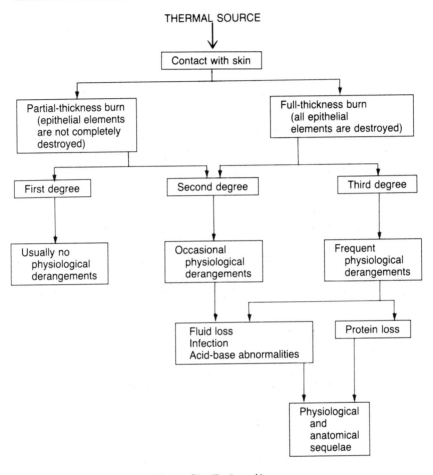

FIG. 1. Classifications of burns.

DIAGNOSTIC PROTOCOL

First Degree

The diagnosis is made on clinical grounds and no specific diagnostic tests are required.

Second Degree (Mild to Moderate)

1. The diagnosis is made on clinical grounds; diagnostic tests are dictated by the extent of the burn.

2. If the second degree burn involves > 10% of the body surface area, hospitalization and further evaluation and treatment are indicated.

3. Hemoglobin, hematocrit, and white blood cell count count: Usually elevated in patients who incur significant burns.

4. Electrolytes, blood urea nitrogen, and creatinine: Assess fluids, biochemical balance, and renal status.

5. Appropriate cultures, as indicated by the patient's condition.

Full-Thickness (Deep Second Degree and Third Degree)

1. Insure an adequate airway: Respiratory arrest is not an uncommon complication of burns, especially if the nares or other portions of the respiratory tract are involved; provide oxygen via an endotracheal or tracheostomy tube.

2. Evaluate the depth and extent of the burn (see Fig. 2).

3. Perform a detailed history and physical examination, looking for other trauma that may not be readily apparent.

4. Evaluate all circumferential burns for the need of early escharotomy (especially of the chest, which may cause respiratory problems, and the extremities).

5. Monitor complete blood cell count, urinalysis, total protein, electrolytes, blood urea nitrogen, creatinine, blood gases, and pH immediately and then every 6 hr.

6. Admit the patient to a burn unit.

7. Monitor vital signs every 30 min initially, then every hour if the patient is stable.

8. Insert a urinary catheter and monitor the urine output, specific gravity, osmolality, sodium content, and look for the presence of hemoglobin.

9. Obtain appropriate bacterial cultures.

TREATMENT PROTOCOL

First Degree

Inpatient management is usually not required for most first degree burns.

Cold water or ice may be placed on the lesion. Butter or greasy substances only make the lesion greasy and do nothing to promote healing.

Second Degree (Mild to Moderate)

1. Intact vesicles and bullae should be left alone and not disrupted.

2. Vesicles and bullae that are disrupted may be debrided.

3. In general, lesions should be left open to air and should be kept clean.

4. Silver sulfadiazine may be applied to the lesions three times a day.

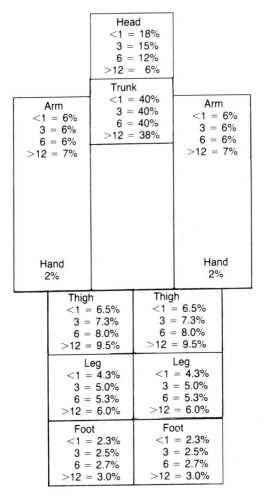

FIG. 2. Estimation of percentage of body surface area burned (ages are expressed in years). Estimates include both anterior and posterior surfaces; if only one surface is involved, the number should be divided by two.

5. Fluid and electrolyte therapy depends on the extent of the burn and the patient's clinical condition.

6. Appropriate antibiotics should be administered when indicated by culture results or the presence of cellulitis.

Full-Thickness (Deep Second Degree and Third Degree)

1. Assure an adequate airway and provide oxygen.

2. Treat shock.

3. The patient's clothes should be removed and the patient should be weighed.

4. The burns should be covered with wet dressings (silver nitrate, 0.5%, silver sulfadiazine, or Sulfamylon® may be used). **Note:** Treatment with silver nitrate causes increased sodium requirements and Sulfamylon® may cause acidosis, requiring bicarbonate administration.

5. Joints should be splinted in physiological position (skeletal traction may be required).

6. Provide appropriate fluids if 10% of the total body surface area is involved with the burn.

    a. Lactated Ringer's (if renal function is adequate): maintenance fluids *plus* 2 cc/percent burn/kg.

    b. Colloid (plasma or albumin) may be required to combat shock if the total protein in the acute phase is <3 g/100 ml, or if the area of the burn is >50% of the total body surface area.

7. Tetanus prophylaxis: 0.5 ml of TT, DT, DPT, or Td (whichever is indicated by the patient's age and immunization status).

8. Assess the patient for permanent or temporary skin cover.

9. Nutrition

    a. 60 Calories/kg/day *plus* 30 Calories/100 cm² burn.

    b. Protein, 3 to 5 g/kg/day.

    c. A liquid diet is usually better tolerated early in the course of treatment; nasogastric feeding may be required.

10. Maintain environmental humidity at approximately 80%.

11. Maintain environmental temperature at 80–85°F.

12. Laminar flow units or rooms should be used.

13. Daily debridement is usually required to remove nonviable tissue and insure approximation of topical antibiotics to viable tissue.

14. Steroids may be beneficial if the respiratory tract is burned (dexamethasone 2 mg/m²).

15. Prophylactic penicillin, 200,000 units i.v. every 6 hr is usually indicated.

16. Maintain the following levels:

    a. Serum protein: 5.5 g.

    b. Hematocrit: 35% to 40% (transfuse if <30%).

    c. Urine output:40 cc/m²/hr (furosemide, 1 to 2 mg/kg may be required).

    d. Urine sodium:20 to 80 mEq/L.

    e. Serum sodium:130 to 140 mEq/L.

    f. Potassium:3.5 to 5.0 mEq/L.

17. If silver nitrate is used, sodium requirement is increased 350 mEq/m^2 of burn/day.

18. If sulfamylon is used, sodium bicarbonate supplementation may be required.

19. If hemoglobinuria is present, the urine should be alkalinized with 0.5 mEq/kg of sodium bicarbonate.

20. Physical therapy.

21. Emotional support for the patient and the family should begin early in the treatment of any burn patient.

Calcium Disorders

Calcium is one of the most important divalent cations in the body. Approximately 99% of it is present in the skeletal system and teeth, with the remaining 1% in the extracellular fluid and blood. Of the relatively small amount of accessible calcium, 40% is protein-bound and 50% is ionized. The remaining 10% is ultrafilterable and unionized. There is a marked consistency to the concentration of ionized calcium in extracellular fluid, and it is this concentration that is essential for the performance of the following bodily functions:

1. Control of cellular membrane activity and coupling of electrical or chemical excitation.

2. Maintenance of cellular adhesion and intercellular connections.

3. Control of the surface permeability of cells.

4. Muscle contraction and production of glandular secretions.

5. Coenzymes in the blood coagulation process.

6. Maintenance of normal neuromuscular irritability.

Extracellular calcium is regulated within very narrow limits. The ionic fraction is regulated by continual movement to and from the extra-cellular fluid. These shifts are closely regulated by parathyroid hormone, calcitonin, vitamin D, and, in a less major way, by thyroid hormone, growth hormone, insulin, and glucagon.

Although calcium is an important cation, only 10 to 40% of ingested calcium is absorbed. This percentage can be increased markedly under conditions of increased available activated vitamin D.

PATHOPHYSIOLOGY

Hypercalcemia

The pathophysiology of hypercalcemia is outlined in Fig. 1.

Hypocalcemia

Refer to the Pathophysiology section of the Rickets chapter.

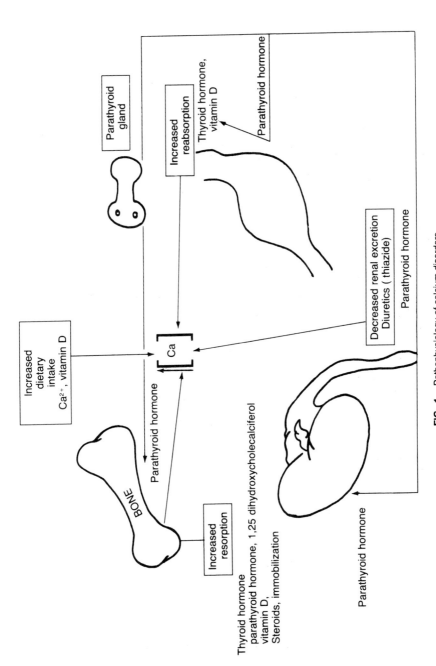

FIG. 1. Pathophysiology of calcium disorders.

SIGNS AND SYMPTOMS

Although the signs and symptoms of hypercalcemia or hypocalcemia often depend on the disease entity causing the chemical imbalance, they have certain similarities. Manifestations of calcium disturbance often consist of central nervous system alterations ranging from tetany to convulsions. Weakness, irritability, and ataxia may occur with hypercalcemia, whereas hypocalcemia more often is associated with paresthesias and muscle cramping.

Renal dysfunction may occur with both extremes of calcium concentration. In hypercalcemic states, however, the renal changes are more clinically apparent; the loss of concentrating ability is associated with polyuria, polydipsia and renal lithiasis. Although children with hypocalcemia may show mental confusion and irritability, bradycardia and electrocardiographic abnormalities (prolongation of the Q-T interval) may be more life-threatening.

DIFFERENTIAL DIAGNOSIS

Hypercalcemia

1. Disorders of calcium intake or administration of calcium-elevating drugs include:
   a. Vitamin D
   b. Vitamin A
   c. Oral or intravenous Ca^{2+} (milk alkali)
   d. Resin Ca^{2+} exchange
2. Endocrine disorders
   a. Hyperparathyroid states:
      (1) Primary
      (2) Secondary associated with renal insufficiency
      (3) Congenital secondary to maternal hypoparathyroid disease
   b. Hypothyroidism and hyperthyroidism
   c. Adrenal insufficiency
3. Idiopathic hypercalcemia of infancy
4. Familial
5. Miscellaneous
   a. Neoplastic bone diseases
   b. Diuretics (e.g., thiazides)
   c. Sarcoidosis
   d. Prolonged immobilization
   e. Hypophosphatasia

Hypocalcemia

1. Disorders of calcium intake or absorption
   a. Dietary deficiency of Ca^{2+} or vitamin D
   b. Malabsorption syndromes or chronic diarrhea
   c. Chronic laxative ingestion
   d. Anticonvulsant medication (e.g., phenytoin, phenobarbital)
2. Renal loss of calcium
   a. Acute or chronic renal failure
   b. Fanconi syndrome
   c. Primary distal renal tubular acidosis
   d. Furosemide (Lasix®) ingestion
   e. Chronic steroid use
   f. EDTA injection
3. Endocrine disorders
   a. Hypoparathyroidism
     (1) Idiopathic
     (2) Secondary to maternal hyperparathyroidism
   b. De George syndrome
   c. Neonatal renal tubular insensitivity
4. Hypoproteinemia
5. Miscellaneous
   a. Hypernatremia
   b. Hypomagnesemia
   c. Acute lymphocytic leukemia

DIAGNOSTIC AND TREATMENT PROTOCOLS

↑ $[Ca^{2+}]_s$ Hypercalcemia

Entity	Diagnostic evaluation	Treatment
Disorders Associated with an Increased Intake or Absorption		
Hypervitaminosis A and/or D	History usually reveals increased intake of vitamins A and/or D, multivitamins, or calcium supplements	Discontinue intake of the substance
Increased dietary calcium	Presence of renal stones, poyuria, hypertension	See Appendix on Vitamin Excesses
Iatrogenic administration (intravenous, exchange resin)	See chart for manifestations of hypercalcemia	Refer to treatment schedule in this chapter

Endocrine Disorders

Parathyroid states of over-activity	Definitive tests to determine primary versus secondary parathyroid disease: e.g., parathyroid homone levels, renal function levels, scan of parathyroid gland	For symptomatic treatment see schedule in this chapter Consider surgical ablation of thyroid gland
Hypo- and hyperthyroidism	See Thyroid Disease chapter	See Thyroid Disease chapter
Adrenal insufficiency	See Adrenal Insufficiency chapter	See Adrenal Insufficiency chapter

Idiopathic

Idiopathic hypercalcemia of infancy (Williams syndrome)	Characteristic elfin facies, failure to thrive, acyanotic congenital heart disease This syndrome reflects exposure of the mother while pregnant to elevated levels of vitamin D	Reduce vitamin D and calcium intake See treatment schedule in this chapter

Familial

Familial hypercalcemia (variant of endocrine disorders)	Multiple varieties, (some seen as genetic dominant multiple endocrinopathies)	For symptomatic treatment see treatment schedule

Miscellaneous

Neoplasm of bone Sarcoidosis Diuretics Prolonged immobilization Hypophosphatasia	Diagnosis is based on the specific entity. The diagnosis of the hypercalcemia can be made using the flow chart. Most entities are reflected in overactivity (activated vitamin D), or increased affect of parathyroid hormone on bone	For symptomatic treatment see section in this chapter

Other Disorders

Many of the disorders associated with hypercalcemia have similar signs and symptoms. This merely reflects that the **body's response is to the hypercalcemia and is limited**, and is not related to the cause of the elevated Ca^{2+} which may or may not cause its own specific symptoms	Medical history
	  Dietary habits
	  Vitamin abuse
	  Prolonged immobilization
	  Prescribed medication, diuretic
	  Maternal illness, i.e., hypoparathyroidism
	  Neoplastic disease
	  Renal calculi
	Laboratory investigations
	  Hematuria
	  Dilute urine and polyuria inappropriate to the patient's condition
	  Calcium, phosphosous, glucose, magnesium, electrolytes, alkalin phosphatase, blood urea nitrogen, and creatinine
	  Acid-base status
	  Ionized calcium and serum protein
	  Urine
	  EKG
		Reduce intake of Ca^{2+}
		Discontinue vitamin D
		Specific treatment directed against the disease entity responsible for the hypercalcemia

Physical examination is not
helpful other than
Hypertension
Depressed reflexes
Bradycardia
Nonspecific behavioral
changes, headache,
irritability

$\uparrow$ [Ca^{2+}]$_s$ **Hypercalcemia**

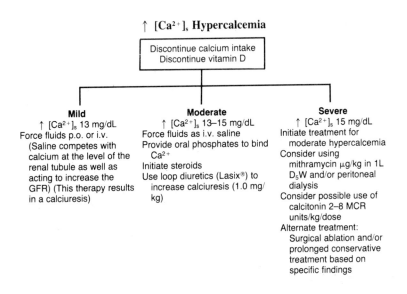

Discontinue calcium intake
Discontinue vitamin D

Mild	**Moderate**	**Severe**
$\uparrow$ [Ca^{2+}]$_s$ 13 mg/dL	$\uparrow$ [Ca^{2+}]$_s$ 13–15 mg/dL	$\uparrow$ [Ca^{2+}]$_s$ 15 mg/dL
Force fluids p.o. or i.v. (Saline competes with calcium at the level of the renal tubule as well as acting to increase the GFR) (This therapy results in a calciuresis)	Force fluids as i.v. saline Provide oral phosphates to bind Ca^{2+} Initiate steroids Use loop diuretics (Lasix®) to increase calciuresis (1.0 mg/kg)	Initiate treatment for moderate hypercalcemia Consider using mithramycin μg/kg in 1L D$_5$W and/or peritoneal dialysis Consider possible use of calcitonin 2–8 MCR units/kg/dose Alternate treatment: Surgical ablation and/or prolonged conservative treatment based on specific findings

$\downarrow$ [Ca^{2+}]$_s$ **Hypocalcemia**

Overview of signs/symptoms and laboratory values common to all hypocalcemia states, regardless of etiology. The serum calcium, as usually measured, includes both Ca^{2+} and undissociated calcium proteinate.

Diagnostic evaluation	Treatment

Pertinent medical history
  Inadequate calcium or vitamin intake (high phosphorous food, especially in the neonate)
  Frequent infections
  Thyroid surgery
  Recurrent or refractory monilial infections
  Rickets
  Maternal hyperparathyroidism
  Chronic renal failure
	Reduce phosphorous intake
	Increase calcium intake and add vitamin D
	Direct treatment against primary disease causing hypocalcemia
	If acidotic, be wary of rapid buffering (potential precipitation of hypocalcemic tetany)
	Refer to treatment chart

Idiopathic seizure disorder
Neonatal insensitivity (relative) to PTH
Physical examination
    CNS dysfunction (e.g., irritability, coma,
      confusion)
    Neuromuscular hyperexcitability, tetany,
      carpopedal spasm, laryngospasm
    Rickets
    Bradycardia
Laboratory investigations
    Calcium, phosphorous, glucose, magne-
      sium, electrolytes, alkaline phospha-
      tase, blood urea nitrogen, and
      creatinine
    Acid-base status
    Ionized calcium and serum protein
    Urinalysis
    EKG

Hypocalcemia
$\downarrow [Ca^{2+}]_s \leq 9.0$ **mg/dl**

| Reduce intake of phosphorous |
| Increase calcium intake |

Mild
$\downarrow [Ca^{2+}]_s \geq 8.0$ mg/dL
Initiate general treatment as above (patient usually has no symptoms)
Supplement calcium intake with calcium gluconate (Neo Calglucon®) 120 ml/m^2/day

Moderate
$\downarrow [Ca^{2+}]_s \leq 8.0$ mg/dL
Initiate general treatment as above
If acutely symptomatic, consider calcium gluconate (10%) solution infusion (rarely needed at this calcium level)
Begin calcium gluconate solution p.o. 120 ml/m^2/day
Consider activated vitamin D

Severe
$\downarrow [Ca^{2+}]_s < 7.0$ mg/dL
Initiate treatment for moderate hypocalcemia (as tolerated)
Infuse calcium gluconate (10%) 0.5–2 ml/kg over 5–10 min (monitor apical heart rate to avoid severe bradycardia)
Maintenance: Initiate calcium gluconate p.o. 120 ml/m^2
Avoid use of calcium chloride as this may cause severe metabolic acidosis

Cardiac Arrhythmias

Although cardiac arrhythmias may be more common in adults than in children, a significant number of children will present with arrhythmias due to cardiac and other disorders. Landtman has reported an incidence of about 2% in a randomly selected group of children. Identification of these arrhythmias, their proper diagnosis, and prompt therapy when indicated, are not only important but also may be lifesaving.

An arrhythmia is present if the patient presents with an abnormal heart rate or heart rhythm, or both, and/or when abnormalities of conduction are observed. Understanding the mechanisms of the genesis of cardiac arrhythmias requires knowledge of the anatomical and electrophysiological properties of cardiac fibers and the cardiac conduction system.

PATHOPHYSIOLOGY

The anatomical and electrophysiological properties of cardiac conduction will be considered very briefly.

All cardiac muscle cells are excitable (i.e., discharge electrically upon the application of an extrinsic stimulus), but the heart has specialized cells collected into the following nodes and conducting tracts.

Sinoatrial (SA) node: Located at the junction of the superior vena cava and the right atrium. It has a vagal and sympathetic nerve supply and is the pacemaker that normally controls the heart rate.

Atrioventricular (AV) node: Located near the coronary sinus and is also supplied by vagal and sympathetic nerves. The AV node receives impulses from the SA node along three pathways known as the anterior, middle, and posterior internodal tracts. The anterior pathway gives a branch to the left atrium, known as Bachmann's bundle. The AV node conducts impulses slowly to allow complete atrial emptying before ventricular contraction.

Bundle of His: Originates in the AV node and passes into the superior and posterior portion of the ventricular septum, giving right and left bundle branches that terminate beneath the endocardium as Purkinje fibers.

In some individuals, the following accessory pathways allow impulses originating in the SA node to bypass the AV node:

Bundle of Kent: Muscular connections across the atrioventricular groove.

James fibers: Connect the internodal tracts to the bundle of His.

Mahaim fibers: Connect the AV node to the ventricular septum. Conduction along these pathways may be anterograde, resulting in preexcitation, or retrograde, resulting in reentry. Both mechanisms are thought to be the cause of many tachyarrhythmias.

Initiation of a cardiac impulse is a spontaneous and repetitive electrophysiological property called automaticity. This property is common to cell nodes and conductive tracts but is not found in myocardial cells; it is the result of spontaneous depolarization of the cellular resting membrane potential. Each depolarized cell acts as a stimulus to adjacent cells, thus allowing for impulse propagation. Changes in action potentials are mediated through ionic changes. Since the rate of diastolic depolarization is increased by catecholamines, fever, hypocalcemia, hypokalemia, anoxia, and acidosis, these changes cause an increased heart rate. The rate of diastolic depolarization is decreased by vagal stimulation, β-adrenergic blockade, hyperkalemia, and drugs such as quinidine and lidocaine, resulting in a decreased heart rate.

Cardiac cells will not initiate a response to another stimulus until they are repolarized. The immediate phase following depolarization is called the absolute refractory period. In the later phases of repolarization, refractoriness is relative and impulses may be propagated, but at a slower rate.

Since in the healthy heart the SA node has the fastest rate of impulse formation, it serves as the usual pacemaker. Distal nodes and tracts have lower rates and hence are normally suppressed by the SA node (Table 1).

Cardiac arrhythmias result from abnormalities of impulse formation (disorders of automaticity) or impulse conduction (conduction disorders), or a combination of both and are classified accordingly (Table 2).

CLASSIFICATION

Disorders of Automaticity

Depression of the SA node: This condition results in escape beats from other areas of the conduction system. These may be atrial escape beats, AV junctional escape beats, or ventricular escape beats. The ectopic rhythm will persist if the SA node does not regain control. Ectopic beats are recognized by longer than normal R-R interval, abnormal P waves or no P waves, or short P-R interval.

TABLE 1. *Relationship of heart rate to age*

Age	Tissue		
	SA node	AV node	Ventricles
<1–1 month old	100–180/min	80–90 min	50–70/min
1-yr-old	110–180/min	—	—
5-yr-old	60-120/min	—	—
10-yr-old	55-110/min	—	—
Adult	50–100/min	50–70/min	35–50 min

TABLE 2. *Classification of arrhythmia disorders*

Automaticity
  Sinus tachycardia
  Sinus bradycardia
  Ectopic atrial, AV junctional, and ventricular premature beats
  Atrial flutter
  Atrial fibrilliation
  Atrial tachycardia
  AV junctional (nodal) tachycardia
  Ventricular tachycardia
  Ventricular fibrillation
  Sick sinus syndrome
  Wandering atrial pacemaker
  Atrial and ventricular escape rhythm
Conduction
  AV block (first, second, and third degree)
  Interventricular block (right bundle and anterior or posterior
    division of the left bundle)
Combined
  AV dissociation
  Parasystole
  Reciprocal tachycardias
  Preexcitation syndromes

Depression of automaticity in all the specialized conductive tissues may lead to ventricular standstill. Some investigators suggest that ventricular standstill is more frequent than ventricular fibrillation as a cause of sudden death after an acute myocardial infarction.

Enhancement of automaticity: This condition may result in various tachycardias. If other than the SA nodes are involved, there may be premature discharges. Atrial or AV junctional foci will result in morphologically normal QRS complexes, whereas ventricular premature discharges will result in wide and bizzare QRS complexes followed by T waves of opposite polarity and a full compensatory pause (interval between the sinus beat is twice the normal R-R interval). Supraventricular ectopic beats with aberrant conduction may also produce wide and bizarre QRS complexes, but they are followed by an incomplete compensatory pause.

Occasionally, enhanced automaticity in areas such as the bundle of His may cause a more rapid impulse formation than that of the SA node; hypokalemia, digitalis, and catecholamines may cause such enhanced automaticity.

Conduction Disorders

Slow or blocked impulse propagation and concealed conduction: Several factors, including weak impulses, reduced excitability of fibers (refractory fibers), or interruption of the pathway interfere with impulse propagation. Reduced excitability of fibers (increased refractory period) may be the result of intrinsic disease, or it may be secondary to interference from other impulses.

Concealed conduction, which may be present after an interpolated (very early) premature ventricular beat, is an example of how such impulses could have a secondary effect on conduction. In this condition, a retrograde impulse enters the AV junction and depolarizes it, but it cannot enter the atrium, which is still refractory from the previously conducted SA impulse. The new SA impulse, reaching the AV node, finds its refractory period increased because of the premature ventricular beat, so the impulse passes through the AV node very slowly, causing the normal QRS complex following the premature ventricular beat to be preceded by a long P-R interval. The long P-R interval is evidence of concealed retrograde conduction. Another example of interference would be in cases of early premature atrial beats followed by P waves that may not be conducted because the AV node and ventricles are still refractory.

Fusion beat: If a premature ventricular (or atrial) beat starts while part of the ventricle (or atrium) is already normally depolarized, a fusion beat will result, combining the characteristics of a normal beat and a premature beat.

Atrioventricular block: Delays of conduction across the AV node produce AV block.

1. First-degree AV block: Prolonged P-R interval, but all beats are conducted.

2. Second-degree AV block: Some sinus beats reach the ventricles and some are not conducted (no fixed relationships).

   a. Mobitz type I AV block (Wenckebach phenomenon): There is transient depression of the AV node characterized by progressively longer P-R intervals ending in a dropped beat. The R-R interval becomes progressively shorter until the dropped beat occurs (the R-R interval at this time appears to be unusually long, indicating that a QRS complex did not occur, but it is less than twice the shortest R-R interval).

   b. Mobitz type II AV block: QRS complexes drop out without prior shortening of the P-R interval.

3. Complete (third-degree) AV block: No beats are conducted to the ventricles, and the ventricles are driven by a junctional or ventricular focus. The QRS rate is slower than the atrial rate.

Organic AV block versus functional AV dissociation: Of the group of patients with bradycardia, it is clinically important to distinguish organic AV block from functional AV dissociation due to physiological refractoriness. Functional AV dissociation may be secondary to slowing of the SA node or due to inappropriate acceleration of a subsidiary pacemaker, or a combination of both (e.g., bradycardia of the athlete in whom junctional beats escape and in turn interfere with P-wave conduction). Complete AV block implies organic disease of the AV junction with consequent failure of ventricular conduction. Such conditions can be congenital or acquired (e.g., ischemic heart disease, primary degenerative disease, digitalis intoxication). The more prolonged the QRS complex, the lower is the focus (below the bundle of His) and the more serious is the situation.

Aberrant conduction: Changes in the excitability of the AV node may be such that it may allow some impulses to pass but will conduct them in an aberrant fashion. This problem may occur in cases of premature atrial beats, supraventricular tachycardias, or prolonged Q-T interval, where impulses reach the AV node in its relative refractory period. Since the right bundle has a longer refractory period than the left bundle, these impulses will be conducted slowly through the right bundle, giving a pattern of right bundle branch block in V_1 and a normal initial vector.

Combined Disorders

Combined disorders are cardiac arrhythmias that result from combined disturbances of impulse formation and conduction in a localized region of the myocardium.

Parasystole: Parasystoles are ectopic beats that are continuously discharging at a slow rate. The QRS complexes have the same morphology, but the interval between the normal QRS complex and the ectopic beat is variable (variable coupling interval) and the intervals between the ectopic beats are the exact multiples of the shortest interectopic interval. The abnormality of conduction (entrance block) allows the parasystolic focus to exist. The presence of an exit block establishes the parasystolic rhythm by not allowing all the impulses to be conducted.

Preexcitation syndromes: These syndromes are characterized by the presence of accessory pathways that allow impulses originating in the SA node to reach the ventricles through two pathways. Delays of the impulses in the AV node allow rapid transmission of the impulses via the accessory pathway, producing a short P-R interval and the slow early part of the QRS complex referred to as the delta wave. The presence of the two pathways allows impulses descending through the AV node to reenter via the abnormal connection, causing reentrant tachycardias.

Several of these syndromes have been described.

a. Wolff-Parkinson-White (WPW) syndrome—type A: A pattern in which the anomalous connection is a left-sided bundle of Kent, recognized by a short P-R interval (<0.12 sec), a positive delta wave in V_1, and a prominent R wave.

2. Wolff-Parkinson-White syndrome—type B: A pattern seen when the anomalous connection is a right-sided bundle of Kent, causing a short P-R interval, a prominent S wave, and a negative delta wave in V_1.

3. Lown-Ganong-Levine syndrome: A pattern seen when the impulses pass through the James fibers, bypassing the AV node and producing a short P-R interval. Since the depolarization of the ventricles follows the normal pattern, no delta waves are seen.

Atrioventricular dissociation: This condition is produced by an accelerated focus (other than the SA node) that is no longer under the control of the SA node, coupled with conduction delays. Atrioventricular dissociation will occur if the SA node fails to capture the ventricles because of increased refractoriness of the AV node and if the AV node fails to capture the atrium via retrograde conduction. The ventricular rate will be equal to or higher than the atrial rate. If the rates are equal but the P-R intervals are too short for a normal sinus rhythm, it is termed isorhythmic dissociation.

Fibrillation: Fibrillation does not represent a single electrophysiological entity, and its manifestation depends on the presence of several factors involving unifocal or multifocal impulse formation, shortened refractory periods, asymmetric slowing of conduction, and reentry. The presence of these factors allows a stimulus to be conducted in depolarized areas and to be blocked in other areas, causing an irregular wave front of excitation and chaotic contraction.

These factors may be fulfilled by hypoxia, ischemia, electrolyte disturbances, or drugs. If the chaotic contraction occurs in the atria, it is referred to as atrial fibrillation. If it occurs in the ventricles, it is referred to as ventricular fibrillation. The fibrillation-sustaining factors may be different from the initiating factors.

DIAGNOSTIC PROTOCOL

The most important aspect of cardiac arrhythmia is proper identification. Appropriate therapy is possible only if the anatomical origin of the arrhythmia (supraventricular or ventricular) and the discharge sequence are correctly identified. The following diagnostic approach is one of several that may be used.

Medical History

1. Palpitations: Identify the frequency, duration, and rate of the arrhythmia

2. Mode of onset: Sudden onset and sudden termination indicate a supraventricular origin

3. Associated symptoms: Syncope suggests asystole or ventricular fibrillation

4. Drug intake or ingestion (manifestations depend on the drug)

5. Alcohol, coffee, tea, or tobacco use: May cause premature contractions

6. Cardiac surgery: Procedures involving the atria cause atrial arrhythmias; ventriculotomies cause bundle branch blocks; procedures involving the septum may cause AV blocks

Associated Disorders

1. Hypoxia: Causes premature contractions

2. Anemia: Causes sinus tachycardia

3. Infection or inflammation: Fever causes sinus tachycardia; myocarditis may be accompanied by disorders of impulse formation (e.g., nodal tachycardias and atrial flutter); viral diseases (coxsackie B virus, ECHO 9 virus) can also cause supraventricular tachycardias; rheumatic fever causes atrial fibrillation or conduction disturbances (e.g., first-degree or second-degree AV blocks)

4. Myocardial involvement by a variety of disorders may cause arrhythmias

    a. Neuromuscular diseases: Friedreich's ataxia, dystrophies, and the polyneuritis syndromes may be associated with various degrees of AV blocks

    b. Collagen diseases: All collagen diseases are capable of producing various degrees of AV block, bundle branch block, or atrial conduction disorders

    c. Storage diseases: Pompe's disease (type II glycogen storage disease), myocardial hemochromatosis, and amyloidosis may cause conduction disturbances; glycogen storage diseases may cause a short P-R interval

    d. Infiltrative diseases: Metastatic and primary cardiac tumors, especially rhabdomyoma, are associated with conduction disturbances *e.* Neurological disease: Head trauma and increased intracranial pressure may cause tachycardia; ventricular tachycardia, fibrillation, syncope, and atrial tachycardias may occur in children with congenital deafness and prolonged Q-T interval

f. Endocrine disease: Hypothyroidism causes sinus bradycardia; hyperthyroidism causes supraventricular tachycardia and atrial fibrillation; myxedema is associated with escape beats and AV blocks

5. Electrolyte disturbances: May cause a variety of arrhythmias, the most lethal of which is ventricular tachycardia and fibrillation caused by hyperkalemia.

6. Associated heart disease: Some forms of congenital and acquired heart disease are associated with specific arrhythmias

a. Atrial septal defect: Associated with ectopic pacemaker and first-degree AV block, as well as right bundle branch block

b. AV canal malformation: Associated with left axis deviation of the QRS complex and AV blocks

c. Ebstein's disease (displaced tricuspid valve into the right ventricle): associated with first-degree AV block and WPW syndrome

d. Prolapsed mitral valve: Associated with reentrant tachyarrhythmias

e. Corrected transposition of the great vessels: Associated with AV blocks and abnormal P-wave axis

f. Asplenia and polysplenia: Associated with an abnormal P-wave axis and ectopic rhythm

7. History of prematurity: Associated with sinus bradycardia and nodal rhythm, especially in the first two weeks of life

8. History of prenatal infections: Congenital infections (e.g., cytomegaloviral diseases) may cause severe conduction disturbances

Physical Examination

1. Vital signs: Determine the blood pressure, pulse rate, respiratory rate, and adequacy of peripheral circulation; vital signs are important if the patient is in distress leading to arrhythmia or caused by the arrhythmia.

2. General examination: Documents the presence or absence of associated conditions and determines the hemodynamic state (e.g., rule out congestive heart failure).

3. Specific examination (see Table 3): Locate the site of the arrhythmia; determine the rate and rhythm of the pulse; observe the jugular venous pulsations for giant A waves or absent A waves; irregular pulse rate and loss of A waves occur in atrial fibrillation.

Laboratory Investigations

1. Complete blood cell count: Determines presence or absence of anemia, polycythemia, and infection

TABLE 3. *Measurements that aid diagnosis*

1. Determine the atrial rate
2. Determine the ventricular rate
3. Make sure that **all** QRS complexes are preceded by a normal P wave and followed by a normal T wave
4. Measure the P-R intervals over several cycles
5. Measure the QRS intervals
6. Measure the Q-T interval
7. Determine the R-R interval
8. Measure the interval between the sinus beat preceding and the sinus beat following an ectopic beat (compensatory pause)
9. Measure the ectopic-to-ectopic interval
10. Measure the shortest interectopic interval
11. Measure the P-R interval of the sinus beat following the premature ventricular contraction (PVC)

2. Erythrocyte sedimentation rate and C-reactive protein: Rules out inflammatory conditions

3. Urinalysis: Rules out associated conditions (e.g., dehydration, ketosis)

4. Blood chemistry: Blood urea nitrogen, creatinine, and electrolytes; electrolyte disturbances commonly cause arrhythmias

5. Arterial blood gases and pH: Hypoxia and acidosis can cause arrhythmias; prolonged arrhythmias associated with decreased cardiac output and hypotension may cause hypoxia and acidemia, which propagate the arrhythmia

6. Chest radiograph: Rules out associated cardiac problems or confirms the presence or absence of cardiomegaly, congestive heart failure, and lung edema

7. Other studies: (as indicated by medical history and physical examination): Serological testing for infection, viral titers, ASO titers; collagen battery; thyroid and other endocrine studies; blood levels of ingested drugs

8. Confirmation studies

   a. Electrocardiogram (ECG): Complete (12-lead) ECG and rhythm strip. The complete ECG is important to rule out heart disease or associated problems and to determine the P, QRS and T-wave axis. The rhythm strip should be recorded from a lead that shows good P waves, usually lead II or V_1. Lead II alone is not enough unless the axis is normal. An adequate rhythm strip should be a continuous strip for at least 1 min (3 feet long). A multichannel ECG allows vectorial analysis of the electrical complexes. If the routine ECG does not capture the suspected arrhythmia, or if there is a need to correlate specific symptoms to the arrhythmia, prolonged ECG recording may be necessary. In such situations, the Holter monitor, a transistorized ECG tape recorder, may be used to record for 12 to 24 hr; analysis of the data is performed at the end of the recording period.

   b. Exercise ECG: Many arrhythmias are modified (become apparent or abolished) by exercise. The exercise ECG may be used in older children and adolescents, but should be preceded by the routine ECG and rhythm strip.

c. Intracardiac electrocardiography (His bundle electrogram): This procedure, with or without atrial and ventricular pacing, involves the introduction into the heart of an electrode catheter under fluoroscopic control; it yields the most satisfactory results regarding the anatomical site of the arrhythmia, the atrial discharge sequence, and the conduction sequence. Indications for this procedure are frequent episodes of tachycardia with a wide QRS complex, complete AV block, 2 to 1 AV block with a normal P-R interval, or preexcitation syndrome with recurrent tachycardia.

TREATMENT PROTOCOL

1. Correct the possible precipitating factors (e.g., hypoxia, acidosis, electrolyte imbalance, hyperthyroidism, drug reactions.)

2. Start with one mode of therapy or drug; therapeutic combinations are not usually advisable.

3. Follow by serial ECG tracings and/or monitoring and serum drug levels.

4. Antiarrhythmic agents: The most common drugs used for treating cardiac arrhythmias are listed in Table 4 and Table 5.

5. Cardioversion: Application of an external current sufficient to convert the arrhythmia into sinus rhythm is used in the treatment of atrial and ventricular tachyarrhythmias only after drugs have failed or if the situation is life-threatening; digoxin should be discontinued 3 days before the use of elective cardioversion.

TABLE 4. *Classification of antiarrhythmic drugs*[a]

Class I
  Decreases the rate of rise of phase 0 of the action potential
    Ia: Prolong action potential duration. Examples: Quinidine, procainamide, dysopyramide and 'imipramine
    Ib: Shorten the action potential. Examples: Lidocaine, phenotoin,[b] aprinidine,[b] ethmozin and [b]tocainide
    Ic: Do not effect the action potential. Examples: [b]Encainide, [b]flecainide and [b]propophenone
Class II
  Competitive inhibitors of beta-adrenergic receptor sites. Example: Propranolol
Class III
  Prolong the action potential with no effect on phase 0. Examples: [c]Amiodarone (has Class I effects also) and [c]bretylium
Class IV
  Selectively block the calcium channel. Example: Verapamil
Note:
  Knowledge of the underlying mechanisms of an arrhythmia is not sufficient to predict the success of the antiarrhythmic drug and trial of several drugs may be necessary
  Electrocardiographic and electrophysiologic follow up as well as blood levels are important in determining therapeutic and/or toxic effects

[a]Classification is based on the drugs' effects on the action potential of normal tissue.
[b]Investigational.
[c]Investigational - shown to be very effective in the maintenance therapy of supraventricular tachycardia associated with W-P-W resistant to other drugs. Dose: 10–15 mg/kg P.O. daily for 4–14 days. Maintenance dose: 5 mg/kg/day P.O. May cause hypothyroidism and enhance digoxin toxicity.

TABLE 5. *Treatment of arrhythmias*

Ventricular Arrhythmias

Acute therapy
Lidocaine (do not use in the presence of complete heart block)
0.5–1.0 mg/kg i.v. bolus. Repeat in 30–60 minutes
0.5–1.0 mg/kg/hour constant i.v. drip; therapeutic serum level is 1–5 mcg/ml
Procainamide (highly effective for ventricular tachycardia) i.v. use only in adults
Bretylium (highly effective for drug-resistant tachycardia and ventricular fibrillation)
Chronic preventive therapy
Quinidine: 15–60 mg/kg p.o. in 4 doses
Follow up the QRS duration and QT interval. Therapeutic serum level is 2–6 mcg/ml
Procainamide: 15–50 mg/kg/day in 4 or 6 doses
Therapeutic serum level is 3–10 mcg/ml
Dysopyramide
Propranolol (drug of choice in arrhythmias associated with prolonged QT interval, digitalis
    toxicity, exercise induced arrhythmias and arrhythmias associated with mitral valve
    prolapse)
0.2–4.0 mg/kg p.o. in 4 doses
10–20 mcg/kg over 10 minutes i.v.
Therapeutic serum level is 20–150 mg/ml
Phenotoin (drug of choice in arrhythmias due to digitalis toxicity)
2–5 mg/kg/day in 3 doses p.o.
3–5 mg/kg over 5 minutes i.v.
Therapeutic serum level is 5–18 mcg/ml

Supraventricular Arrhythmias

Wolff-Parkinson-White syndrome with atrial fibrillation or flutter
Cardioversion: Do not attempt if patient is on digoxin 1.2 Watt-sec/lb bodyweight
Amiodarone
Further treatment requires electrophysiological investigation
Wolff-Parkinson-White syndrome with reciprocating tachycardia (paroxysmal atrial
    tachycardia)
Digoxin: See chapter on Heart Failure
Verapamil: 5–10 mg/kg/day p.o. in 4 doses (max dose 240 mg/day)
Propranolol: 1–2 mg/kg/day in 4 doses
Phenylephrine: 0.005–0.01 mg/kg/ i.v. (monitor blood pressure)
Atrial flutter-fibrillation
Digoxin
Quinidine (for maintenance after conversion)
Sinus tachycardia
No treatment
Propranolol if the cause is hyperthyroidism
Sinus bradycardia
No treatment unless cardiac output is low
Atropine 0.01–0.02 mg/kg i.v.
Sinus arrhythmia: No treatment
High degree (3rd degree AV block)
Atropine 0.01–0.02 mg/kg i.v. (temporary measure)
Isoproterenol 0.1 mcg/kg/minute (temporary measure)
Cardiac pacemaker: Definitive therapy

6. Pacemaker therapy: Used primarily in symptomatic AV block when the ventricular rate is <40/min and if sympathomimetic drugs fail to accelerate the rate; the type of pacemaker is determined by the patient's age, general condition, and cardiac disease.

Child Abuse

Child abuse and neglect have occurred throughout the history of mankind, with a reported incidence directly proportional to societal sensitivity and recognition of children's rights. In spite of its established historical presence, it was not until Dr. Henry Kempe discussed the battered child syndrome at a meeting of the American Academy of Pediatrics that the medical profession formally recognized this entity. Since then, the diagnosis has broadened to include not only the physical battering of children but also molestation, safety neglect, and medical neglect (Fig. 1). In the United States, now, each state has a statute requiring the reporting of child abuse to a mandated state agency, which is charged with making disposition on that case.

SIGNS AND SYMPTOMS

Clinical features of child abuse are highly variable and depend almost entirely on the type of abuse. Therefore, the manifestations may tend to parallel the functional categories:

1. Physical abuse
    a. Battered child syndrome
    b. Sexual molestation (with or without collusion of parent)
2. Neglect
    a. Medical
    b. Safety
    c. Emotional
    d. Caloric
    e. Educational
3. Abandonment

DIFFERENTIAL DIAGNOSIS

1. Physical abuse (battering and/or sexual abuse).
2. Categories of neglect.
3. Genetic musculoskeletal disorder (e.g., osteogenesis imperfecta).
4. Inborn errors of metabolism.

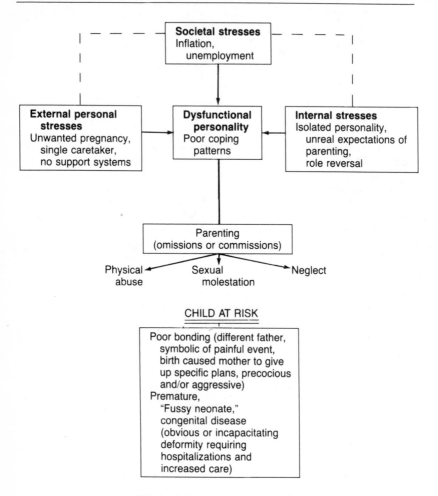

FIG. 1.   Pathophysiology of child abuse.

5. Vitamin deficiency (e.g., scurvy).

6. Vasculitis (e.g., leukocytoclastic).

7. Cultural idiosyncrasies (e.g., "Vietnamese coin rubbing").

8. Bleeding diatheses or coagulopathies.

9. Collagen-vascular disease.

10. Congenital malformations (e.g., CNS, arteriovenous malformation).

SUSPICIOUS EVENTS

The following events are not in themselves diagnostic of child abuse, but they should provide a stimulus for further questioning of the child's caretaker.

1. Delay in seeking treatment for injury.

2. Injury not compatible with child's medical history and/or developmental status.

3. Unrelated person seeking care of child.

4. Injury ascribed to sibling.

5. Multiple prior injuries.

6. Inappropriate affect of caretaker regarding injury of child.

7. Vague description of injury's occurrence.

8. Special child [low birth weight (LBW), premature, handicapped, precocious].

9. Caretaker relates how child is bad and acts in purposefully annoying ways.

10. Doctor or hospital shopping.

11. Caretaker cannot provide basic information about child.

DIAGNOSTIC PROTOCOL

Battered Child Syndrome

1. Caretaker personality characteristics (dysfunctional) are similar to those seen in nonorganic failure to thrive and often involve a "special" child.

2. Caretaker: Abused as a child, poor self-image, apathy and futility may be a prevalent emotion, poor job history, sexual dissatisfaction with mate, frequent power struggles with child and caretaker, child expectations of role reversal.

3. Child: Special problems (e.g., LBW, congenital deformity, mental retardation).

Physical Examination

1. Dermatologic lesions:

    a. Bruises of various ages.

    b. Grab or pinch marks.

    c. Genital bruises.

    d. Slap marks (capillaries ruptured by tips of fingers).

    e. Belt loop or tie marks.

    f. Burns: Doughnut-shaped, symmetrical burns (cigarette burns).

2. Fractures: Spiral (rarely occur spontaneously until child walks), multiple healed and/or healing bucket handle, (pulling injury), periosteal tears.

3. Cranial injuries: Spontaneous bleeding (possible whiplash injury), bruises, black eyes, subdural hemorrhage.

4. Abdominal: Rupture of viscous from blunt trauma.

5. Genitals: Bruises, tears, burns (see Sexual Abuse).

6. Chest and breast: Bruises, hemothorax, pneumothorax.

TREATMENT PROTOCOL

Battered Child Syndrome

1. Provide **immediate** protection and medical care: Hospitalization, relative's home, foster home, protective custody.

2. Treat specific injury or disease.

3. Involve support services: Child-life worker, infant stimulation program, psychiatrist, dietician (see Child Abuse or Neglect and Sexual Abuse).

4. Document all information in the medical chart and notify mandated state agency.

5. Obtain social service consultation to develop liaison with mother while infant is hospitalized and to determine needs of mother when and if child returns home.

6. Develop plan for outreach services: Day care, homemaker service, economic assistance, psychiatric assistance, Parents Anonymous, hot lines.

7. Court plan, if necessary.

8. Potential program for abused child: Parents Anonymous is setting up self-help groups for abused teenagers.

9. Life-skills training: Provides skills to help child avoid sexual abuse; to learn about being touched (e.g., good, bad, forced) and how to obtain assistance.

10. Parenting education: Teaches teenagers about demands of parenting (e.g., egg project, in which high school students provide daily "child" care, care for an egg as if it were a child).

CHILD ABUSE OR NEGLECT

1. Report the case to the mandated state agency, as required by local regulations; report should be made by the examining physician, nurse, or other health professional, as required by state law; record the date and time of the report and the name of the person to whom the report is made.

2. Complete a written case report, as required by local regulations, using the appropriate format.

3. Admit the child to the hospital if there is any question about the child's home environment or safety.

4. Obtain social services consultation.

5. Obtain psychiatric consultation: Advisable in most cases of child abuse or neglect, but mandatory in sexual molestation or emotional deprivation, and in any child exhibiting questionable behavior.

6. Obtain occupational therapy consultation for developmental screening in young children.

7. Perform skeletal survey and/or radionuclide bone scans: Mandatory for physical abuse and any history of accidental or intentional trauma.

8. Obtain obstetrical and gynecological consultation: Mandatory in cases of sexual molestation or genital trauma from rape (see Sexual Abuse).

   a. VDRL testing for syphilis.

   b. Vaginal or penile, rectal, and oral cultures for gonorrhea or chlamydial infections.

   c. "Wet mount" preparation to identify trichamonas.

9. Obtain photographs, as soon as possible, of any manifestations of physical injury (e.g., burns, lacerations, bruises, old scars) or deteriorating conditions (failure to thrive, neglect, malnourishment, severe dehydration); while awaiting photographic documentation, place in the medical chart representative drawings of the lesions and a pertinent narrative on the initial medical history and physical examination.

10. Obtain recreational therapy consultation for behavioral assessment, play therapy with anatomically correct dolls, or infant stimulation.

11. In cases of known or suspected substance ingestion, obtain urine, emesis, and blood screening for the known or suspected substance.

12. Failure to thrive

   a. Record weight, height, and head circumference at admission and plot on appropriate growth charts.

   b. Record birth weight, birth place, and prenatal and postnatal conditions.

   c. Record the name of other hospitals, clinics, or physicians who have provided care.

   d. Record accurate daily weight.

   e. Obtain dietary consultation.

Sexual Abuse

The treatment protocol for sexual abuse is intended to supplement the protocol on general child abuse (see Child Abuse or Neglect).

1. The patient and accompanying family members (caretakers) should be escorted immediately to a private room for the ensuing interview and physical examination.

2. The senior pediatric resident should see all sexually abused children and should assume primary responsibility for their care; an attending staff pediatrician should be notified as soon as possible.

3. Obtain obstetrical and gynecological and social services consultations; psychiatric consultation is often needed immediately as a diagnostic and therapeutic modality for both the child and caretakers.

4. Obtain medical history from the patient alone, if possible, and then from both the patient and the caretakers conjointly, using quotations, when available, supplemented by the child's drawings (the sequence of interviews will vary with the presentation).

5. The initial physical examination should be brief; note any abnormalities, especially of the genital area (obtain vaginal or penile, rectal, and oral cultures and serological testing in all cases of suspected sexual abuse). If genital abnormalities are noted, perform a more complete examination, ranging from simple aspiration of vaginal contents with an eye dropper to a complete pelvic examination with the "rape kit."

6. The pediatric resident and social worker should discuss the findings with the victim and the caretakers in a meaningful manner (avoid unnecessary confrontations).

7. Counsel adolescents about the alternatives to potential pregnancy and the risks of possible venereal disease; treatment should be case specific and individualized (not all cases of child molestation will require use of antibiotics).

8. Advise caretakers about potential personality disturbances in the child (e.g., anxiety manifestations, phobias, sleep difficulties, regression).

9. A police report is usually required, as well as a report to the local or state agency responsible for child abuse.

Coma

The word coma is derived from the Greek word *koma*, which means deep sleep. It is a state of profound unconsciousness from which an individual cannot be aroused. It may have a variety of causes. The etiology may be endogenous, such as a seizure disorder, or exogenous, such as drug ingestion or trauma. Accurate and early diagnosis and management have significant influences on the outcome of coma. A rigidly adhered to diagnostic and treatment protocol is essential to appropriate management. The history is especially important and will provide much diagnostic information.

SIGNS AND SYMPTOMS

The signs and symptoms of coma are generally related to the state of unconsciousness, the level of coma, and other signs and symptoms related to the primary etiology. The Maryland coma scale attempts to classify the level of coma as it relates to cerebral (cortical and subcortical) functioning.

INITIAL DIAGNOSTIC PROTOCOL

1. Evaluate the initial status of the patient. Assure that the vital signs are stable and that there is adequate cardiovascular and respiratory function (if not, resuscitate as necessary).

2. Obtain the medical history and rapidly perform a physical examination.

   a. Search for a history of trauma, drug ingestion, and/or previous illnesses (e.g., diabetes mellitus, seizures).

   b. Look for signs of trauma and/or penetrating wounds (be sure to look at the patient's back).

   c. Search the patient for a medical alert bracelet, necklace, or card.

3. Draw blood for initial laboratory evaluations and administer intravenous fluids.

   a. Administer 50% glucose, 1 mg/kg i.v. push; if the patient responds, the diagnosis of hypoglycemia is established.

   b. Obtain complete blood cell count, electrolytes, blood urea nitrogen, creatinine, blood glucose, liver function tests, blood toxin screening, and typing and crossmatching of whole blood.

   c. Obtain urine toxin screening, urinalysis, and urine ferric chloride testing.

Eye Opening:
Spontaneously 3
To sound 2
To pain 1
None 0
Untestable U

Orientation:
Time, place, person 3
2 of the 3 2
1 of the 3 1
None 0
Untestable U

Pupil, Corneal &
Caloric Reflexes
& Grimace:
Normal 2
Decreased or
  abnormal 1
Absent 0
Untestable U

Stimulus:
Voice 3
Shake or shout 2
Pain 1
Central pain 0

Verbal Response:
Oriented 4
Confused 3
Inappropriate 2
Incomprehensible 1
None 0
Untestable U

Leg Motor Response:
Normal 2
Abnormal or
  extensor 1
None 0
Untestable U

Arm Motor Response:
Dextrous and strong 5
Paretic 4
Localizes 3
Abnormal flexion 2
Extension 1
None 0
Untestable U

DATE												
TIME												
SEDATION MEDS												
PARALYTIC AGENTS												
SEIZURES												
BP												
HR												
RESP												
TEMP												
EYE OPENING												
ORIENTATION												
PUPILS (R/L)												
CORNEALS (R/L)												
FACIAL GRIMACE (R/L)												
CALORICS (R/L)												
STIMULUS												
VERBAL RESPONSE												
ARM MOTOR (R/L)												
LEG MOTOR (R/L)												

FIG. 1. The Maryland coma scale. (From Salcman, Schepp, and Ducker, 1981: Calculated recovery rates in severe head trauma. *Neurosurgery*, 8:301, with permission.)

4. Complete the physical evaluation, paying close attention to the neurological examination (especially the respiratory pattern, pupillary reflex, muscle tone, and deep tendon reflexes).

INITIAL TREATMENT PROTOCOL

1. Resuscitate the patient and stabilize the vital functions, as needed.

2. Begin intravenous fluids and administer 50% glucose, 1 mg/kg, as previously stated.

3. After the initial therapeutic regimen begins, treatment depends on the diagnosis established.

SPECIFIC DIAGNOSTIC AND TREATMENT PROTOCOLS

Table 1 gives diagnostic and treatment protocols for various types of comas (once the origin of the coma has been determined).

TABLE 1. *Coma: Diagnostic and treatment protocols*

Diagnosis	Treatment
Central Nervous System Infection	
Fever, somnolence, lethargy, irritability, nausea, vomiting, and seizures may occur	Treat the underlying infection
The cerebrospinal fluid (CSF) will show pleocytosis, the culture is usually positive, and the Gram stain may be positive for the organism (if the patient has not been taking antibiotics)	Treat cerebral edema, if present
	Treat inappropriate secretion of antidiuretic hormone, if present
Diabetic Ketoacidosis	
Medical history may or may not be positive for diabetes	See Diabetes chapter
Polyuria, polyphagia, and polydipsia may be present	
Nausea, vomiting, abdominal pain, dehydration, and tachypnea are usually found	
Seizures may occur	
Drug- or Poison-Induced	
Medical history may or may not be positive for ingestion of drugs or poisons	See Poisonings chapter
Barbiturates, tranquilizers, alcohol, opiates, and morphine derivatives are commonly involved in coma secondary to substance ingestion	
Head Trauma	
Medical history may or may not be positive for head trauma	Identify and treat the underlying disease or disorder
Neurological signs and symptoms may or may not be present	
Diagnosis of concussion may be made if the patient is unconscious for any amount of time after the trauma or if there is retrograde or anterograde amnesia for the event	
CT scan may help to rule out intracranial bleeding	
Hypoglycemia	
Medical history may be positive for diabetes mellitus and the patient may be taking insulin; hypoglycemia is usually due to insulin overdosage	Administer 50% glucose, 1 mg/kg i.v.
Tachycardia, diaphoresis, and tachypnea occur; disorientation and seizures may also be present	Provide a diet adequate in carbohydrates
Blood glucose is diagnostic	Adjust insulin dosage appropriately

TABLE 1. *(Continued)*

Diagnosis	Treatment
A reagent strip (Dextrostix®) may give rapid information about the presence of hypoglycemia	

Ketotic Hypoglycemia

Diagnosis	Treatment
Affected children are between 18 months and 10 years of age; the first episode of hypoglycemia usually occurs before 5 years of age There is usually an antecedent or concurrent illness Medical history is usually positive for a period of fasting Other symptoms of hypoglycemia are usually present (seizures may occur)	Treat the hypoglycemia as stated above Provide a diet high in carbohydrates Prohibit periods of fasting

Reye's Syndrome

Diagnosis	Treatment
Medical history may be positive for a preceding illness, such as influenza or varicella There is unexplained vomiting SGOT and other liver function tests are abnormal Blood ammonia level is high	See Reye's Syndrome chapter

Seizures

Diagnosis	Treatment
Medical history may be positive for a seizure disorder Major motor manifestations need not be present Other neurological manifestations may be present	See Seizure Disorders chapter

Congenital Infections

A certain group of congenital infections of the newborn are known collectively by the name "torches." The diseases are toxoplasmosis, congenital rubella syndrome, cytomegalovirus disease, herpes simplex disease, and syphilis. They are either acquired in utero or contracted from the birth canal during parturition (Fig. 1). Each may cause a devastating syndrome in the neonate, resulting in permanent disability or death.

DIFFERENTIAL DIAGNOSIS

1. Toxoplasmosis
2. Congenital rubella syndrome
3. Cytomegalic inclusion disease
4. Disseminated herpesvirus infection

5. Congenital syphilis
6. Erythroblastosis fetalis
7. Neonatal septicemia or meningitis

SIGNS AND SYMPTOMS

These congenital infections are grouped together because of similar clinical presentations in many patients. The torches syndrome is characterized by premature delivery, anemia, thrombocytopenia, petechiae or purpura, hepatomegaly, splenomegaly, jaundice, CNS abnormalities, microcephaly, intrauterine growth retardation, or intrauterine death.

The presentation is variable and depends on the extent of involvement. Each agent also may present other manifestations, which may point to a specific etiology.

INITIAL DIAGNOSTIC PROTOCOL

1. Complete blood cell count with platelet count.
2. Examination of the urine sediment for cytomegalovirus.
3. Serologic studies for torches organisms (IgM).
4. IgM level and IgM-specific antibodies.

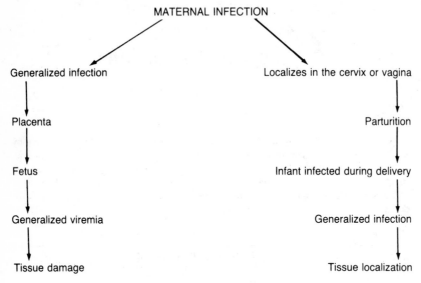

FIG. 1.   Pathophysiology of congenital infections.

5. Viral cultures.

6. Bacterial cultures (septic evaluation).

7. Tzanck smear of vesicular fluid (if present) for herpesvirus.

DIAGNOSTIC AND TREATMENT PROTOCOLS

Table 1 gives diagnostic and treatment protocols for a variety of infections.

TABLE 1. *Torches syndromes: Diagnostic and treatment protocols*

Diagnosis	Treatment
Cytomegalovirus	
Urine examination (sediment) may reveal intracellular inclusion bodies	There is no specific treatment; efforts should be symptomatic and supportive (e.g. transfusions for anemia, anticonvulsants for seizures)
Identification of the virus in tissue culture of the urine or of the gastric aspirate	Antibiotics are not indicated unless there is a concurrent bacterial infection
Serological identification: Indirect fluorescent antibodies, neutralization antibodies, and complement-fixing antibodies	
Liver biopsy may reveal inclusion bodies	
CNS calcifications occur and are characteristically **periventricular** in location	
Microcephaly is not uncommon	
Most infants are infected natally and exhibit sensorineural hearing loss, mental retardation, or hyperkinesis; transplacental infection occurs but is uncommon	
Herpes Simplex	
Mild infections may occur, with vesicular skin lesions as the only clinical manifestation; the neonate may not appear ill; however, disseminated disease occurs in more than half of these infants	Adenine arabinoside, 15 mg/kg/day i.v. over a 12-hr period for 10 days
Infection is usually natally acquired	Supportive and symptomatic treatment
Symptoms appear within the first week of life	Brain biopsy is recommended before beginning treatment
Lethargy, fever, vomiting, and poor feeding are common presenting findings; septicemia may be considered	Treat variations in the intracranial pressure; increases are common
Seizures and coma represent CNS involvement (meningoencephalitis)	
Keratoconjunctivitis and/or gingivostomatitis may be present	
Active herpetic lesions may be present in the mother	
Multinucleated giant cells and intranuclear inclusions from mother's secretions or from the infant suggest the diagnosis	
Viral cultures: Herpesvirus will generally grow in 3 to 4 days	

TABLE 1. *(Continued)*

Diagnosis	Treatment
Congenital Rubella Syndrome	
The major manifestations of the syndrome are commonly present	Treatment is supportive and symptomatic
Other manifestations include cataracts, peripheral pulmonary artery stenosis, "salt and pepper" retinitis, patent ductus arteriosus, blueberry muffin appearance to the skin due to ectopic erythropoiesis	Prevention of the illness through widespread immunization programs is extremely important; all women of childbearing age should be adequately protected against rubella to prevent the possible development of the syndrome in offspring
Sensorineural hearing loss (appears later in childhood and is the most common manifestation of the syndrome)	
Mental retardation is common	
Learning disability	
Cerebral palsy may occur	
Syphilis	
Variable manifestations of the torches syndrome; mid-trimester abortions are common	Aqueous penicillin units G, i.m. 50,000 to 100,000 units/kg/day i.m. in two divided doses for 14 days
Prematurity and/or intrauterine growth retardation are common	The remainder of the therapeutic regimen is supportive and symptomatic
Persistent rhinitis (snuffles) is common	
Radiographs of the long bones show metaphyseal involvement	
Fluorescent treponemal antibody absorption (FTA-ABS) test, and RPR are positive	
Total Igm level is usually elevated	
Cerebrospinal fluid evaluation should be performed	
Later manifestations (e.g., saber shins, Hutchinson's teeth, rhagades) are modified by treatment	
Toxoplasmosis	
Variable manifestations of the torches syndrome	Treatment is supportive and symptomatic
Chorioretinitis is common	Sulfadiazine and pyrimethamine have been used, but they are not known to significantly affect the prognosis of the disease
Hydrocephalus, microcephaly, or intracranial calcification may occur	
Seizures, mental retardation, blindness, deafness, and/or hydrocephalus are common sequelae	
The Sabin-Feldman dye test may be positive	
IgM-specific fluorescent antibody titer is elevated	

Congestive Heart Failure

Congestive heart failure (CHF) is a clinical syndrome characterized by inability of the heart to maintain an output capable of meeting individual metabolic needs. Heart failure may be caused by either volume or pressure overload or because of myocardial (pump) damage. Congestive heart failure occurring in infancy is most commonly caused by congenital heart disease. Iatrogenic fluid overload is also responsible for a large percentage of infants with CHF.

PATHOPHYSIOLOGY

The major determinants of cardiac output are the stroke volume and the heart rate. In any condition leading to decreased cardiac output, the heart attempts to compensate by increasing the heart rate (tachycardia) and by increasing the stroke volume (dilatation to increase the end diastolic volume), which leads to cardiomegaly. Tachycardia and cardiomegaly are almost always present in all CHF states except with restrictive diseases, such as constrictive pericarditis or obstruction to pulmonary venous drainage, where lung edema occurs without cardiomegaly. Because of the nature of the causes of heart failure in infants, it is seldom pure right-sided or left-sided failure. It is usually a combination of both. Therefore, the infant almost always presents with tachypnea. The presence of tachypnea, tachycardia, and cardiomegaly are essential for the diagnosis of CHF in infants. While hepatomegaly and systemic edema (manifestations of right heart failure) also occur, evidence of lung edema may be lacking early in the disease process. Not infrequently, lung edema may present clinically as wheezes, and CHF must be ruled out in any infant who presents with wheezing. Because of high pulmonary vascular resistance at birth, left-to-right shunts such as atrial septal defect (ASD), ventricular septal defect (VSD), and patent ductus arteriosus (PDA) seldom cause heart failure before the age of 6 to 8 weeks, even if they are of large size. They may, however, produce CHF if the pulmonary vascular resistance is nonexistent (the premature infant with a PDA) or if it drops unexpectedly early in life (premature decrease of the pulmonary vascular resistance). This knowledge helps explain the etiological factors that lead to CHF (Table 1).

SIGNS AND SYMPTOMS

The signs and symptoms of CHF in childhood are variable (Fig. 1). Symptoms may relate to the underlying disease. Tachypnea is often the earliest sign. Tachycardia is usually present concomitantly. Pulmonary congestion and edema (manifested by rales, rhonchi, and/or wheezing) and hepatomegaly (or hepatosplenomegaly) also occur. Cyanosis may or may not be present.

TABLE 1. *Etiological factors in congestive heart failure*

Age	Volume overload	Pressure overload	Myocardial disease
At birth	Hydrops fetalis Acute blood loss (or gain)	Premature closure of PDA or patent furamen ovale (PFO)	
1 day to 1 week	Iatrogenic fluid overload Tricuspid atresia Ebstein's disease PDA in premature infant Pulmonary venous obstruction Arteriovenous (A-V) fistula (brain) Respiratory distress syndrome	Hypoplastic left heart syndrome (aortic stenosis, fetal circulation, mitral atresia) Severe pulmonary stenosis	Arrythmias Tumors Diabetic myopathy Infectious myopathy
1 week to 1 month	Total anomalous pulmonary venous return Transposition of the great vessels with ventricular septal defect (VSD)	Coarctation of the aorta	Myocardial storage diseases
>1 month	Any congenital or acquired heart disease causing significant pressure or volume overload; conditions such as myocarditis, inflammatory cardiac diseases, toxic cardiac drugs, thyrotoxicosis, anemia, collagen, or neuromuscular diseases can also cause CHF.		

DIAGNOSTIC PROTOCOL

1. Congestive heart failure must be treated aggressively, regardless of its cause. Because CHF is a clinical syndrome, any infant or child who has tachypnea, tachycardia, and/or cardiomegaly should be diagnosed as having CHF until proven otherwise.

2. Congestive heart failure must be suspected in any infant who has respiratory distress, wheezing, peripheral cyanosis, acidosis, apnea, feeding difficulties, and/or unusual sweating.

3. Medical history should be evaluated for the following:

   a. Previous evidence suggestive of congenital heart disease.

   b. Symptoms of CHF (e.g., cyanosis, feeding problem, sweating).

   c. Fluid intake.

4. CHF may be suggested by the following signs and symptoms on physical examination:

   a. Wheezing.

   b. Heart murmurs.

   c. Accurate resting heart and respiratory rates.

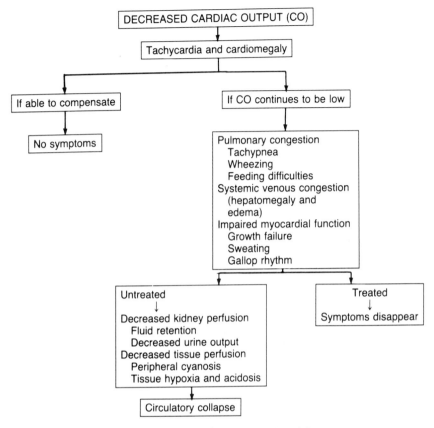

FIG. 1. Pathophysiology of congestive heart failure.

    d. Hepatomegaly.

    e. Eyelid, scrotal, or peripheral edema.

5. Evaluate heart size and pulmonary vasculature on chest radiographs (radiographs taken in expiration may reveal false cardiomegaly).

6. Note evidence of arrhythmias on electrocardiogram (ECG).

7. Monitor arterial blood gases, blood glucose, blood urea nitrogen, electrolytes, complete blood count, and urinalysis.

8. Other tests as indicated to rule out infection, thyrotoxicosis, CNS or neuromuscular disorders.

9. Echocardiogram may be helpful in revealing structural causes, effusions, and myocardial tumors.

TREATMENT PROTOCOL

1. Admit patient to pediatric intensive care unit for continuous monitoring.
2. Allow nothing by mouth if in severe failure; otherwise, allow diet appropriate for age.
3. Semisitting position (cardiac chair for infants).
4. Complete bed rest.
5. Vital signs, including accurate respiratory rate, heart rate, blood pressure at rest.
6. Weigh infant daily.
7. Accurate intake-output measurements.
8. Oxygen by tent or mask.
9. Intravenous fluids for maintenance; accurately monitor the fluid and salt intake (need not be severely restricted if there is adequate renal function and may even be harmful).
10. If the infant or child is severely ill, is not improving, or is in a postoperative state, central venous pressure (CVP) monitoring should be instituted, and an arterial line for systemic pressure monitoring should be inserted.
11. Medications

    a. Digoxin

        (1) Digitalizing doses: 0.03 to 0.04 mg/kg p.o. (infant or child) or 0.02 to 0.03 mg/kg p.o. (premature infant).

        (2) Maintenance doses: One-fourth of digitalizing dose.

        (3) Digitalization: One-half of total dose immediately, *then* one-fourth of dose 6 to 8 hr later, and *then* one-fourth of dose 6 to 8 hr after second dose.

        (4) Monitor ECG before third dose to rule out toxicity.

        (5) Monitor digoxin therapy with ECG (serum digoxin levels are not an adequate substitute), and obtain serum potassium levels.

        (6) Maintenance therapy: One-fourth of total dose given in two doses 12 hr apart; start 8 to 12 hr after last digitalizing dose.

        (7) In the not-so-very-sick infant, it may be possible to start with maintenance doses directly; monitor renal function (digoxin is excreted by the kidney).

    b. Diuretics

        (1) Furosemide (Lasix®), 1 to 2 mg/kg i.v. over a 1-min period (may be repeated every 8 hr) *or* 2 to 3 mg/kg/day p.o.

        (2) Ethacrynic acid (Edecrin®). 1 mg/kg i.v. over a 1-min period *or* 2 to 3 mg/kg/day p.o.

        (3) Monitor fluids and electrolytes, especially potassium; other diuretics may be used.

c. Antiarrhythmic drugs as needed.

d. Medications to treat the primary condition (e.g., infection, hypertension, thyroid disease).

e. Sodium bicarbonate to correct acidosis.

12. Most patients will improve with the described measures; some will have resistant failure and additional measures are needed, especially if there is peripheral circulatory collapse (high CVP and low systemic arterial pressures requiring treatment).

a. Isoproterenol (Isuprel®), 0.1 mg/kg/min, *or* dopamine, 5 to 10 mg/kg/min.

b. Careful but adequate fluid replacement to allow adequate tissue perfusion.

13. If the patient does not respond to the above regimen and does not have intracardiac shunts, the following regimen should be employed.

a. Sodium nitroprusside, 0.5 to 10 mEq/kg i.v. in the acute state.

b. Isosorbide dinitrate, 0.25 to 1.0 mg every 6 hr for continuous management.

c. These drugs decrease the peripheral vascular resistance and end-diastolic pressures and increase the cardiac output; their use necessitates arterial pressure monitoring.

14. If patient shows no improvement and if pulmonary edema is one of the principal manifestations, use the following measures.

a. Positive pressure breathing to keep alveolar pressure above capillary pressure.

b. Peritoneal dialysis.

c. Emergency operation to correct intractable CHF due to congenital heart disease with obstruction to left ventricle or CHF complicating infective endocarditis.

Note: CHF in infants secondary to congenital heart disease is an indication for cardiac catheterization and angiography. If peritoneal dialysis is to be used, the indication must be clear: for lung edema, use hypertonic solution; for electrolyte fluid imbalance, the usual isotonic solution is suitable. Use 50 ml/kg of the dialyzing fluid (7% glucose in balanced solution) and administer slowly over a 10 to 15-min period. Leave for 10 min before allowing to drain by gravity. The hypertonic solution should not be used more than once in any 12-hr period.

Connective Tissue Diseases

Disorders of the connective tissues in children are similar to their counterparts in adults. In certain disorders, however, there are some very different age-related variations in both clinical and laboratory features (e.g., systemic lupus erythematosus). The broad category of connective tissue disease includes at least nine discrete disorders, which often overlap in their presentations and diagnostic evaluations. A single serological fluorescent antibody test may indicate major changes in therapy. In general, the musculoskeletal system, the renal system, and the central nervous system, are the most prominent organ systems affected by these disorders. Their natural history shows that significant morbidity and mortality are due to renal and central nervous system involvement.

It is important to recognize that the distinctions between many of these diseases are more often theoretical than practical and that, most often, these diseases have significant commonalities, which makes the differentiation of one from the other difficult. It appears that the ultimate clinical feature may not be based on the laboratory findings and/or the clinical signs and symptoms, but on the size of the blood vessels affected by the underlying disease process (Fig. 1).

DIFFERENTIAL DIAGNOSIS

The results of laboratory studies in connective tissue disease are often helpful in the differential diagnosis (Table 1). The distinction between the following diseases and disorders is important.

1. Rheumatoid arthritis

2. Rheumatic fever

3. Systemic lupus erythematosus

4. Dermatomyositis

5. Polymyositis

6. Scleroderma

7. Vasculitis syndromes (polyarteritis nodosa, infantile polyarteritis nodosa)

8. Mixed collagen-vascular disease

9. Chronic active hepatitis

10. Complement deficiencies (hereditary or acquired)

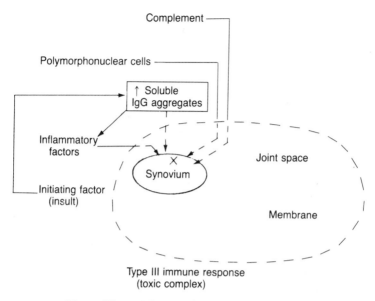

FIG. 1. Differential diagnosis of connective tissue diseases.

DIAGNOSTIC PROTOCOL

Juvenile Rheumatoid Arthritis

1. Incidence peaks between 1 and 3 years of age and again at puberty.

2. Definitive diagnosis requires five of the criteria defined by the American Rheumatoid Association (see Table 2).

3. Three general modes of presentation: systemic, polyarticular, and pauciarticular.

4. Systemic (20–25%)

    a. Medical history: Male predominance, abrupt presentation, acute illness, evanescent pink migratory rash, abdominal pain.

    b. Clinical manifestations: High spiking fever, generalized lymphadenopathy, hepatosplenomegaly, pleuritis, pericarditis, myocarditis, pneumonitis, minimal joint complaints initially.

5. Polyarticular (40–50%)

    a. Medical history: Female predominance, often insidious onset, antecedent complaints of weight loss, lethargy, anorexia, and irritability.

    b. Clinical manifestations: Involves more than five joints, often symmetrical, rare acute illness, small joints affected.

TABLE 1. *Laboratory results in connective tissue diseases*

	Complement deficiency	Systemic lupus erythematosus	Polyarteritis nodosa	Juvenile rheumatoid arthritis	Mixed connective tissue disease	Scleroderma
↑ ESR		+++	+++	+++	+++	+
ANA titer/anti-DNA	+/A	+++/+++ (↑)	+/A	+/A	+++/+	++-+++/+
ANA pattern	*	Diffuse/speckled	A	*	Speckled	*
↓ THC/C3/C4	THC↓	+++/+++/+++	~+/+/+	*	+++/+/+++/++	*
LE preparation/anti-Sm	*/A	+++/+	A/A	A/A	+/A	*/A
Rheumatoid factor	*	+	*	+	+++	+
Joint pain	++	+++	++	+++	+++	*
Coagulopathy	*	+	*	*	*	
Anemia	*	++~+++	++	++~+++	A	+
Hemolytic anemia	*	+		x		A
Leukopenia	*	++	+	*	+++	A
Thrombocytopenia	*	+	*		+++	
Adenopathy	*		+++	+++ (varies)	+++	+*
↑ Gamma globulin	*	+++	+	+++	++	+++
Muscle weakness	+	+		+	+++	++
Renal insufficiency	+	+++ (↑)	+++ (↑)	+	+++	
Skin rash	+~++	+++	+	+++	+++	+
Special studies	Variable, depending on deficiency	Renal, liver, muscle, skin biopsy	Renal and mesenteric angiography; renal biopsy	Radiographs; synovial fluid complement; slit lamp examination	Renal biopsy; ENA against ribonucleoprotein (+++)	Pulmonary function studies; esophageal dysmotility; digital plethysography

Frequency of occurrence: +++ ≥ 70%; ++ ~ 50%; + ≤ 30%; A, absent; *, not usually present (also, not usually tested or not diagnostic).

TABLE 2. *Preliminary criteria for classification of juvenile rheumatoid arthritis*[a]

Morning stiffness
Pain on motion or tenderness
Swelling in at least one joint
Swelling in more than one joint (a symptom-free interval before involvement of a second joint may not exceed 3 months)
Symmetrical joint involvement
Subcutaneous nodules
Radiographic changes typical of rheumatoid arthritis
Positive rheumatoid agglutination reaction
Poor mucin clot formation in joint fluid
Biopsy findings in synovium consistent with rheumatoid arthritis
Biopsy findings in a nodule consistent with rheumatoid arthritis

[a]Developed by the American Rheumatism Association. A definite diagnosis of rheumatoid arthritis can be established if five of the criteria are present along with joint symptoms that have persisted for at least 6 weeks; a probable diagnosis can be made if three of the criteria are present for 4 weeks together with the joint symptoms.

6. Pauciarticular (33%)

　　a. Medical history: Female predominance, often insidious onset.

　　b. Clinical manifestations: Involves one to four joints, rare acute illness, large joints affected (especially knees), frequent iridocyclitis (25%).

Systemic Lupus Erythematosus

1. Incidence is highest from 11 to 15 years of age.

2. May occur in neonates by passive transfer of antibodies or de novo as a new disease.

3. Diagnostic criteria are shown in Table 3.

4. Medical history: Female predominance (88%), often behavioral changes (e.g. emotional lability), lethargy, malaise, weight loss, cold intolerance, manifested by vasomotor instability, nonspecific arthralgias, photosensitivity, ingestion of medication known to produce lupuslike symptoms.

TABLE 3. *Preliminary criteria for classification of systemic lupus erythematosus (SLE)*[a]

Facial erythema (butterfly rash)	Chronic false-positive serological
Discoid lupus	test for syphilis (STS)
Raynaud's phenomenon	Profuse proteinuria
Alopecia	Cellular casts
Photosensitivity	Pleuritis or pericarditis, or both
Oral or nasopharyngeal ulceration	Psychosis or convulsions, or both
Arthritis without deformity	Hemolytic anemia, leukopenia,
LE cells	and/or thrombocytopenia

[a]Developed by the Diagnostic and Therapeutic Criteria Committee of the American Rheumatism Association. A diagnosis of SLE can be established if four or more signs or symptoms are present during any interval of observation.

5. Clinical manifestations: Spiking fever, arthritis, arthralgias, skin rash (e.g., butterfly distribution on face), seizures, neuropathies, psychoses, pneumonitis, carditis, pleuritis, pericarditis, hepatosplenomegaly and/or lymph node enlargement, renal involvement.

Scleroderma

1. Rare in children.

2. Two major forms of presentation: Focal and progressive systemic sclerosis.

3. Focal (may progress to systemic sclerosis)

   a. Medical history: Male predominance, local skin color changes, joint stiffness near affected area, often positive serological tests.

   b. Clinical manifestations: Isolated patches of discolored skin, areas of subcutaneous atrophy.

4. Progressive systemic sclerosis

   a. Medical history: Tightness and hardness of skin, dysphagia, cold and heat intolerance.

   b. Clinical manifestations: Various skin pigment changes, Raynaud's phenomena, joint stiffness and swelling, renal insufficiency, pulmonary sclerosis and hypoxia.

Dermatomyositis and Polymyositis

1. Incidence is highest in the early school years.

2. Polymyositis is very unusual in children and is often associated with a visceral malignancy.

3. Medical history: Female predominance, insidious onset, muscle pain and weakness (especially in proximal muscles of extremities, trunk, and neck flexors), rash on upper eyelids (Helitrope sign) and forehead, dysphagia and regurgitation.

4. Clinical manifestations: Pain and tenderness of affected muscles, subcutaneous edema or brawny induration, heliotropic discoloration of upper eyelids, malar area, and forehead, scaly rash over extensor surfaces of knees and elbows and dorsal aspect of hands, subcutaneous calcification.

Vasculitis Syndromes

1. Represent a wide spectrum of syndromes, ranging from Henoch-Schönlein purpura to the more severe polyarteritis nodosa.

2. Henoch-Schönlein purpura

   a. Medical history: Male predominance, abdominal pain, joint pain, macular purpuric skin rashes on lower extremities, occasional behavioral changes, commonly recurrent, renal disease (ranging from mild microscopic hematuria to proliferative glomerulonephritis with nephrotic syndrome.

   b. Clinical manifestations: Macular and/or urticarial purpuric rash on buttocks and lower extremities, significant arthralgias and arthritis, abdominal pain with a rare intussusception, CNS involvement in older children.

3. Polyarteritis nodosa

   a. Medical history: Infrequent among children, severe hypertension and renal insufficiency.

   b. Clinical manifestations: Severe refractory hypertension with congestive heart failure and/or renal failure, suggesting involvement of the middle, medium-sized, arteries; marked progressive renal insufficiency and hypertension overshadow most other features.

Rheumatic Fever

See Rheumatic Fever chapter for diagnostic protocol.

Complement Deficiencies

1. Acquired and hereditary.

2. Medical history: Manifestations depend on the specific deficiency of the complement system and the hereditary pattern, recurrent pyogenic infections, angioedemalike symptoms, findings compatible with severe combined immune deficiency diseases.

3. Clinical manifestations: Virtually indistinguishable from systemic lupus erythematosus, with exacerbations and remissions; various forms of pyogenic infections, septicemia, gonococcemia, Raynaud's phenomenon, and angioedemalike pictures predominate.

TREATMENT PROTOCOL

Juvenile Rheumatoid Arthritis (JRA)

Differentiate between rheumatoid arthritis, septic arthritis, and rheumatic fever. This distinction is more difficult between pauciarticular rheumatoid arthritis and septic arthritis. In septic arthritis, the inflammation often extends beyond the joint, with induration, heat, redness, and cellulitis, whereas in JRA, pain may be less and redness of the joint minimal. A therapeutic trial of salicylates may be used to distinguish the various entities. The response to salicylates will be very prompt in acute rheumatic fever, delayed in JRA, and absent or minimal in septic arthritis.

1. Salicylate therapy

   a. Salicylates, 45 mg/lb (<60 lb) or 30 mg/lb (>60 lb), every 6 hr.

   b. Maintain blood salicylate level of 20 to 25 mg/dL.

   c. Salicylates, although of limited effectiveness, are helpful in the relief of joint pain and fever. When used as the first drug in the treatment of a newly diagnosed case of JRA, they must be given a trial of at least 6 weeks. Some patients will fail to show an immediate response, even with adequate blood salicylate levels, but if the dosage is continued for several more weeks, there will usually be an excellent response. Control of fever and other symptoms and signs of arthritis and normal erythrocyte sedimentation rate indicate successful therapy. Alternative drugs all have significant higher toxicity than salicylates, so every attempt should be made to obtain and maintain therapeutic control with salicylates.

2. Alternative drug therapy

   a. Ibuprofen (Motrin®), indomethacin (Indocin®), chloroquine, or, occasionally, gold.

   b. Consult pediatric rheumatologist on use of these drugs.

3. Corticosteroid therapy

   Dramatic positive effects of corticosteroids make their use as primary drug therapy tempting, but most often this is both unnecessary and harmful. JRA is usually a chronic disease, with periods of remission and exacerbation, and the long-term use of corticosteroids is fraught with difficulty. When used to control iridocyclitis, myocarditis, pericarditis, or other polyserositis associated with JRA, it is extremely important to reduce the steroid dosage as soon as possible to minimize withdrawal symptoms, osteoporosis, peptic ulceration, immunosuppression, and other adverse effects.

4. Physical therapy

   a. Motion plays a vital part in the management of JRA; permanent joint deformity is avoided only by maintaining joint mobility.

   b. Moist heat from whirlpool baths, simple emersion baths, and application of moist pads to affected areas is effective; the moist heat should be applied after exercise.

5. Psychological rehabilitation

   a. Potential problems of the child, as well as family, friends, and other interacting individuals, should be anticipated. The child's reaction to the chronic illness and insight into peer reaction are important.

   b. The issue of overprotection of the child must be addressed early in the child's illness.

6. Prognosis

   a. Aside from intermittent complications, more often induced by iatrogenic or secondary phenomena (e.g., side effects of corticosteroid therapy), the most serious effects tend to be the result of pericarditis or myocarditis.

   b. The prognosis is based not on mortality but on morbidity, and is almost directly proportional to the patient's outcome at the end of the first year.

Systemic Lupus Erythematosus (SLE)

1. The course of SLE is variable and not totally predictable, with significant initial and late mortality that tends to be related to infection and/or renal failure.

2. Therapeutic aggressiveness should be based on objective physical findings, serological studies (low complement levels, anti-DNA levels), and evidence of impending or ongoing renal damage. Adequate histopathological evaluation is important, including renal biopsy.

3. Mild complaints, such as arthralgia, occur early in the course of SLE, and in the absence of severe renal involvement or threatening serological findings, a course of salicylates is reasonable treatment at this stage.

4. During much of the course of SLE, corticosteroids, 1 to 2 mg/kg/day, will be the drug of choice. Maintenance doses should continue for 3 to 6 weeks, followed by tapering of the dose to a lower maintenance level that controls the disease.

5. Antimalarial drugs are sometimes used to obtain a therapeutic effect and maintain steroids at the lowest possible level.

6. Consultation early in the course of SLE is necessary. The choice of therapy (steroids, antimalarials, or other immunosuppressive drugs) should be based on an overview of the serological and clinical findings, including the rate of progression of symptoms.

Scleroderma

1. Although laboratory findings in the focal form of scleroderma are impressive in their similarity to those of SLE, there is no specific treatment for scleroderma. The pruritis of the focal form may be treated with topical steroids.

2. Physical therapy is used to maintain and improve the range of motion.

3. Some studies have shown benefits from other immunosuppressive drugs, as well as penicillimine.

4. Consultation with a pediatric rheumatologist is essential.

Dermatomyositis and Polymyositis

1. Although early reviews of childhood dermatomyositis described a poor prognosis, recent reports have been more encouraging, due in part to the use of corticosteroid therapy.

2. Prednisone, 1 to 2 mg/kg/day, over a period of several weeks, followed by tapering while monitoring muscle weakness and enzyme tests, appears to be practical treatment.

3. Physical therapy plays a significant role in improving muscle strength, maintaining range of motion, and preventing contractures.

Vasculitis Syndromes

1. Henoch-Schönlein purpura

   a. Therapeutic intervention is most often a tincture of time and support.

   b. Corticosteroid therapy may be indicated for CNS dysfunction and abdominal bleeding.

2. Polyarteritis nodosa

   a. Treatment must be aggressive, with the consultation of a nephrologist and a rheumatologist early in the course of the disease.

   b. Immunosuppressive therapy is used while attempts are made to stabilize blood pressure and renal function.

    c. Prognosis in polyarteritis nodosa is significantly worse than in Henoch-Schön-lein purpura.

Rheumatic Fever

See Rheumatic Fever chapter for treatment protocol.

Complement Deficiencies

A description of intervention in these acquired or hereditary deficiencies is beyond the scope of this chapter, but treatment focuses on the symptoms and attempts to provide therapeutic modalities available through current research; unfortunately, synthetic complement factors are not yet available.

Treatment is directed toward anticipated complications.

Crohn's Disease

Crohn's disease is a chronic inflammatory disease of the bowel characterized by transmural involvement of the intestine. It affects the entire bowel and is not limited to the ileum, although the ileum is the most common portion of the bowel involved. The disease usually begins in the preadolescent period.

SIGNS AND SYMPTOMS

The clinical presentation and course of Crohn's disease are usually characterized by intermittent crampy abdominal pain, alternating diarrhea (occasionally bloody) and constipation, weight loss or failure to thrive (which may be the most striking symptom), and anemia. Anal fistulas and fissures and perianal disease are characteristic. Other associated symptoms and signs may include arthritis, stomatitis, erythema nodosum, and digital clubbing. Occasionally, abdominal masses may be palpable, especially in the right lower quadrant (Fig. 1).

DIFFERENTIAL DIAGNOSIS

1. Appendicitis
2. Functional abdominal pain
3. Ulcerative colitis
4. Tuberculosis
5. Anorexia nervosa
6. Hodgkin's disease
7. Lymphosarcoma

DIAGNOSTIC PROTOCOL

1. Complete blood cell count may show iron deficiency anemia or anemia secondary to blood loss.
2. Erythrocyte sedimentation rate: Elevated in approximately 50% of affected patients and extremely nonspecific.
3. Serum protein level: Usually shows hypoproteinemia.
4. Albumin-to-globulin ratio: Usually shows a reversal.
5. Barium enema and small bowel radiographs may show mucosal irregularities, thickening of the bowel wall, fistulas, and skip lesions.

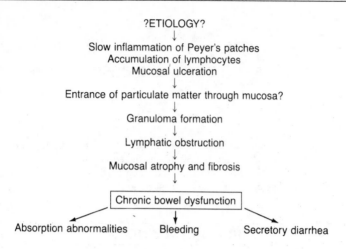

FIG. 1.   Pathophysiology of Crohn's disease.

6. Endoscopy: May show presence of inflammatory lesions and provide a route for obtaining biopsy tissue.

7. Rectal biopsy for pathological confirmation of the diagnosis.

TREATMENT PROTOCOL

1. Supportive care is essential in the acute and chronic management of patients with Crohn's disease.

2. A diet low in oxalate and fat may be beneficial in patients with oxaluria and stone formation.

3. Prednisone, 2 mg/kg/24 hr in four divided doses.

   a. Remission usually occurs within 1 week.

   b. Steroids may be given intravenously in severely ill patients.

   c. Prednisone should be tapered after remission occurs (taper at the rate of 5 mg/day/week).

4. Sulfasalazine (Azulfidine®): 50 mg/kg/24 hr.

   a. Begin when the prednisone dose is 50% of the starting dose.

   b. Continue indefinitely during remissions.

   c. If a relapse occurs, sulfasalazine should be discontinued and prednisone restarted.

5. Total parenteral alimentation is indicated in patients who fail to respond to

steroids and sulfasalazine (70% of patients with involvement of the ileum and colon will respond to parenteral alimentation).

6. Surgical intervention is indicated in massive bleeding, perforation, megacolon toxicity, and intractable symptoms unresponsive to steroids, sulfasalazine, and total parenteral alimentation.

Cyanosis

Cyanosis is a bluish color of the skin and mucous membranes; it is usually due to arterial oxygen unsaturation and hypoxemia. Although it may not be associated with hypoxia, its presence suggests the possibility of a life-threatening illness. Prompt diagnosis and therapy are mandatory. As a reflection of the state of oxygenation of the blood it becomes visible to the naked eye when the oxygen saturation is less than 75%. The degree of cyanosis is dependent on the hematocrit, the pH, the state of the peripheral circulation, and the infant's temperature.

PATHOPHYSIOLOGY

Central Cyanosis

Skin and mucous membrane are bluish.

Central Cyanosis Due to Arterial Hypoxemia

1. Congenital heart disease
   a. Right-to-left shunts (intracardiac or intrapulmonary)
   b. Decreased pulmonary blood flow
2. Pulmonary disease
   a. Acute (pneumonia, embolism, atelectasis, pneumothorax)
   b. Chronic obstructive or restrictive (asthma, emphysema)
3. Decreased atmospheric pressure or oxygen tension

Central Cyanosis Without Arterial Desaturation:

1. Hemoglobin abnormalities (methemoglobinemia, sulfhemoglobinemia)
   a. Congenital
   b. Acquired
2. Polycythemia

Peripheral Cyanosis

Peripheral cyanosis affects the exposed surfaces of the skin; the arterial saturation is normal.

Reduced Cardiac Output

1. Congestive heart failure
2. Shock

Impaired Peripheral Blood Flow

1. Shock
2. Exposure to cold (including Raynaud's phenomenon)
3. Nervous tension
4. Arterial obstruction
5. Venous obstruction

Other Causes of Cyanosis

Other causes of cyanosis may or may not be associated with arterial desaturation.

1. Central nervous system disease
   a. Severe infections
   b. Seizures
   c. Intracranial hemorrhage
2. Neonatal hypoglycemia
3. Neonatal hypocalcemia
4. Neonatal sepsis
5. Infants with apnea
6. Infants with extrapulmonary disease (may compromise pulmonary function)
   a. Tracheal obstruction secondary to vascular rings
   b. Diaphragmatic hernia

SIGNS AND SYMPTOMS

Cyanosis may be associated with either cardiovascular or pulmonary disease. Depending on the etiology, other symptoms may be present. Often, differentiation between cardiovascular and pulmonary etiologies is impossible on clinical grounds alone.

It is important to remember that peripheral cyanosis may be normal immediately after birth. Some infants, even with arterial desaturation, appear to be pink. Bluish skin discoloration may be secondary to lighting, wall coloring, polycythemia or hypothermia.

CYANOTIC INFANT OR CHILD

Resuscitate and stabilize before diagnostic evaluation

History and physical examination

Arterial blood gases on room air (Use right radial or right and left radial arteries.
If the infant has venous and arterial umbilical lines, obtain samples from each **plus** the right
radial artery)

Normal Po₂ and O₂ saturation
Central cyanosis without hypoxia
Peripheral cyanosis

Decreased Po₂ and O₂ saturation
Central cyanosis with hypoxia

Chest radiograph
Evaluate lungs, heart, diaphragm,
and pulmonary vasculature

Abnormal lung
Normal heart

Normal lung
Large heart

Normal lung
Normal heart

Pulmonary disease
Respiratory distress
  syndrome
Aspiration
Pneumothorax
Pneumonia

Increased pulmonary vasculature
Hypoplastic heart
Truncus
Large VSD
A-V canal
Alveolar hypoventilation

Decreased pulmonary vasculature
Pulmonary atresia
Tricuspid atresia
Ebstein's disease
TOF
Fetal circulation

Transposition
  without VSD
Severe pulmonary stenosis
Total anomalous
  PVR

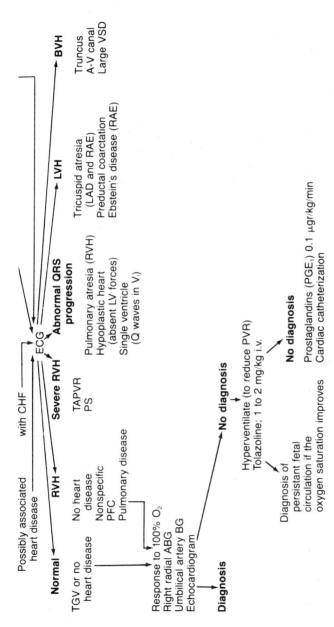

FIG. 1. Diagnostic protocol following initial impression of cyanosis in an infant or child. PVR, pulmonary venous return; VSD, ventricular septal defect; TOF, tetralogy of Fallot; TGV, transposition of great vessels; TAPVR, total anomalous pulmonary venous return; PS, pulmonary stenosis.

DIAGNOSTIC PROTOCOL

1. Obtain a complete medical history, including the time of onset of cyanosis and associated or precipitating factors; check for exposure to cold and/or history of phlebitis, trauma, or immobilization.

   a. Cardiac: Heart murmurs, squatting, syncope, palpitations, and chest pain are suggestive of a cardiac etiology.

   b. Pulmonary: Cough, fever, respiratory distress syndrome, dyspnea, respiratory therapy, oxygen therapy, and complicated prenatal history and delivery suggest a pulmonary etiology.

   c. Hematologic: Family history of hematological problems or ingestion of drugs or toxic substances (e.g., aniline dyes, nitrates, quinones, sulfonamides, phenacetin) suggest a hematological etiology.

2. Perform a complete physical examination. Check for cardiac disease by looking for cyanosis, tachypnea or normal respiratory rate, heart murmur (may be absent), and/or adequate peripheral pulses (absent in the femoral arteries in cases of coarctation). The presence of dyspnea, rales, retractions, and wheezing (wheezing may be the only sign of lung edema secondary to congenital heart disease) or the absence of breath sounds suggest a pulmonary etiology. If peripheral cyanosis is present, check the patient for hypotension, decreased pulses, tachycardia, moist, clammy, cold extremities, evidence of other disease processes, such as scleroderma or systemic lupus erythematosus (SLE), and evidence of arterial or venous obstruction.

3. After the initial impression is formed, the schematic (Fig. 1) may be followed.

4. If electrocardiogram shows no abnormalities, allow infant to inhale 100% oxygen for 15 min and repeat arterial blood gases (ABG). A rise of Po_2 above 100 Torr virtually excludes significant cyanotic heart disease and points toward pulmonary disease. In cyanosis secondary to congenital heart disease, the Po_2 should not increase more than 10 to 15 Torr after oxygen inhalation.

5. If newborn infant is very cyanotic and hypoxic and has required resuscitation measures, a diagnostic therapeutic trial of *tolazoline*, 1 to 2 mg/kg i.v. push, for 5 to 10 min may help to rule out persistent fetal circulation; if this fails and shunt-dependent cyanotic heart disease is suspected, prostaglandins may be tried and will keep the ductus arteriosus patent until further testing is done.

TREATMENT PROTOCOL

1. Cyanotic heart disease

   a. Stabilize the patient's condition.

   b. Treat congestive heart failure.

   c. Immediate cardiac catheterization and angiography.

   d. Surgical intervention: Total correction or palliative.

2. Pulmonary disease: Treat specific condition.

3. Methemoglobinemia: methylene blue, 1 to 2 mg/kg i.v. as a 1% solution; repeat in 4 hr, if necessary.

4. Congestive heart failure (see Congestive Heart Failure chapter).

5. Shock (see Shock chapter).

6. Metabolic problems: Treat specific condition.

7. Raynaud's disease:

  a. Adequate clothing to keep warm.

  b. Tolazine (Priscoline®) 0.5 mg per kg 4 times per day (maximum adult dose is 25–50 mg 4 times per day) with or without reserpine 0.1–0.25 mg daily p.o.

  c. Surgical sympathectomy in very severe cases.

8. Arterial and venous obstruction:

  a. Surgical intervention.

  b. Treat underlying condition.

CYANOSIS IN THE NEWBORN

Table 1 gives diagnostic and treatment protocols for cyanosis in the newborn.

TABLE 1. *Cyanosis in the newborn: Diagnostic and treatment protocols*

Diagnosis	Treatment
General Evaluation and Management	
Medical history and physical examination	Resuscitate, if necessary
Insert a nasal catheter	Maintain temperature
Insert an umbilical artery catheter	Support respiration, nutrition, and fluid intake
Arterial blood gases (right radial and umbilical)	Gentle suction
Administer 100% oxygen for 10 to 15 min and repeat blood gases (used to differentiate pulmonary and cardiac etiology)	Oxygen by hood
	Allow nothing by mouth
Chest radiograph: Evaluate heart, lungs and diaphragm	Assisted ventilation, if necessary
Electrocardiogram	Antibiotics: Ampicillin and gentamicin
Echocardiogram (if cardiac etiology is suspected)	Treat underlying etiology
Cultures: cerebrospinal fluid, blood, urine, nose, throat, umbilicus	
Hemoglobin and hematocrit	
Transilluminate the skull (normal circle of illumination beyond the edge of the transilluminator is 1.5 cm in full-term newborn and 2.0 cm in premature infant	
CT scan and/or ultrasonography if CNS hemorrhage is suspected	

TABLE 1. *(Continued)*

Diagnosis	Treatment

Hyperviscosity

Specific etiological considerations: Feto-fetal, maternal-fetal, or placental-fetal transfusion, small for gestational age, postmaturity, toxemia, maternal diabetes, hyperthyroidism, adrenal hyperplasia, Down's or Beckwith's syndromes

Clinical manifestations:
Respiratory distress, congestive heart failure, seizures, tachypnea, pulmonary infiltrates and oxygen dependency, poor feeding, lethargy, and poor perfusion

Diagnosis is substantiated by the following laboratory results:
Hemoglobin < 21 g%, venous hematocrit > 65%, increased viscosity index, decreased platelets, increased circulating nucleated red blood cells, jaundice, hypocalcemia, and hypoglycemia

Treat respiratory distress and CNS symptoms
Monitor hemoglobin, hematocrit, blood glucose, and calcium
Urinalysis for red blood cells
Partial exchange transfusion using fresh frozen plasma; volume exchange (in ml) = observed hematocrit − desired hematocrit × blood volume ÷ observed hematocrit (blood volume = 80 ml/kg)
Repeat hematocrit after 1,3, and 24 hr

Methemoglobinemia

Etiological considerations: Congenital toxins such as aniline dyes from diapers, sodium nitrate, bismuth subnitrate, benzocaine, and sulfonamides
Laboratory evaluation: Expose one drop of blood to air; it becomes dark brown; hemoglobin electrophoresis

Methylene blue, 1 to 2 mg/kg i.v. as 1% solution in normal saline, for acquired cases **or** ascorbic acid, 300 mg/kg/24 hr p.o., **or** ascorbic acid, 100 mg/kg/24 hr i.v.

Persistent Fetal Circulation

Etiological considerations: Increased pulmonary resistance and R-L shunt across PFO or PDA secondary to hypoxia, severe lung disease, polycythemia, meconium aspiration, intrauterine growth retardation
Clinical manifestations: Tachypnea, cyanosis and pulmonary hypertension in first 8 hr of life, cor pulmonale, hypoxia and acidosis, severe cyanosis, nonresponsive to oxygen, and murmur of tricuspid insufficiency
Laboratory evaluation: If the R-L shunt is across a patent ductus arteriosus the right radial artery Po_2 will be normal, but desaturated in umbilical artery; [if R-L shunt is across a PDA;] echocardiogram shows normal pulmonary artery and valve but abnormal right systolic time intervals

Oxygen to increase arterial Po_2
Ventilate
Tolazoline, 1 mg/kg/hr i.v. as loading dose and then 1 mg/kg i.v. every 4 hr
Treat associated conditions

APPENDIX 1. *Diagnostic approach to cardiac disease with cyanosis*

Disease	Medical history	Physical examination	Chest radiograph	Electrocardiogram	Comments
Transposition of great vessels without VSD	Cyanosis at birth Large baby	Severe cyanosis Tachypnea only initially progressing to severe respiratory distress within days No specific murmur Single S_2	Enlarged egg-shaped heart with narrow base Increased pulmonary vasculature	Normal or mild right ventricular hypertrophy	Arterial P_{O_2} is extremely low (usually < 40 Torr)
Transposition of great vessels with VSD	Mild or no cyanosis at birth Cyanosis in first few weeks of life	Moderate cyanosis Tachypnea Tachycardia Hepatomegaly (CHF) Murmur of VSD Single S_2	Enlarged heart Increased pulmonary vasculature	Biventricular hypertrophy	Because of adequate mixing across the VSD, the cyanosis is not so marked
Pulmonary atresia (severe tetralogy of Fallot)	Pink at birth (due to PDA) Cyanosis appears when the ductus closes (few days after birth)	Murmur of PDA, if still patent; if closed, there will be severe cyanosis and no murmurs Single second heart sound	Normal or slightly enlarged heart Normal or decreased pulmonary vasculature (increased if ductus is patent)	Right axis deviation Abnormal QRS progression in chest leads Right ventricular hypertrophy	Early in tetralogy of Fallot, the infant may not be cyanotic due to VSD and L-R shunt. As the pulmonary stenosis becomes more severe, a R-L shunt develops and the infant becomes cyanotic usually by 1 year of age

APPENDIX 1. (continued).

Disease	Medical history	Physical examination	Chest radiograph	Electrocardiogram	Comments
Severe pulmonary stenosis	Severe cyanosis at birth; moderate respiratory distress (but no tachypnea initially)	Murmur of pulmonary stenosis Intense cyanosis Possible murmur of tricuspid regurgitation	Normal size heart Poststenotic dilatation of pulmonary artery Decreased pulmonary vasculature	Right axis deviation Severe right ventricular hypertrophy	
Tricuspid atresia	Cyanosis at birth	Cyanosis CHF	Enlarged heart Normal pulmonary vasculature Prominent RA	Left axis dev. ($+60°$ to $+30°$) LVH RAE	
Ebstein's disease	Cyanosis at birth	Cyanosis CHF Murmur of tricuspid insufficiency	Enlarged heart Prominent RA	RAE RVH Arrhythmias	
Total anomalous pulmonary venous return	Cyanosis shortly after birth	Cyanosis; tachypnea; no significant murmurs; CHF	Mild cardiac enlargement Increased PBF Picture of lung edema and small heart if there is obstruction	Right ventricular hypertrophy	Very difficult to diagnose Po_2 in all sites (arteries and veins may be the same)
Persistent fetal circulation	Cyanosis at birth Respiratory distress	Cyanosis Respiratory distress No significant murmurs Loud P_2	Normal or slightly enlarged heart Prominent pulmonary vasculature	Right ventricular hypertrophy	If the R–L shunt is at the ductal level, Po_2 is normal in right radial and decreased in left radial or umbilical artery

VSD, ventricular septal defect; S_2, second heart sound; PDA, patent ductus arteriosus; RA, right atrium; LVH, left ventricular hypertrophy; RAE, right atrial enlargement; PBF, pulmonary blood flow; RVH, right ventricular hypertrophy.

APPENDIX 2. Findings in various diseases or disorders causing cyanosis

Cause of cyanosis	Medical history	Physical examination	Laboratory studies						
			CBC	Blood glucose	BUN	Electrolytes	Chest radiograph	ECG	Blood gases
Congenital heart disease	Cyanosis at or after birth Syncope Squatting Dyspnea	Cyanosis Evidence of CHF Evidence of RVH Murmurs Clubbing	↑ Hgb	Normal	Normal	Normal	Abnormal	Abnormal	↓ P_{O_2} ↑→ P_{CO_2} →→ pH
Acute pulmonary disease	Acute onset of respiratory distress Sudden cough Sudden dyspnea Fever Wheezing Foreign body aspiration	Retractions Rales, rhonchi, wheezing Decreased breath sounds	↑ WBC or normal	Normal	Normal	Normal	Abnormal	Normal	↓ P_{O_2} ←↑ P_{CO_2} →↓ pH
Chronic pulmonary disease	History of pulmonary disease Cough Dyspnea Wheezing Hemoptysis	Rhonchi, harsh breath sounds, wheezing Decreased breath sounds Thoracic deformity	↑ Hgb	Normal	Normal	Normal	Abnormal	Occasional RVH	→pH ↓ P_{O_2} ↑↓ P_{CO_2}
Hemoglobin abnormalities	Cyanosis since birth Exposure to chemicals	Cyanosis No clubbing	Normal	Normal	Normal	Normal	Normal	Normal	Normal
Decreased peripheral perfusion	Exposure to cold Evidence of loss of blood Septic fever History of Rheumatic fever and RHD History of surgical intervention	Discoloration of organs Absent pulse Hypotension Thready pulse Tachycardia Clammy skin Varicose veins Mottling of skin	Normal except in hemorrhage ↓ Hgb	Normal or ← (diabetic)	May be ↑ or Normal	Abnormal in shock	Normal	Normal tachycardia or arrhythmia	Normal

Cystic Fibrosis

Cystic fibrosis (mucoviscidosis) is an autosomal recessive disease caused by dysfunction of the exocrine (mucous) glands. It is manifested clinically by pancreatic insufficiency (in 80% of cases), progressive pulmonary obstructive disease, and elevated sweat concentrations of sodium and chloride (>60 mEq/L). Genitourinary (vas deferens), submaxillary gland, and Wolffian duct abnormalities are also common, but less serious, sequelae.

Although every ethnic group is susceptible to cystic fibrosis, its incidence is highest among Caucasians (1 in every 2,000 live births), with affected children often being blond and fair in complexion. Cystic fibrosis occurs only one-tenth as often in blacks, and is rare in Orientals. There does not appear to be any sexual or socioeconomic predominance, although affected males appear to outlive affected females.

The carrier rate is estimated at 1 in 30 persons. Carriers are usually asymptomatic, and no test is presently available to detect carriers or to diagnose this disease in utero. In homozygotes with cystic fibrosis (CF), the iontoelectrophoretic sweat test is reliable and exquisitely valid as a diagnostic technique, even in the neonates, if performed correctly (Fig. 1).

SIGNS AND SYMPTOMS

Clinical manifestations of CF vary with the age of the child's presentation. Ten percent of newborns with the disease will present with intestinal obstruction due to viscous meconium (meconium ileus). Frequent, foul-smelling stools containing excessive fat, poor growth in spite of good caloric intake, and/or recurrent pulmonary infections are commonly seen in infants and older children with CF.

DIFFERENTIAL DIAGNOSIS

1. Asthma
2. α_1-Antitrypsin disease
3. Bronchiectasis
4. Failure to thrive
5. Chronic diarrheal diseases
6. Immune deficiency diseases
7. Malabsorption syndromes
8. Chronic pulmonary infection
9. Cirrhosis
10. Emphysema
11. Pneumothorax or pulmonary hemorrhage
12. Pulmonary foreign body
13. Recurrent abdominal pain

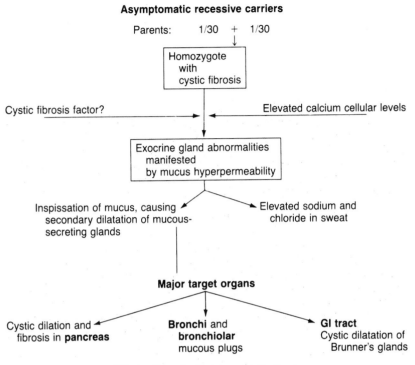

FIG. 1.   The pathophysiology of cystic fibrosis.

DIAGNOSTIC PROTOCOL

1. Medical history
   a. Meconium ileus
   b. Rectal prolapse
   c. Recurrent pneumonia
   d. Chronic cough
   e. Atelectasis
   f. Hemoptysis
   g. Chronic diarrhea
   h. Cirrhosis
   i. Hypoprothrombinemia
   j. Organic failure to thrive
   k. Sinusitis or nasal polyps

l. Family history of cystic fibrosis

m. Heat prostration

n. Hyponatremia

o. Metabolic alkalosis

2. Gastrointestinal tract investigation

   a. Clinical findings: Rectal prolapse, nasal polyps, edema.

   b. Gastrointestinal manifestations: Malabsorption, duodenal drainage to quantify presence of trypsin, liver function tests (elevated serum alkaline phosphatase and/or decreased prothrombin time), ancillary studies (gastrointestinal radiographic series, stool trypsin evaluation).

3. Iontoelectrophoretic sweat sodium and chloride test (>60 mEq/L)

   a. Neonates have poor sweating mechanisms; thus, elevated sweat sodium or chloride level may be missed

   b. Abnormal sweat electrolytes may also be seen in adrenal insufficiency, ectodermal dysplasia, hereditary nephrogenic diabetes insipidus, hypothyroidism, malnutrition, edema, inborn errors of metabolism (e.g., glucose 6-phosphatase deficiency, mucopolysaccharidosis, fucosidosis).

4. Respiratory tract investigation

   a. Clinical findings: Clubbing of fingers, nasal polyps, sinusitis

   b. Pulmonary manifestations: Radiographic evidence of hyperinflation, atelectasis, mucous plugs; hemoptysis or bronchiectasis (bronchoscopy or surgery)

TREATMENT PROTOCOL

A multidisciplinary team approach is essential, including liberal consultation with a pulmonologist and/or gastroenterologist.

Acute (Symptomatic) Treatment

1. Pneumonia: *Staphylococcus aureus* and *Pseudomonas aeruginosa* are most commonly involved; recommended treatment is with parenteral aminoglycosides (e.g., amikacin, tobramycin) and postural drainage (see Pneumonia chapter).

2. Heat prostration: Reduce temperature with a cooling blanket; replace electrolytes rapidly.

3. Bronchospasm or asthma with mucous plugs.

4. Sinusitis: *Hemophilus influenzae* (often ampicillin resistant), *Streptococcus pneumoniae, Staphylococcus aureus*, and *Streptococcus pyogenes* are most commonly involved.

Maintenance Therapy

1. Multidisciplinary team (specialty-oriented nurse, social worker, physical and respiratory therapists) for support, education, and therapy

2. Dietary and nutritional support

  a. Regular diet supplemented by Pancrease EC®

  b. Vitamin supplementation: Multivitamins (double the usual amount), vitamin K, and vitamin E

  c. Progestamil® or Neutramagin® in infants

  d. Adequate salt intake, especially in warm weather

3. Physical fitness

  a. Physical exercise and postural drainage, with moist environment at night

  b. Routine, frequent physical examinations, with sputum cultures and sensitivity tests

  c. Periodic chest radiographs and yearly blood chemistry evaluations, including blood cell counts and liver function tests

4. Prophylactic vaccinations (e.g., influenza vaccine)

5. Continuous antibiotic therapy (dicloxicillin or other antistaphylococcal agent)

Complications

1. Cor pulmonale

2. Diabetes mellitus

3. Hemoptysis or bronchiectasis: Medical treatment as long as possible before resection or shunting procedures

4. Cirrhosis, portal hypertension, hepatic failure, hypersplenism, hypoprothrombinemia, or esophageal varices

5. Adrenal insufficiency

Developmental Problems and Related Disorders

Human physical and psychosocial development follows a clearly defined pattern. Individual variations are minor. Because deviation from the expected human pattern of development may be caused by a variety of factors, diagnostic evaluation of developmental disorders requires the involvement of professionals in many disciplines (occupational therapists, language and speech pathologists, psychologists, social workers, neurologists, psychiatrists, as well as pediatricians). This multidisciplinary approach to the diagnostic evaluation of developmental disorders does not, however, preempt the role of the primary physician, who must continue to bear the burden of performing the developmental assessment, seek out the specific cause of the developmental abnormality, and plan further evaluations and management. Since development is a continuous process, two or more evaluations, at successive ages, may be necessary to determine the presence or absence of developmental problems.

PATHOPHYSIOLOGY, SIGNS AND SYMPTOMS, AND DIFFERENTIAL DIAGNOSIS

The pathophysiology, signs, symptoms, and differential diagnosis of developmental disorders are closely related and depend on the specific process involved in the developmental abnormality. Causative factors include environmental influences (familial, cultural), infection, intoxication, trauma, metabolic disorders, tumors, chromosomal abnormalities, idiopathic, psychological influences, sensory deficits, neuromuscular disorders, chronic illness, developmental deviation, primary speech and language problems, and mental retardation syndromes.

Failure to Thrive

Failure to thrive is a clinical syndrome produced by an external event or group of events that interfere with the child's normal developmental processes, affecting both mental and physical states. Failure to thrive is considered to be present if the child's height and weight are consistently below the third percentile, or if the child presents with significant weight loss, general lag in physical growth, apathy, and depression. Most cases present as infants who have failed to gain weight. For a detailed discussion of the subject, see Failure to Thrive chapter.

Growth Disorders

Disorders of growth are those conditions that affect the somatic size of the child. In general, they are characterized by failure to gain weight, short or tall stature, and obesity.

Disorders of Motor Function

Muscle Weakness

Upper motor neuron lesions cause spastic paralysis of the opposite side of the body. Affected patients have exaggerated deep tendon reflexes and Babinski reflex on the affected side.

Lower motor neuron lesions cause flaccid paralysis and muscle wasting. They may result from primary muscle disorders (muscle dystrophies) or peripheral nerve diseases with generalized weakness, especially of the distal musculature (e.g., polyneuritis).

Anterior horn cell diseases may be symmetrical or asymmetrical. Clinically, there is atrophy, hypoactive deep tendon reflexes, and normal plantar responses.

Ataxia

Ataxia results from cerebellar involvement and is characterized by unsteady, un-coordinated voluntary movements, poor balance during sitting and standing, unsteady gait, and poor hand function. Many causes are defined: congenital cerebellar defects (e.g., ataxic form of cerebral palsy), acute acquired ataxia (e.g., intoxication, exanthems, and nonspecific infections), episodic ataxia (e.g., vertiginous epilepsy, vestibular neuronitis), chronic acquired ataxia (e.g., increased intracranial pressure, brainstem tumors, ataxia-telangectasia, Friedreich's ataxia, inborn errors of metabolism).

Abnormal Muscle Movements

Chorea, sudden, irregular jerky movements, may be caused by rheumatic fever, encephalitis, hypoparathyroidism. Athetosis, slow writhing movements of the muscles of the extremities, may result from kernicterus. Dystonia causes involuntary sustained spasms of the muscles of the neck, trunk, and extremities that result in abnormal posturing. Tremors with basal ganglia disease occur at rest; those of cerebellar origin occur only during volitional movements. Psychogenic disturbances may lead to tics or habit spasms.

Speech and Language Disorders

Delayed speech (absence of word production by 2½ years of age), voice defects, articulation disorders, dysrhythmias, cluttering, and/or stuttering all represent disordered speech or language (see Table 1).

Learning Disabilities

Learning disabilities are defined as failure to achieve the level of academic performance and potential expected in relation to intellectual capacity. Children with

TABLE 1. *Causes of delayed speech*

Hearing loss
  Effect of hearing loss on language development is dependent on age of deafness
Hypoacusis
  Associated with incorrect articulation; hearing loss may involve high frequency sounds only;
    requires audiological evaluation
CNS dysfunction
  Mental retardation is the commonest form of CNS dysfunction associated with a language
    disorder
Maternal deprivation or lack of stimulation
  Lack of parent-child interaction, with a history of diminished affect, decreased motivation, and
    insatiable appetite
Infantile autism
  Lack of interaction between the child and the environment
Elective mutism
  Lack of communication between the child and the environment under certain circumstances
Familial delay
  Family history of delayed speech
Bilingual household
Socially disadvantaged
Histidinemia
Twins
Voice defects (dysphonia)
  Usually a functional process, but may be due to structural defects (e.g., laryngeal papilloma);
    may evolve into an organic process with the formation of vocal cord nodules
Articulation disorders (omissions, distortions, substitution)
  Physiological: Defects in the brain and cranial nerves that innervate the lips, tongue,
    and palate; inadequate velopharyngeal closure from cleft palate, velar paresis, or removal
    of adenoids; hypoplasia of the mandible and failure of fusion of the upper lips
  Environmental: Replication of faulty speech and faulty articulatory sounds
Dysrhythmia
  Lack of normal tongue fluency (undue prolongation of words, hesitation, or unnecessary
    repetition); may be due to interference in control of respiratory mechanisms during speech;
    may be a normal physiological variation before 4 years of age
Cluttering
  Rapid, nervous speech with omissions; may be caused by dissociation between thinking
    and speaking
Stuttering
  Disturbance of rhythm and fluttering; may be psychological or organic; persistence after 5
    years of age may indicate pathological dysfunction

learning disabilities should be distinguished from mentally retarded, emotionally disturbed, or physically handicapped children. The disability may manifest in imperfect ability to listen, think, speak, read, write, spell, or do mathematical calculations.

The neurological examination and laboratory procedures such as the electroencephalogram have uncovered a neurological basis for this academic failure. The current concept is based on the observation of deficits in speech, language, perception, and memory that result from acquired brain disease, which is often minimal and difficult to determine. Affected children are characterized by near normal or above normal intelligence, hyperactive, purposeless, random and disruptive behavior in 75%, short attention span, distractibility, impulsiveness, incoordination, perceptual impairment, and disorders of memory and concept formation. Specific abnormalities include dysgraphia (inability to express thought by handwriting), dyslexia (difficulty in reading), dyscalculia (difficulty in number concepts), dysdiadochokinesia (difficulty with forearm movements), contractures of the Achilles tendon, hyperreflexia or asymmetry, graphanesthesia, dyspraxia (disordered movements in hopping or gait), and delayed cerebral dominance (high incidence of left or mixed laterality, 10% as compared with 4% in the unaffected population).

Pathophysiologically, this syndrome is thought to be due to one or more of several mechanisms, such as actual destruction of specific areas of the brain, hormonal stimulation, nutritional factors (e.g., allergies), or deficiencies in trace metals (e.g., zinc, copper, arsenic), genetic factors, and/or biochemical disturbances.

Mental Retardation

Mental retardation refers to significantly subaverage general intellectual functioning existing concurrently with deficits in adaptive behavior and manifested during the developmental period. Traditionally, persons have been labeled mentally retarded if their performance has fallen two standard deviations below the mean on a standard intelligence test. Different tests, however, measure different aspects of cognitive functioning and are not error free.

Psychosocial Disorders

Psychosocial disorders include abnormal psychosocial response, reactive disorders, developmental deviations, psychoneurotic disorders, personality disorders, psychotic disorders, and psychophysiological abnormalities.

DIAGNOSTIC PROTOCOL

Growth is defined as change in size, development, and maturation of organs and organ systems, acquisition of skills, and the ability to adapt and express. Thus, developmental diagnosis requires examination of growth, the quality of function, and the integration of behavior.

The child's behavior must be appraised in terms of the true chronological age. The behavior may prove to be normal, retarded, or deviated. The optimal age of evaluation is 40 weeks, when all parts of the body have come under some degree of voluntary control. Evaluation may be performed at any age, however, and as early as four weeks of age or as late as the early years of adulthood.

Historical Information

1. Maternal medical history: Pregnancy, labor time, delivery, weight gain pattern, radiation, infections, medications, threatened abortion, toxemia, prenatal care, sedation, fetal presentation.

2. Patient's medical history: Apgar score, neonatal anoxia, neonatal jaundice, sleep pattern, feeding problems, activity level, seizures, fevers, trauma, infections, general nutrition, previously acquired developmental skills, behavioral patterns, previous illnesses, complaints.

3. Social history: Family members and relationships, socioeconomic background, methods of interaction, stimulation, discipline.

4. Academic achievements: Academic performance, teacher's comments and reports, interaction in the classroom and among peers.

5. Family history: Heredofamilial disorders and mental retardation.

Physical Examination

1. Measure height, weight, head circumference and plot on growth curve charts.

2. Perform a complete physical examination and record any abnormal physical features.

3. Transilluminate the skull.

4. Examine vision, with funduscopic examination.

5. Perform a complete neurological examination for evidence of CNS dysfunction:

   a. Poor coordination of gross or fine motor skills.

   b. Delay in motor skill acquisition.

   c. Poor ability to plan and execute a motor task (dyspraxia).

   d. Impaired ability to inhibit movements; mirroring and fidgeting.

   e. Immature neurological signs (e.g., persistent tonic neck reflex, poor equilibrium, and fidgeting reaction).

   f. Impaired sensory-motor perception as shown by tests of proprioception stereognosis, 2-point tactile discrimination graphesthesia, or finger identification when touched.

   g. Poor visual-motor integrative skills assessed by geometric figure drawing, catch-a-ball test, imitation of gestures.

   h. Poor understanding and processing of auditory input (assessed informally or by having the child repeat digits).

   i. Hyperactivity.

   j. Hemiparesis.

   k. Hyperactive deep tendon refelxes, tight heel cords, ankle clonus.

   l. Poor eye tracking and poor control of tongue or oropharyngeal musculature.

   m. Nonspecific symptoms: Impulsivity, distractibility, emotional irritability, poor attention span, delayed language development.

Developmental Screening

Administer the Denver Developmental Screening Test (DDST) and/or the Developmental Screening Inventory (DSI), which examine the different areas of behavior (gross motor, fine motor, language, adaptive, and personal-social). The use of the DSI allows measurement of the development quotient (DQ):

$$DQ = (MA/CA) \times 100$$

where MA is maturity age and DA is chronological age.

Maturity age corresponds to the patient's actual performance and can be obtained for each area of behavior. The DQ can thus be obtained for each area of behavior.

The DQ in the early years of life corresponds to the intelligence quotient (IQ), which can be measured at school age.

The IQ must be used cautiously. Developmental evaluations do not attempt a direct measurement of intelligence as such, but aim at clinical estimates of intellectual potential based on analysis of maturity status.

Special Developmental Testing

1. Testing visual-motor and sensory integration and perception (these tests may be performed by an occupational therapist trained in developmental disabilities).

    a. Developmental Test of Visual-Motor Integration for children 2 to 15 years of age (Berry and Bukenica).

    b. Frostig Developmental Test of visual perception.

    c. Ayres Southern California Sensory Integration Testing with subtests for space visualization, figure ground perception, position in space, kinesthesia, manual form perception, finger identification, graphesthesia, localization of tactile stimuli, double tactile stimuli perception, crossing midline of body, bilateral motor coordination, right-left discrimination, standing balance, motor accuracy, dot-to-dot drawing.

    d. Kephart's Purdue Perceptual Motor Survey.

    These tests may be performed on any child with developmental delay, but are indicated in all children with learning problems. Any deviation from normal is significant and organic brain damage must be considered, especially if the Ayres test reveals defects in stereognosis, motor accuracy, and standing balance. Because it is possible to derive the standard deviation from the mean or age equivalents when the Beery-Buktenica, Frostig, and Ayres tests are used, the severity of the problem may be assessed as well.

    If motor dysfunction is suspected, the Milani-Comparetti test (developmental reflex testing) and muscle tone assessment should be performed. Both tests are indicators of neuromotor maturation and are particularly useful in patients with cerebral palsy.

2. Testing speech and language

    a. A complete developmental evaluation of language disorders is indicated because there are no specific tests for primary disorders.

    b. Evaluate hearing, auditory comprehension, oral formulation, and articulation.

    Within the areas of auditory comprehension, oral formulation, and articulation, evaluate phenology, semantics, syntax, and pragmatics.

    Tests should be administered by an experienced speech and language pathologist.

3. Psychological testing

    a. 2 to 5 years of age

    (1) Stanford-Binet Intelligence Scale: Examine total score and pattern of subtests. If the results reveal poor performance in all areas, the patient is mentally retarded. Organic brain damage is manifested by poor performance in some areas and good performance in other areas.

(2) Wechsler Preschool and Primary Scale of Intelligence (WIPPS): Organic brain damage is present if there are large differences between subtest scores (scatter).

b. 5 to 16 years of age

(1) Bender Visual-Motor Gestalt: Use of the developmental scoring system permits evaluation of perceptual-visual-motor problems. Use of the emotional indicators scoring system permits evaluation of emotional problems.

(2) Wechsler Intelligence Scale for Children (Revised WISC-R): Total IQ score permits evaluation of intelligence (intellectual potential). Large differences between verbal and performance scores are indicative of organic brain damage.

c. >16 years of age

(1) Bender Visual-Motor Gestalt: Use the Pascal scoring system to determine organicity.

(2) Wechsler Adult Intelligence Scale (WAIS): Consider the total scores (intellectual potential) and the differences between verbal and performance scores. Large differences are indicative of brain damage.

(3) Halstead-Reitan Neuropsychological Test Battery: A comprehensive (8-hr) test to determine severity and location of the organic brain damage.

(4) Vineland Social Maturity Scale: Used to corroborate the IQ results for mental retardation.

(5) Leiter International Performance Scale: A nonverbal test for IQ, used for ages 2 years to adulthood (18 years).

(6) Wide Range Achievement Test and Peabody Individual Achievement Test: These tests measure academic achievement rather than IQ, which reflects potential. They may be used without IQ determinations.

d. Learning problems may be evaluated through IQ tests, Bender Visual Motor Gestalt, Draw-A-Person clinical interpretation, House-Tree-Person clinical interpretation, hyperactivity index (questionnaire given to parents and teachers and has a scoring system), Vineland Social Maturity Scale, achievement tests.

e. The diagnosis of a psychopathological disorder and childhood psychosis depends on the patient's approach to the administered tests; the diagnosis is based on the following clinical observations:

(1) Impairment of interpersonal relationships (aloofness, reduced eye-to-eye contact)

(2) Deficits in the development of social behavior (self-care skills, cooperative play)

(3) Stereotyped behavior (self-stimulation, repetition)

(4) Impairment of intellect and reduced school performance

(5) Deficits in speech (mutism, echolalia, delayed development)

4. Measurement of motor activity

  a. Hyperactivity index

  b. Actometer

  c. Pedometer

  d. Stabilimetric cushion

  e. Grid-marked floor

5. Educational assessment

  a. Educational evaluation is concerned with the assessment of specific difficulties (e.g., in reading, writing, or mathematics).

  b. Achievement evaluation indicates the level of instruction in the subject.

  c. Error profiles 0 indicate the specific knowledge that the child lacks.

  d. Intelligence profiles and developmental profiles indicate the intellectual content and the manner in which the child must be instructed.

Laboratory Tests

The tests administered depend on medical history and physical examination.

1. First-stage orders

  a. Complete blood cell count; differential and peripheral smear evaluation

  b. Urinalysis

  c. Urine analysis for reducing substances, phenyl pyruvic acid, and amino acids

  d. Fasting blood glucose and 2-hr postprandial blood glucose

  e. Blood urea nitrogen

  f. Serum amino acid screen

  g. Serum calcium, phosphorous, and magnesium

  h. Serum trace metals (e.g., zinc, copper, lead)

  i. Thyroid function studies

  j. Bone age studies

  k. Skull radiographs

  l. Electroencephalogram

  m. Brain scan

  n. Chromosomal studies

2. Second-stage orders (depending on findings of aforementioned tests)

  a. Serum enzymes

  b. Antibody titers and serological tests

  c. Immunoglobulins

> *d.* Inclusion bodies
>
> *e.* Metachromasia

3. Third-stage orders (with evidence in favor of a specific diagnosis)

   a. Pneumoencephalogram and cerebrospinal fluid studies

   b. Carotid angiogram

   c. CT scan

   d. Electromyogram

   e. Muscle biopsy

   f. Brain biopsy

TREATMENT PROTOCOL

Therapy should be individualized, depending on the diagnosis and etiological factors. One or more of the following therapies may be necessary and will require the involvement of more than one professional:

1. Individual and/or family psychotherapy (counseling)

2. Behavior modification

3. Special educational placement or institutionalization

4. Educational therapy

5. Speech and language therapy

6. Occupational therapy

7. Environmental manipulation and modification

8. Pharmacological intervention using such psychotropic drugs as chlorpromazine (Thorazine®), thioridazine (Mellaril®), methylphenidate (Ritalin®), pemoline (Cylert®), or dextroamphetamine (Dexedrine®)

9. Nutritional advice and therapy

Diabetes Mellitus

Juvenile diabetes mellitus is a disorder of carbohydrate metabolism characterized by hyperglycemia and inadequate insulin production. The most serious complication is diabetic ketoacidosis (Fig. 1). The goal of therapy is to keep the patient as close as possible to the normoglycemic state, prevent episodes of hyperglycemia and ketoacidosis (and hypoglycemia from insulin overdose), and permit normal growth and development. Hyperglycemia (and hypoglycemia) may be life-threatening and must be treated vigorously.

SIGNS AND SYMPTOMS

The most striking symptoms of diabetic ketoacidosis are vomiting, hyperventilation, and dehydration. Children present with variable CNS manifestations, ranging from minimal sensorium changes to complete obtundation. In the absence of a previous diagnosis of diabetic ketoacidosis, these presenting signs and symptoms may be confused with other disease entities. Rapid differentiation is essential for the successful management of the patient. Ketoacidosis may be precipitated by infection, and symptoms related to this may also be present. Usually, a history of polyuria, polydipsia, and/or polyphagia can be elicited.

DIFFERENTIAL DIAGNOSIS

1. Reye's syndrome
2. Hypernatremic dehydration
3. Salicylate intoxication
4. Alcohol intoxication
5. CNS infection
6. Trauma
7. Gastroenteritis

DIAGNOSTIC PROTOCOL

1. Blood glucose: To detect hyperglycemia.
2. Blood ketones: To determine quantitatively the degree of ketosis.
3. Urine glucose and ketones: To determine renal clearance of glucose and to detect the presence of ketonuria.

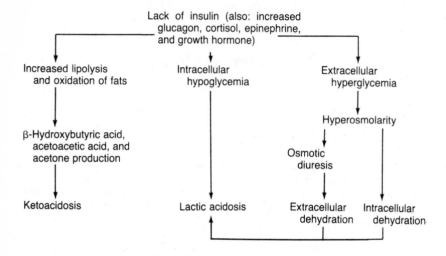

FIG. 1. Pathophysiology of diabetic ketoacidosis.

4. Diagnosis confirmed (presence of hyperglycemia and ketosis in the absence of other causes).

   a. Assess circulatory status and degree of dehydration.

   b. Electrolytes, blood urea nitrogen, and creatinine: To obtain a base-line potassium concentration, to assess the renal status of the patient, and to assess the state of hydration.

   c. Blood gases and pH: To determine the presence and severity of acidosis and to assess respiratory status.

   d. Blood lipid levels: To identify hyperlipidemia (if present, electrolyte concentration will appear factitiously low).

   e. Complete blood cell count, urinalysis, and cultures: To identify a precipitating infection.

   f. Electrocardiogram and cardiorespiratory monitoring: To assess cardiovascular status (also a good guide to the actual extracellular potassium status).

   g. Continuous monitoring of urine output: To estimate urinary fluid loss.

5. Diagnosis unconfirmed (other causes are suspected).

   a. Assess circulatory status and treat dehydration and acidosis.

   b. Electrolytes, blood urea nitrogen, and creatinine: To evaluate electrolyte balance and renal status.

   c. Blood gases and pH: To evaluate the acid/base status and respiratory status.

   d. NH_3, SGOT, SGPT: If Reye's syndrome is suspected (hypoglycemia is usually present in this syndrome).

e. Salicylate and ethanol levels: If ingestion of these substances is suspected.

f. Drug screening: If ingestion of other toxic substances is suspected.

g. Blood, urine, and stool cultures: To identify causative organism if infection is suspected.

h. Lumbar puncture: If CNS infection is suspected.

TREATMENT PROTOCOL

Diabetic Ketoacidosis

1. Correct fluid and electrolyte balance (assume fluid deficit of 10% to 15% of the total ideal body weight if acidosis is severe).

   a. Normal saline, 20 to 30 cc/kg, for the first hour (plasma or albumin should be used if the patient is in shock).

   b. Add potassium as soon as the patient urinates; use 2 to 3 mEq/kg/24 hr as a guide for administration.

   c. Normal saline 10 to 20 cc/kg, for the second hr.

   d. Half-normal saline, 10 cc/kg, for the next 6 hr.

   e. Change fluids to half-normal saline in 5% dextrose in water when blood glucose level falls to 300 mg/100 ml.

   f. Administer the remainder of the calculated 24-hr fluids over the next 16 hr.

   g. If continuous infusion of insulin is used and the patient is not ketone free when the blood glucose level reaches 250 mg/100 ml and continues to fall, increase the dextrose concentration until the patient is ketone free.

2. Treat the metabolic abnormality.

   a. Continuous insulin infusion

      (1) Regular insulin, 0.1 unit/kg i.v. bolus, then 0.1 unit/kg/hr as a continuous i.v. drip (the solution is made by placing 50 units of regular insulin in 250 cc of normal saline, resulting in 1 unit/5 cc of fluid).

      (2) The rate of fall of blood glucose should be approximately 100 mg/100 ml/hr.

      (3) Insulin infusion is continued until the blood glucose level falls below 250 mg/100 ml; it may be discontinued if the patient is acetone free; if ketonemia persists, the infusion is continued at 0.02 to 0.05 unit/kg/hr along with 2 to 4 g of glucose per unit of insulin to prevent hypoglycemia until the ketones are cleared.

      (4) Regular insulin, 0.5 to 1.0 unit s.c., is given after the infusion is discontinued and every 4 to 6 hr thereafter.

      (5) Intermediate-acting insulin may be started 48 hr later in a dose two thirds of the 24-hr regular insulin dosage.

b. Intermittent therapy

(1) Regular insulin, 1.0 to 2.0 units/kg, as i.v. bolus, then 1.0 unit/kg s.c. every 1 to 2 hr.

(2) When the blood glucose reaches 300 mg/100 ml and ketonemia is decreasing, a sliding scale may be used:
   3 + to 4 + and no acetone, add 2 to 4 units/ +
   3 + to 4 + and acetone, add 4 to 5 units/ +

(3) After stabilization, intermediate-acting insulin may be substituted at two thirds of the 24-hr regular insulin dose.

Bicarbonate administration only if pH is <7.15, regardless of regimen.

Appropriate treatment of precipitating infections is essential in either regimen.

Education and dietary management is the basis of long-term therapy.

Diarrhea

Diarrhea is an extremely common condition among children. It is most often nonspecific, self-limited, and benign, requiring only simple supportive care. Usually, diarrhea can be evaluated and treated on an outpatient basis. Simple viral infections, dietary intolerances (indiscretions), and transient enzyme deficiencies (secondary to infections) are the most common causes.

Diarrhea may be a symptom related directly to the gastrointestinal tract, or, in the younger patient, it may be a symptom of systemic disease (Fig. 1). In general, the younger the patient, the more significant the diarrhea becomes. Resultant dehydration and/or malnutrition pose serious immediate dangers. Dehydration and septicemia are the most significant complications of infectious diarrhea. Nutritional disorders, metabolic disorders, and failure to thrive may result from diarrhea as symptoms of a more significant systemic disease process, and other symptomatology may occur concurrently (Fig. 2).

DIFFERENTIAL DIAGNOSIS

Acute Diarrhea

Infectious

1. Systemic disease

    a. Septicemia

    b. Urinary tract infection

    c. Otitis media

2. Gastrointestinal

    a. Viral

    b. Bacterial

    c. Parasitic

Noninfectious or Questionably Infectious

1. Dietary

2. Hemolytic uremic syndrome

3. Inflammatory disease

    a. Ulcerative colitis

    b. Crohn's disease

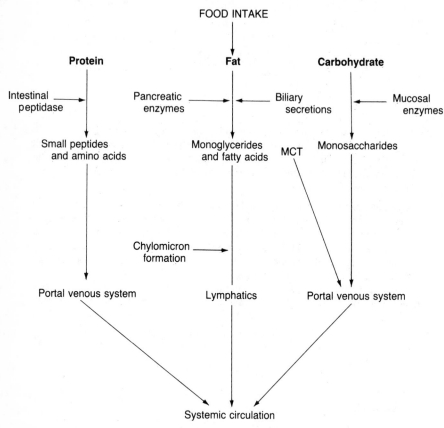

FIG. 1. The pathophysiology of diarrhea may involve abnormalities of single or multiple phases of digestion. MCT, medium chain triglycerides.

Chronic Diarrhea

Gastrointestinal

1. Viral
2. Bacterial
3. Parasitic

Inflammatory Disease

1. Ulcerative colitis
2. Crohn's disease

Chronic Nonspecific Diarrhea

1. Idiopathic

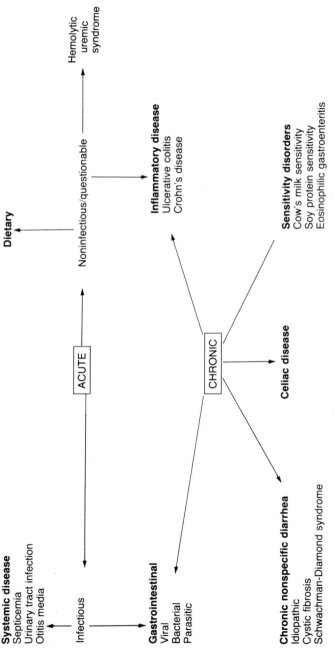

FIG. 2. Differential diagnoses of diarrhea.

Systemic disease
Septicemia
Urinary tract infection
Otitis media

Infectious

Gastrointestinal
Viral
Bacterial
Parasitic

ACUTE

Noninfectious/questionable

Dietary

Hemolytic uremic syndrome

Inflammatory disease
Ulcerative colitis
Crohn's disease

CHRONIC

Chronic nonspecific diarrhea
Idiopathic
Cystic fibrosis
Schwachman-Diamond syndrome

Celiac disease

Sensitivity disorders
Cow's milk sensitivity
Soy protein sensitivity
Eosinophilic gastroenteritis

2. Cystic fibrosis

3. Schwachman-Diamond syndrome

Celiac Disease

Sensitivity Disorders

1. Cow's milk sensitivity

2. Soy protein sensitivity

3. Eosinophilic gastroenteritis

DIAGNOSTIC AND TREATMENT PROTOCOLS

Table 1 gives diagnostic and treatment protocols for various types of diarrhea.

TABLE 1. *Diarrhea: Diagnostic and treatment protocols*

Diagnosis	Treatment
Antibiotic-Induced	
Most often occurs with lincomycin or clindamycin, but has also been reported with tetracycline, chloramphenicol, and ampicillin Diagnosis is made on clinical grounds with the appearance of explosive bloody diarrhea, abdominal distension, abdominal pain, and toxicity 3 days to 1 week after initiation of antibiotic therapy Syndrome may resemble chronic ulcerative colitis or shigellosis **Note: Although ampicillin-induced colitis is rare, diarrhea occurs in approximately 20% of children receiving the drug**	Treatment is supportive and symptomatic Discontinue the offending antibiotic Vancomycin, 50 mg/kg/day p.o. in six divided doses for 7 days Sulfasalazine, cholestyramine, and corticosteroid enemas have been suggested
Bacteria-Induced: Campylobacter	
Septicemia presentation: Fever, malaise, cephalgia, weight loss, abdominal pain, and CNS symptoms may be present; patient usually appears to be ill Enteritis presentation: Blood-streaked diarrhea and abdominal pain are typical; vomiting occasionally occurs; dehydration is rare Diagnosis is made by isolation of the organism in the stool	Septicemia: Chloramphenicol, aminoglycosides, or tetracycline are recommended Enteritis: Symptomatic and supportive treatment (erythromycin is suggested as being potentially effective, but indication for antibiotics is still undefined; drugs may not improve the clinical course)
Bacteria-Induced: Salmonella	
The stool is occasionally bloody and mucoid Stool evaluation: Sheets of white blood cells are frequently found in the stool; guaiac test is frequently positive; culture and sensitivity tests are positive for the organism	If the patient is not systemically ill, only symptomatic and supportive treatment is indicated Antibiotics may prolong excretion time of the organism If the patient is systemically ill or the

Diagnosis	Treatment

diarrhea is intractable, antibiotic therapy is indicated

Ampicillin, 200 mg/kg/day i.v. in four divided doses *or* chloramphenicol, 100 mg/kg/day i.v. in four divided doses

Treat associated dehydration and/or electrolyte abnormalities

Bacteria-Induced: Shigella

The stool is usually bloody and mucoid

Seizures are not uncommon

Stool evaluation: Sheets of white blood cells are frequently found in the stool; guaiac test is frequently positive; culture and sensitivity tests are diagnostic

Ampicillin, 50 to 100 mg/kg/day i.v. in four divided doses

Treat associated dehydration and electrolyte abnormalities

If seizures occur, appropriate evaluation and treatment for febrile seizures are indicated

Bacteria-Induced: Yersinia

Clinical features: Fever, nonbloody diarrhea, erythematous rash, psuedoappendicitis, Reiter's-like syndrome

Diagnosis is made by isolation of the organism in the stool

Trimethoprim, 6 to 12 mg/kg p.o., **and** sulfamethoxazole, 30 to 60 mg/kg/day p.o., every 12 hr for 5 days

Alternative drugs: Chloramphenicol, 50 to 100 mg/kg/day i.v., **or** kanamycin, 15 mg/kg/day i.v., **or** tetracycline, 10 to 20 mg/kg/day i.v., 25 to 50 mg/kg/day p.o.

Celiac Disease

There is usually a history of bulky, foul-smelling stools that may be associated with abdominal pain and distension

Patient is irritable and usually fails to thrive; muscle wasting of the gluteal and prescapular muscles is seen; clubbing of the fingers and abdominal distension are also common findings

D-Xylose absorption test: D-Xylose level <20 mg/100 ml at 1 hr after the loading dose is diagnostic of mucosal malabsorption

Sweat test: To rule out cystic fibrosis

Jejunal biopsy reveals absent villi

Complete blood cell count, urinalysis, stool culture, and stool examination for ova and parasites

A gluten-free diet yields clinical improvement; gluten challenge causes exacerbation of the symptoms

Gliadin antibodies (experimental in U.S.)

A gluten-free diet is required

A secondary lactase deficiency is common and a lactose-free formula should be prescribed for the first months of treatment

Multivitamin supplement should be provided

A gluten challenge is required for confirmation of the diagnosis

A gluten-free diet should be maintained for life

Chronic, Nonspecific

Diagnosis is made by medical history and physical examination; a pattern of the dysfunctional family usually emerges and stress is common; there are usually multiple efforts at dietary manipulation; physical examination shows no abnormalities, and failure to thrive and malnutrition are absent

Upper and lower gastrointestinal series and small bowel radiographs are occasionally indicated to rule out other abnormalities

Reassurance and psychosocial intervention are mandatory

Hospitalization is sometimes required if outpatient management fails and the diarrhea is intractable

TABLE 1. continued

Diagnosis	Treatment

Cow's Milk Sensitivity

Diagnosis is usually made on clinical grounds; frequently a history of irritability, colicky abdominal pain, and failure to thrive; occasionally a history of edema; with systemic reactions (anaphylaxis), wheezing may occur; age at onset of symptoms is usually 6 months

Complete blood cell count reveals a hypochromic microcytic anemia

Serum iron and iron binding capacity

Total protein and albumin

IgE level is usually normal (except in patients with anaphylactic reactions)

Radio allergo sorbant test (RAST) is usually normal (except in patients with anaphylactic reactions)

Endoscopy with biopsy may be indicated

Stool evaluation: Positive for blood

Milk should be totally avoided until the patient reaches the age of 2 years

Milk may be reintroduced for a challenge to confirm the diagnosis (this should be performed before the patient reaches 2 years of age and should not be done on patients exhibiting anaphylactic-like reactions to milk)

Multivitamin and iron supplements should be provided

Crohn's Disease

Diarrhea may be intermittent and associated with other systemic signs and symptoms

See Crohn's Disease chapter

Cystic Fibrosis

The stools are usually bulky and foul smelling (steatorrhea)

Sweat test is diagnostic

See Cystic Fibrosis chapter

Extraintestinal Infections

Diarrhea may occur as a nonspecific manifestation of an extraintestinal infection, especially if the child is younger than 2 years of age

Dehydration and electrolyte abnormalities may occur and be the predominant presenting symptoms

Common infections: Septicemia, urinary tract infections, otitis media; loose stools are not uncommonly associated with illnesses causing profuse rhinorrhea

Diagnosis is usually based on clinical grounds and high index of suspicion; laboratory examinations are guided by the presence of concomitant signs and symptoms

The extraintestinal infection should be appropriately treated

Dehydration, acid-based abnormalities, and electrolyte abnormalities should be appropriately treated

Hemolytic Uremic Syndrome

Diagnosis is made by presence of the clinical triad of hemolytic anemia, thrombocytopenia, and acute renal failure

Onset of the syndrome is usually preceeded by diarrhea, which may be bloody

Diagnosis	Treatment

Lactose Intolerance: Primary

Diagnosis is suggested by the medical history and physical examination, which reveals recurrent abdominal pain and/or watery diarrhea; family history may be positive for similar conditions; the most common ages are 3 years (blacks) to 5 years (whites). Physical examination usually shows no abnormalities
Stool culture: Negative
Stool for ova and parasites: Negative
Reducing substances: Positive
Lactose tolerance test and lactose breath test are occasionally indicated for an accurate diagnosis

Remove lactose from the diet
Multivitamins and calcium supplement should be provided
Lact-Aid® may be beneficial for some patients

Lactose Intolerance: Secondary

Transient lactase deficiency may occur after gastroenteritis from many causes (e.g., viral, bacterial) and other entities that disrupt the intestinal villi
Prompt resolution with removal of lactose from the diet
Usually occurs in infants and children <3 years old

Remove lactose from the diet
Since the deficiency is transient, lactose may be reintroduced to the diet after 3 to 6 weeks; symptoms do not recur

Parasite-Induced: *Endamoeba histolytica*

Stools are usually loose and watery, and may contain blood
Stool evaluation: Guaiac test is usually positive; culture is negative for bacteria; ova and parasite examination may be positive for the organism

Metronidazole, 7 to 10 mg/kg/day in three divided doses for 10 days
Treat associated dehydration or electrolyte abnormalities

Parasite-Induced: *Giardia lamblia*

Stools are loose and watery; blood is usually absent
Stool evaluation: Guaiac test is usually negative; culture for bacteria is negative, ova and parasite examination may be positive for the organism
Duodenal aspirates may be positive for trophozoites

Supportive and symptomatic care should be provided
Quinacrin, 2 to 3 mg/kg/day in three divided doses, **or** metronidazole, 3 to 5 mg/kg/day in three divided doses for 7 days. **(Metronidazole is not recomended by the FDA for the treatment of intestinal giardiasis)**
Treat associated dehydration or electrolyte abnormalities

Soy Protein Intolerance

Diagnosis is usually based on clinical grounds and is similar to cow's milk sensitivity
Occurs in approximately 10% of patients with milk intolerance
Complete blood cell count shows hypochromic, microcytic anemia
Total protein and albumin
IgE and RAST are negative
Biopsy, sigmoidoscopy, and soy challenge

Remove soy protein from the diet
Provide multivitamin and iron supplements

TABLE 1. *(continued)*

Diagnosis	Treatment

Ulcerative Colitis

Diagnosis	Treatment
Diarrhea is usually mucoid and bloody; it may be associated with abdominal pain or other systemic symptoms	See Ulcerative Colitis chapter

Viral Gastroenteritis

Diagnosis	Treatment
Diagnosis is usually made on clinical grounds; frequent and/or loose watery stools; patient does not appear to be ill	Bowel rest through dietary modification (e.g., clear liquid diet)
The stool may or may not contain mucus and usually does not contain blood or significant leukocytes	If the diarrhea is severe and dehydration is imminent or present, hospitalization is indicated; allow nothing by mouth and administer intravenous fluids
No specific diagnostic tests are required	Treat associated dehydration and electrolyte imbalances

APPENDIX 1. *Testing for malabsorption*

Test	Indications	Procedure	Interpretation
D-Xylose absorption test	To detect mucosal absorption abnormalities	Patient should fast for at least 6 hr before testing Orally administer 500 mg of xylose/lb body weight (maximun dose, 25 g); total bolus should be ingested within 5 min to insure accuracy of timing Draw blood at 30, 60, 90, and 120 min after dose is given	Normal: >20 mg/100ml 60 min after dose Low absorption of xylose: Diseases causing malabsorption, overgrowth of bacteria in small intestine, parasitic infection (especially *G. lamblia*), and viral gastroenteritis
Duodenal aspiration	To recover *Giardia lamblia* trophozoites; usually done in conjunction with a peroral jejunal biopsy	Insert a nasogastric tube past the pylorus into the duodenum and aspirate fluid. Send fluid to laboratory for microscopic evaluation; concomitantly obtain bacteria cultures	Normal: No parasites
Fat excretion test (72-hr)	To detect fat malabsorption (steatorrhea); best indicator of a malabsorption defect	Orally administer a charcoal marker, then again 72 hr later; discard the first marker when it appears in the stool; save all stool specimens thereafter, including the second marker when it appears Send the 72 hr stool sample to the laboratory for evaluation of fat Amount of fat in patient's diet must be consistent (100 g/day is usually required)	In children <1 yr old, amount of fat in stool should be <15% of the intake In children >1 yr old, amount of fat should be <5% of the intake
Jejunal biopsy	To detect mucosal disease	Allow nothing by mouth 6 hr before procedure Sedate patient with chlorpromazine (1 mg/kg) and pentobarbital (4 mg/kg for children 6 months to 6 years of age) approximately 30 min before procedure Biopsy capsule is passed by mouth into the jejunum, and guided by fluroscopy to obtain specimen Send specimen to the laboratory for tissue evaluation and biochemical studies (lactase, sucrase, maltase)	Normal: Normal tissue sample and normal biochemical findings Flat or absent villi suggest the cause of the malabsorption state

APPENDIX 1. (continued)

Test	Indications	Procedure	Interpretation
Stool cultures	To detect enteropathogenic bacteria in the stool. Culture must be done on a fresh specimen		
Stool guaiac	To detect occult blood in the stool		
Stool for ova and parasites	To detect ova and/or parasites in the stool; evaluation must be done on a fresh specimen		
Stool pH	Used as a screening test for malabsorption		Normal: pH 4.4 to 8.0 High meat diet will cause stool to be alkaline A large amount of fat in the stool yields an acid pH
Stool reducing substances	To detect carbohydrate intolerance		Reducing substances in the stool suggest disaccharidase deficiency
Stool white blood cells	To screen for invasive infections	Stool is stained with Wright's stain	Neurophils in the stool suggest bacterial inflammation or colitis
Sweat test	To evaluate for cystic fibrosis	Pilocarpine iontophoresis is performed to stimulate sweating Collect sweat on a preweighed gauze or filter paper Do not touch gauze or filter paper on which sweat is collected, since the volume of sweat must be accurately weighed; sweat from fingertips during handling can invalidate the results; handle filter paper or gauze with tweezers or forceps 100 mg of sweat is required to insure accuracy Evaluate sample for sodium concentration	Normal: <45 mEq/L Equivocal: 45 to 60 mEq/L (further investigation is required) Abnormal: >60 mEq/L (diagnostic of cystic fibrosis)

APPENDIX 2. *Gastrointestinal function tests*

Test	Reason for test	Preparation	Performance	Interpretation
Disaccharide absorption tests Lactose (galactose + glucose) Sucrose (fructose + glucose) Maltose (glucose + glucose)	Malabsorbtion of sugars	Fasting for 4 to 6 hrs	Sucrose, 2.0 g/kg, **or** lactose, 2.0 g/kg, **or** maltose, 1.0 g/kg Measure blood glucose level at 0, 30, 60, 90, and 120 min after dose **Do not do disaccharide tolerance tests on successive days on the same patient** **Do not repeat test that yields abnormal results in patients who become symptomic while the test is being done**	An increase in blood glucose of <20 mg/100 ml suggests disaccharide malabsorption
Fecal fat	Fat malabsorption	Fixed long-chain fat diet for 3 days before test Assure intake of >25 g/day in infants, >50 g/day in 2 to 5 year olds, and >100 g/day in >5 year olds	Keep record of all intake Give activated charcoal marker p.o. at time zero Give fat diet for 72 hr Give second charcoal marker 72 hr after the first marker When the first marker appears in the stool, discard it, and then collect all subsequent stools, including the second marker	Coefficient of absorption of fat = $\dfrac{\text{g fat ingested} - \text{g fat excreted}}{\text{g fat ingested}} \times 100$ 6 months to 1 year: >87% (≤4.3 g/day) 1 to 2 years: >93% (≤3.1 g/day) >2 years: >95% (≤5.0 g/day)
pH (stool)	Sugar malabsorption	None	Dilute one part stool with one part distilled water Test supernatant with litmus paper	pH <5.0 indicates the possibility of excess sugar in the stool
Reducing substances (stool)	Sugar malabsorption	None	Dilute one part stool with one part distilled water (use 1 N HCl if sucrose malabsorption is considered; sucrose is not a reducing sugar) Place Clinitest® tablet in a clean test tube and add 15 drops of stool solution	Compare the color of the solution to the Clinitest® chart for urine interpretation Normal: 0.25% Questionable: 0.25% to 0.50% Abnormal: >0.50%

APPENDIX 2. (continued)

Test	Reason for test	Preparation	Performance	Interpretation
D-Xylose absorption test	Absorptional integrity of the duodeno-jejunal mucosa (the test is abnormal in celiac disease, idiopathic steatorrhea, Crohn's disease of the upper small bowel, starvation, short bowel syndrome, and blind loop syndrome)	8-hr fast (4 to 5 hr for young children)	5% D-Xylose, 0.5 g/kg p.o. (may be given via nasogastric tube or instilled directly into the duodenum) Serum xylose is measured at 0, 30, 60, 90, and 120 min after dose Urine xylose may be measured, but is less reliable than serum values	Serum xylose level >25 mg/100 ml at any time is normal If serum xylose level is <20 mg/100 ml, a small bowel biopsy is indicated

Drowning and Near-Drowning

Drowning is the second leading cause of unintentional traumatic death in children younger than 15 years of age. More than 8,000 water-related fatalities occur each year. Approximately 2,700 of the fatal drownings involve children, with more than 200 drownings in backyard swimming pools. Other bodies of water involved are rivers, creeks, lakes, oceans, bathtubs, pails, and puddles. No volume of water should be considered childsafe.

The most important aspect of drowning accidents, as with all unintentional trauma or injury, is their prevention. A respect for water should be taught to both parents and children; this education should begin with the mother prenatally and continue after the birth of the baby.

Adequate and constant adult supervision is the sine qua non of drowning prevention. Epidemiological reports verify the fact that drownings rarely, if ever, occur when adequate supervision is present. **Parents should never leave a child unattended in a bathtub, even for the short time it takes to answer the doorbell or telephone.** Enough water can be aspirated in the first few moments of an immersion incident for death to occur. Backyard swimming pools should be securely obstructed to access by infants and toddlers. Life jackets should be provided for all boat passengers, and nonswimmers should wear them constantly. Swimming areas in lakes, rivers, and streams should be supervised and their access obstructed when supervision is not available. Quarrys and excavations should be obstructed with physical or natural barriers. Warning signs do not provide sufficient deterrent to the curious child.

No infant or child should be considered water safe. Early swimming instruction and water survival training are available, but not enough data are yet available on their efficacy in decreasing drowning accidents (most efficacy data are anecdotal). It is also not known if short-term or long-term psychological complications arise from swimming instruction that begins too early (most classes are accompanied by much screaming and resistance). In general, children are ready to learn to swim when they are old enough to hold their breath on command.

PROGNOSIS

Water temperature plays a major role in the prognosis of drowning or near-drowning. Warm water ($>20°C$) immersion injury carries a significantly poorer prognosis than injury from cold water immersion. Coma and fixed dilated pupils accurately predict death or permanent brain damage (Fig. 1). Submersion or immersion in cold water involves different physiological processes and the prognosis is good when adequate cardiopulmonary resuscitation and rewarming techniques are provided. Cold water

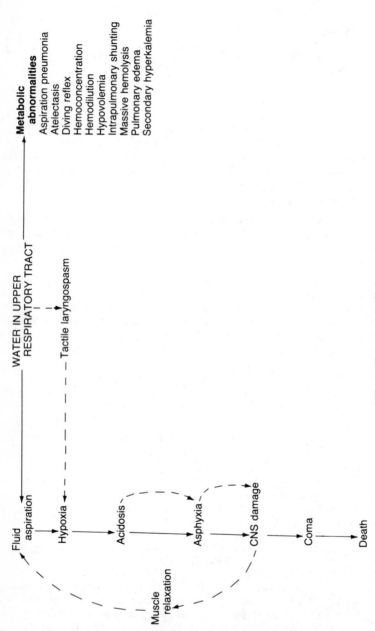

FIG. 1. Pathophysiology of drowning.

near-drowning patients may initially appear clinically dead, but they frequently respond well to therapeutic intervention. Therefore, resuscitative efforts should be vigorous, regardless of the presenting clinical condition.

Metabolic abnormalities are variable; patients should be evaluated and treated according to their individual presentation, regardless of whether the insult was caused by salt water or fresh water.

DIAGNOSTIC PROTOCOL

1. Evaluate the patient for other associated injuries that may have occurred (e.g., head trauma, cervical spine injuries).

2. Blood gases: Po_2, Pco_2, pH.

3. Serum electrolytes: Sodium, potassium, chloride.

4. Blood urea nitrogen and creatinine.

5. Serum calcium.

6. Blood glucose.

7. Complete blood cell count.

8. Chest radiograph: Infiltrates may or may not be present on the initial film.

9. Electrocardiogram.

10. Culture and sensitivity tests of tracheal secretions.

11. Urinalysis (accurately monitor urine output and specific gravity).

12. Repeat the above tests at appropriate intervals as dictated by the patient's condition.

TREATMENT PROTOCOL

Immediate Treatment at the Scene

1. Resuscitation should be attempted regardless of the immediate condition of the patient (especially in cold water immersions).

2. Establish and maintain an adequate airway, assist ventilation, and perform external cardiac massage, if necessary (see Resuscitation chapter for a complete discussion of cardiopulmonary resuscitation).

3. If significant laryngospasm is present, tracheotomy may be required to establish an airway.

4. Water should be drained from the lungs only if it does not interrupt or delay other resuscitative efforts.

5. Provide 100% oxygen, if available.

6. All patients with immersion injuries should be hospitalized regardless of their condition at the scene.

7. Summon transportation.

Hospital Treatment

1. The airway should be maintained, 100% oxygen given, cardiopulmonary resuscitation continued, and an intravenous line established.

2. Give sodium bicarbonate, 1 to 2 mEq/kg i.v.

3. The sine qua non of the treatment of immersion injuries is intensive respiratory care: Mechanical ventilation may be required if respiratory failure is present or imminent; positive end expiratory pressure (PEEP) may be required to insure adequate oxygenation and/or to treat pulmonary edema.

4. If bronchospasm is present, theophylline preparations may be required.

5. Treatment is supportive and symptomatic; plasma colloid may be required to treat hypovolemia, or whole blood may be required if massive hemolysis is present; the treatment is independent of the type of water causing the injury and individual symptoms should be treated as they occur. CNS resuscitation and preservation of adequate CNS function are essential.

6. Antibiotics may be required if infection occurs; fever commonly occurs in drowning victims in the absence of infection and is not an indication for antibiotic therapy.

Encephalitis

Encephalitis is inflammation of the brain. Its causes vary from direct infection of CNS tissues to inflammation secondary to various antigenic stimulations (Fig. 1). The encephalitides are frustrating entities for the practitioner. In most cases, whether or not the diagnosis is established, the treatment is, at best, supportive and symptomatic. Antiviral agents are recommended for use only in documented herpes encephalitis.

SIGNS AND SYMPTOMS

Symptoms of encephalitis vary from mild, nonspecific findings, such as fever and headache, to severe manifestations, such as seizures and coma. Other symptoms consistent with encephalitis are disorientation, somnolence, nausea, vomiting, behavioral changes, inappropriate change in moods, ataxia, dysarthria, meningismus, peripheral neuropathy, papilledema, and weakness.

The patient's medical history may reveal a concurrent infection (e.g., rubeola, mumps), a past infection (e.g., varicella), or a recent immunization, especially with a killed vaccine. The clinical diagnosis of encephalitis is difficult in most cases. Spinal fluid examination is often confusing and of no help. Pleocytosis may or may not be present. The antigen is not frequently recovered from the spinal fluid, especially in patients with postinfectious or noninfectious etiologies.

DIFFERENTIAL DIAGNOSIS

1. Bacterial meningitis
2. Toxic encephalopathy (e.g., lead poisoning)
3. Metabolic encephalopathy (e.g., Reye's syndrome)
4. Space-occupying intracranial lesions
    a. Malignant neoplasms (primary or metastatic)
    b. Expanding arteriovenous malformations
    c. Intracranial abscess
5. Cerebrovascular accident
6. Drug abuse
7. Psychiatric illness (acute schizophrenia)

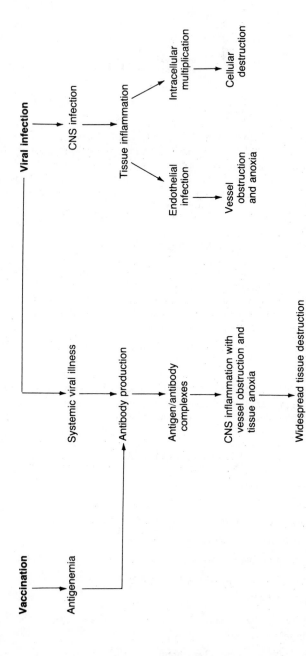

FIG. 1. Pathophysiology of encephalitis.

ETIOLOGICAL DIAGNOSIS

1. Vaccinal
   a. Pertussis
   b. Oral polio vaccine
   c. Influenza vaccine
   d. Rabies vaccine
   e. Yellow fever vaccine
2. Infectious and/or postinfectious
   a. Herpes simplex I
   b. Enterovirus
   c. Rabies virus
   d. Arbovirus
   e. Rubeola
   f. Rubella
   g. Mumps
   h. Varicella
   i. Epstein-Barr virus
   j. Cytomegalovirus
   k. Adenovirus
   l. Herpes zoster
   m. Rickettsia
   n. Spirochete
   o. Protozoan

DIAGNOSTIC PROTOCOL

1. Obtain the medical history and perform a complete physical examination.
2. Complete blood cell count.
3. Urinalysis and urine culture for bacteria.
4. Blood cultures for bacteria.
5. Counterimmunoelectrophoresis on urine.
6. Viral cultures: Blood, urine, cerebrospinal fluid (CSF), stool, throat, nasopharynx.
7. CT scan if increased intracranial pressure or a space-occupying lesion is suspected.
8. CSF examinations: Cell count, glucose and protein levels, viral titers and cultures, counterimmunoelectrophoresis and *Limulus* lysate testing, bacterial cultures, Gram stain.
9. Blood lead level.
10. Toxin screening: If toxic encephalopathy is suspected.
11. SGOT, SGPT, and ammonia levels: If Reye's syndrome is suspected.
12. Electrolytes, blood urea nitrogen, creatinine, glucose, and calcium.
13. Urinary sodium excretion, urine osmolality, and blood osmolality: If inappropriate secretion of antidiuretic hormone is suspected.
14. Cerebral arteriography may be indicated if intracranial bleeding or an arteriovenous malformation is suspected.

15. A brain biopsy and culture are occasionally indicated in patients with suspected herpetic encephalitis.

16. Corneal scrapings may be indicated if rabies is suspected.

TREATMENT PROTOCOL

1. The treatment for encephalitis is supportive and symptomatic care.

2. Assure stability of the patient's vital signs and monitor the patient's condition for deterioration.

3. Neurological signs should be monitored closely, watching for signs of increased intracranial pressure.

4. Intracranial pressure should be monitored closely and significant elevations should be treated vigorously with dexamethasone and/or mannitol.

5. Hypothermia may be indicated to decrease cerebral edema and metabolic rate of the cells; shivering may be suppressed with chlorpromazine (0.25–0.50 mg/kg).

6. An intravenous line should be established, but fluids should be administered carefully so as not to exacerbate cerebral edema and elevated intracranial pressure.

7. The patient should be monitored for the inappropriate secretion of antidiuretic hormone; treat appropriately and restrict fluids.

8. Seizures may be controlled with phenobarbital, 5 mg/kg/day; a loading dose of up to 15 mg/kg may be required to rapidly reach a therapeutic blood level.

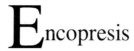
Encopresis

Encopresis is a nonspecific symptom characterized by withholding stool and fecal soiling. The stool retention often begins as early as infancy. It is more serious than enuresis and occurs most commonly in boys.

PATHOPHYSIOLOGY

Encopresis manifests in different children for different reasons. Generally, affected children fall into two groups:

Developmental Failure

Inadequate neuromaturational development and failure to develop conditioned control of the external anal sphincter. Soiling continues from infancy, often accompanied by diarrhea.

Psychogenic

As a symptom of regressive behavior or conversion reaction (dominating mother with compulsive attitudes toward cleanliness and bowel training, passive father, soiling occurs not at school but on the way home) or as a symptom of a personality disorder (parents usually have some personality disturbances, they may have, but often have not, attempted bowel training, child has incipient or frank psychosis).

SIGNS AND SYMPTOMS

Encopresis is most often associated with severe organic developmental disorders or severe psychopathology (Fig. 1). Signs and symptoms of the primary process, infrequent stools and fecal soiling, may be present. The soiling may occur at any time during the day or night. Because the stool is commonly withheld for long periods of time (8–10 days) abdominal distention may occur.

DIFFERENTIAL DIAGNOSIS

1. Neuromaturational (sphincteric control) disturbances.

2. Psychogenic constipation with encopresis, characterized by frequent and irregular involuntary seepage of stools rather than by fecal withholding, may be treated by removing the fecal impaction (manually or by enema), administering mineral oil in orange juice (5–60 ml twice daily) to lead to incontinence, and toilet

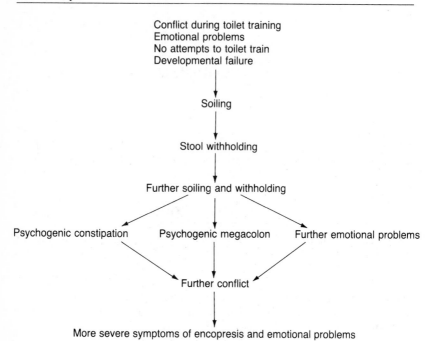

FIG. 1. Encopresis as a symptom of a personality disorder.

retraining of the child while continuing to administer mineral oil in reduced doses. Stool softeners such as docusate sodium (Colace®) may be helpful later, but only after adequate toilet training has been achieved.

3. Aganglionic megacolon.

DIAGNOSTIC PROTOCOL

1. A complete medical history is the most important diagnostic tool in encopresis. The onset of symptoms, toilet training methods and conflicts, current bowel habits, family dynamics profile, and child's personality profile must be documented.

2. The physical examination is usually unremarkable. A relaxed incontinent sphincter, fecal impaction, and empty rectum (signifying aganglionic megacolon) should be searched for.

3. Special procedures: Complete blood cell count to rule out nutritional anemia, urinalysis, evaluation of sphincteric tone, barium enema.

4. A complete psychological evaluation is essential, including family evaluation by a psychologist and an evaluation of the child (personality tests such as the Sentence Completion Test, VMI, or MMPI should be administered). Projective testing should be attempted. Evaluation of the family and the child's social and academic environment by a social worker might be helpful in revealing the foci of stress.

TREATMENT PROTOCOL

1. **Explain** the situation to the family (the most important aspect of therapy).

    a. Resolve the parents' disgust.

    b. Diffuse the parents' anger.

    c. Support parents in not overpressuring or neglecting the symptom.

    d. Obtain adequate psychological or psychiatric support for the child and family.

2. Relief of fecal impaction by manual removal or enema.

3. Immediate therapy

    a. Start toilet training.

    b. Diet plan.

    c. Start the child on mineral oil with orange juice, 5 to 60 ml/day (use judiciously and only if necessary because treatment may be perceived as punitive).

    d. Start psychotherapy.

4. Long-term treatment

    a. Continue psychotherapy as necessary.

    b. Stool softener (Colace®), 5 to 10 mg/kg/24 hr, may be used, but not as a substitute for toilet training.

Enuresis

Enuresis is one of the most common as well as one of the most frustrating disorders of childhood. It is most accurately defined as the involuntary discharge of urine. There are multiple etiologies, both functional and organic. Enuresis is divided into nocturnal enuresis (involuntary discharge of urine during sleep) and diurnal enuresis (involuntary daytime wetting). Enuresis is also classified as primary (children who have never had a significant dry period even though beyond the chronological point in development where most children are no longer wetting) or secondary (children older than 4 or 5 years of age who have had a reasonable dry period, i.e., $\geq$6 months, and have reverted to wetting at least once a week).

The incidence of enuresis is probably factitiously low because many parents are embarrassed and hesitate to admit that their child still wets the bed. Nonetheless, with reporting bias considered, boys predominate at almost all ages, and there appear to be more frequent occurrences among families of lower socioeconomic and educational levels, as well as in institutionalized children.

SIGNS AND SYMPTOMS

In essential enuresis (without an organic basis), the only signs and symptoms may be those of embarrassment and distress on the part of the child and the parents. Quite often, by the time the family seeks help, the intrafamilial dynamics may be causing more difficulty than the enuresis. In evaluating the child for therapy, it is essential to recognize that there is a significant spontaneous cure rate, which has been used in support of the developmental delay theory. In essential enuretics who are treated with tincture of time, 85% of boys and 89% of girls are dry at night by the age of 4½, and 92% of boys and 97% of girls are dry at night by the age of 7 years. The vast majority of children with enuresis will be essential enuretics, with no obvious physical or psychological abnormality, but the basic, noninvasive investigations are indicated to confirm the diagnosis (Fig. 1).

DIFFERENTIAL DIAGNOSIS

1. Neurogenic incontinence (e.g., myelodysplasia)
2. Primary structural incontinence
   a. Exstrophy or epispadius
   b. Ectopic ureter or ureterocele

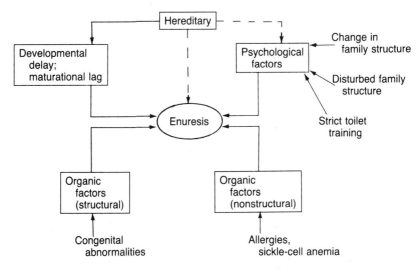

FIG. 1.   Pathophysiology of enuresis.

- *c.* Paradoxical (overflow)
- *d.* Fistula
- *e.* Complex ureteral duplication
3. Secondary structural incontinence
    - *a.* Traumatic
    - *b.* Vaginal reflux
4. Nonstructural incontinence
    - *a.* Uncontrollable detrusor muscle contraction (irritative incontinence) e.g., cystitis, allergy, direct vesical stimulation from foreign body)
    - *b.* "Giggle incontinence"
    - *c.* Occult neurogenic bladder (detrusor-sphincter dyssynergia)
5. Essential enuresis
    - *a.* Primary versus secondary
    - *b.* Nocturnal versus diurnal

DIAGNOSTIC PROTOCOL

Medical History

1. Time of wetting (day, night)
2. Frequency, onset (primary versus secondary)

3. Recent changes or stresses

4. Presence of encopresis

5. Adequacy of the urinary stream, other symptoms referable to the urinary tract (e.g., dysuria, polyuria, frequency, urgency)

6. Birth history

7. Developmental milestones

8. Family history of enuresis, parenting practices (e.g., toilet training)

Physical Examination

1. Growth chart (growth failure may represent renal disease, recurrent urinary tract infection)

2. Hypertension

3. Abdominal masses, palpable bladder or kidneys

4. Neurological examination, especially of lower extremities (gait, strength, reflexes), perineal sensation, anal sphincter tone

5. Careful inspection and palpation of sacral vertebrae

6. Evaluation of the genitalia (e.g., deformities, dripping of urine, type of urine stream)

Laboratory Investigations

Tests depend on medical history and physical examination.

1. Urinalysis

    a. An important procedure; should be performed by an experienced technologist or the physician.

    b. First voided morning urine specimen should be refrigerated until brought for evaluation to minimize possibility of bacterial contamination or breakdown of urine sediment.

    c. Examine urine for unusual constituents, such as particles that might impart an osmotic diuresis (e.g., glucose), significant protein, specific gravity; examine microscopically for red and white blood cell elements or cylindruria; seek evidence of diabetes, urinary tract infection, psychogenic water drinking, glomerulonephritis.

2. Urine culture is indicated in the majority of cases of enuresis, especially in younger children, even if there is no suggestion of infection or anatomical abnormality of the urinary tract; silent, underlying renal disease.

3. Electrolytes and renal function tests (blood urea nitrogen and creatinine) are indicated when findings include any suggestion of growth failure, anatomical abnormalities, family history of genitourinary abnormalities and/or renal disease, inability to concentrate the urine, and mild anemia, or fatigue.

4. Complete blood cell count and eosinophil count (renal compromise or other chronic illness may cause anemia, and various allergic diatheses may cause enuresis).

Radiographic Evaluation

1. The use of radiographic tests in enuretic children without suspected anatomical abnormalities or organic disease is debatable. In findings from several large centers, virtually no radiographic abnormalities were found in children with essential enuresis (as determined by medical history, physical examination, and urinalysis), even with the use of voiding cystourethrograms.

2. In older children with primary or diurnal enuresis, an intravenous pyelogram (IVP), a voiding cystourethrogram (VCU), and urological consultation are indicated.

3. Suspected anatomical defects or other pathological involvement are definite indications for radiographic evaluation.

4. Urological consultation is essential if radiographic studies are nondiagnostic and there is continuing suspicion of structural or nonstructural pathological dysfunction.

Psychometric and Electroencephalographic Testing

Testing depends on medical history and physical examination. It is not routinely recommended.

TREATMENT PROTOCOL

Tincture of time in treatment of enuresis tends to be its own reward. Even though the physician can assure the parents that the child does not have serious life-threatening illness, and the outlook for resolution of the problem without intervention is high, some children require therapy.

Therapeutic intervention may be needed for reasons ranging from an attempt to interrupt escalating family discord to allowing the child freedom to stay overnight at a peer's home (for the child's own sense of well being).

1. Children with anatomical or serious psychopathological involvement should be referred to the appropriate specialist.

2. Counseling (alone or in conjunction with other therapy)

    a. This approach tends to have the most positive, far-reaching effects on the child and parents.

    b. It is important for the parents to recognize that there is a hereditary aspect to this problem (i.e., they themselves may have been bedwetters) and that there is nothing wrong with their child (i.e., they have not produced a defective child).

    c. Address both the parents and the child, individually and together.

   d. Assure the child that he or she is not defective or seriously ill and that, with time, there will be a resolution of the problem.

   e. Parents should understand that there should be no punitive measures taken against the child (e.g., wearing diapers or home restriction).

   f. Counseling tends to be more supportive to the child than actually altering bladder function.

   g. Whether the mode is curative or not, it allows the child to exercise a certain amount of control and to feel an active participant in the treatment process.

   h. The child is requested to retain urine for as long as possible after feeling the urge to void, to increase the interval between voidings, and to practice starting and stopping the stream of urine.

3. Imipramine (Tofranil®)

   a. The drug's mechanism of action is probably related to its anticholinergic properties rather than to any potential effect on sleep processes.

   b. Bladder capacity has been found to increase in children who respond positively to imipramine.

   c. Prescribe 1 mg/kg p.o. 2 hr before bedtime (maximum dose, 25 mg in preadolescents; 50 mg in older children) for 10 to 14 days; double the dosage if there is no response (maximum dose, 50 mg in preadolescents; 75 mg in older children).

   d. If a response occurs, the drug is tapered over a period of several weeks.

   e. A positive response occurs in about half of the children treated, although the efficacy is still controversial and the relapse rate is high.

   f. Side effects include dry mouth, sleep difficulties, constipation, urine retention, and, occasionally, hypotension.

   g. Because enuresis in children with secondary organic defects may respond to imipramine, it should not be used as a diagnostic test to distinguish between organic and nonorganic enuresis.

   h. Accidental or intentional overdosage can lead to serious morbidity or mortality from cardiac arrhythmias and confulsions.

4. Conditioning therapy

   a. This method of therapy has gained increasing popularity in the last decade.

   b. The method is based on use of an alarm system in which a circuit or buzzer (alarm) is activated when the child passes urine.

   c. Theoretically, the child learns by conditioning to awaken before spontaneously voiding and to respond to bladder pressure.

   d. The conditioning device is used for approximately 2 months; the success rate ranges from 50% to 75% (high incidence of relapses and failures).

   e. Burns may be sustained from leakage of the batteries in the alarm unit.

Epiglottitis

Epiglottitis is an infection or inflammation of the epiglottis and is a **medical emergency**. Treatment should begin the moment epiglottitis is the suspected diagnosis. Time should not be wasted in getting the patient to the operating room for intubation. Lateral neck radiographs should be performed to rule out a radiopaque foreign body, but they should not take precedence over transporting the patient to the operating room. If a glottic or tracheal foreign body is present, it must be removed under direct visualization (laryngoscopy, bronchoscopy). If epiglottitis is not present, it will also be noted by direct visualization.

A radiograph that fails to show epiglottitis does not rule out the diagnosis. Infection may begin in the aryepiglottic folds and cause enough edema to lead to obstruction. The entire bulk of the epiglottis does not have to be involved.

The etiology is usually bacterial. *Hemophilus influenzae* is the most common organism causing epiglottitis. Streptococcal, pneumococcal, and diphtheritic infections can cause similar syndromes, but they are extremely uncommon. With appropriate and rapid treatment, the prognosis is excellent. **If there is a delay, the chance for anoxic CNS damage and/or death is great.**

DIFFERENTIAL DIAGNOSIS

1. Acute onset of stridor
    a. Epiglottitis
    b. Diphtheria
    c. Foreign body
    d. Trauma
2. Chronic or recurrent stridor
    a. Tracheal web
    b. Tracheomalacia
    c. Laryngomalacia
    d. Vascular ring
    e. Spasmotic croup
    f. Extrinsic masses or tumors

Clinical differences among the croup syndromes are shown in Table 1.

TABLE 1. Clinical differences among the croup syndromes

	Epiglottitis	Laryngo-tracheobronchitis	Spasmotic croup	Foreign body
Age	2–4 yr	<18 months	<18 months	Any
Onset	Rapid	Slow	Recurrent	Rapid
Fever	High	Low	Absent	Absent
Stridor	Inspiratory	Inspiratory	Inspiratory	Inspiratory, expiratory, or both
Distress	Rapidly progressive	Variable	Variable	Mild to severe
Cyanosis	Frequent	Variable	Absent	Variable
Comments	Patient appears to be quite ill with an anxious facial expression; drooling is common	The onset is slow and, if progressive, it is not rapid, patient usually looks well and may have a croupy cough	Recurrent episodes of stridor and croupy cough are characteristic; cool air and mist usually give rapid relief	A pretracheal slap may be felt; there may be a history of eating small hard candy, peanuts, or playing with a toy with small parts; the episode may be proceeded by laughing, playing, running, and a coughing or choking episode; aphonia may occur

DIAGNOSTIC PROTOCOL

1. The sine qua non of the treatment of epiglottitis is intubation, which effectively controls the airway and prevents complete airway obstruction. The duration of intubation is approximately 48 to 72 hr, until the infection is under control and the edema begins to subside. All patients with epiglottitis should be intubated (it is favored over tracheostomy by most authorities). **The procedure should be done in the operating room under controlled conditions.** A set-up for tracheostomy should be available in the event of a laryngospastic episode and/or inability to pass the endotracheal tube.

2. Visualization of the epiglottis should not be done in the emergency room or the physician's office (unless it can be done without stimulation or manipulation of the oropharynx and unless adequate equipment and facilities are available for appropriate management). The pharynx and larynx of patients with epiglottitis are usually hyperirritable. Stimulation with a tongue blade or laryngeal mirror can cause irreversible laryngospasm, anoxia, and death.

3. Lateral neck radiography is usually done to rule out a foreign body. A swollen, edematous epiglottis may be visualized ("thumb sign," absence of visualization of the laryngeal vestibule). Subglottic narrowing may be seen in patients with laryngotracheobronchitis. Time, however, should not be wasted obtaining radiographs if the clinical condition suggests epiglottitis. Radiographs should be obtained only while waiting for preparation of the operating room or if suspicion of an aspirated foreign body is great. The patient should be accompanied to the radiology department by medical personnel.

4. Other laboratory evaluations should include complete blood cell count, blood cultures and sensitivity tests, β-lactamase testing, and blood gases.

5. After treatment, metastatic hemophilus infections should be checked for (e.g., meningitis, pericarditis).

TREATMENT PROTOCOL

1. Intubation (nasotracheal is the preferred route) under controlled conditions.

2. Administer humidified oxygen. Mechanical ventilation is usually not necessary.

3. Chloramphenicol, 100 mg/kg/day i.v. in four divided doses (if the organism is sensitive to ampicillin and the β-lactamase testing is negative, the patient may be switched to ampicillin for 7 to 10 days).

Failure to Thrive

Failure to thrive (FTT) describes children who are three standard deviations below the mean for weight (on a standard growth curve) and/or who show a persistent downward trend from their own established growth curve. In its severest form, failure to thrive may also affect height and head circumference. The frequency with which a physician encounters this disorder will vary significantly, depending on the location of the physician's practice, institutional capability to provide tertiary care, and community referral patterns. In an inpatient facility providing mainly primary care, failure to thrive will be largely nonorganic in origin. In a tertiary care institution, growth-related disorders will more often have an organic basis.

Although the causes for failure to thrive are multiple, it is important to differentiate between an organic and a nonorganic etiology. A thorough medical history and physical examination will usually provide sufficient clues to allow the examiner to distinguish between these two basic categories, so that in only very rare instances will extensive laboratory tests be required. (An assessment of the maternal-child interaction is an essential and often diagnostic feature of the evaluation.)

In spite of the physician's sensitivity, including adequate use of support services and appropriate testing, the distinction between organic and nonorganic failure to thrive may ultimately be hazy. An initially healthy baby, subjected to caloric deprivation because of lack of tender loving care, especially at critical periods of growth, may ultimately represent a diagnostic dilemma; the baby may display organic difficulties, even though it was a physiologically normal infant.

PATHOPHYSIOLOGY

The pathophysiological mechanisms of failure to thrive are described in a variety of chapters, reflecting both organic causes and nonorganic causes.

SIGNS AND SYMPTOMS

The manifestations of failure to thrive are the result of various potential disease states and pathophysiological mechanisms. The only common denominator may be weight below the third percentile on a standard growth curve. The signs and symptoms may then be a reflection of the child's constitution and the environmental variables to which the child is exposed. Most studies on failure to thrive show that central nervous system disease and gastrointestinal disorders are the most prevalent states involved in organic failure to thrive. These are followed closely by abnormalities of the genitourinary and endocrine systems. Therefore, many children with failure to thrive secondary to these disease states would show physical stigmata compatible with these disorders. Emotional deprivation may not be as obvious if the usual criteria for medical disease is narrowly applied. Emotionally deprived children demand greater sensitivity and interest from the area of developmental pediatrics, since often their interactions with other children, with their caretakers, or with their toys will be of far greater significance to the observant physician than the ensuing physical examination. Sills' evaluation of 185 patients below 3 years of age showed that with a thorough medical history and physical examination, virtually no laboratory tests were needed to separate organic from nonorganic failure to thrive.

DIFFERENTIAL DIAGNOSIS

1. Nonorganic failure to thrive (70%)

   a. The Bare Cupboard syndrome (the cause in <1% of cases until recently): A poverty related condition wherein there are insufficient funds in the household to provide sustenance for the child.

   b. Accidental: Errors in judgment by the caretaker concerning feeding techniques, i.e., incorrect reconstitution of formula (extreme dilution of formula, resulting in water intoxication).

   c. Nutritional or caloric deprivation: An interactive subset wherein the provision of inadequate calories is overshadowed by the dysfunctional relationship between the child and the mother, who may be depressed, apathetic, and often overwhelmed.

2. Organic failure to thrive (30%)

   a. CNS diseases and gastrointestinal disorders are the most common abnormalities.

   b. Cardiovascular disease.

   c. Endocrine disorders.

   d. Renal disorders.

3. Constitutional short stature: Children three standard deviations below their standard growth curve who have had no change in growth velocity and are paralleling their growth curves; these children, other than having growth retardation, appear to be healthy and happy; a family history of genetic short stature will usually be present.

4. Shifting linear growth: Alludes to genetic patterns of growth, as the child, at 6 to 9 months of age, shifts his or her growth velocity to one of the parent's midgrowth channels.

DIAGNOSTIC PROTOCOL

Nonorganic Failure to Thrive

Medical History

1. Dysfunctional parent
   a. Role reversal.
   b. Inappropriate expectations of child for age and ability.
   c. Inability to appreciate when help is needed.
   d. Inability to recognize infant's needs or distress.
   e. Overwhelmed.
   f. Poor parenting ability and coping skills.
   g. Few resources (material or interpersonal).
   h. Social isolation.
   i. See Pathophysiology in Child Abuse chapter.
   j. Statements by mother that the baby's behavior is a personal attack.
   k. The child is described as bad.

2. Parent's history (or absence) of baby's feeding pattern; the feeding history will often provide information about the nurturing ability of the caretaker and her knowledge of feeding skills, and baby's biological needs.

3. Sleeping, crying, and toilet habits of child may give obvious clues to potential organic states, as well as to parent's investment in child.

4. Family history of heights; caretaker's child-rearing experience and conceptions of nuclear and extended family.

5. Social history may reveal recent traumatic events, as well as the degree of anxiety (or absence of anxiety) the caretaker has toward child's failure to thrive.

Physical Examination

1. See Short Stature chapter, for tests and examinations in children with short stature.

2. General appearance of the child: Dysmorphic features, disproportionate limb sizes, lack of eye contact, facial expressions (classic radar or wary gaze).

3. Vital signs.

4. Measurement of arm span, upper and lower segment proportions.

5. Musculoskeletal and neurological examinations.

Laboratory Investigations

Laboratory investigations are similar to screening tests for suspected organic failure to thrive.

1. Complete blood cell count with a peripheral smear and reticulcyte count.
2. Urinalysis and urine culture.
3. Electrolytes, blood urea nitrogen.
4. Bone age.
5. Stool examination for ova and parasites.
6. Tuberculosis test.
7. Consider sweat sodium and chloride test.
8. Stool test for reducing substance.

Organic Failure to Thrive

Medical History
1. Complicated antenatal course.
2. High-risk pregnancy (e.g., young single mother, limited antenatal care).
3. Difficult labor and delivery.
4. Low birth weight.
5. Neonatal sepsis.
6. Neonatal seizures or current seizure activity.
7. Chronic diarrhea.
8. Recurrent or chronic vomiting (regurgitation).
9. Family history of genetic disease or inborn error of metabolism.
10. Primary growth disorder (e.g., intrauterine growth retardation).

Physical Examination
1. Poorly responsive infant with questionable vision and hearing.
2. Disproportionate head size.
3. Pathoneumonic dermatological lesions (phakomatoses).
4. Neuromuscular abnormalities.
5. Congenital abnormalities.

Laboratory Investigations
   See chapters on diseases implicated in failure to thrive for specific laboratory tests.

TREATMENT PROTOCOL

Nonorganic Failure to Thrive

1. Admit the child to the hospital if there is any question of compliance or ability to evaluate the child.

2. Place the child in an environment where there will be as much stimulation as possible.

3. Assign one person on each shift to feed and interact with the child.

4. If possible, parents should feed the child early in the hospital course so that the maternal-child interaction may be assessed.

5. The same nutritional constituents that the child was getting at home should be provided in the hospital; very accurate measurements must be made of day-to-day growth on this comparable routine.

6. Infant stimulation and/or child-life workers should be involved both diagnostically and therapeutically.

7. Developmental testing should be done initially and at various intervals during hospitalization; 90% of children with nonorganic failure to thrive will manifest delays in development, as well as deprivational behavior.

8. Any significant observation regarding maternal-child interaction, the child's development, or mother's knowledge (appropriate and inappropriate) should be documented in the medical chart.

9. If nutritional neglect is suspected, a report should be made to the appropriate state agency so that hospital and agency may work together early on in the case.

10. If failure to thrive is a poverty-related phenomenon, the state agency and other authorities must arrange for financial assistance as well as outreach services to assure continued access to health care and nutrition.

11. If failure to thrive is a result of accidental or inadequate knowledge of feeding, provide education, guidance regarding good nutrition, and general parenting skills; outreach services and weekly homemaker or visiting nurse service should be planned before discharge.

12. If failure to thrive is caused by caloric or emotional deprivation, the problems are more complex; both child and parent will need outreach services and intensive socialization to provide caretaker with nonthreatening helpful role model in parenting and other social skills; close liaison with social service and community service is essential; the modalities used in the other causes of failure to thrive should be instituted; do not discharge the child until the mother is able, ready, or equipped externally for positive environmental interaction with baby.

Organic Failure to Thrive

See chapters on diseases implicated in failure to thrive for specific treatment plans.

Fever of Unknown Origin

Fever of unknown origin (FUO) is defined as an unremitting fever of greater than 101°F, lasting more than 2 weeks, for which no cause can be found clinically. Fever of unknown origin should be differentiated from a fever of undetermined etiology, which is usually present for less than 2 weeks (acute onset) with no localizing signs or symptoms.

Fevers of unknown origin in children do not carry the same significance as they do in adults. In adults, they have a high association with malignancy, but in children, the etiology is usually infectious, most often viral. The younger the child, the more likely is the etiology to be trivial, except in the neonate.

There is a significant variation in the etiology of FUO between children and adults. There is also an age variation among children (Fig. 1). In one study, infections were responsible for 65% of the fevers of unknown origin in children younger than 6 years of age (Pizzo, 1975). Eighty percent of the children with collagen-vascular disease and all of the patients with inflammatory bowel disease were older than 6 years. Infections accounted for only 38% of the children older than 6 years. Thirty-three percent of the children older than 6 years had a collagen-vascular disease as the etiology of the fever.

DIFFERENTIAL DIAGNOSIS

1. Acute onset of fever > 101°F in neonate
    a. Septicemia
    b. Meningitis
    c. Urinary tract infection
    d. Viral syndromes
    e. Pneumonia
    f. Other bacterial infections
2. Acute onset of fever > 101°F in infant >6 weeks old
    a. Viral infections (respiratory, gastrointestinal)
    b. Bacterial infections (otitis media, tonsillitis)
    c. Miscellaneous
3. Chronic fever in child <6 years old
    a. Infections—52% (viral, urinary tract, meningitis, pneumonia, other)

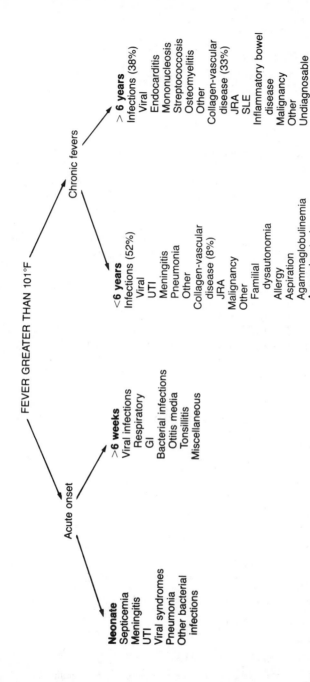

FIG. 1. Differential diagnosis of fever of unknown origin.

b. Collagen-vascular disease—8% (juvenile rheumatoid arthritis)

c. Other (familial dysautonomia, allergy, aspiration, agammaglobulinemia, agranulocytosis)

d. Undiagnosable

4. Chronic fever in child >6 years old

    a. Infections—38% (viral, endocarditis, mononucleosis, streptococcus, osteomyelitis, other)

    b. Collagen-vascular disease—33% (juvenile rheumatoid arthritis, systemic lupus erythmatosus)

    c. Inflammatory bowel disease

    d. Malignancy

    e. Other

    f. Undiagnosable

INITIAL DIAGNOSTIC PROTOCOL

1. Medical history and physical examination: Suggests the diagnosis of the fever in more than 60% of the patients.

2. Complete blood cell count with differential count: Significance is variable; not specifically diagnostic unless there are cells present in the peripheral smear that are peculiar to the disease process (e.g., Downey cells in mononucleosis, lymphoblasts in leukemia).

3. Urinalysis: Presence of protein and/or red blood cells may indicate a collagen-vascular disease or subacute bacterial endocarditis; pyuria may indicate a urinary tract infection.

4. Erythrocyte sedimentation rate (ESR): Usually considered an acute phase reactant; however, an elevated ESR (>30 mm/hr) in the presence of documented FUO usually indicates a more significant underlying disease process and close observation, frequent physical examinations, and/or further diagnostic tests may be indicated.

5. Albumin-to-globulin ratio: A nonspecific laboratory test; a reversal in the presence of a documented FUO usually indicates a more significant underlying disease process.

6. Cultures: Blood, urine, oropharynx, and nasopharynx.

DIAGNOSTIC PROTOCOL

Negative Initial Evaluation

1. If initial evaluations are negative, there are no localizing signs or symptoms, and the patient is clinically well, no further laboratory evaluations are indicated; patient should be followed closely at regularly scheduled intervals.

2. Administration of antimicrobial agents should be avoided.

Positive Initial Evaluation

1. Patient <6 years old:

   a. Patient should be considered a high risk, with close follow-up and frequent medical history and physical examinations indicated; a sign or symptom may suggest specific diagnostic techniques; hospitalization is usually not required unless a specific diagnostic procedure is needed.

   b. Administration of antimicrobial agents should be avoided, unless a specific diagnosis has been made.

2. Patient >6 years old:

   a. Patient should be considered a high risk, with hospitalization and further diagnostic procedures indicated.

   b. Serum complement studies, antinuclear antibodies (ANA), including anti-DNA, rheumatoid factor, lupus erythematosus cell preparation, and HLA-B27 evaluations are indicated because of the high incidence of collagen-vascular disease causing FUO in this age group.

   c. Other diagnostic tests usually include viral titers and cultures, IVP and voiding cystourethrogram (if urinary tract abnormalities are suspected), gastrointestinal radiography with contrast (if inflammatory bowel disease is suspected), gallium scan (if occult abscess is suspected), technetium bone scan (if occult osteomyelitis is suspected), and bone marrow examination (if malignancy, e.g., leukemia, is suspected), but evaluation must be individualized and guided by the medical history and physical examination.

   d. Laparotomy is indicated only in patients with abdominal findings and a negative noninvasive evaluation who are not improving or are worsening; some authorities believe laparotomy should be reserved for patients with fever lasting 6 months or more and associated with abdominal findings and lymphadenopathy.

TREATMENT PROTOCOL

The empirical use of antibiotics should be discouraged.

There is no specific treatment for a fever of unknown origin. The diagnosis must be established and followed by appropriate treatment. In those patients in whom a diagnosis cannot be made (approximately 10% of affected patients), more than half will improve without intervention or sequelae.

Floppy Infant Syndrome

The floppy infant has various degrees of decreased muscle tone, sometimes associated with weakness. A flaccid paralysis and increased range of joint motion may be found.

The age at onset of symptoms is also variable. The decreased tone may be noticeable at birth or may not appear until later in infancy or childhood. The prognosis depends on the etiology. Some children succumb to the disease process early in infancy, whereas others may lead relatively normal lives.

PATHOPHYSIOLOGY

The abnormality may lie in the central nervous system, peripheral nervous system, or end organs (the musculature). Symptoms vary according to the location of the lesion in the neuromuscular axis and also with the various other presenting signs or symptoms that may be associated with the primary disease process (e.g., Down's syndrome, Werdnig-Hoffmann disease, glycogen storage diseases) (Fig. 1).

SIGNS AND SYMPTOMS

Signs and symptoms that suggest hypotonicity are hypermobile or extensible joints, persistence of head lag after the third month of life, lack of head control, and slipping of the patient through the examiner's hands when held in the axillae. Paucity of intrauterine movements, poor sucking, swallowing, or feeding, and lack of movement when left unattended should also alert the practitioner to the possibility of the presence of hypotonia.

Central nervous system disorders can be differentiated from peripheral disorders by checking the patient's reflexes. Central disorders are characterized by brisk reflexes and a positive Babinski sign. There is absence or weak reflexes in peripheral disorders. The electromyogram may also be of help in identifying the location of a lesion.

GENERAL DIAGNOSTIC PROTOCOL

1. Stained fixed-tissue muscle biopsy: Primarily used to differentiate myelopathic or neural atrophy of muscles and primary myopathy. Appropriate handling and staining of the specimen are extremely important (the laboratory should be consulted before the specimen is obtained). Also of vital importance is obtaining the specimen from the appropriate muscle. This should be done in consultation

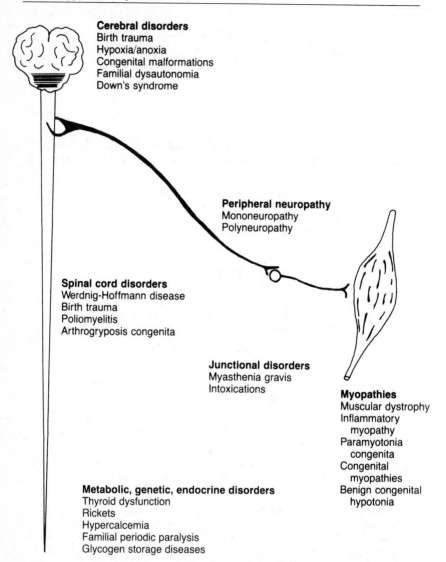

Cerebral disorders
Birth trauma
Hypoxia/anoxia
Congenital malformations
Familial dysautonomia
Down's syndrome

Peripheral neuropathy
Mononeuropathy
Polyneuropathy

Spinal cord disorders
Werdnig-Hoffmann disease
Birth trauma
Poliomyelitis
Arthrogryposis congenita

Junctional disorders
Myasthenia gravis
Intoxications

Myopathies
Muscular dystrophy
Inflammatory
  myopathy
Paramyotonia
  congenita
Congenital
  myopathies
Benign congenital
  hypotonia

Metabolic, genetic, endocrine disorders
Thyroid dysfunction
Rickets
Hypercalcemia
Familial periodic paralysis
Glycogen storage diseases

FIG. 1. Differential diagnosis of the floppy infant.

with a neurologist. Sedation for the procedure may be used (meperidine, 1 mg/kg i.m., and secobarbital, 8 mg/kg i.m.); however, the injection must be given into a muscle distant from the one to be biopsied. Histochemical staining (fiber typing), ultrastructural analysis, and biochemical evaluations (useful in the evaluation of some glycogen storage diseases and lipid storage myopathies) may be performed on the specimen.

2. Electromyography (EMG): Primarily used to differentiate neuropathic and my-opathic processes. Fibrillation potentials and positive sharp waves are usually characteristic of denervation but are occasionally normal in the distal muscles of infants. Muscle disease usually shows reduced amplitude and duration of action potentials and short polyphasic potentials.

3. Nerve conduction testing (NCT): In addition to differentiation of neuropathic and myopathic disease, NCT may differentiate anterior horn cell disorders from peripheral neuropathies. Slow conduction time (usually due to deficiencies in myelinization) are characteristic of peripheral nerve disease. Normal nerve conduction velocities vary with age; the younger the child, the slower the conduction. The most often utilized nerves for NCT are the median nerve and the peroneal nerve.

4. Serum enzyme determination: Creatine phosphokinase (CPK) is the most useful; SGOT, SGPT, lactic dehydrogenase, and aldolase are nonspecific and may be elevated in liver and/or heart disease. CPK levels are usually highest in the muscular dystrophies (Duchenne's and Becker's), but may be normal in several forms of muscular dystrophy.

5. Myoglobinuria: Present where muscle destruction is acute.

6. Skeletal radiographs: If osteogenesis imperfecta or disorders of calcium metabolism are suspected.

7. Serum electrolytes, calcium, and glucose.

8. Erythrocyte sedimentation rate: If a collagen-vascular disease is suspected.

9. Cerebrospinal fluid (CSF): Elevated protein is seen in polyneuropathy.

10. Electrocardiogram (ECG): If conduction abnormalities are suspected; frequently abnormal in the Duchenne's type of muscular dystrophy.

DIAGNOSTIC AND TREATMENT PROTOCOLS

Table 1 gives the diagnostic and treatment protocols for a variety of floppy infant syndrome disorders.

TABLE 1. *Hypotonia: Diagnostic and treatment protocols*

Diagnosis	Treatment
Arthrogryposis Congenita	
Clinical features: Muscular weakness, hypotonia, and congenital fixation of two or more joints; if a neural abnormality is present (e.g., atrophy), localized diminished or absent anterior horn cells can be seen	There is no specific treatment, and a multidisciplinary approach should be provided
Benign Congenital Hypotonia	
Clinical features: Generalized weakness, limpness, and hypotonia at birth, which	There is no specific treatment, and a multidisciplinary approach should be provided

TABLE 1. *(continued)*

Diagnosis	Treatment
characteristically improve with time; sitting and standing are delayed; deep tendon reflexes are variable; respirations are rarely involved EMG: Excessive polyphasic and short duration potentials Muscle biopsy: May be normal	

Birth Trauma

Most children with cerebral disorder (spastic or flaccid) secondary to birth trauma initially present with hypotonia; spasticity occurs with time; the history may reveal a complicated gestation, labor, and/or delivery CT scan: May be helpful in identifying patients with intracranial bleeding and congenital malformations Spinal radiographs: To help rule out trauma to the spinal cord	Treatment depends on the extent and type of trauma; the location of the disorder is also of importance in determining the best method of therapy Long-term follow-up, physical therapy, and occupational therapy are usually required

Congenital Malformations

Congenital CNS malformations may be apparent at birth (e.g., anencephaly, encephalocele) or may appear later in infancy (e.g., porencephalic cysts) Head circumference: May be helpful in identifying hydrocephalus Transillumination of the skull CT scan: May be helpful in identifying the presence, type, and position of a malformation	Treatment depends on the type of malformation and its location

Congenital Myopathies

Clinical features: Onset early in infancy or childhood of progressive proximal muscle weakness, flaccidity, and decreased deep tendon reflexes; myopathic facies and temporalis muscle atrophy are common
Nemaline myopathy
  Uncoordinated gait, dysmorphic facies, and high arched palate are common
  Serum enzymes are normal or mildly elevated EMG reveals myopathic changes
  Muscle biopsy reveals nemaline bodies (dense rod-like structures)
Central-core disease
  Gross motor development is delayed and deep tendon reflexes are normal
  Serum enzymes are normal
  EMG shows myopathic changes
  Muscle biopsy reveals amorphous central core material
	Treatment is supportive and symptomatic; multidisciplinary approach is required

Diagnosis	Treatment

Down's Syndrome

Hypotonia and weakness are characteristic; other stigmata of Down's syndrome are usually present

Chromosome studies reveal trisomy 21

A multidisciplinary approach is required

Special education is extremely important in the management of patients with Down's syndrome

Genetic counseling

Maternal Drugs

A history of drug abuse may be elicited; hypotonia and respiratory depression occur when the mother has taken the drug close to the time of delivery; chronic abuse usually results in the neonatal narcotic withdrawal syndrome

Narcotic analgesics used during labor and/or delivery can cause hypotonia and CNS respiratory depression

Naloxone, 0.005 mg/kg i.m. or i.v., for narcotic analgesic depression (repeat every 2 to 3 min to maximum of two or three doses if required) **or** nalorphine, 0.1 mg/kg i.m. or i.v.

Familial Dysautonomia (Riley-Day Syndrome)

Clinical findings: Poor suck and swallow; gagging and aspiration often occur, increased pulmonary secretions and frequent pulmonary infections, which commonly result in chronic pulmonary disease; lack of tears, excessive secretions and salivation, incontinence, labile hypertension, recurrent fevers, decreased sensation, decreased reflexes, corneal ulcerations, and mental retardation

Chest radiograph shows infiltrates and chronic disease

Mecholyl test: Positive (instill 2% solution of mecholyl into the conjunctival sac of one eye and a solution of normal saline into the other as a control; pupillary constriction within 10 min is a positive test)

Histamine challenge: Positive (inject 0.05 cc of 1:1000 solution of histamine intradermally; the test is positive if there is no flare reaction or pain

Urine homovanillic acid level: Elevated

Urine vanillylmandelic acid level: Decreased

Adequate treatment of pulmonary infections and adequate pulmonary toilet to mobilize secretions is essential

Artificial tears should be given to prevent corneal damage from drying

Protect the patient from traumatic injuries secondary to the loss of pain sensation

Genetic counseling

Glycogen Storage Diseases

Clinical characteristics: Usually severe cramping and fatigue, which are increased by exercise

Little or no increase in lactic acid levels during ischemic exercise testing (e.g., McArdle's disease, phosphofructokinase deficiency)

Muscle biopsy: Increased glycogen and the specific enzyme defect may be identified by doing direct enzyme analysis on the specimen

Treatment must be individualized and depends on the specific diagnosis

TABLE 1. *(continued)*

Diagnosis	Treatment

Hypoxia

Clinical findings: May be a history of a complicated pregnancy, labor, and/or delivery; meconium staining may be present if the insult occurred in utero; cyanosis may be present

Other signs and symptoms depend on the degree of hypoxia and injury and when the insult occurred

Head circumference: May indicate increases in intracranial pressure or hydrocephalus

CT scan: May reveal anoxic/hypoxic damage, congenital malformations, or intracranial bleeding

Blood gases: May detect ongoing hypoxia

Oxygen administration, if hypoxia is still present; assisted ventilation may be necessary

Close follow-up to observe for sequelae, which should be treated only if and when they appear

Inflammatory Myopathies (Dermatomyositis)

Muscle involvement: Proximal muscle weakness (hip/pelvic girdle and shoulder girdle)

Cutaneous manifestations: May be violaceous eyelids, malar maculopapular rash, thickening of the skin over the proximal interphalangeal joints, scaly extensor surface plaques, and telangectasia of the nail beds

There is no specific evaluation for the inflammatory myopathies; laboratory evaluation should be the same as for other collagen-vascular diseases; anti-DNA antibody test is positive

Prednisone: 60 to 100 mg/m^2, initially for 6 to 12 weeks, decreased to 2.5 to 10 mg/day; every-other-day therapy may be required

Intoxications

Usually the insecticides malathion or parathion are the responsible agents

Clinical features simulate a myasthenic crisis: Weakness, bulbar involvement, difficulty in handling secretions, and respiratory distress

Antidotes: Atropine and 2-pyridinaldoxime methiodide (PAM)

Muscular Dystrophy

Clinical findings (Duchenne's type is the most common type): Onset usually between 3 and 6 years of age; clumsiness and falling are common; pseudohypertrophy of the gastrocnemius and deltoid musculature; progressive proximal muscle weakness of the shoulder and pelvic girdles; most patients have difficulty on standing from a supine position (positive Gowers sign), toe walking, and difficulty in climbing stairs; deep tendon reflexes are usually absent

CPK: Markedly elevated

Muscle biopsy with histochemical staining: Can support the diagnosis

ECG: Myocardial involvement is common

Duchenne's type is X-linked recessive and genetic counseling is essential

The therapeutic approach to children with muscular dystrophy is multidisciplinary. Physical therapy, occupational therapy, orthopedic surgery, neurological consultation, special education must be coordinated

The treatment is supportive; there is no specific treatment

Diagnosis	Treatment

Myasthenia Gravis

Three forms are described: **Transient neonatal** (onset is within the first 24 hours of life, the mother is myasthenic, and the symptoms resolve in 3 to 6 weeks; early treatment is required to prevent death in the first few weeks of life); **congenital** (the onset is usually later in infancy and the symptoms do not resolve); **juvenile** (onset at 5–10 years of age)

Clinical manifestations: Bulbar weakness with ophthalmoplegia, ptosis, expressionless facies, weak suck and swallow, weak cry, and respiratory distress; generalized muscle weakness after inactivity, lack of movement, weak grasp reflex, poor Moro reflex, poor rooting reflex; deep tendon reflexes are usually present

Confirmation test: Tensilon® (edrophonium chloride), 0.2 mg/kg i.v. or i.m., is rapidly followed by improvement in the patient's clinical condition

EMG: Progressive decrease in amplitude of action potentials with repetitive stimulation

Neostigmine, 2 mg/kg/day p.o. in six to eight equally divided doses (dose usually requires modification) or pyridostigmine, 7 mg/kg/day p.o. in five to six equally divided doses

Supportive and symptomatic care

Observe the patient closely for myasthenic crisis

The need for thymectomy is controversial

Steroids or ACTH may be required if there is resistance to anticholinesterase medications

Paramyotonia Congenita

Clinical features: Flaccidity and myotonia, especially of the facial muscles and the muscles of the hand; symptoms appear after exposure to cold

Potassium and calcium: Normal

EMG: Myopathic potentials

Autosomal dominant disorder

Treatment is supportive and symptomatic

Patients should avoid exposure to cold

Periodic Familial Paralysis

Clinical features: Acute onset of diffuse muscle weakness, difficulty breathing, and mobilization of secretions after exercise and/or a high carbohydrate meal

Potassium: Elevated, decreased, or normal

ECG: Reflects changes in potassium levels

Autosomal dominant characteristic

Avoid vigorous exercise

Avoid high carbohydrate meals

Provide potassium supplements for patients with the hypokalemic form

Poliomyelitis

Clinical findings: Development of asymmetric flaccid weakness of the muscles, preceded by a mild upper respiratory tract or gastrointestinal tract infection; if the cranial nerves are involved, abnormalities in sucking and swallowing, hoarseness, and stridor can occur

CSF: Pleocytosis may occur

The virus may be cultured from the CSF and the urine

The treatment is supportive and symptomatic

The patient must be closely observed for respiratory involvement

The most important aspect of the treatment of polio is its prevention

TABLE 1. *(continued)*

Diagnosis	Treatment

Polyneuropathy (Guillain-Barre syndrome)

Clinical findings: Distal muscle weakness and pain preceded 10 to 21 days by an upper respiratory tract infection or a gastrointestinal infection; weakness may ascend and involve the muscles of respiration; difficulty in swallowing signifies bulbar involvement; deep tendon reflexes are markedly decreased or absent; duration of the illness is 4 to 6 weeks

CSF: Marked elevation in the protein content, without pleocytosis

EMG: Neuropathic changes and fibrillation potentials

NCT: Decreased

Treatment is supportive and symptomatic

Corticosteroids or ACTH may be of value if given early in the course of the illness

Assisted ventilation may be required if respiratory paralysis occurs

Thyroid Dysfunction

Weakness is common with both hyperthyroidism and hypothyroidism; other clinical features may be present to alert the examiner to the diagnosis

T_4 and thyroid-stimulating hormone determination may be indicated

Werdnig-Hoffmann Disease (Infantile Spinal Muscle Atrophy)

Clinical findings: Marked hypotonia and weakness (especially proximal), absent deep tendon reflexes, fasciculations of the tongue when the baby is at rest (i.e., not crying), and a normal sensory system; pectus excavatum and aspiration pneumonia are common

Serum enzymes: Normal

EMG: Fasciculation potentials

NCT: Normal

Muscle biopsy: Characteristic group atrophy

Type I disease: Onset at <3 months of age

Type II disease: Onset between 3 months and 1 year of age; delayed motor development; patients can usually roll from side to side, but rarely are able to sit without support; resting tremors of the fingers

Type III disease: Onset between 1 and 2 years of age; delayed muscle development; patients can usually sit without support, but can rarely walk without assistance; marked proximal muscle weakness

Type IV disease: Onset between 2 and 5 years of age; there is extreme proximal muscle weakness which mimics Duchenne's muscular dystrophy

The treatment is supportive and symptomatic

Infections (especially pulmonary) should be expected

Occupational and physical therapy should be provided; a multidisciplinary approach is essential

Counseling should be provided

Fluid and Electrolyte Imbalances

GENERAL PRINCIPLES

Renal Function

Glomerular filtration rate and renal blood flow are relatively depressed in infants and do not approximate adult levels until about 18 months of age. Other physiological peculiarities exist in infancy; for example, salt excretion tends to be greater than expected for age. Renal blood flow tends to be less, and renal plasma flow tends to be less than values corrected for surface area. There is an inability to tolerate either a water load or a salt load. Physiologically, the condition is called **glomerulotubular imbalance.** At birth, the glomeruli are relatively complete, but the tubular system is not mature. With time, the newborn child develops increasing tubular length and competence.

Fluid and Volume Physiology

Newborn infants tend to have a body water volume of 70% to 80% of their body weight. The volume falls as the infant matures and reaches approximately 60% in childhood. During the first few days of life, as much as 7% of the body water is lost.

Body Water Compartments

Body water compartments represent about 70% of the lean body mass. They are composed of the extracellular fluid compartment (30% of the body water in infants and 20% in adults; 15% is interstitial and 5% is intravascular). The intracellular fluid constitutes approximately 40% of the body water in both infants and adults.

Turnover Rates

Extracellular fluid is turned over much more rapidly in infants and newborns than in adults. Newborns and infants turn over their extracellular fluid approximately four times as rapidly as adults.

Regulatory Mechanisms

The kidney tends to regulate the homeostatic mechanisms of the body by varying three modalities: the amount of water, the osmolality of the fluids, and the distribution of the water through retention and/or excretion of sodium.

Osmolality

Osmolality refers to the number of osmotically active particles dissolved per unit volume. The following formula will allow approximation of the serum osmolality:

$$Osm = 2(Na) + BUN/2.8 + glucose/18$$

where sodium (Na) is given as mEq/L and blood urea nitrogen (BUN) and glucose concentrations are given in mg/100 ml.

Sodium, urea, and glucose are the major osmotically active particles in solution. The osmolality may be raised by any osmotically active products that are endogenous (e.g., abnormal proteins in dysproteinemias) and/or exogenous (e.g., extrinsic particles ingested in intoxications).

Third Space

The third space refers to the compartments wherein fluids, electrolytes, and drugs are outside of the normal fluid spaces and thereby contribute very little to effective volume (e.g., peritoneal fluid, pleural fluid, effusions).

Electrolyte Physiology

Sodium

Sodium is the principal volume regulator and accounts for approximately 85% to 90% of the extracellular cationic osmolality. It is important to note that 1 g of sodium is very different than 1 g of salt. Salt contains both sodium and chloride, therefore, 1 g of salt is equal to 18 mEq of sodium.

Serum sodium levels may be factitiously low when there are elevated levels of osmotically active particles (e.g., glucose) or lipids. This factitious dilution occurs because fluid is drawn from the intracellular compartments. For every 100 mg of glucose above physiological levels, the sodium level is depressed by 2.0 to 2.5 mEq/L.

The requirements for sodium probably range from 40 to 60 mEq/m^2/24 hr (2–3 mEq/kg/day).

Potassium

Potassium is the principal cation of the intracellular fluid. Ninety-eight percent of the body potassium resides within the intracellular compartment. Its main functions are maintenance of cell membrane integrity and intracellular tonicity. Measurement of intracellular potassium is difficult, and there is no practical quantitative estimate of total body potassium for routine therapeutic replacement purposes.

There is an obligatory loss of potassium in the urine since tubular reabsorption of potassium does not seem to be as efficient as reabsorption of sodium (with sodium restriction, it is possible to find less than 0.5 mEq/L of sodium per day in the urine, but it is most unusual to find urinary potassium levels below 10 mEq/L). As with sodium, potassium salt contains chloride, and 1 g of potassium salt equals 13.40 mEq of KCl.

Maintenance requirements for potassium probably range from 30 to 40 mEq/m^2/24 hr (1–2 mEq/kg/day).

Chloride

Chloride is the principal anion of both the intravascular fluid and gastric juices. Chloride tends to undergo active renal tubular transport, probably within the loop of Henle; in the proximal tubule, it behaves in a passive manner, following the flow of sodium. The requirements for chloride tend to parallel those for sodium and potassium. In times of abnormal losses, it is possible to see a paradoxical aciduria, occurring when there is a chloride deficiency in conjunction with dehydration. In an attempt to conserve volume, sodium is retained and there is rejection of hydrogen ions into the urine.

Calcium

Calcium exists in the serum in both ionized and unionized forms. The ionized fraction constitutes approximately 40% of the total serum calcium. It is partially protein bound, mainly to albumin. Changes in the serum albumin of approximately 1 g/L lower the measurable calcium by approximately 0.8 mg/dL. The ionized portion of the total calcium varies according to the acid-base status of the body. The level of ionized calcium tends to reflect the various clinical situations. For example, a low total serum calcium level is often present in patients with nephrotic syndrome, but symptoms of hypocalcemia are absent. If the acidosis is corrected, causing less ionizable calcium to be present, the patient may become symptomatic.

Magnesium

Magnesium is primarily an intracellular ion and is affected by the plasma pH in a manner similar to calcium. Magnesium deficiency states are clinically similar to those of calcium.

Bicarbonate

Plasma bicarbonate levels tend to fall within a narrow range (23–25 mEq/L). Newborn infants usually exhibit a lower serum bicarbonate concentration because of their glomerulotubular imbalance.

DEHYDRATION

Dehydration is defined as loss of total body water. Hypovolemia refers only to decreased intravascular volume. In treating fluid and electrolyte abnormalities in children, it is assumed that there is some degree of hypovolemia. In lesser degrees of dehydration, compensation may take place by shifts of fluid from the extravascular space to the intravascular space, maintaining vital functions. In greater degrees of dehydration, symptoms of hypovolemia usually appear.

Tonicity of the body fluids is important in classifying the type of dehydration (Fig. 1). Sodium tends to be the main regulator of osmolality (tonicity) and the maintainer of the vascular compartment. It is reasonable, therefore, to divide the states of dehydration into isotonic (normonatremia), hypotonic (hyponatremia) and hypertonic (hypernatremia), as shown in Table 1.

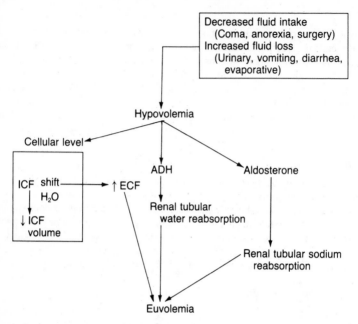

FIG. 1. Pathophysiology of dehydration. ADH, antidiuretic hormone; ECF, extracellular fluid; ICF, intracellular fluid.

TABLE 1. *State of tonicity (osmolality) in dehydration*

	Hypotonic[a] (serum sodium level <130 mEq/L)	Isotonic[a] (serum sodium level 130–150 mEq/L)	Hypertonic[a] (serum sodium level >150 mEq/L)
Skin turgor	Severely decreased	Decreased	Fair
Mucous membrane	Decreased	Decreased	Parched
Urinary frequency	Severely decreased	Decreased	Decreased
Fontanelle	Severely sunken	Sunken	Flat
Sensorium	Lethargy or coma	Lethargy	Irritability or lethargy
Pulse			
Orthostatic (upright position)	Severely increased	Moderately increased	Normal or increased
Supine	Severely increased	Moderate increased	Normal or increased
Blood pressure			
Orthostatic (upright position)	Severely decreased	Decreased	Normal or decreased
Supine	Severely decreased	Decreased	Normal or decreased

[a]Osmolality is clinically related to serum sodium levels and mild (isotonic), moderate (hypotonic), and severe (hypertonic) degrees of dehydration.

TABLE 2. *Signs and symptoms of dehydration*

	Degree of dehydration[a]		
	Mild	Moderate	Severe
Tears	Decreased or absent	Absent	Absent
Mucous membrane	Dry	Dry	Parched
Urinary frequency	Decreased (by history)	Decreased (by history)	Severely decreased
Skin turgor	Decreased	Tenting	Severely decreased
Fontanelle	Flat	Sunken	Sunken
Eyeball	Normal	Sunken	Sunken
Pulse			
Orthostatic (upright position)	Normal or increased	Increased	Weak
Supine	Normal	Increased	Weak
Sensorial changes	Absent or slight lethargy	Lethargy	Lethargy
Blood pressure			
Orthostatic (upright position)	Normal or decreased	Decreased	Decreased
Supine	Normal	Normal	Decreased

[a]Based on weight loss: Mild (5% in infants, 3% in older children), moderate (10% in infants, 6% in older children), severe (15% in infants, 9% in older children).

Signs and Symptoms

The signs and symptoms of dehydration are shown in Table 2.

Diagnostic Protocol

1. Medical history

    a. Length of illness

    b. Vomiting or diarrhea

    c. Weight change

    d. Decreased urine output

    e. Attempts to replenish lost fluid

2. Physical findings: Degree of dehydration is expressed as mild, moderate, or severe, reflecting the degree of weight loss (see Tables 1 and 2)

3. Laboratory investigations (Table 3)

    a. Hemoglobin, hematocrit

    b. Blood urea nitrogen, creatinine

    c. Serum and urine electrolytes (urinary sodium level is usually <20 mEq/L in dehydration; higher levels may indicate renal disease)

TABLE 3. Results of laboratory tests in dehydration

Mechanism of dehydration	Blood									Urine		
	Hgb	Na$^+$	K$^+$	Cl$^-$	BUN	CO$_2$	Glucose	Cr	Osm	Osm	Sp gr	Na$^+$
Increased fluid output												
Urinary loss	↑	↑↓	↑↓	↑↓	↑	↑↓	N	↑	↑↓	↑↓	↑↓	↑↓
Adrenal insufficiency	↑	↓↑	↑	↑	↑	↓	↑↓	↑	↑	↑↓	↑↓	↑
Diabetic ketoacidosis	↑	↑↓	↑	↑	↑	↓	↑	↑	↑	↑↓	↑↓	↑↓
Central or nephrogenic diabetes insipidus	↑	↑	N	N	↑	↑	N	↑	↑	↓	↓	↓
Polyuric (e.g., acute renal failure)	↑	↑↓	↑	↑	↑	↓	N	↑	↑	↓	↓	↑
Vomiting or obstruction (e.g., pyloric stenosis)	↑	↑	↑↓	↓	↑	↑	N	↑	↑	↑	↑	↓
Evaporative or sweat loss (e.g., cystic fibrosis)	↑	↑↓	N	↑↓	↑	↓	N	↑	↑	↑	↑	↓
Diarrhea												
Hypotonic	↑	↓	↑	↑	↑	↓	N	↑	↑↓	↑	↑	↑↓
Isotonic	↑	N	↑	↑	↑	↓	N	↑	N	↑	↑	↑↓
Hypertonic	↑	↑	↑	↑	↑	↓	N	↑	↑	↑	↑	↓
Decreased fluid intake												
Coma or surgery	↑	↑↓	↓	↑	↑	↑	↑↓	↑	↑	↑	↑	↓

Hgb: hemoglobin; BUN: blood urea nitrogen; Cr: creatinine; Osm: osmolality; Sp gr: specific gravity; N: normal.

d. Serum and urine osmolality plus urine specific gravity (specific gravity $\geqslant 1.016$ reflects ability to preserve volume in dehydration; low specific gravity may indicate renal disease)

e. Blood and urine glucose

Treatment Protocol

1. Severe dehydration is associated with severe orthostatic changes, hypotension, tachycardia, and progressive sensorial changes. A well-thought-out approach is of importance in treating these severely ill patients.

2. Weigh the patient, if possible.

3. Most often the patient will be oligoanuric and have evidence of hypotension. Administer a fluid challenge (20 to 30 ml/kg i.v. of normal saline over a 30 min period). Monitor vital signs closely to detect any signs of impending cardiac decompensation.

4. If the vital signs are still stable, but no significant urine output has occurred ($>$1–1.5 ml/kg/hr), continue further infusion of normal saline (10 ml/kg/hr) until the shock is reversed and urine production occurs.

5. **It is most important that the vital signs be monitored closely** so that overly vigorous resuscitation does not result in further debilitation in the patient with an unstable cardiovascular system or parenchymal renal damage.

6. **Obtain laboratory studies immediately**; if a severe hypotonic state exists, alter the infusion to provide a more hypertonic solution (e.g., 3% saline solution).

7. It is of utmost importance that perfusion be restored to the brain, kidneys, and gastrointestinal tract. Lactated Ringer's solution should be avoided; although physiological, it also contains lactate and potassium, neither of which are helpful when the kidneys are poorly perfused and/or the liver tends to be compromised.

POTASSIUM IMBALANCE

Potassium balance tends to be reasonably stable despite continuous and often wide variations in intake and output. The stability of the body's potassium level depends on regulation of its excretion primarily by the kidneys. While the kidney is concerned mainly with extracellular levels of potassium, concurrent mechanisms regulate its intracellular distribution. Only a small fraction of the total body potassium remains in the extracellular compartment. In most normal states, transfer of ingested potassium into cells takes place so rapidly that no change can be measured in the serum potassium concentration. These transcellular shifts are controlled by insulin and aldosterone. However, the mechanisms that handle potassium are not nearly as efficient as the mechanisms that handle sodium. Maximal efficiency during changes in sodium intake may occur within a matter of hours, whereas with potassium changes, it may not be achieved for days or weeks. Secretion of potassium into the urine tends to be facilitated when serum potassium levels are high, and diminished when levels are low.

Complex networks involved in potassium homeostasis ensure that the levels in the extracellular compartment are kept between 4 and 5 mEq/L and 150 mEq/L in the intracellular compartment. As noted, however, there are limits to the ability of the body to deal with potassium fluxes. Renal regulation of potassium is not as exquisitely sensitive as that of sodium, and a urine potassium concentration of 10 to 15 mEq/L may signify near maximal renal conservation even when serum potassium levels are decreased.

Repair of potassium deficits must be made with great care since there is no practical method to measure absolute potassium deficits in the body. As inexact as it is, the serum potassium level must be the factor monitored for replacement. Since any administered potassium must first cross the extracellular compartment to reach the depleted cells, transient hyperkalemia may occur even with large potassium deficits. In healthy adults, an abrupt oral dose of even 50 mEq of potassium, representing a small fraction of the normal body stores, may transiently elevate the serum potassium concentration by 0.5 to 1 mEq/L.

The clinically important manifestations of potassium imbalance relate to its interference with the electrophysiological events underlying muscle contraction (Fig. 2). It is not the absolute serum level of potassium that dictates the complications or manifestations, but the gradient (ratio) of intracellular to extracellular potasssium that results in altered transmembrane potentials. Two groups of symptoms are prevalent at both extremes of potassium levels:

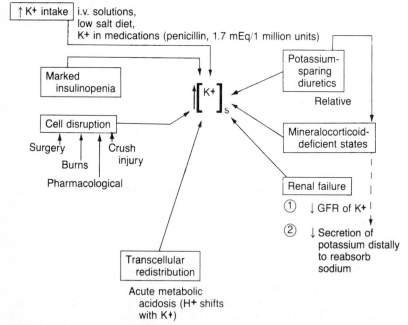

FIG. 2. Pathophysiology of hyperkalemia. $[K^+]_s$, potassium concentration; GFR, glomerular filtration rate.

Neuromuscular Effects

Early complaints may involve paresthesias and/or weakness followed by heaviness and paralysis. Smooth muscle dysfunction is more common in the hypokalemic state, reflected as paralytic ileus and gastric dilatation, but these manifestations may also be seen with hyperkalemia. In addition, myoglobinuria or hemoglobinuria from marked cellular damage is not uncommon in severe hypokalemic states.

Cardiac Toxicity

The human heart is exceptionally vulnerable to states of potassium flux through both conduction tissue and muscle fibers. In hyperkalemic states, by a rule of thumb, there is a relationship between the magnitude of the hyperkalemia and cardiotoxicity, but the rate at which the elevated potassium develops is also an important factor. Because progression to fatal toxicity may be unpredictable and swift, the presence of any changes mandates immediate treatment. Other signs and symptoms of hyperkalemia and hypokalemia are discussed in the following sections.

Signs and Symptoms of Hyperkalemia

See Fig. 2 for the pathophysiology of hyperkalemia.

1. Mild hyperkalemia (serum potassium level 5.0–6.0 mEq/L)
   a. Mild paresthesias
   b. No electrocardiographic abnormalities; mild T-wave peaking or elevation
2. Moderate hyperkalemia (serum potassium level 6.0–7.0 mEq/L)
   a. Paresthesias, mild weakness
   b. No electrocardiographic abnormalities; T-wave peaking or elevation, or P-wave abnormalities
3. Severe hyperkalemia (serum potassium level >7.0 mEq/L)
   a. Possible CNS symptoms
   b. Electrocardiogram shows widening of QRS complex and/or loss of P-waves

Differential Diagnosis

1. Increased potassium load
   a. Dietary (e.g., salt substitute)
   b. Iatrogenic (e.g., excess potassium in i.v. solutions)
   c. Cell breakdown
2. Reduced excretory ability
   a. Acute or chronic renal failure
   b. Hyporeninemia or hypoaldosteronism
   c. Adrenal insufficiency
   d. Potassium-sparing diuretics

  e. Kidney transplant (rejection, infarction)

  f. Severe dehydration

  g. Shock

3. Cellular shifts

  a. Acid-base abnormalities (e.g., acute metabolic acidosis)

  b. Diabetes mellitus

  c. Exercise

  d. Familial hyperkalemic periodic paralysis

Hyperkalemia: Diagnostic Protocol

Medical history	Physical examination	Laboratory investigations
Increased Potassium Load: Dietary		
Increased use of salt substitutes or other potassium-containing products (e.g., low sodium diet)	Clinical manifestations relate to interference with the electrophysiologic events underlying muscle contractions: Neuromuscular changes (parasthesias followed by weakness, feeling of heaviness, flacid paralysis) Electrocardiographic abnormalities in heart rate and rhythm	In general, electrocardiographic abnormalities showing symmetrical peaking of T wave, widening of the QRS complex, lengthening of PR interval. first degree and second degree heart blocks, loss of P waves, prolonged ventricular conduction, merging of the QRS with T wave, ventricular fibrillation
Increased Potassium Load: Cell Breakdown		
Antineoplastic drugs, crush injury, toxins	Reflects entity responsible for the injury (e.g., trauma resulting in crushed tissue)	Nonspecific findings of hyperkalemia as well as uric acid abnormalities and possible renal failure indices following a crush injury or cell breakdown, possible elevated phosphates level, myoglobin and hemoglobin abnormalities
Reduced Excretory Ability: Acute Renal Failure		

Please refer to Renal Failure chapter

Reduced Excretory Ability: Hyporeninemia/Hypoaldosterone States

Nonspecific or compatible with potassium-sparing diuretic, diabetes mellitus, chronic pyelonephritis, possibly sicle cell disease	Nonspecific, tends to reflect the disease entity with which it is involved	Rare coupling of hyperkalemia with hypoaldosteronemia; somewhat paradoxical

Reduced Excretory Ability: Adrenal Insufficiency

Ambiguous genitalia or chronic tuberculosis	Compatible with the entity causing the adrenal disease	Please refer to appropriate chapter

Cellular (Trans-cellular) Shifts: Acid-Base Abnormalities

Acute change in acid-base condition (e.g., acute metabolic acidosis)	Nonspecific, unless a discrete entity is involved	Compatible with the general hyperchloremic and hyperkalemic acidosis

Hyperkalemia: Treatment Protocol
$[K^+]_s > 5.0 \sim 5.5$

Signs and symptoms	Treatment

Mild Elevation: $[K^+]_s > 5.0 - 6.0$ mEq/L

Patient is without symptoms, **or** sensorium clear and only mild parasthesias are present, **and/or** EKG is normal or shows mild T wave changes (peaking or elevation)	Discontinue exogenous sources of K^+ (salt substitutes, medications and i.v. infusion with K^+, potassium-sparing diuretics) Liberalize salt intake as tolerated Repeat K^+ level ASAP to detect trend and confirm initial result If levels continue to rise institute treatment for moderate hyperkalemia regardless of signs or symptoms

Moderate Elevation: $[K^+]_s > 6.0 - 7.0$ mEq/L

Patient is without symptoms **or** shows parasthesias, mild weakness, **and/or** EKG is normal or shows T waves peaking/elevation, **and/or** P waves abnormality	Institute treatment for mild hyperkalemia [a]Administer an ion exchange resin such as sodium polystyrene sulfonate (Kayexalate®) 0.5–1.0 g/kg p.o. or by enema every 4–6 hr as needed (enema should be retained for approximately 30 minutes); $[K]_s$ fall is usually $\sim$ 0.5 mEq/L after 45 min Initiate an infusion of 25% glucose, 0.5 to 1.0 g/kg to run at 0.5–0.8 g/kg/hr (this will raise the glucose $\geq$ 250 mg/dl); begin with a bolus of the chosen solution, e.g., 1 ml/kg of 25% glucose Monitor serum K^+ level

Severe Hyperkalemia: [K]$_s$ ≥ 7.0 mEq/L

| Presence or absence of CNS symptoms, **and/or** EKG shows widening of QRS complex and/or loss of waves | Initiate treatment to reverse cardiac effects immediately: 10% calcium gluconate 1.0 ml/kg i.v. slowly (monitor heart rate for bradycardia) **and/or** NaHCO$_3$ infusion 1-2 mEq/kg i.v. If etiology is in doubt or episodes repeat continue searching for etiology |

[a]If at any point the K$^+$ is rising in disproportion to expectations or symptoms are progressive, make immediate preparation for dialysis while instituting drug regimen to reverse electrophysiologic effects for membrane.

K, Potassium.

Signs and Symptoms of Hypokalemia

See Fig. 3 for pathophysiology of hypokalemia.

1. Mild hypokalemia (serum potassium level 3.0–3.4 mEq/L)

    a. Slight weakness

    b. Flattening of T waves on electrocardiogram

2. Moderate hypokalemia (serum potassium level ≤2.5 mEq/L)

    a. Weakness, ileus, gastric distention

    b. Flat or changing T wave patterns on electrocardiogram

3. Severe hypokalemia (serum potassium level <2.5 mEq/L)

    a. Profound weakness, possibly affecting striated and smooth muscle

    b. Prolonged Q-T interval and widening of QRS complex on electrocardiogram

    c. Possible cardiac arrhythmias

Differential Diagnosis

1. Decreased potassium intake (e.g., surgery or food preferences)

2. Increased renal excretion

    a. Diuretics

    b. Acid-base disturbance [e.g., exogenous alkali load, diabetic ketoacidosis (DKA)]

    c. Mineralocorticoid excess: (1) Cushing's syndrome; (2) Primary hyperaldosteronism

    d. Edema-forming states

    e. Malignant hypertension

    f. Bartter's syndrome

    g. Magnesium deficiency

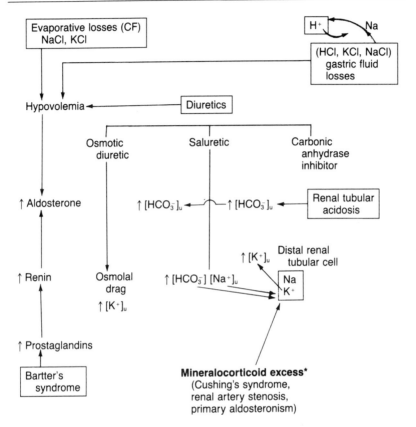

FIG. 3. Pathophysiology of hypokalemias. CF, cystic fibrosis; $[HCO_3]_u$, urine bicarbonate concentration; $[Na^+]_u$, urine sodium concentration; $[K^+]_u$, urine potassium concentration. These entities make use of the important mechanism of Na^+-K^+ exchange in conditions of ↑ Na^+ delivery to the distal tubules. ($NaHCO_3$ may also be exchanged.)

3. Extrarenal losses

   a. Gastric losses

   b. Profuse sweating

   c. Large intestinal losses

Hypokalemia: Diagnostic Protocol

    The medical history and physical examination in each of the differential diagnostic entities will often reflect metabolic alkalosis associated with secondary hyperaldosteronism; signs and symptoms of this state include increased respiratory rate, mild hypovolemia or dehydration, increased frequency of urination, increased amount of urine (compatible with potassium nephropathy and lack of concentrating ability), hypertension (possibly renin-aldosterone-induced associated with muscle weakness, paresthesias, sensorial changes, glucose imbalances, and cardiographic abnormalities).

Medical History	Physical examination	Laboratory investigations
Decreased Potassium Intake: Surgery, Food Fads		
Changes in dietary habits, recent surgery with prolonged administration of solutions containing minimal amounts of potassium, and/or drugs that interfere with potassium absorption or enhance excretion	Recent surgical scar may be present Parasthesias and/or weakness Paralytic ileus or gastric dilation	Elevated blood urea nitrogen, slightly elevated CBC, increased bicarbonate and decreased chloride levels indicate hypovolemia Urinalysis:May or may not reflect concentrated urine depending on the extent of potential potassium nephropathy; glucose may be present reflecting glucose intolerance; Occult blood may indicate rhabdomyolysis or myoglobinuria; urine sodium and chloride levels may be low
Increased Renal Excretion: Diuretic-Induced		
Change in medication or addition of new medication accompanied by increased excretion of dilute-appearing urine	Usually, no specific findings, possible glaucoma suggesting a carbonic anhydrase inhibitor	Nonspecific findings as in decreased potassium intake, electrocardiogram may show T wave flattening or reversal, depression of S-T segments, increased U wave voltage
Increased Renal Excretion: Diabetic Ketoacidosis		
Diabetes Mellitus chapter		
Increased Renal Excretion: Mineralocorticoid Excess (Cushing's Syndrome and Primary Hyperaldosteronism)		
Recent weight gain Change in fat distribution Growth retardation Possible ambiguous genitalia History of increased licorice ingestion Possibly nonspecific signs and symptoms of hypertension	Ofen severe, nonlabile hypertenion Renal artery bruit Presence of buffalo hump, skin striae, trunkal obesity	Urine and plasma studies for specific steroid considered, diurnal cortisol levels, aldosterone secretion rates, angiography

Increased Renal Excretion: Bartter's Syndrome

Growth retardation nongenetically induced, possible seizures	Short stature, normotensive, weak	Nonspecific laboratory tests as in decreased potassium intake, elevated renin and aldosterone levels, elevated levels of certain prostaglandins[a] No specific tests

Edema Forming States

Compatible with the specific edema-forming state	Congestive heart failure, cirrhosis, nephrotic syndrome	No specific tests

Extrarenal Losses: Profuse Sweating (Cystic Fibrosis)

Cystic fibrosis in the family Please refer to Cystic Fibrosis chapter	Failure to thrive Hypertrophic osteoarthropathy Foul smelling stools	Positive iontoelectrophoresis

Extrarenal Losses: Gastric Losses (Pyeloric)

Protracted vomiting	Nonspecific or compatible with obstructive lesion Small child with nonspecific findings	Nonspecific findings of metabolic alkalosis and contraction; positive upper GI series for obstruction

Extrarenal Losses: Congenital Alkalosis and Diarrhea (Chloride-losing)

Persistent and refractory in first few weeks of life Familial disorder (usually in patients of Scandinavian extraction)	Small child with nonspecific findings	Nonspecific as with other metabolic alkaloses Elevated stool chloride (above 50 mEq/L) Minimal urine chloride (less than 10 mEq/L)

[a]Definitive treatment of this disorder has been noted with prostaglandin synthetase inhibitors such as indomethacin and aspirin.

Hypokalemia: Treatment Protocol
$[K^+]_s < 3.5$ mEq/L

Signs and Symptoms	Symptomatic treatment
Mild Decrease: $[K^+]_s \geq$ 3–3.4 mEq/L	
Patient is without symptoms **or** has slight weakness **and/or** early flattening of T waves	Correct underlying defect Discontinue any means of iatrogenic K^+ loss Initiate K^+ replacement (p.o. preferred) 3–4 mEg/kg Monitor $[K^+]_s$ as well as urine K^+ levels to determine renal ability to conserve concentrate $[K^+]_u$

Moderate Decrease: $[K^+]_s \geq 2.5$ mEq/L

Patient is weak **and/or** ileus and/or gastric distention are prominent **and/or** EKG shows flat or negative trends	Institute treatment for mild hypokalemia Administer potassium chloride, in a concentration of 30 to 40 mEq/L, as an i.v. infusion (maximum K^+ dose, 20 mEq/hr) If condition shows no improvement, **cautiously** increase K^+ dose until desired effect, with monitoring of electrocardiogram and $[K^+]_s$ level

Severe Decrease: $[K^+]_s \leq 2.5$ mEq/L

Weakness may be profound, increasing affect on striated and smooth muscle EKG may show prolonged Q-T interval and widening of the QRS complex Cardiac arrhythmias may occur	If cardiac or muscle disturbances are severe infusions of K^+ may be increased to 30–40 mEq/L hr with frequent serum and cardiac monitoring

SODIUM IMBALANCE

Sodium is the most prevalent cation in extracellular fluid. It is actively extruded from the intracellular to the extracellular compartment in an effort to maintain the serum sodium concentration at a constant level. In addition, sodium levels in the extracellular fluid are maintained relatively constant by fluctuation in vasopressin release, with its concomitant water uptake. The body is also well adapted to handling maximal changes in sodium intake within a period of hours to days, whereas comparable mechanisms for potassium compensation require days to weeks.

Sodium salts are handled primarily by renal excretion (filtration and tubular reabsorption). Aldosterone is the major regulator of urinary sodium excretion. It exerts its action in 30 to 60 min by the induction of an intracellular or membrane-bound protein in the distal tubular area. A "phantom" factor called natriuretic hormone has continued to elude investigators. There is consensus, however, that this factor acts in a more immediate manner than aldosterone and provides a rapid saluretic response to volume expansion.

Because sodium does not have the same electrophysiological effect on muscles as potassium, alterations in serum sodium levels are often not as dramatic clinically. Pulmonary edema, hypernatremic dehydration, or hyponatremic seizure activity may occur with significant alterations in the serum sodium level. Vomiting, diarrhea, and dehydration are often present. Fever may or may not be present. The symptoms of dehydration are often exacerbated in patients with hyponatremia and are not as evident in patients with hypernatremia at the same levels of total body water loss.

Hypernatremia

Figure 4 gives the pathophysiology of hypernatremia.

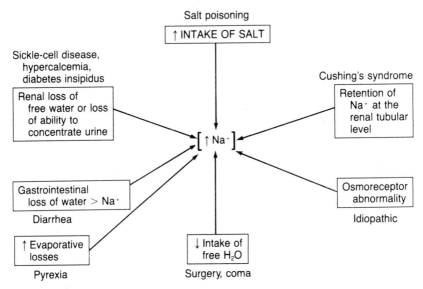

FIG. 4.   Pathophysiology of hypernatremic states. [Na$^+$], sodium concentration.

Differential Diagnosis

Total body increase in sodium:

1. Cushing's syndrome

2. Conn's syndrome

3. Salt poisoning

4. Salt infusion during abortion or resuscitation

Normal total body sodium:

1. Renal losses of water

    a. Nephrogenic diabetes insipidus

    b. Central diabetes insipidus

    c. Hypercalcemia

2. Extrarenal losses (respiratory and evaporative)

Total body decrease in sodium:

1. Renal losses (osmotic diuretic)

2. Extrarenal losses

    a. Excess sweating

    b. Diarrhea

Hypernatremic dehydration:

1. Diabetic ketoacidosis
2. Reye's syndrome
3. Acute abdomen
4. Increased intracranial pressure
5. Intoxications (especially salicylism)

Hypernatremia: Diagnostic and Treatment Protocols

Diagnostic and treatment protocols for hypernatremia are given in Fig. 5.

Hyponatremia

Figure 6 shows the pathophysiology of hyponatremia.

Differential Diagnosis

Normal or slight increase in extracellular fluid volume:

1. Syndrome of inappropriate ADH secretion
2. Myxedema
3. Drugs (nicotine, cyclophosphamide, indomethacin)
4. Sick-cell syndrome (resetting of "osmostat" to a lower level)
5. Primary polydipsia

Expanded extracellular fluid volume:

1. Congestive heart failure
2. Nephrotic syndrome
3. Acute or chronic renal failure
4. Portal hypertension

Decreased extracellular fluid volume:

1. Renal sodium losses
   a. Addison's disease
   b. Drug abuse
   c. Salt-losing nephropathy
   d. Osmotic diuresis
2. Extrarenal losses
   a. Gastrointestinal
   b. Burns
   c. Third spacing of fluids

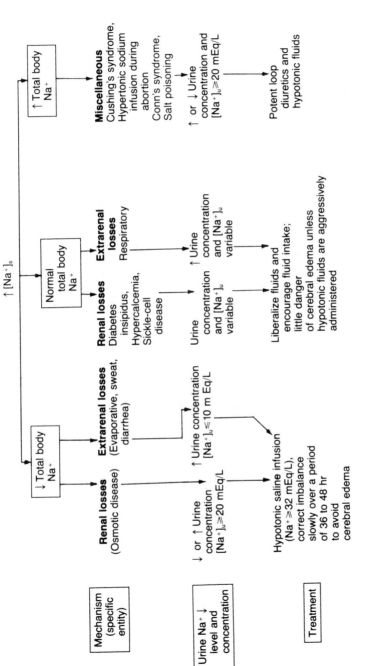

FIG. 5. Diagnostic and treatment protocols for hypernatremia. [Na$^+$]$_s$, serum sodium concentration; [Na$^+$]$_u$, urine sodium concentration. (Modified from *Kidney International*, with permission.)

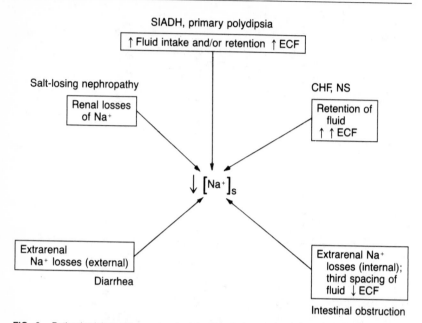

FIG. 6. Pathophysiology of hyponatremic states. $[Na^+]_s$, serum sodium concentration. CHF, congestive heart failure; NS, nephrotic syndrome; ECF, extracellular fluid; SIADH, syndrome of inappropriate antidiuretic hormone secretion.

Hyponatremia: Diagnostic and Treatment Protocols

Figure 7 gives the diagnostic and treatment protocols for hyponatremia.

APPENDIX 1
Fluid Requirements for Hospitalized Children with No Ongoing Fluid Losses

---

Normal urine output (≥ 1 ml/kg/hr) is assumed for all fluid requirements. Urine output of less than 1 ml/kg/hr is considered oliguric and fluid requirements should be adjusted accordingly. Daily obligatory water loss by the kidneys is proportional to their concentrating ability and to the amount of solute brought to the kidneys. For each 100 calories metabolized, 15 to 25 mOsm are developed.

$$\text{Urine volume} \; \frac{\text{mOsm}}{\text{Urine concentration}}$$

Surface Area

Fluid requirements tend to correlate best with body surface area. This method of calculating fluid requirements works most efficiently for children who weigh 8 to 10 kg (usually older than 13 to 14 months of age). By this method, the normal fluid requirement is approximately 1,500 ml/m²/24 hr. See Table 1.

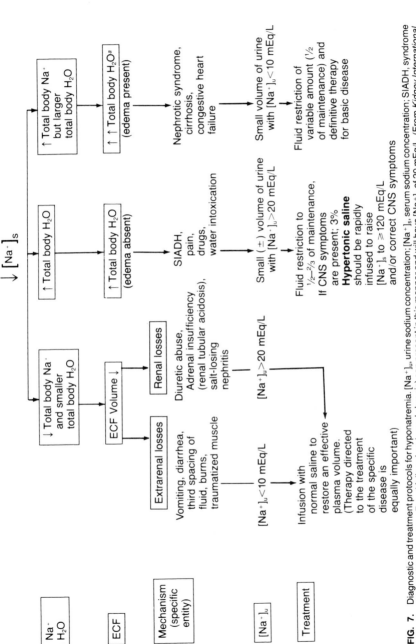

FIG. 7. Diagnostic and treatment protocols for hyponatremia. [Na+]u, urine sodium concentration; [Na+]s, serum sodium concentration; SIADH, syndrome of inappropriate ADH secretion. aRenal failure (acute and chronic) can present in this manner and will have [Na+]u of 20 mEq/L. (From *Kidney International,* with permission.)

Calories Expended

Fluid requirements are extrapolated from metabolic needs. By this method, the normal fluid requirement is 100 to 150 ml/100 calories metabolized.

Body Weight

This is the simplest but probably the least exact way of measuring fluid requirements. This method should be mastered by resident pediatricians before they attempt to use the more finite methods described above. This method presupposes fluid requirements of 100 ml/kg for the first 10 kilograms of body weight, 50 ml/kg for the next 10 kilograms of body weight, 20 ml/kg for the remaining kilograms of body weight. This method of calculation should not be used in neonates. (See Table 2.)

TABLE 1.

Age	Weight (kg)	Surface area (m²)
Newborn	2.5–4.0	0.20–0.23
1 week–6 months	3.0–8.0	0.30–0.35
6–12 months	8.0–12.0	0.35–0.45
1–2 years	10.0–15.0	0.45–0.60

TABLE 2.

Weight (kg)	24-hr Water requirement
2.5–10.0	100 ml/kg
>10.0–20.0	1,000 ml + 50 ml/kg over 10 kg
>20.0	1,500 ml + 20 ml/kg over 20 kg

APPENDIX 2. *Fluid and electrolyte concentrations in body fluids*

	Normal	Hypoperfusion (functional injury)	Fixed injury (parenchymal)	Excess ADH
Urine output	>1–2 ml/kg/hr	↓	↓ or ↑	↓
$[Na^+]_u$	Varies with salt intake, state of hydration	<20 mEq/L	>50 mEq/L	>20 mEq/L
$[Osm]_u$	Varies with salt intake, state of hydration	>500 mOsm	~300 mOsm	>300 mOsm
FE_{Na}	~1%	<1%	>2%	>2%
$[Osm]_u/[Osm]_s$ ratio	Varies, but usually >1.0	>1.5	<0.8–1.2	>2.0
BUN/Cr	10/1	>20/1	Progressive increase	Variable

$[Na^+]_u$: Urine sodium concentration; $[Osm]_u$: Urine osmolality; FE_{Na}: $[Na]_u \times [Cr]_s / [Cr]_u \times [Na]_s$ = amount of $[Na^+]_u$ relative to $[Na^+]_s$ that would have been excreted if all glomerular filtrate were excreted; $[Na^+]_s$: Serum sodium concentration; $[Cr]_u$: Urine creatinine concentration; $[Cr]_s$: Serum creatinine concentration; $[Osm]_s$: Serum osmolality.

APPENDIX 3. *Electrolyte concentrations in various oral solutions*

	Na (mEq/L)	K (mEq/L)	Cl (mEq/L)	HCO_3 (mEq/L)	Calories/L
Milk	22	36	28	30	670
Coca Cola®	0.4	13	—	13.4	435
Pepsi®	6.5	0.8	—	7.3	480
Orange juice	0.2	49	—	50	540
Lytren®	~25	25	30	20	280
Gingerale	3.5	0.1	—	3.6	360
Breast milk	7	13	11	—	666
Infant formula	6.7	19	16	—	666

APPENDIX 4. *Electrolyte concentrations in various intravenous solutions*

	Na (mEq/L)	K (mEq/L)	Cl (mEq/L)	HCO_3 (mEq/L)
Saline	154	—	154	—
3% Saline	513	—	513	—
Ringer's lactate	130	4	109	(±28)
25% Albumin (human)	130–160	—	—	—
Plasma	146	5	105	25

Foreign Bodies

Aspiration or ingestion of foreign objects is a common pediatric problem. A rapid and accurate diagnosis is essential for appropriate management. Some incidents may be relatively benign and require no therapeutic intervention (e.g., the ingestion of a penny by a 3-year-old child). However, ingestion of benign foreign objects should alert the practitioner to the possibility of future ingestion incidents or pica and may indicate the need for special and specific health education and laboratory screening tests (e.g., complete blood cell count and lead level).

SIGNS AND SYMPTOMS

Signs and symptoms of ingested, aspirated, or inserted foreign bodies vary with location. The diagnosis is most often made on the basis of clinical evaluation; few laboratory tests are needed. A high index of suspicion is required for the diagnosis to be made.

Various normal developmental landmarks predispose children to ingestion, aspiration, or insertion of foreign objects. An insatiable curiosity plus oral stimulation and gratification in exploration of the environment, along with an increasingly accessible environment as ambulation is achieved, are responsible for many incidents. Depending on the location of the foreign body and the age of the child, abuse and/or neglect should be a consideration in some patients, especially those with genital trauma.

DIAGNOSTIC AND TREATMENT PROTOCOLS

Diagnostic and treatment protocols for incidents of foreign body ingestion are given in Table 1.

TABLE 1. *Foreign bodies: Diagnostic and treatment protocols*

Diagnosis	Treatment
Gastrointestinal	
Clinical evaluation: The history may be positive for the ingestion; signs and symptoms vary from none to those of an acute abdomen (acute obstruction and/or perforation); larger gastrointestinal foreign	Unless the foreign body is large, is causing obstruction, or is capable of lacerating or perforating the bowel, no treatment is necessary; observation is all that is required

Diagnosis	Treatment

bodies may cause obstruction at the level of the cricoid cartilage, the cardio-esophageal junction, the pylorus, the ligament of Treitz, the ileocecal valve, or the anal canal (areas of physiological narrowing of the lumen)

Dysphagia and vomiting may occur with esophageal foreign bodies

Radiographs: Radiopaque foreign bodies will visualize on a plain film (a swallowed coin will usually appear full face in the esophagus and on end in the trachea on a posterior/anterior film; the opposite is true on lateral films)

Complete blood cell count

Blood lead level

Esophageal foreign bodies may be extracted endoscopically

Surgical intervention may be required if there is obstruction of the lumen of the bowel or if there is perforation

Genitourinary

Clinical evaluation: There may be dysuria, urgency, frequency, incontinence, hematuria, pyuria, or urethral discharge; foul-smelling vaginal discharge suggests a vaginal foreign body

Urinalysis

Abdominal radiograph: May reveal a radiopaque foreign body

Radiographs with contrast: May reveal the (radiolucent) object by the presence of a filling defect or obstruction

Cystoscopy: Diagnostic and therapeutic

A vaginal foreign body may be palpated on a rectal examination

If appropriate, the child should be evaluated for suspected abuse or neglect

Cystoscopy: Usually used for diagnostic purposes, but might be used to remove small foreign bodies

Surgical removal: Frequently required for the removal of larger objects

Antibiotic therapy: May be required if infection is present, which is not unusual with the presence of a GU foreign body; the choice of antibiotic should be guided by the culture results and the organism's sensitivity pattern

A vaginal foreign body can frequently be removed by "milking" through the rectum; if this is not possible, and vaginal removal is required, general anesthesia may be necessary

Parental counseling and close follow-up

Nasal

Clinical evaluation: Unilateral profuse, foul-smelling discharge along with unilateral nasal obstruction suggests a nasal foreign body

Direct visualization

Radiographs with or without contrast: Contrast may be required if there is a posterior radiolucent obstruction

Culture and sensitivity of the discharge: Secondary infection is common

Removal of foreign bodies from the nose must be done under controlled conditions; young children often require sedation (Demerol®, 2 mg/kg; Phenergan®, 1 mg/kg; and Thorazine®, 1 mg/kg)

Appropriate instruments and lighting are necessary

Care must be taken not to inadvertently push the object deeper into the nose, making extraction more difficult or creating a pharyngeal foreign body that may be aspirated

If anterior removal is impossible, intentional creation of a pharyngeal foreign body with subsequent removal under controlled conditions to avoid aspiration may be required

Secondary infections should be treated with appropriate antibiotics

TABLE 1. *(continued)*

Diagnosis	Treatment
Ocular	

Clinical findings: Vary with the type, location, and depth of penetration

A conjunctival foreign body may cause local irritation or unilateral generalized conjunctivitis

Corneal foreign bodies usually cause intense pain, decreased vision, and circumcorneal flush

Fluorescene staining: May be required to delineate the location or presence of the object

Slit lamp examination

Unless conjunctival and superficial, ocular foreign bodies should be treated by an ophthalmologist

Lavage with normal saline may remove a loose conjunctival foreign body

The affected eye should be patched during transport of the patient to the ophthalmologist

Otic

Clinical findings: Otalgia and/or foul-smelling purulent otorrhea are suggestive of a foreign body in the ear; commonly inserted objects are paper clips, small clips, rubber bands, corn, peas

Direct visualization: Usually reveals the object in the external auditory canal

No specific diagnostic tests are required; pneumo-otoscopy, tympanography, and audiography may be required after extraction

Attempts to remove otic foreign bodies should be done under controlled conditions

Lavage of the external canal may dislodge the object; care must be taken not to lavage small dehydrated objects (e.g., small vegetables), since they swell with rehydration and become more difficult to remove

Sedation may be required (see Nasal foreign bodies and Appendixes for sedation protocols)

If removal is difficult, it should be done by an otolaryngologist; care must be taken not to be too vigorous in attempting to remove an otic object, since it may be pushed deeper into the canal, making extraction more difficult and causing tympanic membrane disruption or ossicular disruption

Pulmonary

Clinical findings: Acute onset of choking or coughing and respiratory distress in a previously normal child; distress varies from minimal to severe with complete obstruction; wheezing may be the only symptom; presentation depends on the location and size of the object aspirated

The foreign body is usually a small toy or other object that can be held in the mouth; the episode is most often preceded by laughing, playing, or running while holding the food or toy in the mouth

Chest radiograph: A plain film may show a radiopaque object, hyperinflation, or it may be normal

Inspiratory and expiratory radiographs: The film taken on inspiration may be normal; the film taken on expiration may show unilateral hyperinflation and a mediastinal shift away from the side of the foreign body

Heimlich maneuver for laryngeal foreign bodies causing complete airway obstruction; rapid firm pressure exerted over the epigastrium with two fingers for an infant or clenched fists in the older child or adult frequently causes forced expulsion of the object

Tracheal and bronchial foreign bodies are most often removed bronchoscopically with the patient under general anesthesia

Bronchodilators and postural drainage are ineffective in removal of bronchial foreign bodies and are contraindicated in the management of aspiration incidents

The Heimlich maneuver should not be attempted as the primary treatment in smaller children and infants; four sharp blows to the back with the heal of the hand with the patient in a head down position are recommended

Diagnosis	Treatment
Fluoroscopy: Asymmetrical excursions of each hemithorax Bronchoscopy: Diagnostic and therapeutic A missed foreign body should be suspected when a patient presents with recurrent wheezing and/or a persistent infiltrate on radiograph	

Frostbite

Frostbite is a thermal injury resulting from exposure to extreme cold. Soft tissue freezes and necrosis occurs (Fig. 1). Environmental factors that affect tissue injury are temperature, wind velocity, relative humidity, and duration of exposure. The areas most commonly affected are the tips of the ears, fingers, toes, exposed areas of the legs, and the cheeks or nose. Slapped cheek appearance sometimes occurs in winter months in children who are well protected from the cold except for the face.

SIGNS AND SYMPTOMS

Paresthesias and numbness are the first signs of frostbite. The overlying skin is red, then becomes pale, white, or obviously cyanotic. Vesiculation and bullae formation may occur.

DIAGNOSTIC PROTOCOL

1. The diagnosis of frostbite is made on the history of exposure to cold and the clinical appearance of tissue.
2. No specific laboratory tests are required for the diagnosis.
3. Secondary infection and gangrene may occur. Cultures of the affected areas may be indicated.

TREATMENT PROTOCOL

1. The affected areas should be rapidly rewarmed.
   a. Mild frostbite or very small areas may be rewarmed by covering the tissue with warm hands.
   b. Severe involvement or large areas may be rapidly rewarmed by immersion in a controlled temperature (103–107°F) bath. The time varies with the depth of injury (usually 20 min to 60 min is adequate).
2. The following procedures are **contraindicated.**
   a. Rewarming frostbitten area if refreezing is possible.
   b. Dry heat.
   c. Rubbing affected areas with snow or ice.

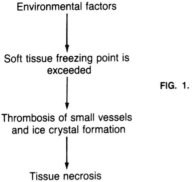

Environmental factors

↓

Soft tissue freezing point is
exceeded

FIG. 1. Pathophysiology of frostbite.

↓

Thrombosis of small vessels
and ice crystal formation

↓

Tissue necrosis

3. Analgesics may be required for pain.

4. Local therapy is essential.

    a. Keep frostbitten areas clean; Phisohex® or Betadine® may be required.

    b. Bullae should be left intact.

    c. Avoid pressure on the frostbitten areas.

    d. Surgical debridement of necrotic tissue.

    e. Amputation should be delayed as long as possible; recovery is common, even
with severe injury.

5. Physical and occupational therapy, if necessary.

6. Antibiotics may be required if secondary bacterial infection occurs.

Gait Abnormalities

Gait abnormalities may be acute in onset or chronic in nature. It is essential to determine, early in the evaluation, the exact time of onset. The type of gait abnormality must also be determined by historical information (i.e., a description of how the disturbance began) and, most importantly, by direct observation of how the patient walks. The practitioner should observe the patient walking for approximately 20 feet in a straight line. Important historical information includes the presence or absence of pain (with active or passive motion of the extremities), time of onset, progression, type of shoes worn, the presence or absence or antecedent trauma, fever, or other concurrent symptoms.

The basic types of gait abnormalities include atalgic (limp), ataxic, waddling, and equinus (toe walking). Steppage, shuffling, and other types of gait abnormalities are usually associated with central or peripheral nervous system disease and are rare. The more common types of gait abnormalities are discussed in this chapter.

PATHOPHYSIOLOGY

The pathophysiology of gait abnormalities is directly dependent upon the underlying disease.

SIGNS AND SYMPTOMS

The diagnostic and therapeutic protocols are determined by the type of abnormality present. The type of abnormality can be described by observing and recording the characteristics of the gait style.

Atalgic Gait (Limp)

This type of gait abnormality is characterized by a short steppage phase on the affected extremity. There is most often pain or weakness present. Other signs and symptoms relate to the underlying etiology. If the limp is secondary to weakness (asymmetrical weakness signifying central or peripheral nervous system abnormality), pain and tenderness will be absent.

Ataxic Gait

An ataxic gait is unsteady and uncoordinated. It is often described as "drunken." The steps are uncertain and the patient has difficulty keeping balance. The symptoms may be exacerbated by (or the patient may not be able to perform) tandum walking, standing with feet together, hopping on one foot, or other coordinated alternating movements. The origin of the disturbance may be vestibular, cerebellar, or proprioceptive. A patient with generalized symmetrical weakness may also appear to be ataxic.

Equinus Gait

Equinus gait is toe walking. Affected children walk on the anterior metatarsal surfaces and toes. The heel does not touch the floor. It may be normal in young children first learning to walk, but also may be a sign of hypertonicity, spasticity, and/or shortening of the Achilles tendon.

Hemiplegic Gait

A hemiplegic gait is similar to an equinus gait, but there is associated flexion of the hips and knees when the patient walks. The upper extremities may be held in flexion.

Scissors Gait

A scissors gait is characterized by each step crossing the midline. It is usually associated with hypertonicity and spastic states.

DIAGNOSTIC PROTOCOL

Atalgic Gait Abnormalities

1. Most often associated with musculoskeletal abnormalities.

2. Asymmetrical weakness may result in a limp.

3. Possible external etiologies (i.e., tight fitting shoes, foreign bodies located in the foot or shoe).

4. Possible trauma or infection.

5. Evaluate hip, knee, ankle, and foot, as well as the long bone.

6. Radiographs of the hip, knee, ankle, and/or foot, depending on the physical findings.

7. Aspiration of the joint for a septic process within the joint space.

8. Nucleotide scans for possible bone infection.

Ataxic Gait Abnormalities

1. Generally associated with CNS disease or intoxications.

2. Associated with several metabolic and storage diseases.

3. Neurological evaluation.

4. Possible ingestion of a medication or poison.

5. Toxicology screening of blood and urine.

6. CT. scan for suspicion of a space occupying lesion.

7. Lumbar puncture for suspicion of infection or infiltrative process.

TREATMENT PROTOCOL

Atalgic Gait Abnormalities

The treatment is determined by the underlying cause.

1. Trauma is the most common cause of atalgic gait in childhood.
2. Joint disease or dysfunction (foot, ankle, knee, hip, pelvis).
3. Muscle pain or disease.
4. Tumors.
5. Infections (bone, joint, muscle, and soft tissue).
6. Osteochondritis.
7. Other less common neurological, orthopedic, and/or muscular abnormalities.

Ataxic Gait Abnormalities

The treatment is determined by the underlying cause.

1. Cerebellar ataxia (familial or primary).
2. Friedreich's ataxia.
3. Cerebral palsy.
4. Encephalitis.
5. Tumors or abscesses (cerebellar).
6. Guillain-Barré syndrome.
7. Lead poisoning.
8. Hydantoin poisoning.
9. Phenothiazine intoxication.
10. Degenerative CNS diseases.

Gastroesophageal Reflux

The symptom of regurgitation or vomiting is common in infancy. Frequently, it is due to gastroesophageal reflux, which results from a free retrograde passage of stomach contents into the esophagus. The presence of reflux is generally benign and will spontaneously resolve by the age of 18 months in approximately 60% of affected patients (Herbst, 1981). However, persistence of regurgitation and/or vomiting occurs in up to 30% of these patients. The remaining 10% will have significant sequelae (e.g., esophageal strictures or death) (Fig. 1).

SIGNS AND SYMPTOMS

The usual age at which the onset of symptoms is recognized is 6 weeks. Regurgitation and vomiting occur in almost all affected patients. Frequently, the vomiting is forceful and variable in relation to the time of feedings. Failure to thrive may occur because of the persistence of vomiting and the loss of calories and essential nutrients. There may be associated pylorospasm and symptoms associated with it.

Pulmonary symptoms are common. Vomiting need not occur for pulmonary disease to be present. Aspiration is thought to be the most likely cause of the pulmonary manifestations. Wheezing and bronchospasm are common and the patient may appear asthmatic.

Berquist and colleagues (1981) reported that 49% of patients with recurrent pneumonia and/or clinical asthma had concomitant gastroesophageal reflux. They found that the pulmonary disease improved in most of the patients who underwent antireflux management. Of those patients who were not helped by medical management, 92% improved or became asymptomatic after fundoplication.

Esophagitis may be manifested by chronic irritability. These patients frequently improve with antacid therapy. Hematemesis, melena, anemia, and esophageal stricture formation may also result from the esophagitis, caused by chronic reflux of gastric acid.

Unusual symptoms include Sandifer syndrome, rumination, and finger clubbing (Herbst, 1981).

DIFFERENTIAL DIAGNOSIS

1. Pyloric stenosis
2. Gastrointestinal atresias or webs
3. Partial small bowel obstruction
4. Electrolyte abnormalities

265

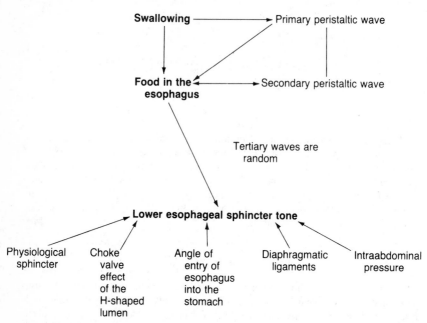

FIG. 1. Physiology of the esophageal sphincter. All of these factors participate in lower esophageal sphincter tone for the prevention of reflux. Variabilities in one or all will upset balance and may result in reflux.

5. Chronic renal disorders

6. Metabolic abnormalities

7. Systemic infections

8. Intoxications

9. Reye's syndrome

10. Gastrointestinal infections

DIAGNOSTIC PROTOCOL

If the baby is otherwise healthy and thriving, medical therapy may be instituted without diagnostic evaluation.

If failure to thrive is present or the symptoms are severe, further evaluation is indicated prior to instituting a therapeutic regimen.

Barium swallow (esophagogram) may show reflux and uncoordinated esophageal peristalsis and will rule out certain anatomical abnormalities; the volume of barium used is important and should approximate the volume of a normal feeding.

If the medical history and radiographic tests suggest gastroesophageal reflux, aggressive medical therapy should begin.

If there are inconsistencies between the medical history and radiographic studies, or if surgery is being considered, further diagnostic tests are indicated. The agreement of any two tests generally confirms the diagnosis.

1. Acid-reflux testing (Tuttle test): Tests for acid stomach contents in the esophagus. A pH probe is placed in the esophagus 3 cm above the sphincter; an acidic solution is placed in the stomach; the pH is monitored for 30 min; two episodes of pH <4.0 are considered diagnostic of reflux and treatment should begin; sensitivity of the test is >85%.

2. Esophageal manometry: Measures sphincter pressure (which is usually variable) and does not measure reflux; a difficult test to perform.

3. Endoscopy: Confirms the presence of esophagitis or its complications; usually requires general anesthesia or significant sedation.

4. Biopsy: Usually performed during the course of endoscopy; tissue may show changes consistent with gastroesophageal relfux (e.g., patches of columnar epithelium, increased basal epithelial layer thickness, and increased dermal peg size).

5. Extended pH monitoring: Esophageal pH is monitored over an 18- to 24-hr period, looking for frequency and length of reflux and the occurrence of reflux in various positions while child is awake and asleep.

6. Esophageal nucleotide scan: Detects reflux, volume of reflux and aspiration of gastric contents into the lungs; a sensitive test.

TREATMENT PROTOCOL

Medical Therapy

The approach is determined by the severity and type of presenting symptoms; the regimen should be individualized.

1. Counseling on feeding techniques: Do not overfeed the patient, burp frequently, no vigorous play after feeding, maintain upright position for 15 to 45 min after meals.

2. If simple modifications of feeding techniques fail, **strict positional therapy is indicated.**

    a. Place the child prone on a 30° incline plane after feedings and while awake; a special padded board is required (see Herbst, 1981).

    b. Small frequent feedings should be provided (in severely ill patients, continuous gavage feedings may be required).

    c. Thicken feedings with cereal.

3. If strict positional therapy fails, drugs may be required.

    a. Antacids and/or cimetidine may be indicated if esophagitis is present.

    b. Bethanechol, 8.7 mg/m^2, may be given in three divided doses; usually reserved for patients with severe symptoms.

Surgical Intervention

If medical therapy fails, fundoplication is the surgical procedure of choice; it will control the symptoms in approximately 95% of affected patients. Surgery is indicated in the following circumstances.

1. Severe life-threatening complications.

2. Intensive medical therapy has been attempted for at least 6 weeks without improvement of symptoms.

3. The patient is older than 18 months of age (the natural history of the disease shows improvement by that age).

H eadache

Headache is a symptom that must not be dismissed in children, because it is unlikely that it represents a psychogenic disorder in the very young as opposed to adolescents and adults. Deciding on a diagnostic approach is often difficult. The difficulties can be minimized if the diagnostic process is planned around a meaningful medical history, a complete physical examination, and an understanding of the current etiological classification of headaches in children. Whenever there is evidence of increased intracranial pressure or systemic illness, diagnosis should be directed toward the primary disorder.

CLASSIFICATION

Adults

1. Vascular headache

2. Muscle contraction (tension) headache

3. Traction, inflammatory headache

The Temporal Pattern of Headache (Table 1)

1. Single, acute episode of headache

2. Paroxysmal recurrent headache

3. Chronic progressive headache

4. Chronic nonprogressive headache

Each of these four groupings can be subclassified as due to:

1. Extracranial disease

2. Intracranial disease

3. Vascular disease

4. Psychogenic

Etiological

1. Mechanism of pain uncertain

   a. Migraine

      (1) Classical migraine (preceded by focal symptoms)

      (2) Common migraine (lacking prodroma)

      (3) Ophthalmoplegic (associated with transient paralysis of occulo-motor nerves)

      (4) Periodic migrainous neuralgia, cluster headaches, Horton's histamine cephalgia

TABLE 1. *Causes of headache according to the temporal pattern*

Acute extracranial headache
    Sinusitis: Frontal pain only in 13%; associated with cough, allergies, and rhinorrhea; diagnosed by skull radiograph
    Ocular abnormalities: Uncommon causes of headache; frontal; occurs after watching television or after schoolwork
    Dental disorders: Localized pain secondary to malocclusion; temporomandibular dysfunction; caries and abscesses
    Respiratory infections: Pharyngitis and otitis
    Trauma: Localized to area of acute trauma due to tissue injury; protracted trauma (postconcussion syndrome) associated with insomnia, irritability, personality change, memory problems, dizziness; focal signs require full investigation; periodic reevaluation
Acute recurrent headache
    Migraine syndrome: Genetic; intermittent vascular constriction and dilatation; triggered by stress, fatigue, trauma, exercise, illness, diet, menses and birth control pills; unilateral in adults; bilateral in children; vomiting and drowsiness follow attack
    Variants of migraine syndrome
        Classical: With visual aura
        Common: Without visual aura
        Cluster headache: Unilateral, orbital, lacrimation, rhinorrhea
        Ophthalmologic: Eye pain; if third cranial nerve is involved, palsy and/or ptosis may be present
        Hemiplegic: Recurrent paralysis; vascular malformation
        Basilar: Recurrent with paroxysmal ataxia, vertigo, and loss of consciousness
        Paroxysmal vertigo: With inability to maintain posture
        Confusional states: Paroxysmal; differentiate from encephalitis
        Cyclic vomiting: Paroxysmal, usually without headache
        Convulsive equivalent: As an aura (psychomotor seizures) or associated with headache and vomiting and/or electroencephalographic abnormalities
Chronic progressive headache (secondary to increased intracranial pressure)
    Tumors: Frontal or occipital headache exaggerated by cough; present in the morning; associated with vomiting
    Hydrocephalus
    Subdural hematoma
    Brain abscess
    Pseudotumor cerebri: Increased intracranial pressure without obstruction and without a mass lesion; CT scan is negative or may show small ventricles
Chronic nonprogressive (psychogenic)
    Conversion reactions; hysteria; malingering
    Perform psychometric testing

    (5) Hemiplegic migraine

    (6) Episodic facial pain

    (7) Facioplegic migraine

    (8) Retinal migraine (retinal ischemia with recurrent pain)

    (9) Cyclic vomiting

  (10) Convulsive equivalents

  b. Cluster headache (migrainous neuralgia)

  c. Tension headache

  d. Psychogenic headache

2. Muscle contraction

  a. Spasm

  b. Fatigue

3. Pain-sensitive structures (extra- or intracranial)

  a. Traction

  b. Inflammation

  c. Pressure

4. Vascular

  a. Distention of scalp vessels

  b. Arteritis

c. Angioma

d. Aneurysm

e. Hypertension

5. Sinusitis

   a. Infection

   b. Allergic

6. Respiratory

   a. Pressure (cough) headache

   b. Anoxia

7. Infection

   a. Viral or bacterial

   b. Fever

8. CNS disease

   a. Cerebrovascular accidents

   b. Neoplasm (primary or secondary)

   c. Meningitis or encephalitis

   d. Brain abscess

e. Posttraumatic

   (1) Immediate

   (2) Chronic: Subdural hematoma; postconcussion syndrome; postepileptic; neuralgia

f. As an aura in psychomotor seizures or as a convulsive equivalent with postictal state and abnormal electroencephalogram (EEG)

9. Eyes

   a. Eyestrain

   b. Glaucoma

   c. Refractive errors

10. Other

    a. Cervical arthritis

    b. Spondylosis

    c. Other referred pain

SIGNS AND SYMPTOMS

The manifestations of some common types of headache are shown in Table 2.

DIAGNOSTIC PROTOCOL

Because the medical history and physical examination determine the need for further evaluation, they must be as detailed and as accurate as possible.

Medical History

Obtain answers to all the following questions:

1. To determine the temporal pattern

   a. How did the headache begin?

   b. How long has it been present?

   c. How many episodes?

   d. Are the episodes getting worse or the same?

   e. How long does the headache last?

   f. What produces it?

TABLE 2. *Clinical manifestations of various types of headache*

Clinical manifestations	Cluster and migraine	Arteritis	Tension	Vascular	Intracranial disease
Duration of pain	Recurrent, with symptom-free periods	—	Long	—	Short, acute
Location of pain	Unilateral, anterior; common migraine is bilateral; cluster migraine is periorbital	Localized, temporal	Generalized, bi-occipital, band-like	—	Starts as unilateral and then becomes generalized or unilaterally occipital
Quality of pain	Throbbing and pounding	—	Pressing, squeezing	Throbbing and pounding	Explosive and intense
Prodromal symptoms	Euphoria, anorexia, or nausea; scotoma, hemianopsia, or dysphagia	—	—	—	—
Associated symptoms	Prodromal symptoms, transient blindness, lacrimation in cluster headaches	Fever, anorexia	Other psycho-physiological disturbances	—	Seizures, vomiting
Aggravating factors	—	—	Emotional factors	Alcohol, hypoxia, hormonal changes	Changes in head position, Valsalva maneuver, coughing
Characteristics	Migraine occurs at any time and persists for 6-36 hr; cluster headache is nocturnal; persists for 30 min to 1 hr and clinical findings are negative	More frequent in adults and older individuals	Persistent; worsens as the day progresses	—	No specific pattern, but usually persistent and progressive
Family history	Positive in migraine; negative in cluster headaches	—	—	—	Positive in the phakomatosis syndrome
Physical examination	Transient Horner's syndrome; flushed face, rhinorrhea and lacrimation occurs in cluster headaches	Fever, weight loss, anemia	Negative	High blood pressure	Papilledema, bruits, meningeal signs, focal neurological signs[a] or confusional state

[a] In some forms of CNS disease, focal signs may be absent (i.e., chronic subdural hematoma and midline neoplasms).

    g. Can you tell when it is going to happen?

    h. Where does it hurt?

    i. Does it make you stop activity?

    j. What makes it go away?

2. To rule out increased intracranial pressure and CNS disease (focal signs)

    a. Is there any lethargy or drowsiness?

    b. Is there any vomiting or nausea?

    c. Is there any ataxia?

    d. Is there any weakness?

    e. Are there any seizures?

    f. Are there any personality changes?

3. To rule out developmental problems

    a. Prenatal, natal and neonatal history

    b. Past illnesses

    c. Home and social environment

4. To rule out specific etiological disease

    a. History of trauma

    b. Family history of headaches or hypertension

    c. Accompanying symptoms, such as fever, rash, neck stiffness, visual disturbances

    d. Allergies

    e. Cyanotic congenital heart disease

Physical Examination

1. General examination (look for evidence of systemic disease)

    a. Blood pressure

    b. Growth parameters

    c. Inspection of skin (striae or pigmentation, café au lait spots, depigmented areas, petechiae)

    d. Fever

    e. Bruises

2. Eye examination

    a. Visual acuity

    b. Muscle movement (sixth nerve palsy may be a sign of increased intracranial pressure)

    c. Papilledema (acute increase in intracranial pressure)

    d. Optic atrophy (chronic increase in intracranial pressure) *e.* Intraocular pressure

  f. Visual fields

3. Neurological examination

  a. Emotional status

  b. Gait

  c. Head size and shape

  d. Intracranial bruits

  e. Cranial nerves

  f. Muscle strength and symmetry

  g. Reflexes (presence or absence and symmetry)

Laboratory Investigations

  If the medical history and physical examination are negative, no further investigation is warranted.

1. If there is suggestion of an organic cause, the following procedures are indicated:

  a. Complete blood cell count

  b. Urinalysis

  c. Erythrocyte sedimentation rate

  d. Chest radiograph

  e. Skull radiographs (look for erosions, calcifications, fractures, suture separation, sinus disease)

  f. EEG (look for epilepsy or convulsive equivalent, focal or generalized slowing)

  g. CT scan (to evaluate effects of trauma, vascular or degenerative disorders, neoplasms, bleeding, ventricular size, congenital malformations, effects of infection)

2. If any abnormalities are found, consider the following procedures:

  a. Angiography (reserved for progressive or vascular disease; should be preceeded by CT scan, except in emergencies)

  b. Pneumoencephalography (rarely needed except to evaluate the sella turcica or brainstem)

  c. Ventriculography

3. Other studies depend on etiological considerations; lumbar puncture is indicated in subarachnoid hemorrhage, encephalitis or meningitis. It is contraindicated if there is increased intracranial pressure, except in meningitis with papilledema.

TREATMENT PROTOCOL

1. Treat primary disorder, if identified.

2. Acute extracranial headaches

   a. Treat primary cause.

   b. Mild analgesics, such as acetaminophen (Tylenol®) 5 to 10 mg/kg repeated every 4 hr as needed for pain.

3. Migraine headaches

   a. Frequent attacks with aura: Cyproheptadine (Periactin®), 0.2–0.4 mg/kg/day in two or three doses, phenytoin (Dilantin®), 5–8 mg/kg/day in two doses, *or* propranolol (Inderal®), 10–30 mg three times a day prophylactically (Dilantin® and Inderal® should be given cautiously).

   b. Infrequent attacks: Sedatives, antiemetics, and analgesics.

   c. Older children and adolescents: Cafergot®, 1.0 mg at onset of aura and repeated in 30 min if symptoms persist; only two or three tablets may be taken for one single attack; if symptoms persist, continue with Tylenol®.

4. Convulsive equivalents: Dilantin®, 5 to 8 mg/kg/day in two doses, **or** barbiturates, 3 to 5 mg/kg/day in two doses.

5. Psychogenic headache

   a. Family counseling

   b. Psychotherapy

6. Tension headaches

   a. Analgesics

   b. Antianxiety drugs, such as chlordiazepoxide (Librium®), 5 to 10 mg two or three times a day.

   Note: Methysergide is not recommended for children.

Hematuria

The problem of hematuria (blood in the urine) exists in all age groups and therefore concerns the pediatrician, internist, general practitioner, and urologist. Gross hematuria is a symptom that rarely goes unnoticed, but it is usually no more dangerous prognostically than microscopic hematuria. Since gross hematuria is easily noticed and quite alarming, the patient usually seeks rapid medical attention and early treatment.

Even small amounts of blood in the urine may result in macroscopic hematuria. It has been reported that as little as 1 ml of blood added to a 24-hr urine sample of 1,000 ml will result in a gross color change. The passage of red, dark brown, or smokey colored urine may be the earliest clue to the presence of blood; however, it may reflect other substances that discolor the urine in a similar manner, some of which are of no importance.

Evaluating the cause of hematuria is a true challenge (Fig. 1) and requires diagnostic testing that may begin with a simple dipstick test of the urine and end with a renal biopsy. Most testing for blood in the urine is done by using the dipstick method, in which a reagent strip impregnated with a buffered mixture of organic peroxide and orthotoluidine is dipped in urine. The peroxidaselike activity of the hemoglobin, myoglobin, and some of their byproducts catalyzes the oxidation of orthotoluidine, resulting in a blue color. This test is more sensitive to free hemoglobin and myoglobin than to intact red blood cells; therefore, it is possible to have a urine sample with only three to five red blood cells in the high power field and yet have an intense discoloration of the dipstick, reflecting free hemoglobin and myoglobin in the sample. Hemoglobinuria may result from the hemolysis of red blood cells within the circulation; more often it is caused by hemolyisis of the red blood cells in the urine because the urine has not been processed quickly and is alkaline or hypotonic.

Once hematuria has been documented, it is equally important to determine the presence or absence of proteinuria. The association of hematuria and proteinuria is of far greater significance than hematuria alone. Significant amounts of blood in the urine will, in itself, result in a positive test for protein; however, the amount of protein from the hemolyzed red blood cells does not exceed 2–3 + as measured on a protein dipstick.

SIGNS AND SYMPTOMS

The overall incidence of asymptomatic microscopic hematuria in children is less than 1%. The incidence rises in older children, who are more prone to collagen, vascular, and other multisystem diseases. Also, the signs and symptoms of microscopic hematuria are often minimal and may come to the physician's attention only after

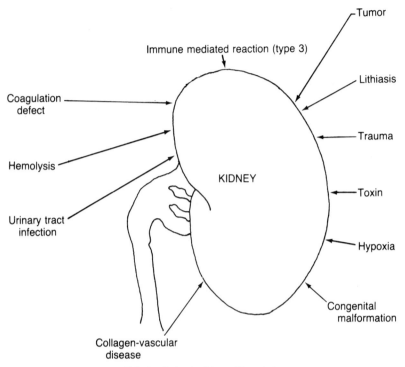

FIG. 1. Pathophysiology of hematuria.

detection during a screening examination. One possible exception to this paucity of symptoms is the anxiety created when there is gross hematuria. Most clinical manifestations are related to the disease causing the hematuria. See Figs. 2 and 3 for evaluating hematuria.

DIFFERENTIAL DIAGNOSIS

1. Conditions simulating hematuria (various substances and conditions cause urine discoloration, which may simulate hematuria): Bilirubin pigment and its derivatives, carotene pigments, pyridium, porphyria, various foods (e.g., beets, blackberries), some vegetable dyes, drugs (phenothiazines and phenytoin), and, occasionally urates

2. Hematuria unrelated to any intrinsic diseases of the urinary tract: Menstruation, coagulation defects, masturbation, exercise, foreign body, meatitis, and vaginitis

3. Myoglobinuria

4. Hemoglobinuria

5. Neonatal hematuria

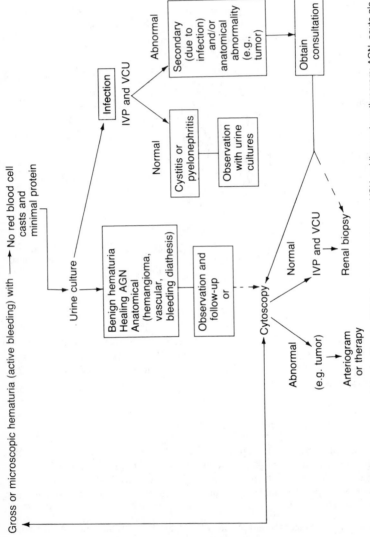

FIG. 2. Hematuria with no red blood cell casts. IVP, intravenous pyelogram; VCU, voiding cystourethrogram; AGN, acute glomerulonephritis.

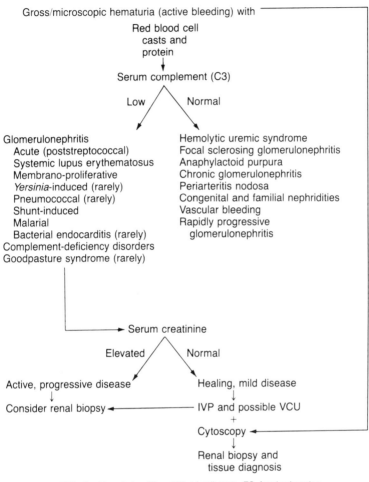

FIG. 3. Hematuria with red blood cell casts. FS, focal sclerosing.

   a. Large kidney hematuria syndrome (renal vein thrombosis, tubular necrosis, uric acid nephropathy, medullary necrosis, and renal artery thrombosis)

   b. Polycystic disease

   c. Obstructive disease

   d. Neoplastic disease

   e. Congenital anomalies (arteriovenous malformations)

6. Hematuria in children

   a. Poststreptococcal glomerulonephritis

   b. Collagen-vascular disease

c. Bacterial endocarditis

d. Trauma

e. Familial congenital disorders

f. Tumor

g. Renal calculi

h. Urinary tract infections

i. Chemically induced (cyclophosphamide, Cytoxan®)

j. Foreign body

k. Idiopathic hypercalciuria

DIAGNOSTIC PROTOCOL

Medical History

1. Birth trauma or asphyxia

2. Hypotension

3. Oliguria

4. Manipulation of genitourinary tract with a foreign body

5. Trauma to the abdomen

6. Familial history of renal disease

7. Renal lithiasis

8. Drug use, especially those known to cause irritation of the bladder or intravascular hemolysis

9. A burn or crushing injury

10. Coagulopathy or vascular abnormality

11. Hemoglobinopathy

12. Metabolic or inborn error of metabolism

13. Urinary stream abnormality

14. Initial or terminal hematuria

15. Allergies

16. Orthostatic component to hematuria

17. Recent infection, especially streptococcus, or exposure to individuals with recent infection

Physical Examination

1. Systolic and/or diastolic hypertension

2. Dermatological lesion and location thereof

3. Edema or anasarca

4. Arthritis and/or arthralgias

5. Cardiomegaly or cardiac sounds (extra sounds, increase or decrease in intensity, murmurs, and/or rubs)

6. Pulmonary system, evidence of effusion or infiltrates, as well as bronchospasm

7. Presence or absence of organomegaly

8. Evidence of any genital lesions

9. Miscellaneous findings: Recent hair loss, intermittent urethral or rectal discharge, musculoskeletal weakness, nuchal rigidity, or headache

Laboratory Investigations

1. Primary screening tests (microscopic hematuria)

   a. Complete blood cell count with peripheral smear, platelets, reticulocyte count, erythrocyte sedimentation rate, electrolytes, blood urea nitrogen, creatinine

   b. Complement levels and antistreptolysin-O titer (Streptozyme® test, if available)

   c. Throat culture

   d. Urinalysis, urine Gram stain and culture

   e. Consider intravenous pyelogram

2. Negative primary screening tests with persistent bleeding and/or progressive symptoms:

   a. Calcium, phosphorus, alkaline phosphatase, uric acid

   b. Antinuclear antibodies test and anti-DNA test

   c. Immunoglobulin levels

   d. Creatinine clearance and urine protein excretion

   e. Australian antigen

3. Macroscopic/microscopic hematuria (see Figs. 2 and 3)

   a. Laboratory tests (as above)

   b. Consultation with urologist

   c. Cystoscopy

   d. Renal biopsy (see Table 1)

TABLE 1. *Contraindications to percutaneous renal biopsy*

Absolute	Relative
Unilateral kidney	Atypical renal position (high, low, rotated)
Coagulation abnormality	Pregnancy
Malignant disease or perinephritis	Severe hydronephrosis
Polycystic disease	Suspected renal vein thrombosis
Uncontrolled hypertension	Renal artery aneurysm
Small kidneys	Uremia (if chronic, kidneys may also be small and the associated bleeding diathesis may cause severe bleeding)

Hepatitis

Hepatitis means inflammation of the liver. The etiologies are varied, ranging from infections and infestations to toxic and/or metabolic processes. The prognosis for the various causes differs, making an accurate etiological diagnosis important (Fig. 1). Regardless of the cause, treatment is generally similar (with minor variations), unless the specific etiological agent is amenable to therapy (e.g., parasitic infestation of the liver).

SIGNS AND SYMPTOMS

The severity of the illness varies from asymptomatic subclinical involvement of the liver manifested only by biochemical changes to acute hepatic failure and death. Fever (usually low grade), anorexia, nausea, vomiting, and abdominal pain are frequently present, making the differentiation from acute gastroenteritis difficult clinically. Clinical jaundice is usually present, but many children may be anicteric throughout the entire illness. Other nonspecific symptoms of hepatitis include weakness, cephalgia, malaise, diarrhea, and/or constipation. Pruritus is uncommon. Acholic stools and dark urine (due to increased urinary excretion of bilirubin) may be seen. Occasionally, patients may present with a bleeding diathesis secondary to deficient production of liver-dependent clotting factors. Hepatomegaly and abdominal tenderness are common. Splenomegaly is present in approximately 15% of affected patients.

Other signs and symptoms of hepatitis depend on the clinical etiology. Generalized adenopathy is usually present with infectious mononucleosis, although patients with infectious hepatitis may also have generalized adenopathy. Conjunctivitis and meningeal signs are commonly present in patients with leptospirosis.

DIFFERENTIAL DIAGNOSIS

Liver abnormalities must be differentiated from entities such as influenza, pneumonia, appendicitis, or acute gastroenteritis, which may present with similar or identical symptoms.

Once liver involvement is established, the following diagnoses must be differentiated:

1. Hepatitis A
2. Hepatitis B
3. Non-A, non-B hepatitis

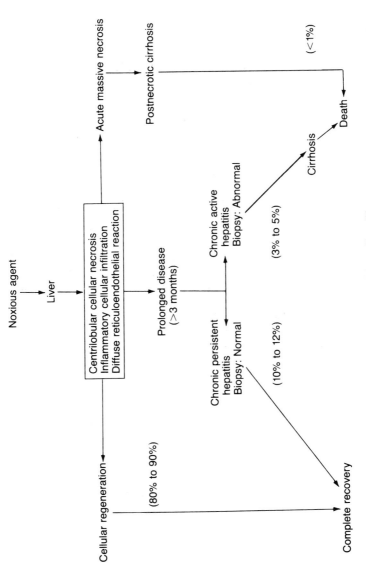

FIG. 1. Pathophysiology of hepatitis.

4. Other viruses: Coxsackie virus, ECHO virus, Epstein-Barr virus, herpesvirus, adenovirus

5. Leptospirosis

6. Chronic liver disease

7. Liver abscesses

8. Hepatic drug reactions (e.g., carbon tetrachloride, toluene, trichloroethylene, mithramycin, chlorpromazine, isoniazid, erythromycin estolate, acetaminophen)

DIAGNOSTIC PROTOCOL

1. Complete blood cell count: Usually normal; may show a relative lymphocytosis and granulocytopenia early in the disease.

2. Urinalysis: Increased urinary excretion of urobilinogen.

3. Serum bilirubin: Increased; the direct reacting fraction is increased early; indirect reacting fraction is elevated during recovery.

4. SGOT and SGPT: Elevated early in the disease; their fall heralds recovery.

5. Prothrombin time (PT) and partial thromboplastin time (PTT): Usually abnormal when there is significant liver disease; if they are prolonged, hospitalization is usually indicated.

6. Viral antigens and antibodies: The most common are HB_sAg, HB_sAb, hepatitis A antibody, Epstein-Barr virus titers, heterophil antibody test (Monospot®), toxoplasma titers, and cytomegalovirus titers.

7. Leptospirosis agglutination test: If there is conjunctivitis and/or meningismus.

8. Toxin screening: If a toxic hepatopathy is considered; include screening for common drugs.

9. Chest radiograph and flat plate radiograph of the abdomen: If pneumonia or an acute abdomen is considered.

10. Liver biopsy: Usually reserved for patients with persistent symptoms or persistent enzyme elevations for more than 3 months.

TREATMENT PROTOCOL

1. There is no specific treatment for hepatitis; care is supportive and symptomatic.

2. Affected patients should be followed closely at 4-week intervals for the appearance of chronic disease.

3. Prophylaxis:

   a. Prophylaxis is required for direct household contacts and school contacts, only in nursery-like situations where the children are in intimate contact (e.g., nap together).

b. Prophylaxis is not required for less intimate contacts (e.g., usual contacts at school or in apartment building).

c. Hepatitis A prophylaxis: 0.02 to 0.04 cc/kg of gamma globulin.

d. Hepatitis B prophylaxis: immune serum globulin, **or** 0.12 cc/kg of gamma globulin.

4. Corticosteroid treatment is contraindicated; steroids increase the incidence of chronicity of the disease.

Hepatosplenomegaly

Although hepatomegaly and splenomegaly may occur independently, they are considered together because they share a common differential diagnosis and a similar diagnostic plan. The involvement of one organ requires investigation of the other organ.

By definition, a palpable spleen is an enlarged spleen. This, however, is not true of the liver. Hepatomegaly is present only if an abnormal liver span is demonstrated on percussion of the upper border (behind the right rib cage) and the lower border (below the right costal margin) of the liver. The normal liver span at various ages is shown in Table 1.

The liver, and not infrequently the spleen, are normally palpable at birth to about 2 cm below the costal margins. Occasionally, this may persist up to the age of 1 year.

PATHOPHYSIOLOGY

The mechanisms of enlargement of the liver and spleen are shown in Table 2.

DIFFERENTIAL DIAGNOSIS

The differential diagnosis of hepatosplenomegaly is shown in Table 3.

DIAGNOSTIC PROTOCOL

Medical History

1. Family history of similar problems.
2. History suggestive of prenatal or neonatal infections.
3. History of jaundice.
4. Associated symptoms.

Physical Examination

Because hepatosplenomegaly is often a reflection of disease in other organs, an accurate physical examination of all systems is indicated (see Table 3).

Laboratory Investigations

Laboratory investigation should be guided by the medical history and physical findings.

TABLE 1. *Normal liver span at various ages*

Age	Liver span (cm)	Age	Liver span (cm)
<5 yr	7 ± 2	10–14 yr	9 ± 2
5–9 yr	8 ± 2	Adult	12 ± 2

TABLE 2. *Mechanisms of liver and spleen enlargement*

Hepatomegaly[a]	Splenomegaly
Inflammation	
Intra- and extrauterine infection, hepatitis, hepatic abscess, parasitic infection, drugs, biliary tract obstruction	Intra- and extrauterine infection, tuberculosis, systemic fungal infections
Hyperplasia	
Sepsis, malignancy, granulomatous reaction	Viral infections (e.g., infectious mononucleosis, cytomegalovirus), endocarditis, sepsis
Congestion	
Congestive heart failure, Budd-Chiari syndrome (venous obstruction)	Portal hypertension seen in chronic hepatitis, cystic fibrosis, Wilson's disease, biliary atresia, infection of umbilical vein, portal vein thrombosis, splenic trauma, sequestration of sickle cell disease
Infiltration	
Tumors, leukemias, and lymphomas, erythroblastosis	Leukemia, lymphomas, metastatic neuroblastoma, histiocytosis
Storage	
Glycogen storage, mucopolysaccharidosis, Gaucher's disease, Neimann-Pick disease, gangliosidosis, α-antitypsin deficiency, amyloid, hepatic porphyrias	Lipid storage diseases (see below)
Accumulation of Fat	
Malnutrition, hyperalimentation, cystic fibrosis, diabetes, galactosemia, Wolman's disease, Reye's syndrome	Tay-Sachs disease, Gaucher's disease, Neimann-Pick disease, metachromatic leukodystrophy, gangliosidosis
Primary Tumor	
Polycystic liver, telangiectasia, hepatoblastoma, hepatoma	Splenic hemangiomas, cysts, and cystic hygroma
Other	
—	Hemolytic disease

[a]A smooth and tender liver suggests acute enlargement seen in congestive hepatomegaly, acute infection, or inflammation; a nodular liver suggests chronic conditions or tumors; ascites or edema indicate chronic conditions; parenchymal liver disease is associated with spider nevi, gynecomastia, palmar erythema, and splenomegaly; hepatic tumors may produce a friction rub over the liver.

TABLE 3. *Differential diagnosis of hepatosplenomegaly*

Condition	Associated findings
Newborn	
Intra-or extrauterine infection	Microcephaly, hydrocephaly, rashes
Erythroblastosis	Jaundice in first day of life
Biliary tract obstruction	Prolonged jaundice
Neonatal hepatitis	Prolonged jaundice
Congestive heart failure	Evidence of heart disease
Hepatitis	Prolonged jaundice
Sepsis	Fever, lethargy, poor feeding
Infants	
Cystic fibrosis	Abnormal breath sounds, abnormal stools, testicular abnormalities
Metabolic (storage disease)	Enlarged spleen and liver; neurological abnormalities, macular degeneration
Histiocytosis	Eczema, chronic otitis, anemia
Hypervitaminosis (vitamin A) and malnutrition	Gingival inflammation; papilledema, craniotabes, carotenemia
Tumors and cysts	Cystic kidney, hematological abnormalities
Children	
Toxic	History of drug ingestion (all drugs should be suspected)
Parasitic (larva migrans)	—
Leukemias	Bleeding tendencies, fever, lymphadenopathy, anemia, and pancytopenia
Congestive	Signs of portal hypertension (e.g., various hemorrhoids), history of umbilical vein catheter and jaundice
Older Children and Adolescents	
Hepatitis	RUQ, pain and tenderness, anorexia, jaundice
Juvenile rheumatoid arthritis	Iritis, erythema nodosum, arthritis, fever
Drugs	Drug ingestion (all drugs should be suspected)
Lymphomas	Lymphadenopathy, fever, weight loss
Wilson's disease	Kayser-Fleischer ring, cataract, gingival inflammation, neurological abnormalities
Porphyrias	—

RUQ = right upper quadrant.

1. First-stage orders

    a. Complete blood cell count with platelet count, reticulocyte count, and smear evaluation.

    b. Urinalysis, routine and for reducing substances.

    c. Urinary bilirubin and urobilinogen.

    d. Liver function tests: Total and direct serum bilirubin, SGOT, SGPT, lactic dehydrogenase, and alkaline phosphatase.

e. Serum chemistry studies, including total protein, albumin-to-globulin ratio, blood urea nitrogen, fasting blood glucose, and cholesterol.

f. Prothrombin time.

g. Purified protein derivative (PPD) test.

h. Upper gastrointestinal series.

i. Chest radiograph.

j. Coombs test.

Suspected Hematological Disorder

1. Serum electrophoresis.

2. Hemoglobin electrophoresis.

3. Bone marrow aspirate.

4. Fragility and autohemolysis tests.

Suspected Infection

1. Appropriate cultures.

2. Appropriate skin tests.

3. Congenital infection ("torch") and other titers.

4. Heterophile antibodies.

5. Skull radiographs.

If the above tests are not diagnostic, further tests are indicated.

1. Second-stage orders

a. Liver and spleen scans.

b. Liver, spleen, gall bladder ultrasound studies (kidneys may be included).

c. Skeletal radiograph survey.

d. Acid phosphatase.

e. Antinuclear antibody tests, including anti-DNA; rheumatoid factor.

f. Sweat chloride.

g. Serum vitamin K, α_1-antitrypsin, serum copper oxidase level.

h. 24-hr urinary excretion of porphyrin and copper.

If there is still no diagnosis, the following procedures are suggested.

1. Third-stage orders

a. Asymptomatic patient with mild hepatosplenomegaly and normal growth and development: Observe and reevaluate periodically.

b. Asymptomatic patient with marked hepatosplenomegaly or symptomatic patient: Lymphangiography, gallium scan, liver and/or spleen scan, and/or lymph node biopsy, skin biopsy, rectal biopsy, laparotomy.

Note: Any of the causes of hepatomegaly may produce direct or indirect hyperbilirubinemia. Albumin is decreased in chronic cases. Liver enzymes may be elevated in any condition. Alkaline phosphatase is highest in infiltrative processes. If the patient is jaundiced (see Table 4).

TABLE 4. *Differential diagnosis of laboratory and clinical findings*

Type of jaundice	Direct bilirubin	Stools	Urine bile	Urine urobilinogen	Alkaline phosphatase	SGOT (IU)
Hemolytic	↑ (>50%)	nl	Absent	Present	nl	nl
Hepatocellular	↑	Acholic	Present	—	<10	>300
Obstructive	↑	Acholic	Present	—	>10	<300

nl = normal.

Histiocytosis

The histiocytosis syndromes (reticuloendothelioses, histiocytosis X) are usually described as distinct disease entities. However, most authorities believe that each descriptive entity is part of a continuum of a single disease process. All are characterized by a common pathological lesion in which there is granuloma formation with histiocytic proliferation. The etiology is unknown. Some describe the lesion as a neoplastic process, whereas others believe it to be a borderline (or quasi) neoplasm (Fig. 1).

SIGNS AND SYMPTOMS

The disease may present in any form or may progress along the continuum and exhibit the entire spectrum of clinical manifestations (see Diagnostic and Treatment Protocols).

DIAGNOSTIC PROTOCOL

Eosinophilic Granuloma of Bone

1. There may or may not be pain and/or swelling of one or multiple sites.
2. The most common age at onset is 4 to 7 years.
3. Radiographs show lytic lesions of the bone.
4. The long bones, skull, and pelvis are the most common sites.
5. Biopsy: Tissue diagnosis is required.

Hand-Schüller Christian Disease

1. Usually multiple bone lesions; mild papuloseborrheic skin lesions (usually mild mucuous), membrane involvement; occasional invasion of the orbit, causing exophthalmos; occasional invasion of the hypothalamic-pituitary axis, causing diabetes insipidus.
2. The most common age at onset is 2 to 3 years.
3. Anemia is common.
4. Biopsy: Tissue diagnosis is required along with clinical correlation.

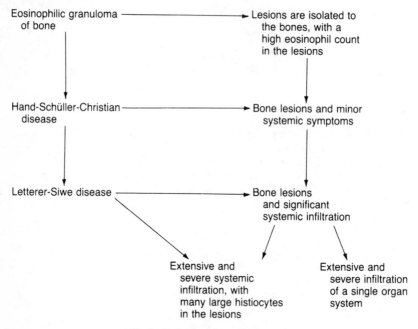

FIG. 1. Pathophysiology of histiocytosis.

Letterer-Siwe Disease

1. This form represents a more extensive systemic infiltration of the pathological process.

2. The age at onset is usually <2 years (the younger the patient, the more fulminant and invasive the disease).

3. Hepatosplenomegaly and generalized lymphadenopathy are common.

4. Thrombocytopenia and anemia reflect bone marrow infiltration.

5. Pulmonary infiltration appears as a miliary, granular, or honeycomb pattern.

6. Severe secondary infections and mucosal involvement occur.

7. Severe skin manifestations (papuloseborrheic eruptions, petechial rashes, and desquamative dermatitis) are present.

8. Bone lesions are present, but are usually not symptomatic.

9. Death is common.

TREATMENT PROTOCOL

Eosinophilic Granuloma of Bone

1. No specific treatment is available.

2. Continuously painful lesions may be successfully treated with low doses of radiation.

3. The lesions usually resolve spontaneously 1 to 2 years after the diagnosis is made.

Hand-Schüller Christian Disease

1. No specific treatment is available.

2. Continuously painful bony lesions, skin lesions, or lymphadenopathic lesions of the lymph system may be successfully treated with low doses of radiation.

3. Low-dose radiation to the hypothalamic-pituitary axis may be required in patients with diabetes insipidus.

4. Vasopressin (Pitressin®) therapy may be required in patients with diabetes insipidus.

Letterer-Siwe Disease

Treatment usually takes the form of one of several chemotherapeutic (anticancer) regimens; antileukemic and antilymphoma regimens are most often used; medications administered alone or in combination include chlorambucil, vinblastine, methotrexate, 6-mercaptopurine, procarbazine, and prednisone.

Hodgkin's Disease

Hodgkin's disease is the third most common malignancy in childhood. More than 60% of affected patients are male (some studies cite a male-to-female ratio of 3:1). The disease is more common in adults, but the most common age range of presentation in the pediatric age group is during adolescence; it is unusual in children younger than 5 years old. Immunosuppressed patients and those with immunologically based diseases (e.g., systemic lupus erythematosus, juvenile rheumatoid arthritis) have a significantly higher incidence of Hodgkin's disease.

PATHOPHYSIOLOGY

The etiology and pathogenesis of malignant transformation are unknown, but the illustrated mechanisms have been postulated (Fig. 1).

SIGNS AND SYMPTOMS

The disease classically presents as painless swelling of a cervical lymph node or group of nodes. Systemic manifestations intially are rare in children unless the disease process is extensive. The lymph nodes in the axillary, inguinal, mediastinal, and retroperitoneal regions may also be involved. When palpable, the nodes tend to feel rubbery, discrete, and firm. The histologic characteristics of the disease are described in Table 1. The characteristic relapsing fever seen in adults (Pel-Ebstein) is usually not seen in childhood.

DIFFERENTIAL DIAGNOSIS

1. Lymphadenitis (infectious)
2. β-Streptococcal pharyngitis
3. Infectious mononucleosis
4. Branchial cleft cyst
5. Toxoplasmosis
6. Cytomegalovirus infection
7. Other tumors
   a. Neuroblastoma
   b. Non-Hodgkin's lymphoma

DIAGNOSTIC PROTOCOL

1. Obtain the medical history and perform a complete physical examination.

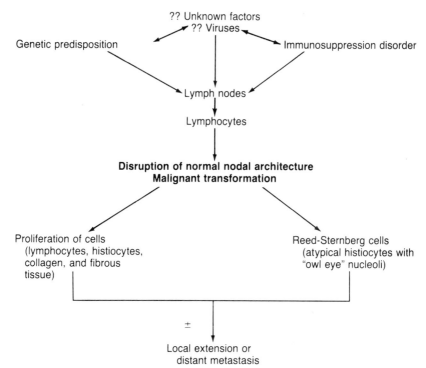

FIG. 1. Postulated mechanisms of malignant transformation in Hodgkin's disease.

2. Search for processes causing lymphadenopathy:

   a. Complete blood cell count

   b. Urinalysis

   c. Monospot® (heterophil antibody) test

   d. Epstein-Barr virus titers

   e. Cytomegalovirus and toxoplasma titers

   f. Throat culture

TABLE 1. *Histologic characteristics of Hodgkin's disease*

Nodular sclerosing
　Occurs in 50% of patients; intermediate prognosis
Mixed cellularity
　Occurs in 25% of patients; intermediate prognosis
Lymphocyte predominance
　Occurs in approximately 20% of patients; best prognosis
Lymphocyte depletion
　Occurs in 5% of patients; extremely fulminant; most ominous prognosis

g. Liver function tests

3. Chest radiograph and purified protein derivative (PPD) test (special attention should be paid to the mediastinum).

4. If initial assessment favors the diagnosis of tumor rather than infection, a lymph node biopsy is essential.

5. Once the diagnosis is established by biopsy, the following procedures should be considered for accurate staging:

   a. Intravenous pyelogram

   b. Skeletal survey

   c. Lymphangiogram

   d. Bone marrow biopsy

   e. Tomography (if mediastinum is involved)

   f. Exploratory laparotomy: Splenectomy, liver biopsy, lymph node biopsy (multiple samples)

TREATMENT PROTOCOL

---

1. Diagnosis and treatment of patients with Hodgkin's disease should be done in consultation with an experienced pediatric oncologist and hematologist

2. Treatment depends on the stage of disease (Table 2):

   a. Stage I: Radiation

   b. Stage IIa: Radiation

   c. Stage IIb: Radiation and/or chemotherapy

   d. Stage III: Radiation and/or chemotherapy

   e. Stage IV: Chemotherapy (nitrogen mustard, vincristine, procarbazine, and prednisone)

3. Administer supportive and symptomatic therapy for complications of the disease and its treatment; some complications of treatment include growth retardation, spinal deformities, myelosuppression, nausea, and vomiting.

TABLE 2. *Clinical or operative staging of Hodgkin's disease*

Stage I: The tumor is limited to one lymph node region or two contiguous anatomical regions on the same side of the diaphragm
Stage II: Malignancy exists in more than two regions on the same side of the diaphragm
Stage III: Malignancy exists on both sides of the diaphragm, but is limited to lymphatic tissue
Stage IV: There is widespread disease, extending beyond the lymphatic system

---

Each stage is divided into substages A and B. Substage A indicates the absence of fever, night sweats, and weight loss >10% of total body weight. Substage B indicates the presence of such findings.

Hypertension

The recognition that hypertension occurs with some regularity in children (1.4% to 11%) and the knowledge that its detection and treatment can prevent or delay many serious sequelae have resulted in a marked interest in the epidemiology, measurement techniques, tracking, and aggressive therapy of hypertensive children. The American Academy of Pediatrics has recently recommended that all children, on attaining the age of 3 years, have their blood pressure measured as part of their routine examinations. As early as the first month of life, infants of hypertensive parents will tend to have higher blood pressure and more recent investigations may soon allow the detection of children at risk by the use of hypertensive markers (Na^+-K^+ red blood cell flux, urine kallikrein). Thus, it may become possible for pediatricians to detect and treat hypertension in its earliest stages (Fig. 1).

SIGNS AND SYMPTOMS

Clinical features of increased blood pressure are so nonspecific and diffuse that only a high index of suspicion allows the diagnosis. In primary hypertension, only exogenous obesity is present often enough to be statistically significant as a physical finding. Unless the blood pressure is inordinately elevated or hypertension is of long-standing duration, a casual examination may be unremarkable. Headaches and nosebleeds are unusual and, if related to blood pressure, indicate markedly raised levels. Signs and symptoms of hypertension, such as blurred vision, convulsions, or congestive heart failure, are quite rare and usually are associated with secondary forms of hypertension. Thus, their presence should direct the examiner to focus on known potential anatomical changes (e.g., abdominal bruits, decreased femoral pulses).

DIFFERENTIAL DIAGNOSIS

1. High normal blood pressure
2. Sustained elevated blood pressure
3. Fixed elevated blood pressure
   a. Primary hypertension (essential)
   b. Secondary hypertension
      (1) Renal disorders (e.g., acute acquired, chronic acquired, congenital structural malformation, tumors, renal vascular abnormalities)
      (2) Cardiovascular abnormalities (e.g., coarctation or hypoplasia of the aorta)

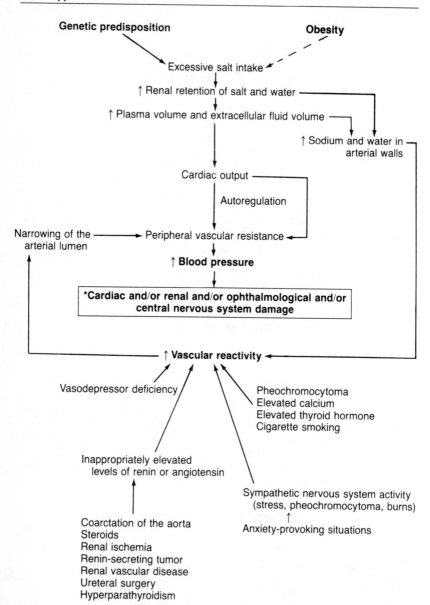

FIG. 1. Pathophysiology of hypertension. *Major potentially affected target organs.

(3) Endocrine disorders (e.g., adrenal, parathyroid, thyroid)

(4) Collagen-vascular diseases (e.g., systemic lupus erythematosus, periarteritis nodosa)

(5) CNS abnormalities (e.g., tumors, trauma, inflammation)

(6) Drugs or toxins (e.g., sympathomimetics, oral contraceptives)

(7) Burns

(8) Orthopedic procedures (e.g., leg lengthening, traction or stretch procedures)

(9) Genitourinary procedures (e.g., ureteral surgery)

(10) Hypercalcemia (e.g., sarcoidosis, immobilization, exogenous administration of calcium)

(11) Porphyria

(12) Dysautonomia

(13) Stevens-Johnson syndrome

DIAGNOSTIC PROTOCOL

High Normal Blood Pressure

1. Definition: The asymptomatic child who, on any casual blood pressure measurement, has a single blood pressure elevation (systolic and/or diastolic) above the 95th percentile for age and sex.

2. Investigations

    a. Comprehensive hypertensive history, including historical information about blood pressure in first degree relatives, renal disease, myocardial infarction, and stroke, blood pressure in siblings, and drug treatment and prior illnesses in patient.

    b. Thorough physical examination, including fundoscopy and abdominal examination.

3. Follow-up: Two repeat blood pressure examinations at 2- to 3-week intervals, by the same examiner and the same equipment, if possible; if both measurements exceed the 95th percentile, the child should be placed in the sustained elevated blood pressure category.

Sustained Elevated Blood Pressure

1. Definition: The asymptomatic child who has blood pressure elevations (systolic and/or diastolic) above the 95th percentile on three separate occasions 2 to 3 weeks apart (the child will not necessarily develop fixed hypertension); if target organ damage is present, the child should be placed in the category of fixed elevated blood pressure.

2. Investigations

a. Medical history and physical examination as in high normal blood pressure.

b. Laboratory tests: Complete blood cell count, urinalysis and culture, electrolytes, blood urea nitrogen, creatinine, cholesterol, chest radiograph, electrocardiogram, echocardiogram.

3. Follow-up: Examinations every 2 to 3 months for 1 year; if repeat blood pressure measurements continue to be elevated, the child should be placed in the category of fixed elevated blood pressure.

Fixed and/or Symptomatic Elevated Blood Pressure

1. Definition: The child with a prior diagnosis of sustained elevated blood pressure, who after follow-up for approximately 1 year, continuously has blood pressure elevations exceeding the 90th percentile, with a majority of the recordings above the 95th percentile (child may or may not be symptomatic) or a newly presenting child who is symptomatic from the elevated blood pressure and usually has blood pressures at least 10 to 20 mm Hg above the 95th percentile.

2. Investigations

a. Medical history and physical examination as in the first two categories.

b. Laboratory tests as in the sustained category plus 24-hr creatinine clearance and protein excretion.

3. Follow-up:

a. If a strong family history of primary hypertension is present, and the child has no symptoms, specific signs, or suggestions of secondary causes, further testing is usually not indicated in children older than 10 years of age.

b. If further procedures are indicated, they should be individualized, but will most often include radionuclide renal studies and a hypertensive intravenous pyelogram.

c. Other tests [e.g., urine assay for vanillymandillic acids (VMA), selective angiography with renal vein-renin ratios, complement and antinuclear antibody studies, aldosterone secretion rate, 17-ketosteroids, Addis count] may be indicated but their need must be evaluated in relation to the statistical likelihood of the presence of specific disorders.

d. A nephrology consultant should be involved early in the diagnosis and treatment of hypertension.

TREATMENT PROTOCOL

Only medical therapy of fixed and/or symptomatic hypertension is discussed, as it is assumed that once a diagnosis of secondary hypertension is made the patient's condition will be stabilized and surgical therapy will be attempted.

Step care is a regimen that calls for initiating therapy with a small dose of an antihypertensive agent and increasing the dose of that drug before adding other drugs, one after another, as needed. Each of these steps should be supplemented by a nonspecific regimen called RISC: relaxation exercises, isotonic exercises (aerobics), salt restriction, and caloric restriction, as applicable.

1. **Treatment is advisable**

   a. Absent or mild symptoms and/or blood pressure 10 mm Hg above the 95th percentile.

   b. Nephrology consultation is warranted if not already obtained.

   c. Step 1: Thiazide diuretic (e.g., hydrochlorothiazide), 2.0 mg/kg/24 hr in a single dose.

   d. A trial of 4 to 6 weeks, with increasing doses every 2 weeks, should be attempted before control is judged inadequate and the step 2 treatment plan is instituted.

2. **Treatment is necessary**

   a. Mild to moderate symptoms and/or blood pressure 15 to 20 mm Hg above the 95th percentile.

   b. Target organ damage may be present.

   c. Step 2: Methyldopa, 10 to 40 mg/kg/24 hr in two to four divided doses, **and/or** propranolol hydrochloride, 0.5 to 1.0 mg/kg/24 hr in three or four divided doses.

   d. A trial of 2 weeks at each new dose and new medication is warranted to obtain control and avoid marked variations in blood pressure.

   e. Inadequate control with maximal drug levels (early side effects may preclude maximal doses) and/or acceleration of disease may necessitate institution of step 3 treatment plan.

3. **Treatment is mandatory**

   a. Moderate to severe symptoms or rapidly accelerating hypertension.

   b. Target organ damage is often present.

   c. Step 3: Hydralazine, 0.75 to 3.0 mg/kg/24 hr in three or four divided doses, **and/or** minoxidil, 0.1 to 0.2 mg/kg/24 hr in two divided doses.

4. **Emergency treatment**

   a. Signs and/or symptoms reflecting encephalopathy, renal failure, or congestive heart failure; the severity and clinical course will determine the aggressiveness of treatment.

   b. Acute clinical hypertension: Hydralazine, 0.1 to 0.2 mg/kg i.v. or i.m. every 6 to 8 hr, **and/or** reserpine, 0.07 mg/kg i.m. (maximum dose, 2.5 mg) every 8 to 12 hr, **and/or** furosemide, 0.5 to 1.0 mg/kg i.v. (not to exceed 5 mg/kg); repeat as needed.

   c. Hypertensive crisis: Diazoxide, 5.0 mg/kg by rapid i.v. infusion, **or** nitroprusside, 1.4 µg/kg/min by continuous i.v. infusion may be used as the initial drugs in hypertensive emergencies; furosemide, 0.5 to 1.0 mg/kg i.v. (not to exceed 5 mg/kg/dose) may be used as adjunctive therapy.

APPENDIX 1.

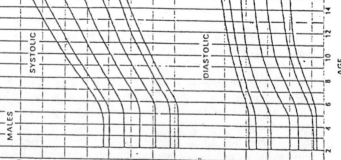

LEFT: Percentiles of blood pressure measurements in female patients (right arm, sitting position). **RIGHT:** Percentiles of blood pressure measurements in male patients (right arm, sitting position). [From National Heart, Lung, and Blood Institute (1977): Report of the task force on blood pressure control in children. *Pediatrics*, 59:797.]

Hypoglycemia

Hypoglycemia is not an infrequent problem in newborns, infants, and children. Significant hypoglycemia is defined as follows:

1. **Preterm newborns:** Blood glucose concentration <25 mg/100 ml on each of two determinations.

2. **Full-term newborns:** Blood glucose concentration <35 mg/100 ml on each determination in the first 72 hr of life and <45 mg/100 ml subsequently.

3. **Older infants and children:** Blood glucose concentration <50 mg/100 ml.

A low blood glucose concentration causes several adverse effects on the brain, even if the patient is asymptomatic. Failure to recognize, diagnose, and treat hypoglycemic episodes promptly may lead to brain damage, especially in newborns. Intravenous glucose administration may be necessary before the diagnosis is made in a very sick infant with nonspecific symptoms, particularly if the patient is at risk for developing hypoglycemia. In infants of diabetic mothers, hypoglycemia may occur as soon as 30 min after birth. In patients small for gestational age, twins, and infants of hypertensive mothers, hypoglycemic episodes usually occur 24 to 48 hr after birth. Such episodes should be anticipated and prevented.

PATHOPHYSIOLOGY

Glucose is derived from a variety of sources through several metabolic pathways, including intestinal absorption, conversion of hexoses such as galactose and fructose, hydrolysis of polyglucoses such as starch and glycogen, and conversion of amino acids. These processes require the presence of adequate hormones and enzymes. Hypoglycemia may occur if any of these processes is interrupted. The various causes of hypoglycemia are listed in Table 1.

SIGNS AND SYMPTOMS

Clinically, newborns present with hyperinsulinism, decreased glucose stores, infection, metabolic disorders, endocrine disorders, and/or asphyxia. The resultant hypoglycemia is indicated by lethargy, floppiness, apnea, tremors, cyanosis, pallor, poor feeding, hypothermia, and/or a weak cry. Associated findings are bulging fontanelle, cardiomegaly, acidosis, low birth weight, or large infants.

Infants and children present with hyperinsulinism, hepatic diseases, endocrine disorders, ketosis, malabsorption, and/or metabolic disorders. These disturbances may

TABLE 1. *Causes of hypoglycemia*

Hyperinsulinism
    Pancreatic beta-cell tumors
    Pancreatic beta-cell adenomatosis
    Pancreatic beta-cell hyperplasia: Infants of diabetic mothers; erythroblastosis (primary and
        secondary; to exchange transfusion); Beckwith's syndrome with macroglossia,
        microcephaly, hepatomegaly, somatic gigantism and omphalocele; leprechaunism;
        panhypopituitarism (hypothalamic) associated with multiple endocrine problems and
        small phallus
    Prediabetes
    Leucine sensitivity
    Maple syrup urine disease
    Functional pancreatic secretory defects
    Functional extrapancreatic tumors, such as teratomas with pancreatic tissue
Hepatic enzyme deficiencies
    Glycogenosis: Glucose 6-phosphatase; amylo-1,6-glucosidase (debrancher enzyme);
        phosphorylase; glycogen synthetase
    Disorders of fructose metabolism: Fructose 1-phosphate aldolase (fructose intolerance),
        fructose 1,6-diphosphatase
    Disorders of galactose metabolism: Deficiency of galactose 1-phosphate uridyl transferase
        (galactosemia)
    Pyruvate carboxylase deficiency: With or without subacute necrotizing
        encephalomyelopathy (Leigh syndrome)
    Maple syrup urine disease and other amino acid disorders, such as cystinosis and
        tyrosinemia
Hepatic damage
    Primary liver disease
    Reye's syndrome
    Toxic liver damage
    Neoplastic infiltrations
Ketotic hypoglycemia
    Most common cause of hypoglycemia in children
    History of small-for-gestational-age at birth
Endocrine disorders
    Pituitary disorders: Growth hormone deficiency; ACTH deficiency with hypo- or
        hyperinsulinism
    Adrenal disorders: Hyper- or hypoplasia; glucocorticoid deficiency; medullary
        unresponsiveness
    Thyroid diseases: Hypothyroidism
    Hypothalamic dysfunction with or without other neurological disorders
Drug-induced
    Ethyl alcohol (ingested or after sponging to reduce the temperature of febrile infants)
    Salicylates or acetaminophen
    Sulfonylureas
    Propranolol
    "Bush tea" ingestion (Jamaican vomiting sickness)
    Hepatic toxicity (e.g., carbon tetrachloride, chloroform)
    EDTA
    Manganese
Other causes
    Malabsorption syndromes
    Renal glycosuria
    Malnutrition: Kwashiorkor; infants on low phenylalanine diets
    Primary neurological disease
    Idiopathic, spontaneous, postprandial
    Chronic diarrhea
    Biotin deficiency with glossitis and dermatitis
Neonatal hypoglycemia (in addition to aforementioned disorders)
    Infants of diabetic mothers
    Small-for-gestational age

Twin pregnancies
Prematurity
Infants delivered by cesarean-section
Erythroblastosis fetalis
Exchange transfusions with acid citrate dextrose blood
Maternal treatment with chlorpropamide
Sepsis and shock
Asphyxia
Hypothermia
Intracranial hemorrhage or any stress, such as respiratory distress
Intrauterine growth retardation and placental insufficiency
Reactive, following discontinuation of intravenous glucose solutions

result in weakness, faintness, headache, sweating, anxiety, incoordination, slurred speech, ataxia, visual disturbances, and/or hyperactivity. Associated findings are acidosis and hepatomegaly.

DIFFERENTIAL DIAGNOSIS

1. Adrenal insufficiency
2. Congenital heart disease
3. Narcotic/drug withdrawal symptoms
4. Hypocalcemia
5. Hypomagnesemia
6. Electrolyte disorders
7. Primary seizure disorders, including pyridoxine deficiency
8. Renal failure
9. Liver failure
10. Sepsis

DIAGNOSTIC PROTOCOL

1. In symptomatic newborns and newborns at high risk, treatment with intravenous and/or oral glucose is more urgent than obtaining a precise diagnosis. Once the treatment has begun, attempt to make an immediate diagnosis of hypoglycemia by blood glucose evaluation (Dextrostix®), Ames eye tone instrument (Ames Co., Division of Miles Laboratories, Inc., Elkhart, Indiana), and immediate and/or fasting blood glucose determination.

2. Medical history and physical examination: The findings may be specific enough to suggest the underlying disorder and thus guide the diagnostic evaluation (e.g., maternal history of diabetes, infections or drug ingestion, history of perinatal complications, and/or family history of hypoglycemia or other metabolic disorders).

3. If the patient presents with hypoglycemia of uncertain etiology, obtain blood samples for the following blood level determinations of glucose, β-hydroxybutyrate, amino acids, insulin, growth hormone, lactate, and ketones, and pH. Freeze some plasma for future tests if indicated, treat the patient if necessary, and proceed with diagnostic protocol.

First-Stage Tests

1. High carbohydrate diet for 3 days; allow nothing by mouth for 12 hr (6 hr for infants); obtain blood samples for fasting blood glucose level, insulin level, liver function tests, and urine for urinalysis.

2. Oral glucose tolerance test: Glucose, 2 g/kg (<2 years old), or 1.75 mg/kg (>2 years old), as corn syrup or as a 20% glucose solution with flavoring (commercial products may be used) using 150 mg/m^2; draw blood samples at 30, 60, 90, 120, and 180 min and at 4 and 5 hr for blood glucose determinations; collect urine at 1 and 2 hr for determination of urine glucose and ketone levels.

3. Intravenous glucose tolerance test: Use 0.6 mg/kg of 20% glucose; collect blood samples every 5 min for 45 min.

4. Following the glucose tolerance test, draw blood samples for determination of serum lactate, β-hydroxybutyrate, ketones, and pH.

5. Glucagon tolerance test: Glucagon, 20 to 30 mg/kg i.v. (maximum dose, 1 g); draw blood samples at 10, 20, 40 min and at 1 and 2 hr. (Carbohydrate function tests should be interrupted if the patient develops symptoms. Always have an intravenous line ready during testing.)

Interpretation and Second-Stage Tests

1. Normal glucose tolerance test: Fasting glucose level is achieved at 120 min and no hypoglycemia occurs at 4 or 5 hr.

2. Normal insulin level: Fasting insulin level is <10 μm/ml.

3. Normal glucagon tolerance test: A rise of glucose by at least 25 mg/dL within 15 to 45 min, and a rise of 10 mg/dL after a 24-hr fast; indicates normal hepatic glycogen and probably normal glycolytic function.

4. Normal β-hydroxybutyrate level: less than 0.5 mmoles/ml.

5. Retrial of fasting for 18 to 24 hr may produce hypoglycemia in ketotic hypoglycemia; if hypoglycemia occurs, do glucagon tolerance test; if there is no response, the diagnosis is ketotic hypoglycemia; if hypoglycemia does not occur, start the patient on a ketogenic diet and/or oral medium-chain triglycerides; in ketotic hypoglycemia, hypoglycemia and ketonuria will be precipitated.

6. If the patient does not have ketotic hypoglycemia but develops ketonuria, consider endocrine function tests, growth hormone, corticoids, and glucagon levels at beginning and end of fast; thyroid function tests; bone age determination; skull radiographs; CT scan.

7. Occurrence of abrupt and significant fall in blood glucose level between 30 and 60 min with normal or high insulin levels, decreased β-hydroxybutyrate, and normal glucagon tolerance test indicates high probability of hyperinsulinism.

8. Tests for hyperinsulinism

    a. Tolbutamide test: Tolbutamide, 20 mg/kg i.v. (maximum dose, 2 g) over a 1-min period; obtain blood samples at 0, 5, 10, 20, 30, 45, 60, 90 and 120 min; measure blood glucose and insulin levels (normally, glucose level falls 20% to 40% within 20–30 min, but in hyperinsulinism, the response is exaggerated).

b. Leucine sensitivity test: L-Leucine, 150 mg/kg p.o. as 2% solution or 75 mg/kg i.v. as 2% solution in 0.45% saline; obtain blood samples at 15–30 min; measure glucose and insulin levels (normally, insulin level increases slightly and glucose decreases by about 10 mg/100 ml; if leucine sensitivity exists, there will be a marked rise in insulin and profound hypoglycemia (in obesity, there may be a marked rise in insulin but glucose will decrease normally).

c. Trial of diazoxide (diagnostic and therapeutic): Diazoxide, 10 mg/kg/24 hr p.o. in two doses (failure to respond suggests a functional pancreatic tumor, e.g., adenoma, and laparotomy should be performed).

9. Occurrence of abnormal (nonspecific) or normal glucose tolerance test with slightly decreased, normal, or mildly increased insulin level, normal β-hydroxybutyrate level, abnormal glucagon level, normal or abnormal liver function tests indicates high probability of hepatic disorders (enzyme deficiencies), glycolytic dysfunction, starvation, or malnutrition.

10. Tests for hepatic disorders (enzyme deficiencies), glycolytic dysfunction, starvation, or malnutrition

a. Glucagon tolerance test with and without fasting: Failure to respond shows glucose 6-phosphatase deficiency; failure to respond when fasting or normal response without fasting shows debrancher enzyme deficiency; normal response when there is no hypoglycemia and an abnormal response during hypoglycemia shows ketotic hypoglycemia).

b. Fructose tolerance test: Fructose, 0.5 g/kg p.o. or 0.25 g/kg i.v. as 10% solution over a 4-min period; obtain blood samples for glucose, phosphate and lactate levels at 0, 15, 30, 45, 60, 90 and 120 min; glucose should be measured by the glucose oxidase method, which is specific for glucose (fructose intolerance or fructose 1,6-diphosphatase deficiency will be indicated by decreased glucose, increased fructose, decreased phosphate, and increased lactate levels).

c. Alanine tolerance test: L-Alanine, 500 mg/kg p.o. or 250 mg/kg i.v.; obtain blood samples at 0, 30, 60, and 90 min (glucose normally increases, but shows no change with fructose 1,6-diphosphatase deficiency; the already increased lactic acid level will increase further).

d. Galactosemia test: Specific enzyme assay; do not use the galactose tolerance test.

e. Liver biopsy.

f. Tissue enzyme assays.

g. Amino acid screen.

h. Flat curve on glucose tolerance test is compatible with malabsorption.

i. Delayed hypoglycemia on glucose tolerance test (at 3 to 4 hr) is compatible with hyperinsulinemia of prediabetes.

j. Delayed hypoglycemia (after 18 to 24 hr fast) is compatible with ketotic hypoglycemia.

TREATMENT PROTOCOL

Newborns

1. Well infant at high risk: Check blood glucose level at 3, 6, 12, and 24 hr of age; start early oral and/or gavage feeding with 10% dextrose every 2 hr until condition is stable.

2. Asphyxiated infant: Intravenous glucose should be given as part of the resuscitation.

3. Symptomatic infant: Dextrose, 0.5 to 1.0 g/kg (25% dextrose 2–4 cc/kg) i.v. push, at the rate of 1 cc/min; continuous i.v. drip, 4–8 mg/kg/min; glucagon, 30 mg/kg i.m.; if infant shows no response to above measures, consult endocrinologist.

Older Infants and Children

1. Start intravenous glucose.

2. Give small, frequent feedings.

3. Establish the cause of the hypoglycemia (glucagon, 1 mg i.m., may be given but there will be no response in patients with glucogenosis, hepatic disease, or ketotic hypoglycemia).

4. Treat the primary disorder.

5. Dietary manipulation may be necessary, depending on the cause of the hypoglycemia.

6. Ketotic hypoglycemia: Give 5 or 6 meals a day; increase protein and carbohydrate intake; in stress situations, give excess carbohydrate in liquid form.

7. Hyperinsulinism: Diazoxide, 10 mg/kg/24 hr p.o. in two doses; if no response, laparotomy is indicated; if no tumor is found, perform subtotal pancreatectomy; if hypoglycemia persists after pancreatectomy, give another trial of diazoxide; if hypoglycemia persists after pancreatectomy and the second trial of diazoxide, use steroids, further surgical intervention, streptozotocin (usually used for treatment of pancreatic carcinoma).

8. If the hypoglycemia has caused seizures, do an EEG; if EEG is abnormal, start the patient on antiseizure therapy.

9. Provide psychological support and further evaluation and follow-up.

Immune Deficiency Syndromes

From the moment a baby enters the world, his (or her) body is bombarded with potentially lethal foreign proteins. The infant's survival depends on his ability to defend himself against these exogenous substances. The immune system constitutes the principal means of defense. Recognition of a material by the immune system as foreign may "turn on" a protective mechanism by which the individual can ward off infection, or it may produce an allergic diathesis. This attempt to eliminate foreign antigens may be positive or may lead to potentially adverse clinical reactions. Thus, an allergy may be thought of as an adverse immune response.

In a predetermined manner, the immune system initially responds to foreign material with a nonspecific response consisting of inflammation and phagocytosis. If the substance is eliminated at this stage, the host response terminates. If the primary response results in the foreign material being "processed," a secondary, more specific, immune response is activated. The secondary response depends on the body's being previously exposed to the foreign substance and involves the B-cell system (the antibody elaborating system) and the T-cell system (concerned with cellular immunity). Although the B-cell and T-cell systems are the major effectors, the complement system, coagulation sequence, and mediator cells, as well as the system of lymphokine secretions from sensitized T cells, function to amplify the immune response.

The specific mechanisms of the immune response are complex and multifaceted and often involve a cascade of events. As expected, the multiple enzymes and cascade systems may present problems (congenital and acquired) that lead to immunodeficiency (Fig. 1).

SIGNS AND SYMPTOMS

Recurrent infections, especially with usually nonpathogenic or exotic organisms, are commonly seen in children with immune deficiency states. Failure to thrive is also commonly noted. A child with multiple upper respiratory tract infections, or other simple viral or bacterial diseases, who is growing well and thriving is unlikely to have an immune mechanism disorder.

The clinical manifestations of any of the immune system dysfunction syndromes are often specifically related to the respective effector mechanisms. The resulting diseases reflect the dysfunction of one or more of the four main mediators of the body's defense: B cells, T cells, phagocytes, and complement.

1. B-cell disorders: B cells are plasma cells which secrete immunoglobulins and are responsible for humoral immunity.

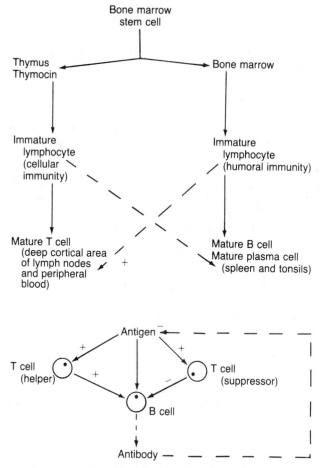

FIG. 1. Pathophysiology of immune deficiency disorders. Step 1: Antigen acts to turn on T-cell helper. Step 2: T-cell helper stimulates B cells (after contact with antigen). Step 3: B cell proliferates and matures and secretes immunoglobulins (antibodies). Step 4: Secreted antibody acts on antigen to cause it to turn on T cell (suppressor). + Indicates turn on of cell function. − Indicates turn off of cell function.

2. T-cell disorders: T cells are responsible for cellular immunity, such as delayed hypersensitivity reactions and immunity to viruses, fungi, and mycobacteria.

3. Phagocytic dysfunction diseases: This type of cellular disease in children usually results in severe pyogenic infections (e.g., chronic granulomatous disease of childhood, Job syndrome).

4. Complement diseases: Complement abnormality syndromes may show manifestations of systemic lupus erythematosus, gonococcemia, or severe pyogenic infections.

In addition to being dysfunctional or absent, any of the defense mechanisms can also be defective in various combinations rather than in an isolated form. Very often, the signs and symptoms produced lead directly to identification of the dysfunction.

DIAGNOSTIC AND TREATMENT PROTOCOLS

Table 1 gives diagnostic and treatment protocols for immune deficiency syndromes of varied origins. The list of disorders is representative of the various diseases and is not comprehensive. The treatment protocols may not be the "state of the art" therapy.

TABLE 1. *Diagnostic and treatment protocols*

Diagnosis	Treatment
Bruton's Disease (Agammaglobulinemia)[a]	
X-linked recessive disorder	Replacement of the humoral antibodies by
Little, if any, humoral antibody response, but delayed cellular immunity is normal	use of gamma globulin, 6 ml/kg i.m. monthly
The number of circulating lymphocytes is normal, but circulating plasma cells are absent	Plasma, 10 ml/kg (via a buddy system), may be tried in patients who do poorly on gamma globulin injections
The thymus appears to be normal, but germinal centers of normal and stimulated lymph nodes are absent whereas paracortical regions are normal	
Affected children appear to be well during the first 6 months of life and then begin developing severe pyogenic infections, most often with *H. influenzae, S. pneumoniae,* or *S. aureus*	
Selective Deficiencies of Immunoglobin Production[a]	
Genetic basis is unknown	As in Bruton's disease, infusions with
Both secretory and circulating IgA may be decreased or absent, slight increase in IgM	gamma globulin from pooled isoimmune human hepatitis or measles globulin; **caution:** gamma globulin from a donor
Humoral responses to antigens are selective	placenta has more IgA than pooled plasma and may cause anaphylactic-type reactions
Cellular immunity responses may be impaired	
The number of circulating lymphocytes is often normal	
The histopathology of the thymus, lymph nodes, respiratory tract, and GI tract is variable and selectively abnormal	
Recurrent episodes of bronchitis and sinusitis associated with enteropathy (malabsorptive)	
Transient Hypogammaglobulinemia of Infancy[a]	
Familial entity (genetic basis is unknown)	Immune serum globulin until about 1½ to
IgG is primarily depressed	2½ years of age, as in Bruton's disease
Humoral responses to most antigens are usually absent or missing, but cellular immunity is normal	
The number of circulating lymphocytes is normal, but the number of plasma cells is	

TABLE 1. *(continued)*

Diagnosis	Treatment

decreased; T helper cells are decreased
Peripheral lymphoid tissue appears to have absent germinal centers
Recurrent pyogenic infections from 6 to 18 months of life but most problematic in the first 6 months of life

Common Variable Immune Deficiency (Variable Onset and Expression)[a]

Diagnosis	Treatment
Immunoglobulins are missing, but the type and degree vary (IgG deficiency is invariably present)	With gamma globulins, as noted above
Humoral deficiency in response to antigens, cellular immune response is appropriate, lymphocytes are normal in number and it appears that either T cells suppress immunoglobulin synthesis or that carbohydrate incorporation is defective	
The thymus is usually normal, but lymphoid tissue varies greatly	
A high incidence of autoimmune disorders and malignancies	
Critical features: Recurrent pyogenic infections, giardiasis, and sinusitis	

Severe Combined Immunodeficiency Disease[b]

Diagnosis	Treatment
Autosomal recessive disorder	Bone marrow transplant (histocompatible)
Antigenic stimulation shows a deficiency in all humoral responses and equally deficient cellular immunity responses to antigens	Fetal thymus or fetal liver transplants may reconstitute T-cell immunity
The number of lymphocytes and plasma cells is extremely low	
The thymus is hypoplastic and the lymph nodes show marked absence or deficiency of lymphocytes	
Affected children do not usually survive infancy	
Particular sensitivity to graft-versus-host reactions	
Death often follows blood transfusions	
Marked deficiency of all immunoglobulins	

Cellular Immunodeficiency with Abnormal Immunoglobulin Synthesis: Nezelof's Syndrome[b]

Diagnosis	Treatment
Autosomal recessive disorder	Bone marrow transplant (rarely)
Immunoglobulins are quantitatively abnormal	Fetal thymus transplant, if possible
Humoral antibody response to stimulation is normal if present, but the quantity is probably somewhat decreased	Aggressive antibiotic treatment
Deficiency in cellular response to antigenic stimulation	Gamma globulin and/or frozen plasma monthly if immunoglobulins are not formed after immunization
The number of lymphocytes is low; the number of plasma cells is normal	
The thymus is hypoplastic and the peripheral lymphocytes are markedly deficient	

Diagnosis	Treatment

Germinal centers of lymph nodes may be normal

Affected children frequently die of viral, fungal or pneumocystis infection

Thymic Aplasia: Di George's Syndrome[b]

No evidence of a genetic mechanism

Immunoglobulins are apparently normal

Humoral antibodies to an antigenic response are deficient and the cellular immunity responses to all antigens are absent

The number of lymphocytes are normal, as are the number of plasma cells

The thymus is absent, with failure of development of the epithelium of the third and fourth pharyngeal pouches; germinal centers in peripheral lymph nodes are present, but the number of lymphocytes are decreased in the paracortical areas

The parathyroids are absent and the syndrome is usually recognized as tetany in the newborn (cardiovascular complications are frequent)

Affected childen usually die in infancy from frequent viral, fungal, or pneumocystis infections

Thymus transplant, with normal restoration of the number of T cells and rosette formation 2 to 3 days later

Skin test reaction should be positive 2 to 4 weeks after transplant

Immune Deficiency with Thrombopenia and Eczema: Wiskott-Aldrich Syndrome[c]

X-linked recessive disorder

Immunoglobulin deficiency is usually present, but the type and degree vary (frequently, low IgM and high IgA), response to humoral antigens is variable, but cellular immunity response is severely deficient

The number of lymphocytes progressively declines, but the number of plasma cells is normal

The thymus appears to be normal, but peripheral lymphoid tissues have decreased germinal centers; progressive decrease of lymphocytes in paracortical areas

T cells may be normal in infancy but decline rapidly

Eczema and thrombocytopenia are common characteristics

Lack of isohemagglutinins

An apparently higher incidence of lymphoreticular malignancy

Frequent pyogenic, viral, or fungal infections

Bone marrow transplant

Bleeding episodes: Treat with platelets (cautiously because of potential presence of autoantibodies)

Transfer factor: Rarely helpful

Thymosin and thymus transplants are experimental

Ataxia-Telangiectasia[c]

Autosomal recessive disorder

Inconsistent humoral response to antigens, but severely impaired response to cellular antigens; the number of lymphocytes is decreased, but plasma cells are usually normal

Gamma globulin and/or frozen plasma administered monthly

Aggressive antibiotic treatment of sinusitis and pulmonary infections

Thymus transplant

TABLE 1. *(continued)*

Diagnosis	Treatment
The thymus lacks cortical and medullary organization and is without Hassall's corpuscles; peripheral lymph nodes show decreased germinal centers; decreased number of lymphyocytes in the paracortical region	
Cerebellar ataxia is progressive, as is telangiectasia, which may appear late; ovarian dysgenesis is frequent; a higher incidence of lymphoreticular malignancy later in life	
Frequent signs of pulmonary infections, especially with low IgA	

Chronic Granulomatous Disease of Childhood[d]

X-linked or autosomal recessive disorder	Antistaphylococcal medication
Certain enteric catalase-positive organisms are phagocytized by leukocytes but are not killed effectively	Incision and drainage, as necessary
This defective killing mechanism is especially poor in reference to staphylococci, *Serratia*, and certain fungi	
A normal increase in oxygen consumption (oxygen burst) is absent after ingestion of these bacteria	
The formation of oxygen radicals appears to be missing	
Some affected patients also lack an antigen on red blood cells (a particular killing antigen) and this may be shared abnormality with the white blood cells in these patients	
Liver abscesses are also common	

Chédiak-Higashi Anomaly[d]

A generalized defect in lysosomal structure	Antibacterial agents, usually antistaphylococcal, as appropriate
Partial albinism (a packaging defect in melanin)	Incision and drainage, as necessary
Skin and bowel infections are particular problems during infancy	
Morphologically abnormal neutrophils	
All immunoglobulins are present in normal amounts	
Normal cellular and humoral immunities	
Should the children survive long enough, they usually develop a disseminated malignancy	

C1 Esterase Deficiency[e]

Autosomal dominant disorder	Largely symptomatic, but fresh plasma may be used in emergencies
Lack of C1 esterase activity leads to spontaneous activation and subsequent destruction of the fourth and second components of complement	
Low C4 levels are diagnostic when C2 levels are normal	

Diagnosis	Treatment
Episodes are intermittent and associated with trauma, menstruation, and infection Because of the frequency of abdominal pain, affected patients often seek surgical consultation Potential mortality because of laryngeal edema On discovery of an index case, the entire family should be studied to determine which members have potential to develop this disease	

C8 Deficiency[e]

Autosomal recessive disorder, with a probable codominant factor Often resembles a disseminated gonococcal infection and/or an SLE-type syndrome	Supportive and symptomatic; no specific treatment

CII Deficiency[e]

Autosomal recessive disorder, with a possible codominant factor SLE-type syndrome Membrane proliferative glomerulonephritis Henoch Schönlein purpura Dermatomyocytis (rarely) accompanied by infections, especially recurrent pneumococcal sepsis	As above

[a]Primary B cell diseases: Immunoglobin deficiency.
[b]Primary T cell diseases: Combined immune deficiencies.
[c]Combined B and T cell diseases.
[d]White blood cell deficiencies.
[e]Complement deficiency disorders.

Increased Intracranial Pressure

Increased intracranial pressure is caused by a variety of insults to the central nervous system. Its manifestations may be silent and/or life-threatening, persistent, or intermittent. All cases are affected by multiple extracranial physiological factors, such as respiratory function, cardiac output, and the state of hydration.

Regardless of its cause, timely recognition of increased intracranial pressure is important. Treatment is often life-saving and may be instituted long before a specific cause is identified.

PATHOPHYSIOLOGY

Modified Monro-Kellie Doctrine

In a fixed-volume container, such as the skull, the pressure varies directly with the volume of the closed space; thus, if the volume increases in one of the compartments, a compensatory decrease must occur in another compartment to maintain a stable pressure.

Figure 1 shows the pathophysiology of increased intracranial pressure.

SIGNS AND SYMPTOMS

Increased intracranial pressure shows a wide variation in its clinical manifestations and may be extremely difficult to recognize if lethargy or coma is present. There are, however, certain commonly manifested classic features. A bulging fontanelle on an infant or an elevated opening pressure in a lumbar puncture is direct evidence of increased intracranial pressure. Papilledema, although occasionally confused with papillitis and other ischemic optic neuropathies, is another direct sign of pressure elevation. Other signs and symptoms in children include cranial nerve paralysis, headache, vomiting, lethargy, personality or behavioral changes, and/or anorexia. Unfortunately, these nonspecific signs and symptoms are common in many childhood illnesses. Radiographic evidence of increased convolutional markings or splitting of the cranial sutures strongly suggest the presence of increased intracranial pressure.

DIFFERENTIAL DIAGNOSIS

1. Acute CNS infection (meningitis, encephalitis, brain abscess)
2. Craniocerebral trauma

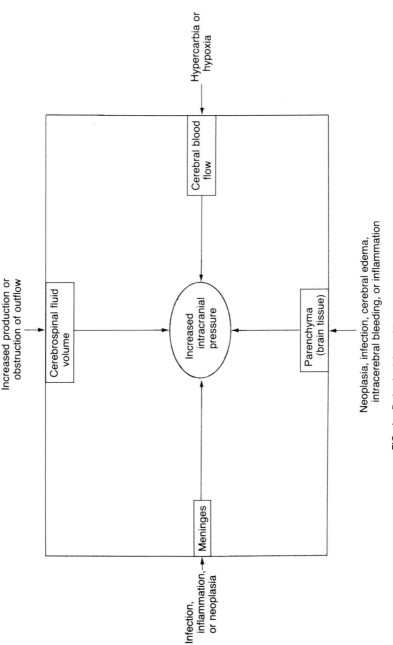

FIG. 1. Pathophysiology of increased intracranial pressure.

3. Hypoxic-ischemic injuries associated with intoxications and/or respiratory arrest

4. Lead poisoning

5. Intracranial hemorrhage, especially in neonates

6. Bulging fontanelle syndrome of infancy (e.g., secondary to tetracycline ingestion, vitamin A intoxication, or vitamin A deficit)

7. Neoplastic disorders

8. Hydrocephalus

9. Cerebrovascular occlusion with sickle-cell disease

10. Pseudotumor cerebri (increased intracranial pressure without other focal neurological signs or CNS abnormalities)

11. Hypoparathyroidism

12. Addison's disease

DIAGNOSTIC PROTOCOL

General Signs and Symptoms

1. Bulging fontanelle (split cranial sutures)

2. Papilledema

3. Cranial nerve findings

4. Altered level of consciousness

5. Headache

6. Vomiting

7. Lethargy

CNS Infections

1. Meningitis or encephalitis

   a. Medical history and physical examination: Often a younger child with a prodromal illness who abruptly becomes pyrectic, irritable, anorectic, and/or lethargic; bulging fontanelle. See Meningitis and Encephalitis chapters.

   b. Laboratory investigations: Lumbar puncture (see Meningitis and Encephalitis chapters).

2. Brain abscess

   a. Medical history and physical examination: Predisposing cause (e.g., congenital heart disease, chronic otitis media, foreign body, open head wound).

   b. Laboratory investigations: Electroencephalogram, CT scan; surgical removal, if possible.

Acute Toxic Encephalopathies

1. Intoxications (e.g., lead)

    a. Medical history and physical examination: General signs and symptoms (as above) or nonspecific symptoms; evidence of pica or lead ingestion.

    b. Laboratory investigations (see Lead Poisoning chapter).

2. Postviral illness (e.g., Reye's syndrome)

    a. Medical history and physical examination: Viral prodrome followed by vomiting and coma.

    b. Laboratory investigations (see Reye's Syndrome chapter).

3. Postimmunization illness (e.g., smallpox, pertussis)

    a. Medical history and physical examination: Recent immunization.

    b. Laboratory investigations.

4. Systemic diseases without meningitis or encephalitis (e.g., hepatic coma)

    a. Medical history and physical examination.

    b. Laboratory investigations.

Vascular Disorders

1. Intracerebral bleeding in neonates

    a. Medical history and physical examination: Low birth weight, asphyxia and/or respiratory distress syndrome, infusion of hypertonic solution.

    b. Laboratory investigations.

2. Coagulation defect, vascular malformation, vasculitis (allergic)

    a. Medical history and physical examination: Evidence of familial disorder, signs of systemic bleeding.

    b. Laboratory investigations.

Congenital or Acquired Hydrocephalus

1. Medical history and physical examination: Complicated perinatal course (e.g., in utero infection, subarachnoid bleeding, neonatal meningitis), associated congenital anomalies, abnormal rates of head growth shown by accurate plots of head circumference over a period of time, delay in psychomotor development.

2. Laboratory investigations: Skull radiographs, CT scan, evaluation for neonatal infection.

Neoplasms

1. Primary CNS tumor

    a. Medical history and physical examination: Nonspecific signs, prior treated neoplastic disease, family history of genetic neoplasia.

    b. Laboratory investigations: Skull radiographs, specific changes in anterior clinoids.

2. Metastatic disease

    a. Medical history and physical examination: Family history of genetic neoplasia (e.g., phakomatoses, predisposing conditions, multiple endocrinopathies), prior or present neoplastic disease.

    b. Laboratory investigations: CT scan, appropriate evaluation for metastatic disease.

Benign Intracranial Hypertension

1. Vitamin A intoxication or deficiency, tetracycline overdosage, Addison's disease, hypoparathyroidism, deprivation dwarfism, severe iron deficiency, rapid brain growth after malnutrition, Guillain-Barré syndrome, roseola infantum.

    a. Medical history and physical examination: General signs and symptoms (as above), most frequent in young obese girls, but occurs in all children, localizing neurological signs are usually absent, except in chronic states, in which visual field defects may occur.

    b. Laboratory investigations: Usually self-limited (distinguish from other causes, which require extensive evaluation and aggressive treatment), CT scan (to exclude mass lesion and evaluate ventricular system), avoid offending agent, lumbar puncture may be both diagnostic (only the pressure is abnormal) and therapeutic.

Craniocerebral Trauma

1. Medical history and physical examination: Determine how injury occurred and localize it anatomically, if possible.

2. Laboratory investigations: Skull radiographs, CT scan, consultation with neurologist.

TREATMENT PROTOCOL

Supervision and Monitoring

Admit or transfer the patient to a facility able to provide close supervision and to intervene medically or surgically immediately should the patient's condition unexpectedly deteriorate. The possibility of the need for continuous monitoring of intracranial pressure and the ready availability of a competent neurosurgical team should influence the decision.

1. Continuous monitoring of intracranial pressure

    a. As a guide to the diagnosis, treatment, and prognosis in an unconscious patient in whom signs of increasing intracranial pressure might not be evident.

    b. As a guide to treatment in a variety of conditions (e.g., metabolic or traumatic).

    c. As the basis for determining volumes of infusions, frequency of treatment, and/or the need for other modes of intervention.

d. As a method of identifying an unexpected and precipitous alteration in pressure so that measures may be instituted to preclude "medullary anemia" (slowing of the pulse and alteration in respiratory rate with a compensatory increase in blood pressure when intracranial pressure exceeds diastolic blood pressure).

2. Lumbar puncture

a. Usually a relatively harmless procedure for the measurement of opening pressures and examination of cerebrospinal fluid, but **should not be performed** in increased intracranial pressure without a thorough understanding of the potential hazards and implications (i.e., tentorial or tonsillar herniation or impaction).

b. If lumbar puncture is necessary (e.g., in meningitis to determine the organism), certain precautions must be taken to minimize the complications:

(1) Perform the procedure immediately after or during infusion of an osmotic diuretic such as mannitol.

(2) Collect spinal fluid slowly with the stylet remaining partially within the shaft of the spinal needle.

(3) Perform the procedure as rapidly and as painlessly as possible to avoid undue stimulation or irritation and concomitant exacerbation of pressure.

3. CT scan

a. A noninvasive technique that reduces the need for invasive studies with a potentially high degree of side effects.

b. Once the child's condition is stabilized, a good quality CT scan may provide information that will allow the neurosurgical team to effect a primary correction of the elevated pressure (e.g., removal of a mass lesion obstructing the ventricles); it may also identify unexpected herniation, subarachnoic hemorrhage, or a brain abscess.

c. Equally important may be the absence of abnormalities on the CT scan, which will allow the neurosurgical and intensive care team to feel confident that a removable lesion was not missed.

Surgical Therapy

1. Removal of primary cause of increased intracranial pressure (e.g., a mass lesion obstructing the ventricles or the evacuation of a large subdural hematoma).

2. A shunting procedure to relieve increased intracranial pressure when the primary cause is surgically untreatable.

3. Lumbar or cisternal puncture, preferably performed with great care by neurosurgical consultants, as a temporizing measure to reduce pressure through direct removal of fluids.

Pharmacological Therapy

1. 20% Mannitol, 1.5 to 3.0 g/kg i.v. every 4 to 6 hr over a period of 45 to 60 min to avoid sudden increase in extracellular fluid and congestive heart failure; onset of action within 20 to 30 min; osmotic diuretic; avoid in case of hepatic or renal insufficiency; intermediate rebound.[1]

2. 30% Urea, 1.0 to 1.5 g/kg i.v. every 4 to 6 hr; onset of action within 15 min; osmotic diuretic; avoid in case of hepatic or renal insufficiency; maximal rebound.[1]

3. Glycerol, 0.5 to 1.5 g/kg i.v. or p.o. (nasogastric tube) every 4 to 6 hr (maximum dose, 4 g/kg/24 hr); onset of action within 30 min; osmotic diuretic; minimal rebound.[1]

4. Dexamethasone, 0.2 to 0.5 mg/kg i.v., i.m., or p.o. (nasogastric tube) every 6 hr; onset of action within 12 to 18 hr; restores blood-brain barrier; minimal rebound.[1]

Mechanical Therapy

Passive hyperventilation, reduce P_{CO_2} to ≤ 30 mm Hg; onset of action immediately; reduces cerebral blood flow; minimal rebound.

Metabolic Therapy

Hypothermia, reduce temperature to 28 to 30°C; onset of action within 1 hr; reduces cerebral blood flow; minimal rebound.[1]

---

[1]Rebound of symptoms on cessation of therapy, caused by changes in osmolality with subsequent influx of fluid.

Infection

The diagnosis of infection is made on clinical examination of the patient and confirmed in the laboratory. Various organisms are responsible for the production of specific definitive syndromes. The nonspecific infections, less common syndromes, and unusual infections are discussed in this chapter; other kinds of infections are covered elsewhere in this volume (see Epiglottitis and Urinary Tract Infection chapters).

Pathogenic bacteria gain entrance to the body by various means. In general, each bacterial organism has a predilection for certain tissues. Organisms may reach target tissues hematogenously, by direct extension, and by penetrating innoculation. The respiratory tract, gastrointestinal tract, and genitourinary tract are common portals of entry.

SIGNS AND SYMPTOMS

The clinical response to infection varies with the type of infecting agent, the age of the patient, and the target tissue involved. Table 1 shows the general characteristics of infection in the uncompromised host. It must be emphasized that the presentation of any illness is extremely variable and evaluation of disease must be individualized.

GENERAL DIAGNOSTIC PROTOCOL

1. Complete blood cell count

2. Urinalysis

3. Buffy coat smear with Gram stain

4. Gram stain and culture of exudate, if present or obtainable

5. Bacterial and viral cultures

    a. Blood: If hematogenous dissemination is considered

    b. Urine: If urinary tract infection is suspected or if the genitourinary system is considered the portal of entry

    c. Stool: If gastrointestinal infection is suspected or if the gastrointestinal tract is considered the portal of entry

    d. Throat: If tonsillopharyngitis is suspected or if the pharynx (nose and throat) is considered the portal of entry

    e. Cerebrospinal fluid (CSF): If meningitis is considered

TABLE 1. *Clinical response to infection*

	Viral	Bacterial	Fungal	Parasitic
Most common portal of entry	Respiratory (gastrointestinal)	Respiratory (gastrointestinal, cutaneous)	Cutaneous (genitourinary)	Gastrointestinal (cutaneous)
Fever	Low-grade to moderate	Moderate to high	Usually none, unless there is systemic invasion	Usually none, unless there is systemic invasion
WBC response	Leukopenia to mild leukocytosis	Leukocytosis	None or mild to moderate leukocytosis	Mild to significant leukocytosis
Usual cellular response	Lymphocyte, monocyte	Polymorphonuclear	Mononuclear	Eosinophil (if systemic)
Sedimentation rate	Increased	Increased	Increased	Increased
Rash	Yes	No	Maybe	No

6. Viral titers: Acute and convalescent titers are required

7. Counterimmunoelectrophoresis: To detect bacterial antigen (hemophilus, pneumococcus, meningococcus, and streptococcus may be detected by this means)

8. *Limulus* lysate: To detect gram-negative endotoxin

DIAGNOSTIC AND TREATMENT PROTOCOLS

Table 2 gives diagnostic and treatment protocols for infections and infecting agents. Table 3 gives the preferred drugs for the resultant diseases and syndromes.

TABLE 2. *Infection: Diagnostic and treatment protocols*

Clinical syndromes and/or features	Diagnosis	Treatment
H. influenzae		
Meningitis (six times more common than the next most common organism causing this disease) Epiglottitis Pneumonia (especially in the presence of a pleural effusion) Otitis media Cellulitis (especially if the overlying skin has a violaceous discoloration) Osteomyelitis (especially of the facial bones) Septic arthritis Orbital cellulitis	Gram stain: Gram-negative pleomorphic rods Culture and sensitivity testing Counter-immunoelectrophoresis (CIE) β-Lactamase testing: In addition to sensitivity testing	Chloramphenicol, 50 to 100 mg/kg/day i.v. in 4 divided doses (best single drug if the resistance pattern of the organism is not known), **or** Ampicillin, 200 to 400 mg/kg/day i.v. in 4 to 6 divided doses (if the organism recovered does not produce penicillinase), **or** Cephalosporins (the currently approved cephalosporins are contraindicated if CNS infection is suspected or considered), **or** Carbenicillin or trimethroprim and sulfamethoxazole (if the organism is resistant to both ampicillin and chloramphenicol) If meningitis is considered or suspected, and laboratory evidence suggests an infection, ampicillin **and** chloramphenicol are used until the organism is confirmed to be sensitive to one or the other
S. pneumoniae		
Pneumonia (pneumococcal pneumonia occurs four times more often than the next most common form, H. influenzae pneumonia) Meningitis (usually acute and fulminant course)	Gram stain (gram-positive, lancet-shaped diplococci; end-to-end orientation) Culture and sensitivity testing CIE	Penicillin G, 100 to 200 mg/kg/day in 4 divided doses (route depends on severity of infection), **or** Cephalosporins or erythromycin (if the infection is nonmeningitic),

TABLE 2. *(continued)*

Clinical syndromes and/or features	Diagnosis	Treatment
Septicemia (especially common in splenectomized patients)		**or** Chloramphenicol (for meningitis if the patient is allergic to penicillin) Multiple drug resistance is rare, but has been reported
	N. meningitidis	
Meningitis and septicemia (especially when the infection is associated with petechiae and/or purpura) Arthritis	Gram stain (gram-negative, kidney-shaped diplococci; opposing concave sides) Petechial Gram stain will frequently yield the organism CIE Culture and sensitivity testing	Penicillin G, 250,000 units/kg/day i.v. in 4 divided doses, **or** Ampicillin, 200 to 400 mg/kg/day i.v. in 4 to 6 divided doses, **or** Chloramphenicol, 50 to 100 mg/kg/day i.v. in 4 divided doses
	S. pyogenes	
Tonsillopharyngitis Peritonsillar abscess Cervical lymphadenitis Acute glomerulonephritis (sequelae of an acute streptococcal infection) Rheumatic fever (sequelae of an acute streptococcal infection) Impetigo Otitis media	Culture and sensitivity testing Antistreptolysin O Antihyaluronidase Anti-DNAase	Penicillin G, 300,000 to 600,000 units i.m. (one dose of long-acting penicillin is usually enough to prevent the sequelae of acute streptococcal infections), **or** Erythromycin, 30 to 50 mg/kg/day p.o. in 4 divided doses (recommended for patients allergic to penicillin)
	S. aureus	
Soft-tissue abscesses Impetigo, including scalded skin syndrome Wound infections Pneumonia, sepsis, and/or meningitis in the compromised host Osteomyelitis Orbital cellulitis Preseptal cellulitis Conjunctivitis	Gram stain Culture and sensitivity testing Coagulase testing	Penicillin G, 20,000 to 25,000 units/kg/day i.v. in 4 divided doses (if the organism is sensitive), **or** Nafcillin, 50 to 150 mg/kg/day i.v. in 4 divided doses, **or** Oxacillin, 50 to 150 mg/kg/day i.v. in 4 divided doses, **or** Methicillin, 100 to 200 mg/kg/day i.v. in 4 divided doses, **or** Cloxacillin, 25 to 50 mg/kg/day p.o. in 4 divided doses, **or** Dicloxacillin: 12.5 to 25 mg/kg/day p.o. in 4 divided doses, **or** Vancomycin: 30 to 40 mg/kg/day i.v. in 4 divided doses

Clinical syndromes and/or features	Diagnosis	Treatment
		(if the organism is resistant to the semisynthetic penicillins), **or** Gentamicin: 3 to 5 mg/kg/day i.m. or i.v. in 2 divided doses, **or** Kanamycin: 15 mg/kg/day i.m. or i.v. in 2 divided doses, **or** Amikacin: 15 mg/kg/day i.m. or i.v. in 2 divided doses
	N. gonorrheae	
Venereal diseases (urethritis, cervicitis, pelvic inflammatory disease) Nonvenereal presentation (arthritis, perihepatitis, septicemia, tonsillopharyngitis, conjunctivitis)	Gram stain (yields gramnegative intracellular diplococci) Culture and sensitivity testing (specimen must be collected on Thayer-Martin medium and stored in a "candle jar" which provides a CO_2-rich medium)	Penicillin G (long-acting), 1.2 million units i.m., along with one dose of probenecid, 25 mg/kg p.o. before administration of the penicillin. Above treatment is for the symptomatic or asymptomatic patient with a localized infection of the genitourinary tract; if the infection is disseminated or localized to an area of the body other than the genitourinary tract, the following treatment is recommended: Pelvic inflammatory disease: Aqueous penicillin G. 20 million units/day i.v. in 4 divided doses Neonatal conjunctivitis: Aqueous penicillin G, 50,000 units/kg i.v. in 2 divided doses for 7 days Arthritis or septicemia: Aqueous penicillin G, 75,000 to 100,000 units/kg/day i.v. in 2 or 3 divided doses for 7 to 10 days Meningitis: Aqueous penicillin G, 100,000 units/kg/day i.v. in 3 or 4 divided doses for at least 10 days If the organism is penicillinresistant or if the patient is sensitive to penicillin, spectinomycin, tetracycline, cefoxitin, or trimethoprim and sulfamethaxazole may be used

TABLE 2. *(continued)*

Clinical syndromes and/or features	Diagnosis	Treatment
Rocky Mountain Spotted Fever		
There is almost always a history of an antecedent tick bite Prodromal period of 3 to 12 days, consisting of cephalgia, anorexia, and malaise Fever (to 104°F) and chills Rash begins on the third or fourth day (centrifugal maculopapular rash with heaviest concentration around the ankles and wrists, progressing centrally and becoming petechial; sometimes hemorrhagic and confluent; the palms and soles of the feet are usually involved; necrosis may occur)	Weil-Felix reaction test: Proteus OX-2 and OX-19 are positive after 2 to 3 weeks Complement fixation test: Usually a rise in the titer by the third week	Chloramphenicol, 50 to 100 mg/kg/day i.v. in 4 divided doses, **or** Tetracycline, 40 to 50 mg/kg/day p.o. in 4 divided doses (may initially be given i.v.) for 14 days
Mucocutaneous Lymph Node Syndrome (Kawasaki Syndrome)		
Fever (usually for 5 or more days) Four of the following five characteristics must be present for the diagnosis to be made: Bilateral conjunctivitis Mucous membrane involvement (dry, cracked lips, strawberry tongue, pharyngitis) Polymorphous centripetal rash Centrifugal desquamation, edema, or discoloration (red to violaceous discoloration of the hands or feet) Cervical lymphadenopathy Absence of other causes (e.g., scarlet fever, mononucleosis, rubeola)	No diagnostic tests	Supportive and symptomatic Salicylates (aspirin), 100 mg/kg/day p.o. in 4 doses, to maintain a therapeutic blood level; used for antiinflammatory properties
Diphtheria		
Sore throat Low-grade fever Rapidly progressive membrane in pharynx (nose or throat) Croup syndrome Cervical lymphadenopathy	**Treatment with antitoxin must be instituted when there is a high index of suspicion on clinical grounds and not on diagnostic confirmation of the infection**	Antitoxin therapy (equine), 10,000 to 60,000 units i.v. (depending on the location and the severity of the disease) Test for hypersensitivity to equine serum before its

Clinical syndromes and/or features	Diagnosis	Treatment
Prostration and tachycardia (out of proportion to that expected by the presence of fever) Unexplained carditis Lack of adequate immunizations	Culture: On blood agar, Loeffler's slant, and tellurite media Virulence testing of the organism	administration: Instill a 1:10 dilution of the serum (in normal saline) into the conjunctival sac. Place the same quantity of normal saline solution into the other eye. If epiphoria and redness occur within 20 min, hypersensitivity to the serum is present. If the patient is sensitive to the equine serum, rapid desensitization may be done using extremely small doses of diluted serum; be prepared for acute treatment of any allergic manifestations Antibiotic therapy (in addition to antitoxin therapy): Aqueous procaine penicillin G, 600,000 units/day parenterally, **or** Erythromycin, 50 mg/kg/day if the patient is allergic to penicillin

Infectious Mononucleosis

Malaise, lethargy, anorexia, fever Exudative tonsillopharyngitis Generalized lymphadenopathy Splenomegaly	Complete blood cell count: Atypical lymphocytosis with true Downey cells, not reactive lymphocytes Monospot® and heterophile agglutination testing Epstein-Barr virus titers	Symptomatic and supportive

Viral Hepatitis

Nausea, vomiting, diarrhea Fever Abdominal pain Hepatomegaly Jaundice History of contact History of blood products or drugs	HB_s antibody and antigen HB_c antibody and antigen SGOT, SGPT Coagulation studies Fecal isolation of the virus If persistent or recurring, liver biopsy may be indicated	Symptomatic and supportive

Poliomyelitis

Prodrome of mild upper respiratory tract infection or gastroenteritis Headache, vomiting Muscle pains (especially back, neck, and limbs) Meningismus Asymmetrical lower motor neuron paralysis (usually of the lower extremities; may be bulbar and compromise respiration)	CSF: Pleocytosis Virus isolation: Throat, blood, feces Neutralizing antibodies: Appear after the first week of the illness Complement fixation test: Positive after 10 to 14 days	Symptomatic and supportive. The main thrust of therapy is prevention by adequate immunization

TABLE 2. *(continued)*

Clinical syndromes and/or features	Diagnosis	Treatment
Infant Botulism		
Constipation Head lag (as manifestation of generalized hypotonia) Weakness, loss of head control Weak cry Difficulty feeding Ptosis; ophthalmoplegia Infant (<1 year of age)	The diagnosis is based on the presence of the clinical syndrome and the recovery of spores in the stool	Supportive and symptomatic Patients treated with antibiotics, especially aminoglycosides, do worse than untreated patients
Influenza Virus		
Upper respiratory tract infection (rhinitis and pharyngitis) Pneumonia Myalgia, cephalgia, malaise Complications (otitis media, bacterial pneumonia, ?Reye's syndrome)	Specific antibody titers	Supportive and symptomatic Prevention: Influenza A vaccine Amantadine hydrochloride: Reserved for severe infections Treat bacterial complications with appropriate antibiotics
Mycoplasma		
Pneumonia (diffuse, especially in school age children and adolescents) Upper respiratory tract infections Tracheobronchitis Many patients are asymptomatic	Mycoplasma titers Cold agglutinins: Occur in 75% of patients with mycoplasma infections	Erythromycin, 30 to 50 mg/kg/day p.o. in 4 divided doses, **or** Tetracycline, 250 mg p.o. 4 times a day (reserved for adolescents)
Varicella-Zoster		
Chickenpox (in children) Herpes zoster (in children and adults)	Usually diagnosed by the presenting clinical syndrome and the appearance and distribution of the vesicular lesions	Supportive and symptomatic Treat bacterial complications Observe for complications (e.g., encephalitis) Ara-A (adenine arabinoside), 10 mg/kg/day over a 12-hr period (reserved for severe life-threatening infections; experimental; FDA consent is required)
Anaerobic		
Organisms encountered *Bacteroides fragilis:* Found in the bowel and the female urogenital tract *Fusobacterium* *Peptococcus,* *Peptostreptococcus* *Clostridia perfringens* *Actinomyces*	Special cultures are generally required for the isolation of anaerobic organisms	Penicillin G, 30,000 to 150,000 units/kg/day i.v. in 4 to 6 divided doses (appropriate for most anaerobes, except *B. fragilis*), **or** Chloramphenicol, 25 to 50 mg/kg/day i.v. in 4 divided doses (*B. fragilis* is usually sensitive), **or** Clindamycin, 8 to 40 mg/kg/day i.m. or i.v. in 3 or 4

Clinical syndromes and/or features	Diagnosis	Treatment
		divided doses, **or** Tetracycline, 20 mg/kg/day i.v. in 4 divided doses, **or** Erythromycin, 30 to 40 mg/kg/day p.o. in 4 divided doses, **or** Metronidazole, 7 to 10 mg/kg/day p.o. in 3 divided doses (*B. fragilis* is usually sensitive)

Pertussis

Clinical syndromes and/or features	Diagnosis	Treatment
Mild upper respiratory infection and cough in adolescents and adults Catarrhal phase: Rhinorrhea and low-grade fever are usually present Paroxysmal phase: Severe cough with audible inspiratory whoop; facial redness or cyanosis, bulging of the eyes, and protruding tongue usually occur during the expiratory phase of the cough; small infants may not have the characteristic whoop; vomiting frequently occurs after the paroxysm; facial petechiae and subconjunctival hemorrhages occur Convalescent phase: Cough and paroxysms resolve	Fluorescent antibody test Organism identification on cough plates or nasopharyngeal swabs Absolute lymphocytosis of 70% to 80% on complete blood cell count	Erythromycin, 40 mg/kg/day p.o. in 4 divided doses (no effect on the course of the disease if administered in the paroxysmal phase, but will prevent spread by eradicating the organism from the pharynx) Supportive and symptomatic Treat complications (e.g., bronchopneumonia)

TABLE 3. *Infection: Drugs of choice*

Disease/syndrome	Organisms	Drug	Daily dose	Divided doses	Route	Duration	Comments and alternate therapy
Abscess							
Brain	Anaerobes (S. aureus)	Penicillin and Chloramphenicol	250–500,000 units 100 mg/kg	6 4	i.v. i.v.	7 days postop 7 days postop	
Lung	Anaerobic streptococci S. aureus Coliforms	Penicillin G Nafcillin Gentamicin	100,000 units/kg 100–150 mg/kg 5 mg/kg	6 4 3	i.v. i.v. i.v.	14 + days 14 + days 7 + days	Chloramphenicol Oxacillin Kanamycin
Peritonsillar	Streptococci S. aureus	Penicillin G Nafcillin	100,000 units/kg 100–150 mg/kg	6 4	i.v. i.v.	10 + days 10 days	Oxacillin, penicillin (if sensitive)
Soft-tissue	S. aureus	Nafcillin	100–150 mg/kg	4	i.v.	10 days	Penicillin (if sensitive)
Adenitis, cervical	Streptococci	Penicillin V	25–50 mg/kg	4	p.o.	10 days	Penicillin G, erythromycin
Amebiasis	Entamoeba histolytica	Diiododhydroxyquin metronidazole plus Diiododhydroxyquin	40 mg/kg 40–50 mg/kg 40 mg/kg	3 3 3	p.o. p.o. p.o.	20 days 10 days 20 days	For mild and asymptomatic patients For severe infections and amebic abscesses
Ascariasis	Ascaris lumbricoides	Pyrantel pamoate	11 mg/kg	1	p.o.	1 dose	Mebendazole, piperazine
Aspergillosis (invasive)	Aspergillus fumigatus	Amphotericin B	30–40 mg/kg (total dose)	—	i.v.	6 weeks	A dose of 0.25 mg/kg is given over 6 hr, and increased by 0.25 mg/kg every 2–3 days with a total dose of 30–40 mg/kg in 6 weeks (see package insert for proper preparation of solution and proper method of administration)
Arthritis, septic	S. aureus	Nafcillin	100–150 mg/kg	4	i.v.	21 days	Oxacillin, penicillin (if sensitive)
	H. influenzae	Ampicillin and Chloramphenicol	150–200 mg/kg 100 mg/kg	4 4	i.v. i.v.	10 days 10 days	Cefamandol (if there is no CNS involvement); choose a single antibiotic after the sensitivity pattern is known

Condition	Organism	Antibiotic	Dosage	No.	Route	Duration	Comments
	N. gonorrheae	Penicillin G	100,000 units/kg	4	i.v.	7–10 days	Miconazole
Candidiasis Topical	C. albicans	Nystatin	Topical	3	Topical	5–7 days	Amphotericin B, miconazole
systemic		Flucytosine	100–150 mg/kg	4	p.o.	7–10 days	Ampicillin (if sensitive)
Cellulitis Orbital	H. influenzae	Chloramphenicol	100 mg/kg	4	i.v.	10 days	Penicillin (if sensitive)
	S. aureus	Nafcillin	100–150 mg/kg	4	i.v.	10 days	Penicillin (if sensitive)
Soft-tissue	S. aureus	Nafcillin	100–150 mg/kg	4	i.v.	10 days	
	Streptococci	Penicillin G	50–100,000 units/kg	6	i.v.	10 days	
	H. influenzae	Ampicillin **and**	200–400 mg/kg	4	i.v.	10–14 days	H. influenzae is common when there is facial or buccal soft-tissue involvement; choose a single antibiotic after the sensitivity pattern is known; cefamandol (if there is no CNS involvement)
		Chloramphenicol	100 mg/kg	4	i.v.	10–14 days	
Conjunctivitis	Virus, staphylococci, H. influenzae, Chlamydia	Sulfacetamide	10% soln	3	Topical	5 days	Neomycin-polymyxin B
Endocarditis	Streptococci group D	Penicillin **and**	100,000 units/kg	6	i.v.	30 days	Penicillin and vancomycin
		Streptomycin	30 mg/kg	2	i.m.	14 days	
	Enterococcus	Ampicillin **and**	200 mg/kg	4	i.v.	10–14 days	Penicillin and streptomycin; Vancomycin and streptomycin
	S. aureus	Gentamicin	5 mg/kg	3	i.v./i.m.	10–14 days	Vancomycin
		Nafcillin	100–150 mg/kg	4	i.v.	45 days	
Enterocolitis (pseudomembranous)	C. difficile	Vancomycin	50 mg/kg	6	p.o.	7 days	
Epiglottitis	H. influenzae	Chloramphenicol	100 mg/kg	4	i.v.	7–10 days	May change to ampicillin if the organism is sensitive
Gastroenteritis	Salmonella species	Ampicillin	100 mg/kg	4	i.v./i.m.	7 days	Most patients do not require antibiotic therapy; it is reserved for those patients with septicemia and those with severe intractable diarrhea
	Shigella	Trimethoprim **and** Sulfamethoxazole	10 mg/kg 50 mg/kg	2	p.o.	5 days	Ampicillin (if sensitive)
	Yersinia	Chloramphenicol	50–100 mg/kg	4	i.v.	5–7 days	Antibiotic efficacy not known; trimethoprim and

TABLE 3. *(continued)*

Disease/syndrome	Organisms	Drug	Daily dose	Divided doses	Route	Duration	Comments and alternate therapy
							sulfamethoxazole, tetracycline
	Campylobacter	Chloramphenicol	50–100 mg/kg	4	i.v.	5–7 days	Antibiotic efficacy not known
Giardiasis	*Giardia lamblia*	Mepacrine	6 mg/kg	3	p.o.	10 days	Metronidazole (15 mg/kg/day, p.o., for 10 days)
Hookworm	*N. americanus, A. duodenale*	Mebendazole	100 mg/kg	2	p.o.	3 days	Pyrantel pamoate
Histoplasmosis	*H. capsulatum*	see Aspergillosis	—			—	
Visceral larva migrans	*Toxocara canis, Toxocara cati*	Thiabendazole	50 mg/kg	2	p.o.	—	Treat until asymptomatic; diethylcarbamazine
Malaria	*P. malariae*	Chloroquine	10–15 mg/kg	1	p.o.	Stat 6 hr, 24 hr, 48 hr later	If chloroquine resistant *P. falciparum*, use a combination of quinine, pyrimethamine, and sulfadiazine
	P. vivax	**then**	5 mg/kg		p.o.		
	P. falciparum	Primaquine	0.3 mg/kg	1	p.o.	14 days	
Mastoiditis	Pneumococci	Penicillin G	250,000 units/kg	6	i.v.	10 days	Oxacillin
	Staphylococci	Natcillin	100–150 mg/kg	4	i.v.	10 days	
Meningitis	Unconfirmed	Ampicillin **and**	400 mg/kg	4	i.v.	10 days	Choose appropriate antibiotic after sensitivity pattern is available
		Chloramphenicol	100 mg/kg	4	i.v.	10 days	
	H. influenzae	Chloramphenicol	100 mg/kg	4	i.v.	10 days	May switch to ampicillin if the organism is sensitive
	Pneumococci	Penicillin G	250,000 units/kg	6	i.v.	10 days	
	Meningococci	Penicillin	250,000 units/kg	6	i.v.	10 days	
	Neonatal	Ampicillin **and**	250 mg/kg	4	i.v.	10+ days	
		Gentamicin	7.5 mg/kg	2	i.m.	7 days	
Osteomyelitis, Acute	*S. aureus*	Nafcillin	100–150 mg/kg	4	i.v.	21 days	Penicillin (if sensitive)
Chronic	*S. aureus*	Cephalexin **and**	100 mg/kg	4	p.o.	6–12 mo	Cloxacillin (p.o.)
		Probenecid	40 mg/kg	4	p.o.	6–12 mo	
Otitis media	?	Ampicillin	50–100 mg/kg	4	p.o.	10 days	Usually the organism is not known; 80% are sensitive to the initial antibiotic and the rest sensitive to alternate drug; cefaclor,

Condition	Organism	Drug	Dose	Doses/day	Route	Duration	Alternative
							amoxicillin, trimethoprim, and sulfamethoxazole
Pericarditis	Pneumococci	Penicillin G	100,000 units/kg	6	i.v.	14 days	
	Staphylococci	Nafcillin	100–150 mg/kg	4	i.v.	21 days	Penicillin (if sensitive)
	Streptococci	Penicillin G	100,000 units/kg	6	i.v.	14 days	
	Meningococci	Penicillin G	100,000 units/kg	6	i.v.	14 days	
	H. influenzae	Ampicillin **and**	200–400 mg/kg	4	i.v.	14 days	Choose one antibiotic after the sensitivity pattern is known
		Chloramphenicol	75–100 m g/kg	4	i.v.	14 days	
Peritonitis, primary	Coliforms	Gentamicin	5 mg/kg	3	i.v./i.m.	21 days	
	Pneumococci	Penicillin G	100,000 units/kg	6	i.v.	21 days	
Pharyngitis	Streptococci	Benzylpenicillin G	25,000 units/kg	1	i.m.	1 dose	Penicillin V
Pinworms	E. vermicularis	Pyrantel pamoate	11 mg/kg	1	p.o.	1 dose	Mebendazole
Pneumocystosis	P. carinii	Trimethoprim **and** sulfamethoxazole	20 mg/kg 100 mg/kg	4	p.o.	14 days	Pentamidine
Pneumonia	Pneumococci	Penicillin G	100,000 units/kg	6	i.v.	10 days	
	H. influenzae	Ampicillin **and**	200 mg/kg	4	i.v.	10 days	Choose one antibiotic when the sensitivity pattern is known; cefamandole
		Chloramphenicol	100 mg/kg	4	i.v.	10 days	
	Mycoplasma	Erythromycin	20–40 mg/kg	4	p.o.	10 days	Tetracycline
	Staphylococci	Nafcillin	100–150 mg/kg	4	i.v.	10 days	Oxacillin
	Legionnaires	Erythromycin	20–40 mg/kg	4	p.o.	10 days	Rifampin
Scalded-skin syndrome	S. aureus	Nafcillin	100–150 mg/kg	4	i.v.	10 days	Oxacillin, penicillin (if sensitive)
Sinusitis	Streptococci	Penicillin V	25–50 mg/kg	4	p.o.	10 days	Erythromycin
Strongyloidiasis	S. stercoralis	Thiabendazole	50 mg/kg	2	p.o.	2 days	Paromomycin
Tapeworms	T. saginata	Niclosamide	1 g <35 kg 1.5 g >35 kg	1	chewed	1 dose	
	T. solium						
Tetanus	C. tetani	Penicillin G	100,000 units/kg	6	i.v.	10 days	Plus antitoxin
Trichomonas	T. vaginalis	Metronidazole	15 mg/kg	3	p.o.	7–10 days	
Trichinosis	T. spiralis	Thiabendazole	50 mg/kg	2	p.o.	—	Treat until symptoms subside
Typhoid fever	S. typhi	Chloramphenicol	50–100 mg/kg	4	i.v./p.o.	14 days	Ampicillin, amoxicillin, trimethoprim and sulfamethoxazole (if sensitive)
Urinary tract infection	Enterobacter	Trisulfapyrimidine	120–150 mg/kg	4	p.o.	7 days	Gentamicin, carbenicillin (if *Pseudomonas*), trimethoprim and sulfamethoxazole
Recurrent		Nitrofurantoin	5–7 mg/kg	4	p.o.	10 days	

Jaundice

Jaundice is generally defined as a yellowish discoloration of the skin secondary to hyperbilirubinemia. Hyperbilirubinemia is defined as a total serum bilirubin level greater than 2 mg/100 ml. Physiological jaundice is not uncommon in neonates and is considered to be secondary to immaturity of hepatic enzyme systems at birth. The bilirubin level in physiological jaundice rarely rises above 12 mg/100 ml in term infants or 15 mg/100 ml in premature infants.

Hyperbilirubinemia in older children may be due to a variety of conditions. The disease may have an acute onset, with the presence of other constitutional or systemic signs and symptoms, or it may be chronic, with a paucity of other findings. The defect causing hyperbilirubinemia may occur at various stages of the metabolism of bilirubin. Knowledge of the metabolism of bilirubin is important in establishing the diagnosis of jaundice (Fig. 1).

Hyperbilirubinemia may be of two types: conjugated and unconjugated. Elevated unconjugated bilirubin may occur from overproduction by hemolysis, impaired uptake by the hepatocyte, and defects in the conjugation process. Conjugated hyperbilirubinemia usually occurs when the excretion of conjugated bilirubin into the bile duct and/or intestine is prevented, causing reflux into the systemic circulation. In neonates, most of the bilirubin is unconjugated (Fig. 2).

SIGNS AND SYMPTOMS

Jaundice is the clinical presentation of hyperbilirubinemia. There is a yellow discoloration of the skin due to deposition of pigment at bilirubin levels between 4 and 7 mg/100 ml. The sclera are usually first involved and noticeable. Kernicterus usually is isolated to the neonatal period and is more common at lower bilirubin levels in more premature infants. Clinical kernicterus is uncommon in older children and adolescents.

Other signs and symptoms of hyperbilirubinemia are related to the specific etiology (e.g., anorexia and hepatomegaly with hepatitis, anemia with hemolytic disease).

DIFFERENTIAL DIAGNOSIS

Neonates

1. First day of life
   a. Rh, ABO, or minor group incompatibility
   b. Intrauterine infection

2. Second or third day of life
   a. Physiological jaundice
   b. Rh or minor group incompatibility

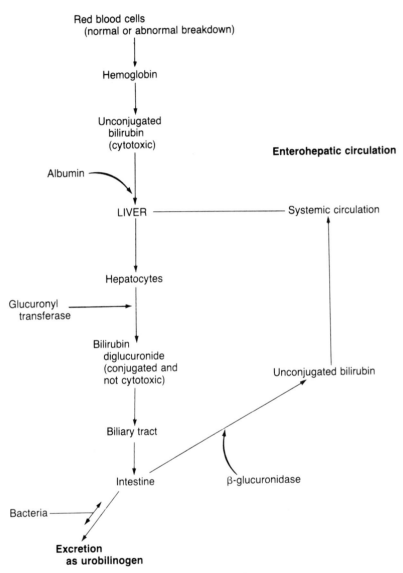

FIG. 1.   Bilirubin metabolism.

c. Gram-negative infections

d. Polycythemia

e. Hemorrhage

f. Respiratory distress syndrome

g. Drug-induced jaundice

h. Abnormal red blood cell morphology

i. Red blood cell enzyme deficiency

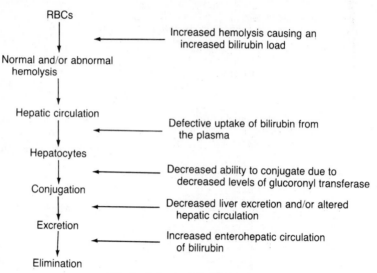

FIG. 2. Pathophysiology of jaundice.

3. Fourth or fifth day of life

   a. Breast feeding

   b. Respiratory distress syndrome

   c. Diabetic mother

   d. Crigler-Najjar syndrome

   e. Gilbert syndrome

4. >1 week of age

   a. Infections (bacterial or viral, especially *H. simplex*)

   b. Pyloric stenosis

   c. Hypothyroidism

   d. Hepatitis

   e. Bile duct obstruction and atresia

   f. Galactosemia

   g. Choledochal cyst

Older Children

1. Infectious hepatitis

2. Systemic infections

3. Drugs and toxins

4. Obstructive causes

   a. Inspissated bile syndrome

   b. Anatomical obstruction (e.g., tumor, gallstone)

5. Hemolytic

   a. Sickle-cell disease

   b. Glucose 6-phosphatase deficiency

c. Autoimmune

d. Hemolytic-uremic syndrome

e. Spherocytosis

f. Transfusion reaction

6. Gilbert syndrome: Similar to Crigler-Najjar syndrome, but bilirubin is not as elevated; occurs predominantly in males; onset at >10 years of age

7. Crigler-Najjar syndrome: Glucuronyl transferase deficiency

8. Rotor syndrome: Defect in excretion of conjugated bilirubin; liver biopsy shows no abnormalities

9. Dubin-Johnson syndrome: Similar to Rotor syndrome, but liver appears to be black on gross examination; pigment granules in the hepatocytes

10. Lucy-Driscoll syndrome: Circulating inhibitor of conjugation

DIAGNOSTIC PROTOCOL

Neonates

1. Total and direct serum bilirubin levels, hematocrit, and hemoglobin.

2. Peripheral smear for red blood cell morphology, platelet count, reticulocyte count (normal: $4.7 \pm 1.9\%$ in full-term infants; 6–10% in premature infants), and nucleated red blood cell count (normal: 0–24/100 white blood cells).

3. Normal direct bilirubin, increased indirect bilirubin, and increased reticulocyte count (hemolytic jaundice): Coombs' test.

    a. Positive Coombs' test: Rh and/or ABO incompatibility; monitor mother's and infant's Rh and ABO, hematocrit, hemoglobin, serial serum bilirubin levels (every 6 hr), total serum protein.

    b. Negative Coombs' test: Abnormal red blood cell morphology, red blood cell enzyme deficiency; evaluate peripheral smear and monitor red blood cell enzyme level, serial hematocrit, and hemoglobin (vitamin K may cause hemolysis in presence of glucose 6-phosphatase deficiency).

4. Normal direct bilirubin, increased indirect bilirubin, and normal reticulocyte count (decreased conjugation): Coombs' test.

    a. Negative Coombs' test: Physiological jaundice (breast milk-induced or con-genital-familial—glucuronyl transferase deficiency); serum bilirubin level rarely rises above 12 mg/100 ml in full-term infants or 15 mg/100 ml in premature infants.

    b. Serum bilirubin level <13 mg/100 ml: Observe; if repeat serum bilirubin levels show a decrease and there are no symptoms, discharge infant.

    c. Serum bilirubin level >13 mg/100 ml: Discontinue breast feeding; obtain cultures; serological testing for intrauterine infection; urine test for reducing substances; blood glucose level (hypoglycemia may be present in galactosemia); thyroid function tests.

5. Increased direct and indirect bilirubin and normal reticulocyte count: Coombs' test.

    a. Negative Coombs' test: Liver disease (hepatitis, galactosemia, glycogen storage disease), diabetic mother, cystic fibrosis, biliary atresia, choledochol cyst, sepsis, annular pancreas.

    b. Obtain cultures: Serological testing for intrauterine infection; urine test for reducing substances.

    c. Evidence of infection: Appropriate antimicrobial therapy.

    d. No evidence of infection: Liver function tests; ultrasound scan for obstructive masses; liver needle or open biopsy; operative cholangiogram.

Older Children

1. Complete blood cell count: May suggest a hemolytic etiology.

2. Urinalysis: To detect urobilinogen in the urine.

3. Electrolytes, blood urea nitrogen, and creatinine: To ensure adequate renal function.

4. SGOT, SGPT, lactate dehydrogenase, alkaline phosphatase: Reflect liver function.

5. Bromsulphalein (BSP) excretion test: Most sensitive test of liver function (clearance and excretion).

6. Serum proteins: Usually decreased in liver disease.

7. Coagulation studies: Liver-dependent factors are decreased in liver disease.

8. α-Fetoprotein: May be elevated in children with hepatic neoplasms.

9. Glucose 6-phosphatase level: If deficiency is suspected by a positive medical history and the presence of hemolytic anemia.

10. Sickle-cell preparation, hemoglobin electrophoresis, osmotic fragility test: If red blood cell abnormality is suspected.

11. Hepatitis markers and other viral titers: To detect hepatic infection.

12. Cholesterol level: Liver disease causes decreased synthesis of lipoproteins and a decrease in serum cholesterol.

13. Liver biopsy: In patients with chronic liver disease and/or unexplained hepatomegaly or jaundice.

TREATMENT PROTOCOL

Neonates

1. Phototherapy: Unconjugated bilirubin may be photo-oxidized in the skin to water-soluble forms that may be excreted in the bile and urine; used most often in newborns with physiological jaundice or mild hemolytic disease; effectively reduces the need for exchange transfusion.

2. Exchange transfusion: Effectively reduces the level of circulating bilirubin in neonates by up to 85% (using a two-volume exchange).

Older Children

Incidence of kernicterus is less than in neonates and higher levels of bilirubin can be tolerated. Establishment of an accurate diagnosis, treatment of underlying disease processes (if amenable to therapy), and provision of supportive care are of major importance.

Joint Pain

Joint pain is a common complaint in children and encompasses both arthritis and arthralgia. Arthralgia is the subjective complaint of joint pain without objective signs. With arthritis, there is usually joint swelling and/or limitation of motion. Heat, pain, and/or tenderness also occur.

Increasing numbers and complexities of recognizable diseases causing joint pain in children are being identified (Fig. 1). Many laboratory tests are being performed, often because the patients are unable to provide a pertinent history.

SIGNS AND SYMPTOMS

Unless the patient is febrile, has had a puncture wound, or has a distended, erythematous, hot joint, the diagnostic dilemma is complex. It should be determined as early as possible whether the joint symptoms are being caused by primary joint disease or reflect a multisystem disease, of which arthralgia is merely the first manifestation. The child who has joint complaints not overtly suggestive of septic arthritis or trauma but accompanied by fever, arthralgia, and/or skin rash has a high likelihood of having an inflammatory or infectious disease; the joint manifestations are only part of the systemic process.

DIFFERENTIAL DIAGNOSIS

1. Infectious (bacterial, fungal, viral)
2. Inflammatory [collagen-vascular (connective tissue) disease, vasculitis]
3. Noninflammatory (trauma, metabolic, neoplastic, reactive, systemic diseases associated with arthritis or arthralgia)

DIAGNOSTIC AND TREATMENT PROTOCOLS

Table 1 gives diagnostic and treatment protocols for a variety of conditions leading to joint pain.

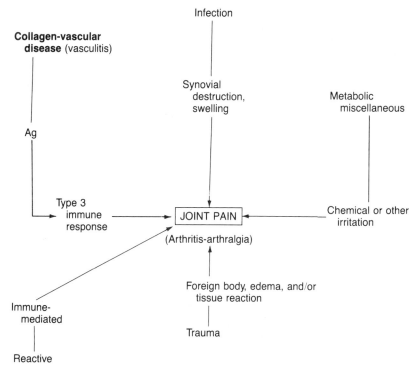

FIG. 1. Pathophysiology of joint pain. Ag, antigen.

TABLE 1. *Joint pain: Diagnostic and treatment protocols*

Diagnosis	Treatment
Septic Arthritis: Bacterial	
Most often a single joint is involved Bacteria-induced: Staphylococcus (in 40% <2 years old, in 50% 2–15 years old), streptococcus (in 25% <2 years old, in 35% 2–15 years old), *H. influenzae* (in 30% <2 years old, in 3% 2–15 years old), *N. gonorrheae* (in 5% 2–15 years old) Medical history may reveal abrupt onset of joint pain accompanied by chills, toxicity, and fever The affected joint is exquisitely tender, warm, distended, and held immobile (often in classic positions). Occasionally, a history of trauma with penetration of the joint space may be elicited	Early treatment is essential to preserve physiological range of motion; a true medical emergency After obtaining appropriate cultures, administer parenteral antibiotics (oral administration produces lower serum levels and depends on gastrointestinal absorption, which is quite variable) Intra-articular instillation may be harmful because of reaction to the antibiotic or its carrier substance The duration of antibiotic therapy varies with the organism causing the arthritis Successful treatment of most bacterial pathogens requires 3 to 4 weeks of therapy

TABLE 1. *(continued)*

Diagnosis	Treatment
Usually an elevated white blood cell count with a shift to the left Erythrocyte sedimentation rate (ESR), although a nonspecific test, is often elevated above 50 mm/hr A radiograph of the affected joint taken with low penetration may show only soft-tissue swelling and a day or two later, repeat radiograph might reveal mild distention of the joint Radionuclide bone scanning is frequently the earliest positive test A positive scan (hot spot) may show up within one to two days of the infection A high incidence of false negative scans occurs in neonates Aspirated joint fluid is usually cloudy with elevated white blood cell count with a majority of polymorphonuclear forms; protein content is usually elevated and glucose depressed; perform fluid culture and Gram stain	Treat gonorrheal arthritis with intravenous penicillin for 3 days, followed by an oral course of therapy for 7 days Along with antibiotic therapy, immobilize the joint to minimize pain and decrease further joint destruction by altering the pressure dynamics within the joint Orthopedic consultation is essential and should be obtained as soon as bacterial infection of the joint is suspected Although the initial arthrocentesis for diagnosis accomplishes a rapid decrease in the intra-articular pressure and lysosomal enzyme activity, ongoing drainage procedures are usually essential for optimal resolution without any limitation of motion; ongoing decompression may be achieved by serial aspirations or open surgical drainage and must be decided by the consultant

Septic Arthritis: Viral[a]

These arthritides may precede, accompany, or follow various viral infections; toxicity, pyrexia, or acuteness of onset is rarely present Physical examination reveals a symmetrical polyarthritic process often involving the smaller joints The arthralgias accompanying these infections tend to be subjectively stronger than the objective signs The white blood cell count may be normal or mildly elevated with a predominance of lymphocytes The ESR is usually normal or slightly elevated A radiograph of the affected joint(s) may reveal soft-tissue swelling and/or mild distention of the joint Radionuclide bone scan is rarely indicated if the course is uncomplicated Joint aspiration should be performed if there is any doubt as to the etiology; aspirated fluid may vary from yellow to cloudy and have an elevated white blood cell count with a predominance of lymphocytic cells; the glucose and protein content tends to be nondiagnostic; the culture and Gram stain are usually negative	Viral arthritides are usually self-limited and resolve without sequelae Treatment is supportive and centered on the relief of pain (which may be considerable); analgesia and joint immobilization are usually adequate therapy for acute attacks

Septic Arthritis: Fungal[b]

Infection of the synovium by fungi is rarely an acute process; more often it is subacute or	Treatment should be handled by an infectious disease consultant in conjunction with an

Diagnosis	Treatment
chronic and results from hematogenous spread (rarely osteomyelitis may involve the joint by direct extension) Travel to an endemic area or antecedent primary focus of infection are significant The involved joint does not appear to be acutely involved and may be associated with a more obvious osteomyelitis or pyodermal lesion White blood cell count, ESR, and joint radiographs are not often helpful; the diagnosis often rests on a needle biopsy of the synovium and arthroscopy for histological and microbiological diagnosis	orthopedic surgeon; it is both complex and chronic

Tuberculous Arthritis

May involve the joints in a chronic progressive fashion but is not usually a primary manifestation of tuberculosis	See Tuberculosis chapter

Reactive Arthritis: Dysentery Illness[c]

Several acute and chronic arthritides are related to infections, but the pathogenesis is unclear (the infecting organism cannot be cultured from the joint fluid or elsewhere); they are grouped in a category of reactive arthritis and share the features of being systemic illnesses, often with a genetic predilection for the presence of HL-A-B27 antigen, and show immune complexes; they often have mucocutaneous, cardiac, ocular and/or gastrointestinal manifestations An arthritis may follow these dysentery illnesses by a period of weeks and is associated with a Reiter's-type disease, but acute polyarthritis may occur without any of the features of Reiter's disease; diagnosis rests on isolation of these organism(s) and in identification of the HL-A-B27 antigen	These entities tend to be self-limited; therapy is supportive and symptomatic

Reactive Arthritis: *Klebsiella* Pneumonia

A high fecal carriage rate of *klebsiella* pneumonia occurs in patients with active ankylosing spondylitis; the identification and association of *klebsiella* pneumonia with the HL-A-B27 cells in ankylosing spondylitis is sufficient to tentatively imply a reactive arthritis due to this organism	

Reactive Arthritis: Venereal Disease[d]

Infection with one of these three organisms and/or the presence of urethritis in the presence of other symptoms of Reiter's disease are sufficient to provide a tentative diagnosis of reactive arthritis due to venereal infection	The arthritis is self-limited and it is unclear whether antibiotic treatment (tetracycline) is efficacious

TABLE 1. *(continued)*

Diagnosis	Treatment

Noninflammatory Arthritis*e*

A history of recent trauma is not always volunteered, making the diagnosis more difficult, but evidence of swelling, discoloration, or puncture wound over the site of pain may be present; unless a complicating infection is present, there may be minimal physical signs (crepitation of motion may be present in the case of a fracture)

Bleeding into the joint should be obvious and there may be cues from the medical history, especially in the case of hemophilia and/or von Willebrand's disease, and in other coagulopathies and blood dyscrasias

Monitor hemoglobin to determine if the patient is losing blood into the lesion and obtain studies of various clotting factors

Soft-tissue and bone radiographs may be helpful to rule out foreign body and/or significant fracture

The treatment of a foreign body is surgical removal with either local analgesia or general anesthesia, depending on the location and the anticipated difficulty in its removal

A fracture in or near the joint should be handled by an orthopedic surgeon, utilizing open or closed reduction followed by immobilization

Hemarthrosis reflecting blood dyscrasias is most often initially treated by aspiration to allow decompression of the joint followed by the addition of specific factors

Collagen-Vascular Disease: Rheumatic Diseases*f*

The rheumatic diseases of childhood are similar to their counterparts in adults

Arthritis or arthralgia in connective tissue disease is only one feature of a multisystem disease and the diagnosis, with the exception of juvenile rheumatoid arthritis, tends to rely on other organ system manifestations and specific laboratory tests

Systemic Diseases with Arthralgias or Arthritides*g*

Unless the arthritis is associated with the systemic illness, the diagnosis is difficult and tends only to be made at the time that the precipitating illness becomes evident

Treatment is entity specific

Neoplastic Disease: Leukemia, Lymphoma, Neuroblastoma

Basic disease almost always occurs before development of joint pain, which is usually caused by pressure within the marrow by the packed cells or ongoing lysis and destruction of the bone by metastatic lesions

Treatment tends to be disease specific

Diagnosis	Treatment

Hereditary and Metabolic Disorders: Varied and Multiple

See specific chapters

---

[a]Hepatitis B, rubella, mumps, mononucleosis.

[b]Coccidioidomycosis, blastomycosis, cryptococcosis, sporotrichosis.

[c]*Salmonella, shigella, yersinia enterocolitica.*

[d]*Chlamydia, mycoplasma, N. gonorrhea.*

[e]Trauma or nontraumatic orthopedic conditions, foreign body, Osgood-Schlatter's disease, slipped capital femoral epiphysis.

[f]System lupus erythematosus, polyarteritis nodosa, monocutaneous lymph node syndrome, scleroderma, dermatomyositis, mixed collagen-vascular disease, systemic vasculitis, anaphylactoid purpura, ankylosing spondylitis, rheumatic fever, rheumatoid arthritis.

[g]Inflammatory bowel disease, e.g., ulcerative colitis or regional enteritis, psoriasis, sarcoid, Stevens-Johnson syndrome.

Lead Poisoning

Lead poisoning is an environmental disease that affects people of all ages, but children are specifically, and severely, affected by its extreme toxicity. The normal blood level of lead is zero. However, in our industrialized society, almost everyone has a detectable blood level of lead.

There are two main portals of entry: the gastrointestinal tract and the respiratory tract. The ingestion of paint chips peeling from interior walls painted with lead-based paint was the most important source of high doses of lead before the 1950s. After the 1950s, lead-based paint was no longer used on interior surfaces, but, in older dwellings, the old paint was just covered with coats of new paint. Peeling of both the new and old paint can occur, still making lead available for children to ingest. Other environmental sources of lead that are considered intermediate dose sources are exterior surface paint, dust and dirt contaminated with automobile emissions, contaminated snow, small baubles and trinkets coated with lead-based paint, glazes fired at temperatures below 2000°F, newsprint, and smelter's dust. Respiratory tract absorption of lead is more complete than gastrointestinal tract absorption, but it is much less common. The amount of lead absorbed from the lungs is also dependent on the particle size.

Children are considered to have an increased body lead burden when they are asymptomatic and exhibit a blood lead level between 30 and 79 μg/100 ml or an erythrocyte protoporphyrine level between 60 and 189 μg/100 ml. Children are considered to have lead poisoning under several circumstances:

1. When the blood lead level is 50 to 79 μg/100 ml and specific symptoms of lead intoxication are present

2. When the blood lead level is 50 to 79 μg/100 ml and there is an abnormality of one or more of the other biochemical tests indicative of lead poisoning

3. When the erythrocyte protoporphyrine level is 110 to 189 μg/100 ml in the presence of specific symptoms of lead intoxication

4. When the blood lead level is greater than 79 μg/100 ml or the erythrocyte protoporphyrine level is greater than 189 μg/100 ml in the symptomatic or asymptomatic child

PATHOPHYSIOLOGY

The basic defect attributable to lead intoxication is the blockage of δ-aminolevulinic acid dehydratase.

SIGNS AND SYMPTOMS

Three systems are primarily affected by lead: the gastrointestinal system, the hematological system, and the central nervous system. Early in the course of toxicity, the symptoms are vague. There may be nausea, vomiting, and abdominal pain. At this point, the symptom complex may appear as an acute gastroenteritis. However, there is usually constipation, rather than diarrhea.

A hypochromic microcytic anemia occurs. The hemoglobin level is usually less than 10 grams and may be associated with pallor.

The central nervous system is significantly affected by increasing total body and tissue lead levels. Lethargy, malaise, ataxia, neuropathy, and behavior changes are not uncommon. Signs and symptoms of increased intracranial pressure may be present. Major motor seizures and coma may occur. Major central nervous system sequelae and chronic seizure disorders are common in 80% of significantly symptomatic patients.

DIAGNOSTIC PROTOCOL

Screening Tests

To detect an increased body lead burden in asymptomatic patients; children between the ages of 1 and 5 years who live in old housing built before the 1950s (especially if the dwelling is poorly maintained) should be screened yearly between May and October.

1. Erythrocyte protoporphyrine level: A good first line screening test; if it is positive (>60 $\mu g/100$ ml), blood lead level should be determined.

2. Blood lead level: A sensitive test, but affected by many external and internal influences; lead is in dynamic equilibrium between the blood and soft tissues; levels >100 $\mu g/100$ ml increase the risk of encephalopathy.

3. A negative blood lead level or erythrocyte protoporphyrine level virtually excludes lead intoxication; a positive test requires further investigation (see Table 1).

Further Diagnostic Tests

1. Complete blood cell count: A microcytic hypochromic anemia is usually present; basophilic stippling in the peripheral blood is extremely variable, but in a bone marrow smear stippling of the normoblasts is common in lead poisoning.

2. Urinalysis: Glycosuria and proteinuria are common.

3. Qualitative urinary coproporphyrine: An intense reaction is usually associated with lead levels >100 $\mu g/100$ ml and is an emergent indication for hospitalization.

4. Quantitative urinary coproporphyrines: >150 $\mu g/24$ hr is abnormal.

5. Urinary excretion of δ-aminolevulinic acid: >20 $\mu g/100$ ml is abnormal.

6. EDTA mobilization test: Only to be performed on asymptomatic patients. Calcium disodium EDTA, 25 mg/kg (maximum dose, 1 g); collect urine for 24 hr.

TABLE 1. *Classification of lead screening results*

Class	Erythrocyte protoporphyrine level (μg/100 ml)	Blood lead level (μg/100 ml)	Comments
I	59	29	Normal; no further evaluation is necessary except normal screening
Ia	60	29	May be normal; treat iron deficiency if present; provide appropriate follow-up
Ib	29	30–49	monthly to ensure that there is no increase in the body lead burden
II	60–109[a]	30–49[a]	Minimal; search for iron deficiency and treat if present; further medical history and testing may be indicated; patients usually do not require treatment other than removing the lead source
III	110–189	50–79	Moderate; further testing is indicated; lumbar puncture should be avoided unless meningitis is suspected; EDTA challenge is indicated in asymptomatic patients; treat the patient in the hospital
IV	190	80	Severe; medical emergency regardless of whether the patient is symptomatic or asymptomatic; risk of encephalopathy is high; hospitalize the patient

[a]Classify as Class IV if symptoms are present.
Modified from Rudolph, *Pediatrics*.

When ratio of micrograms of lead excreted to milligrams of EDTA ingested is >1, lead poisoning is indicated.

7. Flat plate radiograph of the abdomen: To detect radiopaque paint chips or flecks (present in approximately 50% of symptomatic children).

8. Radiographs of the long bones: Lead lines in the metaphyses of long bones are usually present in children 2 to 5 years of age.

9. Urine lead output: If the patient is symptomatic, the excretion of >1.5 mg of lead in 24 hr in the first day of chelation therapy is diagnostic of lead poisoning.

TREATMENT PROTOCOL

Supportive Care

1. Ensure adequate urine flow.

2. Judicious management of fluids; enough hydration to ensure good urine output, but not enough to exacerbate cerebral edema, if present; syndrome of inappropriate secretion of antidiuretic hormone (SIADH) is not uncommon in patients with encephalopathy.

3. Diazepam (Valium®) may be required to control seizures; maintenance with paraldehyde is preferable to phenobarbital or phenytoin (Dilantin®) early in the disease.

4. Mannitol may be used to treat increased intracranial pressure (specific neuro-surgical procedures are usually contraindicated).

5. Specific treatment protocol depends on the extent of elevation of the blood lead level and the presence or absence of symptoms.

Protocol I

All symptomatic patients with or without encephalopathy, and asymptomatic patients with blood lead level >100 μg/100 ml.

1. Dimercaprol (BAL), 4 mg/kg i.m. (it is important to give only BAL as a first dose to prevent the precipitation of acute encephalopathy when the lead is drawn out of bone and soft tissue during chelation).

2. BAL, 4 mg/kg i.m., **and** EDTA, 12.5 mg/kg i.m., in separate sites, 4 hr later.

3. BAL, 4 mg/kg i.m., **and** EDTA, 12.5 mg/kg i.m., every 4 hr for 5 days (usually 30 doses).

4. Penicillamine, 25–40 mg/kg/24 hr divided b.i.d., for 3 to 6 months after initial chelation therapy.

5. Subsequent courses of inpatient chelation therapy are determined by blood lead levels 2 or 3 weeks after the first course. If encephalopathy is present, a second 5-day course is indicated with blood lead levels >80 μg/100 ml. If there is no encephalopathy, but blood lead level is >60 μg/100 ml, a second 5-day course is indicated.

Protocol II

Asymptomatic patients with blood lead levels of 80 to 100 μg/100 ml.

1. EDTA, 50 mg/kg/24 hr deep i.m. in two or three divided doses for 3 to 5 days.

2. Penicillamine, 25–40 mg/kg/24 hr divided b.i.d., for 3 to 6 months.

3. A second 5-day course is indicated if the blood lead level is ≥60 μg/100 ml 2 or 3 weeks after the first course.

Protocol III

Long-term chelation therapy.

1. D-Penicillamine, 30–40 mg/kg/24 hr p.o. in two divided doses for 30 days (an investigational drug in the United States; not licensed for the treatment of plumb-ism; consult the Food and Drug Administration for policy regarding its use).

2. Blood lead level should be monitored monthly; subsequent elevations may be due to continued exposure or continued high body burden.

3. D-Penicillamine is contraindicated in patients with penicillin allergy and those with residual lead in the bowel.

Leukemia

Leukemia is a primary neoplastic disease of the bone marrow. Immature, undifferentiated blast cells replace normal marrow elements. Acute leukemia is the most common malignancy in children, the incidence being 4 cases per 100,000 children below 15 years of age. Approximately 4,000 new cases of leukemia are reported each year. The peak age range is between 2 and 6 years. Males are affected slightly more often than females (1.3:1) and whites are affected more often than nonwhites (2:1).

The leukemias are defined by their predominant cell type: acute lymphoblastic (lymphocytic) leukemia and acute myelogenous leukemia. Acute myelogenous leukemia is subdivided into five types: myeloblastic, promyelocytic, monocytic, and di Guglielmo's syndrome (erythroleukemia). Chronic leukemias are rare in children, accounting for only 2% of the cases. The most common leukemia is acute lymphocytic leukemia (ALL), which accounts for more than 80% of the cases.

PATHOPHYSIOLOGY

The exact etiology of leukemia is unknown, but certain factors appear to be involved or to increase the risk of its development (Fig. 1).

SIGNS AND SYMPTOMS

The onset of leukemia is either explosive or insidious. Symptoms differ widely among patients and none are definitively diagnostic. Signs and symptoms are usually secondary to marrow infiltration and displacement by tumor cells or extramedullary invasion of other organs. Pallor, fatigability, cephalgia, lethargy, and fever are common. A history of easy bruisability and excessive bleeding is often present. Recurrent infections are not unusual. Lymphadenopathy, abdominal distention, bone pain, petechiae, arthralgias and/or priapism may be present. Less common manifestations include Mikulicz syndrome (from leukemic infiltration of the salivary glands) and subcutaneous nodules (leukemia cutis). Central nervous system involvement may cause cranial nerve palsy and/or increased intracranial pressure.

DIFFERENTIAL DIAGNOSIS

1. Idiopathic thrombocytopenic purpura
2. Aplastic anemia
3. Meningococcemia
4. Infectious mononucleosis
5. Rheumatic fever

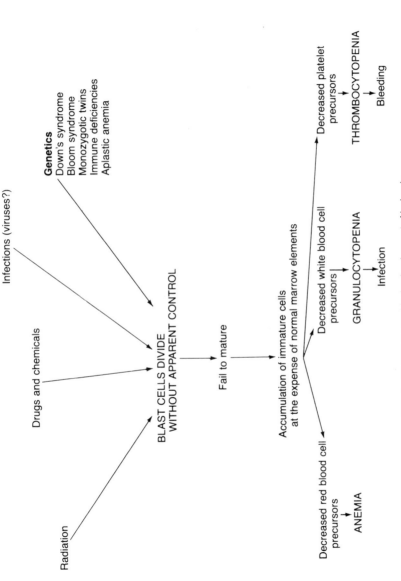

FIG. 1. Factors involved in the development of leukemia.

6. Rheumatoid arthritis

7. Osteomyelitis

8. Hodgkin's disease

9. Non-Hodgkin's lymphoma

10. Other tumors with marrow invasion

DIAGNOSTIC PROTOCOL

1. Obtain the medical history and perform a complete physical examination. The diagnosis of leukemia should be considered in any patient who presents with unexplained bleeding, ecchymosis, petechiae, anemia, and/or hepatosplenomegaly.

2. Complete blood cell count may reveal pancytopenia; massive leukocytosis may occur.

3. Urinalysis.

4. Chest radiograph.

5. Blood cultures and viral titers (if an infection is considered).

6. Blood chemistries: Uric acid (often elevated at the time of diagnosis), calcium (hypercalcemia or hypocalcemia may occur), potassium and sodium (both may be elevated or depressed), blood urea nitrogen and creatinine (to assess renal function), muramidase or lysozyme levels [present in acute myeloblastic leukemia (AML)].

7. Bone marrow aspiration (required for the diagnosis): >50% of the marrow will be replaced with abnormal immature cells; occasionally, the marrow will be difficult to aspirate due to massive infiltration (in such cases, a bone biopsy must be performed).

8. Cerebrospinal fluid examination (if CNS leukemia or infection is suspected).

9. Chromosome analysis (if a genetic predisposition is suspected).

10. Liver-spleen nucleotide scan.

11. Immunological markers (T-cell markers are found in approximately 20% of patients with ALL).

TREATMENT PROTOCOL

1. With early and aggressive management, 90 to 95% of children with ALL will obtain an initial remission (relapse often occurs within 12 to 36 months).

2. Nonspecific measures and general supportive care

   a. Hydrate and assure adequate caloric intake.

   b. Treat any concurrent infection vigorously.

   c. If the patient is significantly anemic, packed red blood cell transfusion(s) may be required.

d. If symptomatic thrombocytopenia is present, or if the platelet count is below 10,000, a platelet transfusion may be required.

e. Treat any identified electrolyte abnormality.

f. If hyperuricemia is present, treat with allopurinol, 10 mg/kg/day in equally divided doses (100–150 mg/m^2/12 hr) **and** sodium bicarbonate, 3 g/m^2/day in divided doses. (Most authorities recommend treatment of patients with ALL prior to antileukemic therapy to prevent hyperuricemic acidosis and uric acid nephropathy.)

3. Specific treatment should always be performed under the direction of an experienced pediatric oncologist and hematologist.

   a. Induction: Vincristine and prednisone.

   b. Radiation to the CNS axis (prophylaxis).

   c. Intrathecal methotrexate is also used in some protocols.

   d. Maintenance therapy is provided with methotrexate and 6-mercaptopurine (some regimens also include cyclophosphamide).

   e. Pulse doses of vincristine and prednisone are also used in some protocols.

Meningitis

In spite of all the advances made in medicine and the newer diagnostic and therapeutic techniques, meningitis is still one of the most serious, life-threatening infections of childhood. Mortality has been reduced substantially by rapid diagnosis and treatment and close monitoring, but a significant number of children recovering from meningitis are left with various gradations of neurological sequelae.

In most instances, the meninges are infected by hematogenous seeding from a distant focus (e.g., lobar pneumonia, bacterial endocarditis). In meningococcal infections, the organisms appear to gain access to the bloodstream via the nasopharynx. Direct extension of infection from the middle ear to the mastoids and then to the meninges (or through a fractured cribriform plate) also occurs (Fig. 1).

Meningeal infections appear to have a seasonal variation. Meningitis due to *H. influenzae* is chiefly an autumn or winter disease, whereas pneumococcal and meningococcal meningitides tend to occur in late winter or early spring. Males seem more predisposed than females to develop meningitis, as do individuals living in areas of high population density and poverty. Meningococcal meningitis is both epidemic (with a periodicity of approximately 10 years) and/or sporadic. Meningococcal and *Hemophilis* meningitis are transmitted from person to person and require prophylactic antibiotic treatment for the close contacts.

SIGNS AND SYMPTOMS

The clinical picture of acute bacterial meningitis is dependent on the age of the patient. The classic signs observed in older children and adults are rarely seen in infants. In general, the younger the child, the more diffuse and confusing the symptoms. The disease may begin with a mild fever accompanied by vomiting and chills. Within a brief period, a moderately severe headache may develop, especially in older children. Occasionally, CNS symptoms may overshadow the initial prodrome and the first sign of illness may be a convulsion. Similarly, the young infant with meningitis may exhibit nonspecific symptoms and reveal no specific signs of meningeal irritation (e.g., irritability, high-pitched cry, fretfulness, poor feeding, bulging fontanelle). In spite of the variation in the presentation, there are several common and classic signs of meningeal irritation:

1. Brudzinski's sign: Rapid flexion of the neck in the supine position results in severe pain and flexion of the knees.

2. Opisthotonos: Hyperextension of the spine.

356

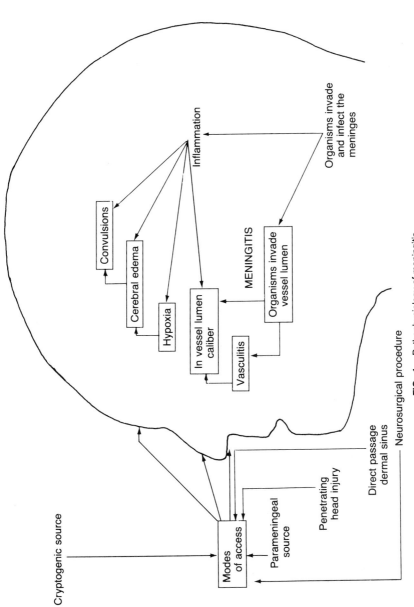

FIG. 1. Pathophysiology of meningitis.

3. Kernig's sign: In the supine position, there is resistance to extension of the knee with the thigh flexed at the hip.

Other nonspecific signs and symptoms, such as photophobia, dysphagia, hypotonia, hypothermia, and various skin rashes (especially with *N. meningitidis*) may be present.

DIFFERENTIAL DIAGNOSIS

The differential diagnosis of meningitis in children focuses on the distinction between meningismus and true meningeal irritation, as well as identification of the specific organism involved. Meningismus is described as meningeal signs without meningitis and may be associated with other acute systemic illnesses (viral or bacterial) that have not directly involved the meninges. Unfortunately, meningismus may precede any obvious signs and symptoms of the disease with which it is associated, and therefore, exacerbate an already confusing situation in an acutely ill child.

The etiology of acute bacterial meningitis varies with the age group considered and the setting under which the infection has occurred. Although many bacteria have been reported to cause meningitis, *N. meningitidis*, *H. influenzae*, *S. pneumoniae*, group A streptococcus, and *E. coli* cause the majority of meningitis in children from birth through 16 years of age (Table 1).

Aseptic meningitis is often benign and has multiple etiologies. It is characterized by headache, fever, vomiting, and meningeal signs. Cerebrospinal fluid (CSF) shows an increase in cells, mainly lymphocytes, and the sine qua non is that there is no bacterial growth in CSF cultures. Recovery is often complete and occurs within 7 to 10 days. Agents that result in aseptic meningitis may give rise to more diffuse involvement of the central nervous system (e.g., meningoencephalitis, encephalitis, encephalomyelitis). The boundary between the various forms of meningitis is quite indistinct. The enteroviruses (poliovirus, Coxsackie virus, ECHO virus) often tend to be associated with aseptic meningitis, but mumps, lymphocytic choriomeningitis, and herpesvirus are not uncommon.

TABLE 1. *Frequency of causative organisms in meningitis by age*

Organism	Newborn–2 months	2 months–3 yr	3–16 yr
E. coli	2	Occasionally	Rarely
Staphylococcus, group A	1	Occasionally	Rarely
H. influenzae	5	1	3
D. pneumoniae	4	2	1
N. meningitidis	—	3	2
S. aureus and species	3	4	Rarely

1, most frequent; 5, least frequent.

The following diseases and disorders must be considered in the differential diagnosis of meningitis:

1. Nonviral, nonbacterial agents
2. Protozoan and fungal infections
3. Postinfectious inflammation (e.g., rubeola, rubella, varicella)
4. Intrathecal medication
5. Leukemic infiltration
6. Hodgkin's disease
7. Metastatic carcinomatosis
8. Benign infectious lymphocytosis
9. Cat-scratch fever
10. Pemphigus
11. Benign myalgic encephalomyelitis
12. Poisons or toxins
13. Reactive inflammation secondary to a contiguous structure
14. Bechet's syndrome
15. Subluxation of the cervical vertebrae
16. Subarachnoid hemorrhage
17. Local irritation secondary to a lumbar puncture
18. Medications
19. Spider bites
20. Early herniation of the cerebellar tonsils
21. Tumor in the cervical or paracervical area
22. Neuroblastoma (medulloblastoma)

GENERAL DIAGNOSTIC PROTOCOL

There are certain findings that are common to bacterial meningitis regardless of the causative organism.

Medical History

1. Infants may show irritability, lethargy, vomiting, lack of appetite, and seizures (neck rigidity may be absent).

2. After 4 months of age, infants may show signs and symptoms similar to those in older children, with a full fontanelle and neck rigidity.

3. Older children experience headaches, vomiting, confusion, and lethargy, which may be followed by seizures.

4. Certain organisms should be suspected because they may follow, complicate, or be associated with other systemic signs:

    a. D. pneumoniae follows ear or sinus infections.

    b. N. meningitidis follows petechial skin lesions and/or arthritis.

    c. H. influenzae is most commonly associated with focal or generalized seizures in meningitis.

Physical Examination

1. Papilledema is distinctly unusual in uncomplicated meningitis in children; if present, consider brain abscess with rupture or an intracranial epidural abscess with extension.

2. Cranial bruits may occur in very young children with purulent meningitis.

3. Bulging fontanelle (increased intracranial pressure) is common in infants with meningitis.

4. Kernig's and Brudzinski's signs represent meningeal irritation, usually in older children (nuchal rigidity occasionally follows otitis media, subarachnoid hemorrhage, upper lobe pneumonia, cervical adenopathy, and retropharyngeal abscesses).

5. Skin lesions may occur in children with sepsis or meningitis, but classically accompany meningococcal meningitis (often manifested as a diffuse petechial or hemorrhagic rash, more pronounced on the extremities and the back); a similar rash may occur in *N. gonorrheae*, and more rarely in *H. influenzae* meningitis; occasionally, a maculopapular rash occurs with ECHO and adenoviruses; *Pseudomonas* septicemia may cause a distinctive rash known as erythema gangrenosum; the rash may accompany disseminated intravascular coagulation.

Laboratory Investigations

1. The white blood cell count is usually elevated with a shift to the left (a count of 20,000 to 30,000 white blood cells is not unusual); leukopenia that persists with severe infection is a poor prognostic sign.

2. Serum glucose level is usually depressed and occasionally elevated in overwhelming sepsis or in meningitis.

3. Serum sodium level may be normal or may reflect mild hyponatremia if the child has been given excess fluid or has the syndrome of inappropriate antidiuretic hormone secretion (SIADH) secondary to meningitis. Conversely, the child may be dehydrated, in which case the electrolytes can manifest as in other conditions associated with dehydration (elevated blood urea nitrogen and creatinine).

4. Recurrent meningitis or repeated significant bacterial infections necessitate evaluation for immune deficiency disease [beginning with immunoglobulins and considering stimulated nitroblue tetrazolium (NBT) tests].

5. If skin lesions are present, it is worthwhile to aspirate or swab the lesion and perform a Gram stain.

6. A skin test for tuberculosis should be strongly considered.

7. Skull and chest radiographs should be performed as soon as the patient's condition is stable to detect evidence of sinusitis, mastoid infection, or congenital or traumatic abnormalities.

8. Urinalysis should be performed to assess urine concentrating ability and to detect abnormal sediment; monitor urine electrolytes if there is any question about hyponatremia and SIADH.

9. C-reactive protein in CSF is a relatively new but promising test; early studies indicate its validity may be greater than the cell count, Gram stain, CSF protein or glucose. Moreover, it can be done with a minimal amount of spinal fluid (absolute amount will vary from laboratory to laboratory).

10. Cerebrospinal fluid examination for definitive diagnosis of bacterial meningitis (Table 2).

   a. The color of the fluid should be inspected (normal CSF is colorless); color tends to change from clear to slightly opalescent when there are approximately 500 cells in the fluid; a larger number of white blood cells are required to produce a turbid or cloudy spinal fluid.

   b. A significant amount of protein in the CSF produces a yellowish color, or haziness, and may cause coagulation if the protein is high enough.

   c. Red blood cells in the CSF may be the result of a traumatic tap or may reflect bleeding within the brain, which communicates with the ventricular system. A basic rule of thumb is that fewer than 350 red blood cells/ml^3 do not cause significant gross changes in the CSF, but at approximately 500 red blood cells/ml^3 a slight discoloration begins to occur and, with increasing amounts of blood, the fluid becomes increasingly discolored. A point of ongoing contention is whether the tap was traumatic or whether the patient sustained a previous bleeding. Rather than focusing on a few crenated cells, it may be worthwhile to centrifuge the sample and examine the supernatant. Red blood cells begin to hemolyze and alter the color of the supernatant only after they have been in the CSF for 4 to 12 hr.

   d. The blood cell count and determination of the particular type of cell are of prime therapeutic importance; it is imperative to note any polymorphonuclear forms and count them accurately.

   e. A Gram stain of the CSF is often helpful in suggesting the causative organism; if the fluid is purulent, centrifuging the specimen prior to the Gram stain may make identification easier.

   f. Countercurrentimmunoelectrophoresis (CIE) of the CSF allows indirect identification of the organism and should be ready within 30 to 60 min after the

TABLE 2. *Characteristics of cerebrospinal fluid in meningitis*

Cerebrospinal fluid	Bacterial meningitis	Viral meningitis	Tuberculous or fungal meningitis
Cell total	>500-1,000	≤500	≤500
Cell type	↑ Polymorphonuclear forms	↑ Lymphocytes	↑ Lymphocytes
Protein	Increased	Increased	Increased
Glucose	Decreased	Normal	Decreased
Organism	Present	Absent	Present

laboratory obtains the fluid; because the method depends on an antigen rather than on actual identification of the organism, it may be positive even with a negative culture.

g. CIE can also be performed on concentrated urine (some reports indicate that the results may be superior).

h. *Limulus* lysate test is controversial for use in children (its greatest efficacy is in identification of endotoxemia and shock in adults).

i. In a majority of previously untreated bacterial infections, the CSF results are diagnostic and classically consist of an elevated opening pressure (180 mm H_2O), a cloudy or purulent fluid, and numerous polymorphonuclear cells.

j. The CSF glucose is usually depressed relative to the serum glucose ($<50\%$); protein content is elevated; the offending organism is often identified tentatively on a Gram stain, allowing selection of antibiotics based on more than just age-specific statistics.

k. In some cases, the CSF findings are not diagnostic; if the child is not very ill, it is not unreasonable to repeat the spinal tap in 4 to 6 hr, based on the theory that the bacterial invasion occurred shortly before the spinal tap was performed and an adequate inflammatory response had not yet occurred.

l. Children who are granulocytopenic or immunosuppressed may have a minimal CSF cellular response, thereby paralleling the course of their white blood cells throughout the rest of the body.

m. Marked serum hyperglycemia may result in spurious interpretation of the CSF glucose.

n. Although viral meningitis usually evokes a lymphocytic response, it is not uncommon that a polymorphonuclear response will occur early in the course and become lymphocytic within several hours; unfortunately, tuberculous meningitis has a similar lymphocytic response; in tuberculous meningitis, the glucose often drops precipitously, whereas in viral meningitides, it may be normal.

o. Another entity which occasionally causes hypoglycorrhachia is subarachnoid bleeding.

p. The mechanism lowering CSF glucose is thought to be due to several interactive processes:

   (1) rapid uptake of glucose by the polymorphonuclear cells, which have undergone an increase in their metabolic rate.

   (2) an increase in the rate of glucose utilization by the brain, and defective transport across the inflamed blood-brain barrier.

q. Specific isoenzymes of lactic dehydrogenase may be elevated in bacterial meningitis; this has been suggested as a distinguishing feature between bacterial and viral meningitis, but the test remains controversial.

r. It is imperative to recognize that there are entities other than bacterial meningitis which cause comparable CSF changes; leukemia and metastatic infiltrates may cause similar cellular response, and it has been postulated that migraine headaches may result in pleocytosis in otherwise normal CSF.

s. One of the greatest concerns to physicians performing spinal taps on children is the possibility that bacteria may be introduced into the meninges, especially if the lumbar puncture is performed during a period of bacteremia. This concern remains more theoretical than factual, and a repeat spinal tap 4, 6, or 12 hr later, depending on the results and clinical condition, is indicated when clinical findings strongly suggest meningitis and CSF from the first spinal tap showed no abnormalities. There is some evidence that repeated taps may yield the best return with meningococcal infections, as early infiltration of the meninges by these organisms may provoke a very limited response.

GENERAL TREATMENT PROTOCOL

1. All children with suspected meningitis should be treated initially intravenously; treatment should not be withheld pending definitive identification of the organism.

2. The choice of antibiotic should be based on the statistical probability of which organism is commonly incriminated in that particular age group (see Table 1).

3. Intravenous fluids should be decreased slightly (two-thirds of maintenance) because of the likelihood of SIADH, which often occurs subclinically.

4. Antibiotics should be administered by intravenous infusion as soon as the lumbar puncture is performed; with a deteriorating condition, they should be administered immediately and then followed by the lumbar puncture within a few minutes (some data show that partial treatment of *H. influenzae* meningitis has little effect on the culture, but meningococcal organisms seem exquisitely sensitive to even one to two doses of penicillin; nevertheless a sick child must be treated).

5. When the diagnosis is obscure, it would seem best to err on the side of conservatism and begin treatment immediately, with the assumption that the child has bacterial meningitis.

6. It is reasonably conventional to begin empirical treatment with two drugs, most often penicillin or a penicillin derivative plus a broad-spectrum antibiotic to cover gram-negative organisms. Because of the increasing number of ampicillin-resistant strains of *H. influenzae*, treatment may consist of ampicillin, 300 to 400 mg/kg/day, **plus** chloramphenicol, 100 mg/kg/day (every 6 hr) for 10 days.

7. Seizures are not infrequent concomitants of meningitis and may be intermixed (focal and generalized), recurrent and prolonged, and/or focal, which should alert the physician to the possibility of a local process.

8. Acute cerebral edema is life-threatening; mannitol (by infusion over a 30-min period) or glycerol (p.o., nasogastric tube) may be used to decrease the cerebral edema; our choice is mannitol.

9. Dexamethasone, 2 to 4 mg i.v. every 4 hr, may be used to reduce cerebral edema.

10. The acute vasculitis of meningitis is treated empirically, most often only by treatment of the acute infection; steroids have been used with varied success.

DIAGNOSTIC PROTOCOL

Hemophilus influenzae

1. Most common cause of bacterial meningitis in children >2 months to 3 years of age (serious infections are rare over 10 years of age).

2. Repeat the spinal tap in 24 to 36 hr if there is any question about the response, especially in view of *H. influenzae* resistance.

3. The disease is more common in the winter months and usually cases of meningitis are from type B influenza.

4. An upper respiratory infection or otitis media often precedes the onset of meningitis.

5. The initial signs of *H. influenzae* meningitis are often more subtle than those of pneumococcal or meningococcal meningitis, which may result in a lack of prompt treatment.

6. Positive CSF cultures are obtained in 60% to 70% of cases.

Neisseria meningitidis

Classification includes groups A–D with various serogroups X, Y, Z, and Z'.

1. Gram-negative cocci often arranged in pairs and thus often referred to as diplococcus.

2. Majority of cases are groups B and C.

3. Antibody formation occurs either with clinical infection or with colonization of the organism in the nasopharynx.

4. Immunity may be acquired in infancy (passively transferred maternal antibody) or later in life through exposure to meningococcal antigen by colonization with nongroupable meningococci, which rarely cause systemic disease but may be a potent stimulus for the production of antibodies against more virulent strains.

5. Manifestations of meningococcal disease are those of septicemia with endotoxins affecting the heart, skin, joints, nervous system.

6. The severity varies, but the disease may be ushered in with joint pain, headaches, and fevers or the rash may be an overshadowing and more prevalent feature (papular lesion to confluent ecchymotic lesions mainly on lower extremities).

7. Cardiac involvement in meningitis is widely recognized and may be the significant feature in the outcome of this disease; pericarditis and pericardial effusion are also associated, and acute cardiac tamponade may cause death.

8. Arthritis may be debilitating and severe but is usually transient and appears to represent immune-complex formation or hypersensitivity rather than actual seeding of the joints with meningococcal organisms.

9. Between 10% and 15% of affected patients develop skin lesions (cutaneous vasculitis) or arthritis, which tends to occur at the end of the first week of the illness and is more closely associated with patients who are more acutely ill on presentation.

10. Ocular manifestations (endophthalmitis, conjunctivitis).

11. Fulminating downhill course and then death may represent endotoxic shock or disseminated intravascular coagulation.

12. Waterhouse-Friderichsen syndrome: Originally thought to represent a form of adrenal failure secondary to hemorrhage, but cortisol levels are often elevated and many patients fail to respond to cortisol therapy; may be caused by inability of the vessels to respond to epinephrine, resulting in peripheral vascular collapse.

13. Disseminated intravascular coagulation: Injury to the endothelium of the blood vessels may result in or trigger a disseminated intravascular coagulation process.

14. Positive CSF cultures are obtained in 60% to 70% of cases, in addition to the other laboratory findings that are nonspecific.

Diplococcus pneumoniae

1. A gram-positive cocci often occurring in pairs with a well-defined capsule.

2. This organism can be divided into more than 75 types on the basis of distinct polysaccharides in the capsule. Fortunately, not all are prevalent in causing meningitis.

3. Pneumococcus is a rare cause of meningitis in neonates, but in children 4 months to 3 years of age it ranks second only to *H. influenzae*.

4. As compared with other forms of bacterial meningitis, pneumococcal meningitis is more often rapid and fulminant in its onset, being ushered in by convulsions and meningeal signs within hours after its initial manifestation.

5. Occasionally, this meningitis occurs without an obvious focus (presumably results from seeding secondary to pneumococcal septicemia).

6. A notable feature is its relative frequency of association with underlying structural defects or systemic illnesses (e.g., defect penetrating the subarachnoid space, head trauma with skull fracture, congenital defect of the cribriform plate, congenital defect of the foot plate of the stapes, and/or a congenital dermal sinus with direct connection to the CSF). These forms of meningitis are often recurrent and an anatomical defect should be suspected in any patient with recurrent episodes of meningitis of any type.

7. Otitis media, paranasal sinusitis, mastoiditis, and paracranial foci have been associated with an increased incidence of pneumococcal meningitis in children.

8. Elective splenectomy, especially when associated with blood dyscrasia, predisposes children to pneumococcal meningitis. Lumbar puncture may be associated

with a paucity of reactive cells, although an overwhelming number of organisms may be seen on Gram stain; the risk of postsplenectomy infection is much less in individuals with splenectomy secondary to trauma than in those with elective splenectomy. One theory here is that after trauma, occasionally niduses are spilled into the abdomen and implant as functional tissue.

9. The hazard of overwhelming infection appears to also be age related with children <4 to 5 years of age at the greatest risk.

10. Patients who have undergone autosplenectomy (e.g., as in sickle-cell disease) are equally at risk for developing overwhelming pneumococcal meningitis and septicemia (pneumococcus is not the only opportunistic organism in these patients).

11. Children with certain systemic illnesses, especially immunodeficiency disorders, are more prone to develop overwhelming pneumococcal sepsis.

Tuberculous Meningitis

1. Tuberculous meningitis has become so uncommon, while viral meningitis has become so frequent, that it is often not even considered as part of the differential diagnosis, resulting in unacceptably delayed diagnosis and treatment.

2. Every child admitted to the hospital should have a tuberculin test performed.

Viral Meningitis

1. The differential diagnosis of viral meningitis consists of a plethora of potential organisms.

2. Isolation of the offending organism or demonstration of titer elevations between acute and convalescent sera.

TREATMENT PROTOCOL

Hemophilus influenzae

1. The frequency of *H. influenzae* meningitis is unchanged, but the antibiotic sensitivity patterns show continued alteration. It is important to know the susceptibility patterns in a specific area, but with reported incidences of 20% resistance in many areas, treatment with penicillin **and** chloramphenicol is suggested when there is any question about the child's response, deteriorating state, or local bacterial sensitivities.

2. See General Treatment Protocol.

3. Chloramphenicol, 100 mg/kg/day every 6 hr, **plus** ampicillin, 250 to 300 mg/kg/day every 6 hr, for 10 days.

4. The oral use of chloramphenicol in meningitis has been successful but greater experience with this route of administration is needed.

TABLE 3. *Treatment of acute complications of bacterial meningitis*

Complication	Treatment
Shock	Volume expansion; corticosteroids digitalis
Cerebral edema	Fluid restriction; osmotic diuretic, mechanical hyperventilation
Hyponatremia	Fluid restriction; hypertonic saline
Recurrent fever	
Phlebitis	Supportive care for phlebitis;
Subdural effusion	Evacuation of effusion or abscess
Abscess	
Convulsions	Anticonvulsant drugs, monitor electrolytes
Disseminated intravascular coagulation	Volume expansion, diuretics, dialysis

Complications (Table 3)

1. Subdural effusion is a common complication; suspect if fever persists after 48 hr of treatment (Table 4).

2. Positive CSF cultures and/or convulsions after 48 hr of treatment may occur (the quantity of fluid is not significant; the organism can readily be grown when a subdural tap is performed).

3. There is a risk of serious infection to intimately exposed adults and children (risk of secondary infection in children <4 years of age is estimated at 2.1%).

4. Mortality rate is 5% to 8%.

5. Sequelae range from very mild to severe and incapacitating (hearing loss and facial nerve deficits are prevalent, but mental retardation, hydrocephalus and seizures occur with alarming frequency).

6. CSF may be obstructed (measure head circumference and follow growth curve during course of illness and for a period of time thereafter).

Neisseria meningitidis

1. See General Treatment Protocol.

2. Aqueous penicillin G, 5 to 8 million units/day i.v. (2 to 5 years old) or 8 to 12 million units/day i.v. (5 to 10 years old) in four to six divided doses, **or** ampicillin,

TABLE 4. *Causes of persistent fever in meningitis*

Ineffective or inappropriate treatment	Subdural effusion or empyema
Phlebitis	Foreign body (e.g., catheter)
Abcess	Tissue necrosis
Superficial	Drug fever
Deep brain parenchyma	

200 to 300 mg/kg/day i.v. every 6 hr (there is some question as to whether ampicillin adequately penetrates into the CSF when the infection is with meningococcal meningitis).

3. If the patient is allergic to penicillin, use chloramphenicol.

4. Initially, half of the daily dose of antibiotic may be given over a 30-min period or as a bolus in smaller quantity (a third of the daily dose over several minutes) in an attempt to avoid the possible complications of meningococcal meningitis.

5. There is still a significant mortality rate of 8.1%.

6. Sequelae ranging from hearing loss through bilateral chronic subdural empyemas, are also significant.

7. Acute sequelae, such as endotoxic shock with fulminating meningococcemia, require early diagnosis and prompt therapy.

Diplococcus pneumoniae

1. See General Treatment Protocol.

2. Aqueous penicillin G, 250,000 units/kg/day i.v. in four to six divided doses, **or** ampicillin, 300 to 400 mg/kg/day i.v. in four divided doses for 3 weeks.

3. Pneumococcal vaccine should be used in patients who are known to be predisposed to infections such as pneumococcus.

4. Therapy should be slightly more prolonged than the usual 10 days to 2 weeks in other forms of bacterial meningitis; a 3-week course of therapy is recommended.

5. Chloramphenicol is an acceptable alternative for patients who are allergic to penicillin.

6. It is generally thought that 2% of children with bacterial meningitis will experience a reappearance of bacteria in the CSF during therapy or a relapse of the meningitis, usually within a month after therapy; these complications are usually seen in patients younger than 2 years of age or patients who have predisposing conditions (Table 5).

7. Repeat spinal taps and/or a search for secondary nidus of infection are warranted if there should be recrudescence of fever or other atypical signs; review of the antibiotic dosage intervals and sensitivity of the organism to the antibiotic is appropriate.

TABLE 5. *Causes of recurrent meningitis*

Congenital	Chronic infections
Dermoid sinus	Apical periostitis
Immune system disorders	Active otitis media
Traumatic	Other
Fracture of the cribriform plate	Vogt-Koyanagi-Harada syndrome
Ventriculostomy	Mollaret's disease

8. It is beyond the scope of this volume to discuss the various modalities used to determine potential anatomical defects for the source of recurrent pneumococcal infection, but a CSF leak is demonstrated by using nasal secretions and reagent strip (Dextrostix®) as well as myelographic installation of dyes.

Viral Meningitis

1. See General Treatment Protocol.
2. Treat the same as bacterial meningitis with the exclusion of antibiotics.

Mental Retardation

Mental retardation is defined as significantly subaverage general intellectual functioning (two standard deviations below the normal) existing concurrently with deficits in adaptive behavior and manifested during the developmental period. The diagnosis is based on subnormal performance on standardized intelligence tests and the inability of the patient to meet the standards of personal and social independence expected for age. Four categories are recognized: mild (IQ 55–69), moderate (IQ 40–54), severe (IQ 25–39), and profound (IQ <25).

Before a child is labeled as mentally retarded, several facts must be considered. If the above definition of mental retardation is accepted, a blind person who has a normal IQ (normal intelligence) may not have adequate adaptive behavior. Conversely, a child who has a low IQ (retarded) may have normal adaptive and social behavior. Therefore, **the I.Q. alone is not enough to establish the diagnosis of mental retardation.** An accurate assessment of mental ability depends on a complete developmental evaluation performed by professionals who are certified to administer and interpret the tests.

Mental retardation is only one cause of a low IQ score. Other causes include seizures, deficiencies in hearing and vision, illness, fever, anxiety or fear during the testing, deficient cultural orientation, and emotional problems.

Before the IQ score is interpreted, all other physiological causes of a low IQ score must be excluded. If in doubt, the tests must be repeated or administered in different settings, or other tests must be utilized.

Once mental retardation is established, other associated problems must be ruled out, including problems related to ambulation, speech, emotional development, vision, toilet training, and hearing. Associated seizures and chronic organic conditions (heart disease, diabetes, obesity, anemia, dental disease, venereal disease, nutritional problems) also must be excluded.

Mentally retarded children often have mentally dull and/or socioeconomically deprived parents (polygenic and environmental factors). It is unlikely that a specific diagnosis will be achieved. Children with a specific chromosomal abnormality (XXY or XXX) may be detected in this group, and a few will have metabolic defects or mild CNS defects.

Although only three conditions associated with mental retardation are treatable—phenylketonuria (PKU), hypothyroidism, and subdural hematoma—and although an etiology may not be readily identified except in 50% to 60% of affected patients, every attempt should be made to establish a diagnosis for obvious genetic and prognostic reasons.

DIAGNOSTIC PROTOCOL

1. Obtain a detailed medical history.

   a. Onset of the problem (prenatal, perinatal, postnatal, or undecided).

   b. Manifestations of the problem (abnormal appearance, abnormal function, and/or obvious neurological dysfunction).

   c. Maternal history of pregnancies, abortions, infections, all drug intake, and/or eclampsia.

   d. Patient's medical history, including neonatal history, presence of fevers, and/or previous trauma.

   e. Family history, including the presence of similar conditions in other family members.

   f. Environmental history (parenting), living conditions, and/or social interactions.

2. Perform a detailed physical examination with special attention to any observed defects (malformations), dysfunction, and/or neurological deficits.

3. Laboratory investigations should not be haphazard and unnecessarily costly; they depend on the age at onset and presumed cause of the disorder (see Table 1); all patients should receive the following evaluations.

   a. Complete blood cell count.

   b. Urinalysis.

   c. Urine ferric chloride test and test for reducing substances.

   d. Buccal smear for the X and Y chromatin.

   e. PKU test.

TABLE 1. *Presumed causes of mental retardation by age at onset*

Prenatal onset
    Single brain defect (e.g., microcephaly, hydrocephaly, neural tube defect)
    Multiple brain defects (e.g., chromosomal syndromes, unknown, nonchromosomal
      syndromes)
Perinatal onset
    Birth trauma (e.g., hypoxia, CNS hemorrhage)
    Metabolic (e.g., kernicterus, hypoglycemia)
    Infection (e.g., sepsis, meningitis)
Postnatal onset
    Environmental
    Metabolic
    Infection
    Other
Undecided age at onset
    Prenatal infection (e.g., rubella, toxoplasmosis, cytomegalovirus)
    CNS disease
    Hypothyroidism
    Unknown

f. Thyroid function tests (PKU and thyroid function tests should be done even if the initial screening tests at birth showed no abnormalities).

g. Blood glucose, blood urea nitrogen and creatinine.

h. Complete ophthalmological examination.

i. Further testing depends on the index of suspicion and may include skull radiographs, electroencephalogram (EEG), CT scan, pneumoencephalogram and arteriogram (in rare cases), bone survey (skeletal series).

4. If a chromosomal abnormality is suspected, perform the following analysis:

a. Banded karyotype analysis using serum lymphocytes.

b. Bone marrow cells may be used to shorten the period for results if chromosomal problems (trisomy 13 or 18) are suspected in a critically ill infant.

5. If a lysosomal storage disease is suspected, test for the following diseases (all have in common a degenerative course, visceromegaly, retinal degeneration, corneal clouding, skeletal dysostosis, positive family history, and/or abnormal facial features).

a. Mucopolysaccharidosis.

b. Lipidosis.

c. Type II glycogen storage disease.

d. Mucolipidosis.

e. Specific tests for the specific enzyme defect suspected should be requested (no screening tests are available).

f. Enzyme assay is done on serum leukocytes, fibroblasts, blood, bone marrow, and urine (frozen samples).

g. Electron microscopy and/or histochemical studies on frozen biopsy specimens from intestine, skin, muscle, liver, and brain (before any specimen is taken for assay or histochemistry studies, the laboratory where the test will be performed should be contacted and the efforts coordinated).

6. If an amino acid disorder is suspected (e.g., phenylketonuria, maple syrup urine disease, propionic acidemia, or urea cycle defects) or if a disorder of renal tubular transport is suspected (e.g., cystinuria, Hartnup disease, galactosemia, tyrosinemia, hereditary fructose intolerance, Lowe's syndrome, or Zellweger's syndrome), the following evaluation should be performed.

a. Allow nothing by mouth for 4 to 6 hr.

b. Patient must not have an infection, hypoglycemia, or be in a state of hyperalimentation.

c. Collect blood and urine samples (24-hr or one voided specimen); a single specimen is adequate if quantitation of amino acids is calculated per gram of creatinine.

d. Single-dimensional paper chromatography may be used for screening.

e. Quantitative analysis using high-pressure ion exchange chromatography or gas chromatography.

f. Gas chromatography and mass spectroscopy (GC-MS) is used for screening ill, acidotic neonates with no diagnosis; may identify amino acid and other types of inborn errors of metabolism.

g. Specific enzyme assays on blood or fibroblasts.

7. If a disorder of carbohydrate metabolism or enzyme deficiency in nonspherocytic hemolytic anemia is suspected, perform the following tests.

a. Blood glucose, lactate, and pyruvate.

b. Urine test for reducing substances.

c. Glucose, galactose, glucagon, and fructose tolerance tests.

d. Enzyme assays on erythrocytes, fibroblasts, amniotic fluid cells.

e. Liver biopsy for definitive diagnosis of hepatic glycogenosis.

8. Other tests:

a. Serum folate (important if the patient has megaloblastic anemia and increased homocystine in the blood).

b. Serum uric acid.

c. Serum copper (kinky hair syndrome).

d. Parathyroid function tests.

e. Serum calcium, phosphorus, and electrolytes.

TREATMENT PROTOCOL

1. Treat the specific cause of the mental retardation.

2. Define the child's needs, including medical, social, emotional, educational, vocational, and domiciliary (institutional or foster care).

3. Provide child and family counseling to help foster acceptance, to provide coping advice, and to prevent physical, sexual, or emotional abuse (the team approach is particularly helpful, with involvement of social worker, occupational therapist, psychologist, psychiatrist, physician, and educational diagnostician).

Mucocutaneous Lymph Node Syndrome

Mucocutaneous lymph node syndrome is a disease first described by Kawasaki in Japan and is of unknown etiology. It was classified by some as an infectious disease, but no specific agent could be isolated. Now, it is most often considered along with vasculitides and other inflammatory diseases or syndromes. The mortality rate is approximately 1%, usually secondary to myocardial thrombosis during the convalescent period.

PATHOPHYSIOLOGY

The exact pathophysiology of mucocutaneous lymph node syndrome has not yet been elucidated. However, most of the symptoms are attributable to a diffuse and intense vasculitis.

SIGNS AND SYMPTOMS

Fever is usually present for at least 5 days. Typically, there is a polymorphous rash with a centripetal distribution, bilateral conjunctivitis, cracking of the lips (or other mucous membrane involvement), cervical lymphadenopathy, and indurative swelling of the hands and feet with a red to violaceous discoloration. During convalescence, there is desquamation of the skin, beginning at the fingertips. Other symptoms that may appear during the acute phase of the illness are abdominal pain and diarrhea, arthritis, encephalitis, aseptic meningitis, hydrops of the gallbladder, myocarditis, congestive heart failure, and jaundice. The acute phase generally lasts 2 to 3 weeks.

Coronary artery aneurysm, thrombosis, and myocardial infarction are the major complications and occur during the convalescent period. They are the major cause of death in affected patients.

DIAGNOSTIC PROTOCOL

1. The diagnosis is based on the finding of the typical symptom complex.

   a. Fever (usually lasting at least 5 days).

   b. Four of five characteristics.

      (1) Conjunctivitis (bilateral).

      (2) Mucous membrane lesions.

      (3) Centripetal rash.

      (4) Cervical lymphadenopathy.

      (5) Centrifugal edema, discoloration, and/or desquamation.

    c. Absence of other etiologies of the syndrome.

2. Complete blood cell count: May show leukocytosis; thrombocytosis may occur during the convalescent phase.

3. Erythrocyte sedimentation rate: Usually elevated.

4. IgE level: Usually elevated.

5. Electrocardiogram: May show changes associated with myocarditis, pericarditis, tamponade, or myocardial infarction.

6. Coronary arteriography: Advocated by some experts; abnormalities in the coronary vessels may be seen, and this procedure would have its greatest effect on the treatment and, more important, the prognosis, but it is still a research procedure.

TREATMENT PROTOCOL

1. There is no specific treatment for the syndrome; supportive and symptomatic care is indicated.

2. Life-threatening cardiac complications are usually treated with prednisone, 2 to 3 mg/kg/day in four equally divided doses. The steroids are continued for approximately 3 days and then tapered over a 2-week period.

3. Aspirin, 110 mg/kg/day in five equally divided doses, is added on the third day; the dose should be adjusted to maintain a blood salicylate level of approximately 25 mg/dL.

4. The salicylates are continued for 5 weeks and then tapered by 25% per week.

5. If life-threatening complications are not immediately present, salicylates, 150 mg/kg/day in six equally divided doses, may be used alone; salicylate levels should be maintained at approximately 25 to 28 mg/dL; when this level is reached, the dose is decreased to 100 to 110 mg/kg/day, continued for 5 weeks, and then tapered by 25% per week.

Muscular Dystrophy

The muscular dystrophies are a group of inherited diseases characterized by progressive skeletal muscle degeneration. They are the most common diseases of muscle in young children and adolescents.

The most common form is the Duchenne type. It is X-linked in inheritance and, therefore, only clinically affects males. The other forms of muscular dystrophy are inherited autosomally and may affect either sex.

PATHOPHYSIOLOGY

Muscular dystrophy is a genetically inherited disease. There is characteristic muscle degeneration, usually of proximal muscle groups, along with pseudohypertrophy of the distal groups (especially with Duchenne's dystrophy). The type of dystrophy is dependent on the mode of inheritance (autosomal or X-linked), the primary muscle groups involved, and the rate of progression of the disease process.

SIGNS AND SYMPTOMS

The signs and symptoms of muscular dystrophy vary with the type of disease encountered and are dependent on the muscle group most affected. The extent and rate of progression of the disease will also affect the presenting signs and symptoms. The cardinal symptom is weakness, usually of proximal muscle groups.

DIFFERENTIAL DIAGNOSIS

1. Werdnig-Hoffmann disease
   (especially the Kugelberg-Welander form)
2. Peripheral neuropathy
3. Guillain-Barré syndrome
4. Myasthenia gravis
5. Inflammatory myopathies
6. Metabolic myopathies

INITIAL DIAGNOSTIC PROTOCOL

1. Complete blood cell count, urinalysis, electrolytes, calcium, renal functions, and liver functions: Normal.

2. Creatine phosphokinase (CPK): Markedly elevated (usually 10 to 100 times normal); enzyme elevation can be found before the clinical appearance of symptoms and is often abnormal in carrier females.

3. Electromyogram (EMG): Reveals characteristics of primary muscle disease; nerve conduction is usually normal.

4. Biopsy: Usually diagnostic, especially if there is a clinical correlation with histochemical studies.

5. The diagnosis is usually made with these laboratory studies and clinical correlation (see Diagnostic Protocol).

DIAGNOSTIC PROTOCOL

Duchenne Type

1. Inheritance: X-linked.
2. Onset of symptoms: 3 to 6 years of age.
3. Signs and symptoms: Difficulty climbing stairs, toe walking, weakness of hip girdle muscles, clumsiness, falling, pseudohypertrophy, difficulty in rising from supine position (Gowers' sign), decreased deep tendon reflexes.
4. Pseudohypertrophy: Prominent.
5. Progression: Rapid; patients are usually wheelchair-bound by 12 years of age.
6. Complications: Myocardial involvement; early flexion contractures.
7. Biopsy/EMG: Usually of the deltoid muscle, but should be guided by a neurologist; the specimen usually reveals muscle degeneration, fat infiltration, and deposition of perimysial and endomysial collagen.

Dreifuss and Hogan Type

1. Inheritance: X-linked.
2. Onset of symptoms: 3 to 5 years of age.
3. Signs and symptoms: Pelvifemoral weakness.
4. Pseudohypertrophy: Absent.
5. Progression: Slow.
6. Complications: Usually benign; myocardial involvement may occur.
7. Biopsy/EMG: Only moderate degenerative changes.

Mabry Type

1. Inheritance: X-linked.
2. Onset of symptoms: 10 to 15 years of age.

3. Signs and symptoms: Proximal weakness beginning in the hip girdle.

4. Pseudohypertrophy: Very prominent.

5. Progression: Slow.

6. Complications: Myocardial involvement is common; flexion contractures are absent.

7. Biopsy/EMG: Fat infiltration with little variation in fiber size; "ring" fibers are common and characteristic.

Becker's Type

1. Inheritance: X-linked.

2. Onset of symptoms: 4 to 20 years of age.

3. Signs and symptoms: Initially, pelvifemoral weakness; symptoms are similar to Duchenne type.

4. Pseudohypertrophy: Present.

5. Progression: Slow.

6. Complications: Cardiac involvement and contractures are usually absent.

7. Biopsy/EMG: Resemble changes seen in Duchenne type.

Facioscapulohumeral Type

1. Inheritance: Autosomal dominant.

2. Onset of symptoms: 7 to 10 years of age.

3. Signs and symptoms: Facial muscle weakness (facial diplegia) causing a characteristic myopathic facies (open mouth expression); shoulder girdle weakness also occurs; CPK may be only mildly elevated or may be normal; hip girdle involvement occurs late in the progress of the disease.

4. Pseudohypertrophy: Absent.

5. Progression: Slow.

6. Complications: Unusual.

7. Biopsy/EMG: Both show changes consistent with a myopathic process (degeneration of muscle fibers and fat replacement).

Limb-Girdle

1. Inheritance: Autosomal recessive.

2. Onset of symptoms: 7 to 10 years of age.

3. Signs and symptoms: Weakness of the hip girdle and shoulder girdle musculature.

4. Pseudohypertrophy: May or may not be present.

5. Progression: Slow.

6. Complications: Variable.

7. Biopsy/EMG: Evidence of myopathic process and primary muscle disease.

Oculopharyngeal Type

1. Inheritance: Unknown.

2. Onset of symptoms: 5 to 15 years of age.

3. Signs and symptoms: Usually isolated to the extraocular muscles with weakness and ophthalmoplegia; ptosis; dysphagia; difficulty in handling secretions.

4. Pseudohypertrophy: Absent.

5. Progression: Slow.

6. Complications: Pulmonary problems may occur secondary to pharyngeal involvement and difficulty in mobilizing secretions.

7. Biopsy/EMG: Extraocular muscles and/or pharyngeal muscles show changes consistent with primary myopathic processes.

TREATMENT PROTOCOL

There is no specific treatment for muscular dystrophy; most regimens are supportive and symptomatic.

1. The major emphasis of the management plan is on establishing the mode of inheritance in order to provide adequate genetic counseling and preventing or delaying complications of the primary disease process, both physical and psychological.

2. The approach is multidisciplinary and involves the primary care physician (as the coordinator of care), neurologist, orthopedic surgeon, geneticist, physical therapist, occupational therapist, psychologist, teacher, and other health care specialists.

3. Continuity of care is essential and the support and services provided by the Muscular Dystrophy Association should be made available to the patient and the family.

Myasthenia Gravis

Myasthenia gravis causes weakness secondary to a disorder of the neuromuscular junction (Fig. 1). Two forms occur in children: a transient neonatal form and a congenital (juvenile) form. The neonatal type occurs in infants born to mothers with myasthenia gravis. The onset is early, usually in the first few hours of life (almost all neonates with this disorder have symptoms within the first 24 hr after birth). Feeding abnormalities, facial muscle weakness, bilateral ptosis, lack of spontaneous movements, weak suck, weak cry, weak grasp, a poor Moro reflex, and generalized hypotonia are characteristic findings in the affected infants. The deep tendon reflexes are usually normal. The critical period is the first 3 days after onset. Treatment is usually required for 3 to 6 weeks. After this time, the symptoms resolve spontaneously and treatment may be discontinued. The congenital form usually begins at 5 to 10 years of age and does not remit. Treatment is required throughout life.

SIGNS AND SYMPTOMS

Bulbar muscular weakness with ptosis, ophthalmoplegias, difficulty swallowing, and difficulty in handling secretions are common. Generalized weakness of the extremities that worsens with activity is also characteristic.

Myasthenic crisis is characterized by an acute explosive onset (or exacerbation) of bulbar muscle weakness with respiratory distress. Rapid diagnosis and treatment are essential. Patients in crisis may require mechanical ventilatory support because respiratory failure may occur.

DIFFERENTIAL DIAGNOSIS

1. Muscular dystrophies (especially oculopharyngeal type)
2. Organophosphorus intoxication
3. Drug reaction (e.g., trimethadione)
4. CNS tumor or infection
5. Guillain-Barré syndrome
6. Werdnig-Hoffmann disease

DIAGNOSTIC PROTOCOL

1. Complete blood cell count, urinalysis, electrolytes, calcium, glucose, and renal and liver functions: Usually normal.
2. Creatine phosphokinase (CPK): Usually normal.

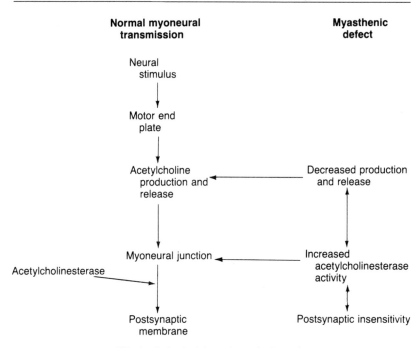

FIG. 1. Pathophysiology of myasthenia gravis.

3. Electromyogram (EMG): Usually characteristic, with a typical decrease in action potential after repetitive stimulations; changes are reversible after the administration of acetylcholinesterase inhibitors.

4. Biopsy: Usually not required or performed.

5. Edrophonium chloride challenge (Tensilon® test).

  a. Edrophonium chloride, 0.2 mg/kg i.m. or i.v. (maximum dose, 1 to 2 mg); a positive test is indicated by prompt reversal of symptoms after administration of the test dose (the change in action potential may be seen on the EMG); the response takes 30 sec if administered i.v. and 2 to 8 min if given i.m.

  b. Edrophonium chloride, 0.05 mg/kg i.m. or i.v., is used for differential diagnosis of myasthenic crisis.

  c. An overdose of edrophonium results in worsening of symptoms.

TREATMENT PROTOCOL

1. Pyridostigmine (Mestinon®), 0.1 mg/kg i.m.; patient is then switched to oral medication (the usual starting dose is 6 to 7 mg/kg/day p.o. in six equally divided doses; the actual dose and frequency must be individualized; modification of the starting regimen is usually required.

or

2. Neostigmine (Prostigmin®), 2 mg/kg/day p.o. in six to eight equally divided doses; modification of dosage and frequency is usually required.

3. Treatment of myasthenic crisis

   a. Edrophonium chloride, 0.05 mg/kg i.v.; if the patient is undermedicated, there will be resolution of symptoms.

   b. Because of the acute onset of bulbar weakness, intubation (or tracheostomy) and assisted ventilation may be required.

   c. Supportive and symptomatic care and counseling should be provided, including genetic counseling.

   d. Patients should be followed closely for worsening of symptoms or overmedication. Overdosage of medication results in worsening of symptoms as the dosage is increased.

Necrotizing Enterocolitis

Necrotizing enterocolitis (NEC) is a severe and often fatal disease that most often affects premature infants. Its incidence ranges from 1% to 10% in low birth weight babies, with a mortality rate as high as 50% to 70% in severely affected infants.

Although the exact etiology of NEC has not been well defined, the infant at risk has a definite profile. The infant is typically premature, has some respiratory distress from asphyxia at or before birth, has a low Apgar score, and often has been exposed to prolonged rupture of the mother's membranes. Also, there is a great likelihood that the infant has been exposed to an exchange transfusion, umbilical or venous catheter, and feeding by nasogastric or transpyloric tube.

SIGNS AND SYMPTOMS

The manifestations of NEC are variable and often confusing (Fig. 1). When the disease is recognized and treated early, the patients may completely recover. Unfortunately, in the majority of patients, very diffuse, nonspecific systemic symptoms precede the well-known gastrointestinal complications.

The infant appears well enough to be fed, but is usually in the recovery stage from some form of stress. Glucose water, cow's milk, or elemental formula is given by bottle or tube. Sometime after feedings begin (an average of 4 days of age), the infant develops lethargy, temperature instability, retention of gastric contents, and abdominal distention. Gastrointestinal bleeding is frequent and may be profuse or occult (noted only by chemical test). If a diagnosis of NEC is not made and appropriate treatment is not begun at the early stages of abdominal distention and occult gastrointestinal bleeding, apnea and bradycardic episodes soon follow and are harbingers of severe metabolic acidosis, disseminated intravascular coagulation, and vasomotor collapse. Radiographic findings are common and helpful in confirming the diagnosis of NEC reasonably early in its natural history. The earliest finding tends to be dilatation of the small bowel, which is rapidly progressive and associated with findings of gas within the bowel wall (pneumatosis intestinalis). Understanding the inciting events may not prevent this disease, but it should preclude a rapid and downhill progression to the infant's death.

DIFFERENTIAL DIAGNOSIS

1. Sepsis
2. Intestinal perforation
3. Intestinal obstruction
4. Electrolyte imbalance
5. Disseminated intravascular coagulation defect
6. Ruptured viscus
7. Congenital malformation

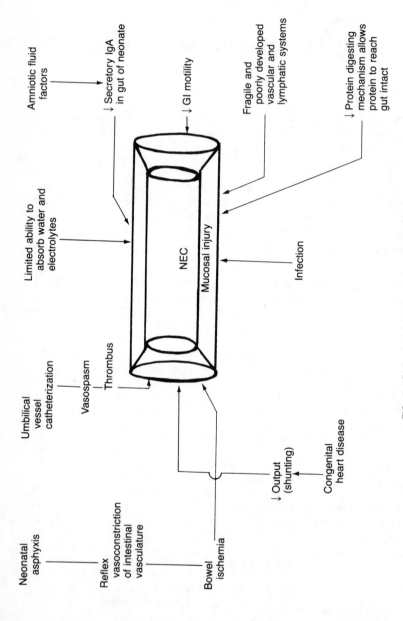

FIG. 1. Pathophysiology of necrotizing enterocolitis.

DIAGNOSTIC PROTOCOL

Medical History

1. Asphyxial episode in the perinatal period.

2. Respiratory distress syndrome.

3. Difficult resuscitation.

4. Hypothermic episodes.

5. Exchange transfusions.

6. Umbilical vein or artery catheterization.

7. Complications of labor and delivery (cesarean section, breech delivery, abruptio placenta).

8. Complications of pregnancy (prolonged rupture of the membranes, preeclampsia, postpartum bleeding, diabetes mellitus, multiple births).

9. Low Apgar scores.

10. Average time prior to diagnosis (4 days of age).

11. Apnea, positive stool guaiac, regurgitation, temperature instability, diarrhea, irritability, constipation.

Physical Examination

1. Abdominal distention, bile-stained aspirate.

2. Bradycardia.

3. Lethargy and irritability.

4. Hypothermia.

5. Hematochezia or melena.

6. Abdominal wall edema.

Laboratory Investigations

1. Abdominal radiographs show pneumatosis intestinalis, hepatic portal venous gas, pneumoperitoneum, and other nonspecific signs (hepatic portal venous gas significantly increases the chance of mortality).

2. Complete blood cell count, platelets, reticulocyte count: Platelets are often reduced, granulocyte count is occasionally reduced (associated with an increased mortality rate).

3. Urinalysis and urine culture.

4. Blood culture: *Clostridium* and *Bacteroides* species isolated tend to colonize the intestines of newborns within several weeks of their birth and an injured friable mucosa appears to be the perfect environment for their growth.

5. Coagulation studies: Disseminated intravascular coagulation is a common event late in the course of the disease.

6. Electrolytes, blood urea nitrogen, and creatinine: Often the electrolytes will be abnormal secondary to third spacing of fluid in the gut and to any effect on the electrolytes of other organ dysfunctions, such as shock or renal dysfunction.

TREATMENT PROTOCOL

1. Treatment must be initiated as soon as there are any signs suggestive of NEC, especially gastric retention and abdominal distention.

2. Discontinue feeding and insert nasogastric tube.

3. Begin intravenous infusion for calories and antibiotics (there is some disagreement about the use of systemic antibiotics in NEC) (see Neonatal Complications chapter).

4. Begin gentamicin by nasogastric tube, 10 to 15 mg/kg every 6 hr, and discontinue suction of nasogastric tube for 1 hr after medicine has been given.

5. Consider infusions of fresh plasma to provide added defense mechanisms against the potential gram-negative invaders.

6. Treat disseminated intravascular coagulation with exchange transfusion or a temporizing transfusion of fresh frozen plasma.

7. Treat shock (considered endotoxic) with steroids.

8. Isoproterenol or other ionotropic agents should be considered if the infant needs further circulatory support.

9. After the first few days, when the situation is no longer quite as critical, administration of appropriate calories must be considered in conjunction with the possibility of hyperalimentation.

10. The possibility of oral feedings should not be considered for approximately 2 weeks.

11. Indications for surgery

    a. Intestinal perforation.

    b. Full thickness necrosis of the bowel wall (radiographic evidence of dilated bowel loops that remain unchanged for several days).

    c. Peritonitis (ascites, abdominal mass, edema, and erythema of the abdominal wall, localized sign of abdominal resistance to palpation).

Neonatal Complications

The practitioner should be well acquainted with the prenatal and perinatal history of the neonate, and potential problems should be anticipated. If complications are not preventable, the practitioner should be prepared to deal with them. Most neonatal mortality occurs within the first 24 hr of life. Personnel trained in neonatal resuscitation must attend all high-risk deliveries so that prompt care can be delivered as soon after birth as possible.

It is important to differentiate between low birth weight infants, premature infants, and infants who are small or large for gestational age. Low birth weight infants weigh less than 2,500 g. Preterm infants have a gestational period of less than 37 weeks. Infants in less than the 10th percentile in weight for the assessed gestational age are considered small for gestational age, and infants large for gestational age are in greater than the 90th percentile. Infants weighing between the 10th and 90th percentile are considered appropriate for gestational age.

Guidelines for the initial assessment, Apgar scoring, management, and nutritional support of newborn infants are shown in Tables 1 and 2. Maternal and fetal factors that may lead to neonatal complications are shown in Table 3, and the management of respiratory depression in neonates is described in Table 4.

NEONATAL INFECTIONS

Etiology

1. Congenital
   a. Rubella
   b. Cytomegalovirus (CMV)
   c. Toxoplasmosis
   d. Varicella
   e. Coxsackie virus, group B
   f. Syphilis
   g. Tuberculosis
2. Acquired at time of delivery
   a. Premature rupture of membranes
   b. Unsterile delivery
   c. Cervical or vaginal herpes simplex or group B streptococci
   d. Infected mother
   e. Gonorrhea
3. Acquired in the nursery
   a. Prematurity
   b. Manipulation
   c. Overcrowding
   d. Infected nursery staff
   e. Gram-negative bacteria (e.g., *E. coli, Pseudomonas*)
   f. Staphylococci

TABLE 1. *Initial assessment and Apgar scoring of newborn infants*

Examination procedure
  Place the newborn infant on a previously warmed resuscitation table with an
    overhead radiant heat source in a 15° Trendelenburg position
  Auscultate the heart and simultaneously gently suction (<15 cm or H_2O pressure)
    the upper airway briefly
  Avoid traumatic physical stimulation and exposure
  Obtain the Apgar score at 60 sec and again at 5 min after birth
Apgar score

	0	1	2
Color	Blue	Acrocyanosis	Pink
Heart rate	0	<100	>100
Reflex irritability	No response	Grimace	Cry
Muscle tone	Flaccid	Flexion of extremities	Active
Respiratory effort	Absent	Slow, irregular	Strong, crying

Apgar score interpretation
  Apgar score 0–3
    Suction and temperature support
    Intubate, using a size 10 or larger Cole endotracheal tube (size 8 in infants
      weighing <1,000 g)
    Inflate the lungs 40 to 60 times per minute at 30 to 40 cm H_2O (reduce
      pressure to 15 cm H_2O after expansion)
    Check breath sounds, heart rate, and color
    If no heartbeat is heard, institute cardiac massage, using two fingers over the
      heart to the left of the sternum; depress the chest ¾ inch 100 to 120
      times per minute
    Naloxone hydrochloride (Narcan®), 0.02 mg/ml maximum dose (1 ml in
      premature infants; 2 ml in full-term infants) if narcotic depression is suspected,
      and/or sodium bicarbonate,
      2 mEq/kg i.v., **and/or** epinephrine, 0.5 to 1 ml i.v., **and/or** calcium gluconate,
      2 ml i.v.
    If no response, cannulate the umbilical artery or vein under sterile conditions,
      using a size 5 or 8 radiopaque umbilical catheter
    Sodium bicarbonate, 2 mEq/kg i.v., immediately
    Plasmanate®, 10 ml/kg i.v.
    Chest radiograph
    Consider other causes of respiratory distress
  Apgar score 4–6
    Suction and temperature support
    Intermittent postive pressure breathing by bag and mask, using 30 to 40 cm
      H_2O at 1.5-sec intervals (40 to 60 per min)
    If normal respirations ensue, observe the infant until its condition stabilizes
      and then transfer it to the newborn nursery
    If spontaneous respiration does not ensue after 2 min, intubate the infant and
      proceed as in the protocol for Apgar score 0–3
  Apgar score 7–10
    When the infant's condition becomes stable, transfer it to the newborn nursery;
      no special procedures are required
    A score of 10 indicates the infant is in the best possible condition

TABLE 2. *Management and nutritional support of newborn infants*

Full-term
  Nutritional support
    Calories, 110 to 130 kg/day
    Protein, 2 to 3 g/kg/day
    Formula or breast feeding
    Supplement: fluoride, 0.25 mg/day, <2 years of age; 0.50 mg/day, 2 to 3 years of age;
      1 mg/day, 3 to 16 years of age
Low birth weight
  Management
    Maintain skin temperature at 97°F and rectal temperature at 98.6°F.
    Use isolette or radiant heat warmer if infant weighs <1,800 g
    Clear airway; monitor vital signs hourly; weigh daily; monitor blood glucose level
      (Dextrostix®) immediately; monitor hematocrit immediately and every 2 weeks
      thereafter; administer vitamins A, C, and D, and iron at 7 days of age; consult social
      services and developmental specialists
  Nutritional support
    Feed orally if infant weighs >1,500 g and gestational age is >34 weeks
    Feed nasogastrically if infant weighs <1,500 g and gestational age is <34 weeks
    5% Dextrose in water for two feedings, 65 ml/kg/24 hr, if tolerated, and then 13 calories
      per ounce of formula four or five times a day for first day, if tolerated; thereafter, 20
      calories per ounce of formula four times a day, if tolerated, and then 24 to 27 calories
      per ounce of formula; increase fluids to 120 to 150 ml/kg/24 hr
    Supplements: Medium-chain triglycerides, 8.3 calories per gram, p.o.; vitamin E after 1
      week of age, 25 to 50 units p.o. (discontinue before discharge); folate, 0.25 to 1 mg/
      day; vitamin K, 0.5 mg/week i.m.; calcium gluconate, 150 mg/kg/day
Small for gestational age
  Management and nutritional support are the same as for low birth weight infant
Large for gestational age
  Management and nutritional support are the same as for low birth weight infant, with the
    following additional evaluations
    Chest radiograph
    Blood and urine cultures
    Blood urea nitrogen, serum electrolytes, total serum proteins, serum calcium, blood
      glucose

Manifestations

Each manifestation may occur as an isolated symptom or in any combination.

1. Hepatosplenomegaly
2. Jaundice
3. Anemia
4. Disseminated intravascular coagulopathy (DIC)
5. Microcephaly
6. Intracranial calcification
7. Chorioretinitis
8. Respiratory distress syndrome
9. Poor feeding
10. Poor cry
11. Hypotonia
12. Hypothermia or hyperthermia
13. Vomiting
14. Abdominal distention, especially with necrotizing enterocolitis
15. Diarrhea, bloody or nonbloody
16. Apnea
17. Cyanosis
18. Evidence of intrapartum infection with *N. gonorrheae* (e.g., ophthalmia, rhinitis, arthritis, anorectal infection, sepsis)

TABLE 3. *Maternal and fetal factors that may result in neonatal abnormalities*

Factors	Potential complications
Maternal Factors	
Alcohol consumption	Congenital abnormalities (especially cardiac), withdrawal symptoms, fetal alcohol syndrome
Breech delivery	Hypoxia, acidosis, aspiration pneumonia, CNS hemorrhage, brachial palsy, fractures
Cesarean section	Prematurity, respiratory distress syndrome
Diabetes	Hypoglycemia, hypocalcemia, congenital heart disease, renal vein thrombosis, electrolyte disturbances, diabetic cardiomyopathy
Eclampsia	Low birth weight, hypoglycemia, hypocalcemia, apnea, hypotension
Infection	Prematurity, death, meningitis, septicemia
Narcotic addiction	Low birth weight, withdrawal symptoms (e.g., twitching, vomiting, irritability, respiratory distress)
Oligohydramnios	Renal abnormalities, hypoplastic lung, hypoplastic kidneys
Polyhydramnios	Tracheoesophageal fistula, intestinal obstruction, bladder extrophy, erythroblastosis, anencephaly, infection, chromosomal abnormality
Premature rupture of membranes	Infections (e.g., septicemia, meningitis, pneumonia)
Rh incompatibility	Erythroblastosis, anemia, heart failure
Smoking	Low birth weight
Fetal Factors	
Prematurity	Respiratory distress syndrome, atelectasis, pneumonia, seizures, CNS hemorrhage, newborn hemorrhagic disease, infection, apnea
Postmaturity	Meconium aspiration, apnea, pneumothorax
Respiratory and/or CNS depression	Hypoxia, apnea, aspiration, hypoglycemia, hypernatremia, pneumothorax, heart failure, hypothermia, CNS hemorrhage, hypocalcemia
Small for gestational age	Hypoglycemia, hypocalcemia, hypothermia, postmaturity, meconium aspiration, congenital anomalies
Large for gestational age	

Diagnosis

1. Serological tests for syphilis, CMV, rubella, toxoplasmosis
2. IgM studies
3. Urine test for CMV inclusion bodies

TABLE 4. *Management of respiratory depression in neonates*

Symptoms	Etiology	Therapy
Initial cry, then apnea; good color following use of resuscitation bag	CNS depression secondary to maternal anesthesia or drugs	Naloxone (Narcan®), 0.005 mg/kg; exchange transfusion if no response
Retractions	Upper airway obstruction and asphyxia (aspiration, clots, meconium)	Suction before positive pressure respiration; intubation
Flaccid; color and heart rate improve following use of resuscitation bag	Asphyxia without airway obstruction (prolapsed cord, breech birth, meconium)	Suction; supportive therapy
Pale and weak, but not edematous	Hypovolemia and shock	Salt-poor albumin, 1 g/kg; Plasmanate®, 20 ml/kg, **or** type O, Rh-negative whole blood, 20 ml/kg
Excessive secretions	Tracheoesophageal fistula	Allow nothing by mouth; immediate surgical intervention; intermittent suction of proximal orophagus
Pale, hydropic, hepatosplenomegaly	Erythroblastosis	Suction; lower central venous pressure (CVP) by modified exchange or with packed cells; exchange transfusion
Unusual facies	Hypoplastic lungs (Potter's syndrome)	Resuscitation; if diagnostic, no need for resuscitation
Ecchymosis and edema of lower extremities	CNS hemorrhage secondary to traumatic delivery (e.g., breech)	Resuscitation
Normal infant with sudden apnea	Aspiration, CNS hemorrhage	Suction; resuscitation
Scaphoid abdomen	Diaphragmatic hernia	Surgical intervention; decompression of the stomach; intubation to expand lungs; correction of shock and acidosis
Cyanotic when quiet, ordinary feedings, pink when crying	Choanal atresia	Surgical intervention
Foul odor	Infection	Resuscitation; antibiotics

4. Skull radiographs for calcifications

5. Long bone radiographs for periostitis and radiolucencies

6. Cultures (nose, throat, blood, cord blood, urine, stool, ears, gastric aspirate, cerebrospinal fluid)

7. Serum bilirubin, calcium, magnesium

8. Serum electrolytes and blood urea nitrogen

9. Arterial blood gases

10. Chest radiograph

11. Abdominal radiograph (ileus, free air, pneumatosis intestinales in cases of necrotizing enterocolitis)

Treatment

1. Supportive

    a. Treat shock.

    b. Intravenous fluid.

2. Complications

    a. Ampicillin, 200 mg/kg/24 hr in two divided doses, **and** gentamicin, 7.5 mg/kg/24 hr in two divided doses, until diagnosis is made, then treat specifically.

    b. Anemia: Whole blood, 10 cc/kg, if hematocrit is <40%.

    c. Seizures, respiratory distress syndrome, heart failure, jaundice: Treat specifically.

3. Toxoplasmosis: Pyrimethamine (Daraprim®), 1 mg/kg/24 hr in two divided doses, **plus** sulfadiazine, 150 mg/kg/24 hr in four divided doses.

4. Varicella: Zoster immune globulin, 0.1 ml/kg i.m. at delivery.

5. Syphilis: Penicillin, 10,000 units/kg/24 hr i.m. for 10 days, if serological tests are positive and infant's titers are higher than mother's or mother is inadequately treated, **or** if there is clinical or radiographic evidence of syphilis in the infant, or if mother is adequately treated, but infant's titers increase or remain high with serological testing every month for 6 months and at 1 and 2 years of age.

6. Tuberculosis

    a. If mother is treated and sputum is negative, keep the infant with the mother; obtain chest radiograph and protein purified derivative (PPD) test at birth and at 6 weeks of age; vaccinate infant with BCG at 6 weeks of age if chest radiograph and PPD test are negative.

    b. If mother is untreated, separate the infant and mother; obtain chest radiograph and PPD test at birth and at 6 weeks of age; vaccinate infant with BCG at 6 weeks of age if chest radiograph and PPD test are negative; return infant to mother 6 weeks after vaccination or earlier if mother's sputum becomes negative.

    c. If PPD test is positive at 6 weeks of age, give isoniazid (INH), 10 mg/kg/24 hr, for 3 months.

    d. If infant is clinically ill, give INH, 10 to 20 mg/kg/24 hr, **and** streptomycin, 40 mg/kg in two divided doses every 2 days.

7. Herpes simplex: Gamma globulin, 10 to 20 ml/24 hr for 10 days, **or** idoxuridine, 600 mg/kg/24 hr i.v. for 5 days.

8. Diarrhea

    a. Close nursery to new admissions, isolate infants with diarrhea, observe all infants, obtain stool cultures on all infants and nursery personnel.

    b. Administer neomycin, 50 to 100 mg/kg/24 hr for 7 days, to carriers and all exposed persons.

    c. Repeat stool culture every 3 days.

    d. Clean the unit before new admissions are accepted.

    e. Treat *E. coli* with kanamycin, *Salmonella* and *Shigella* with ampicillin, *Staphylococcus* with methicillin, *Klebsiella* with gentamicin, and *Candida* with nystatin.

9. Gonorrhea: Penicillin G, 50,000 to 100,000 units/kg/day i.v. in two or three divided doses for 10 days.

10. Necrotizing enterocolitis

    a. Ampicillin, 200 mg/kg/24° i.v. in two divided doses, **plus** gentamicin.

    b. Allow nothing by mouth, discontinue umbilical lines; bowel resection may be indicated; gastrointestinal suction if no improvement.

BIRTH INJURIES

Birth injuries may be anoxic or mechanical. Special attention must be exercised when examining premature infants or infants with a history of unusual presentation, prolonged labor, difficult delivery, or low Apgar score. A birth injury should be suspected if the infant presents with:

1. Superficial bruises and skin lacerations
2. Unusual head shape
3. Lethargy
4. Seizures
5. Cyanosis
6. Inability to move any extremity
7. Irregular breathing
8. Shock

Diagnostic and Treatment Protocols

Table 5 gives diagnostic and treatment protocols for a variety of birth injuries.

SURGICAL PROBLEMS

Any newborn infant presenting with any of the following symptoms should be examined for serious, potentially curable, problems that require urgent and often lifesaving surgical intervention.

1. Respiratory distress

    a. Tracheoesophageal fistula (associated with aspiration)

    b. Diaphragmatic hernia

    c. Paralysis of phrenic nerve and diaphragmatic paralysis

    d. Choanal atresia and other upper airway obstructive disease

TABLE 5. *Birth injuries: Diagnostic and treatment protocols*

Diagnosis	Treatment
Cranial: Caput Succedaneum	
Etiological considerations: Prolonged labor, vertex presentation Clinical manifestations: Edema of scalp extending beyond midline and suture lines, with or without ecchymosis and jaundice Diagnostic measures: Clinical	None
Cranial: Subconjunctival Hemorrhages	
Etiological considerations: Prolonged labor, sudden increase in intrathoracic neck and head pressures Clinical manifestations: Petechial hemorrhages Diagnostic measures: Clinical	None, unless associated with hemorrhagic disease or DIC
Cranial: Cephalhematoma	
Etiological considerations: Subperiosteal hemorrhage Clinical manifestations: Limited to surface of one cranial bone; differentiate from cranial meningocele, which usually pulsates Diagnostic measures: Clinical, skull radiographs	None
Cranial: Skull Fractures	
Etiological considerations: Forceps delivery Clinical manifestations: None, unless associated with intracranial hemorrhage Diagnostic measures: Skull radiographs	Linear: None Depressed: Elevate
Intracranial: Hemorrhage	
Etiological considerations: Trauma, anoxia, hemorrhagic disease, congenital vascular anomalies Clinical manifestations: Hypotonia, lethargy, apnea, pallor, cyanosis, seizures, high-pitched cry, paralysis Diagnostic measures: CT scan, ultrasonography, lumbar puncture	Vitamin K; transfusion of fresh whole blood, 10 mg/kg; prevent hyponatremia; limit fluid intake; dexamethasone, 10 mg/m^2 initially and **then** 5 mg/m^2 every 6 hr; follow-up for hydrocephalus; treat seizures
Intracranial: Spinal Cord	
Etiological considerations: Breech delivery, manipulation Clinical manifestations: Paralysis, respiratory depression, hypotonia, areflexia; differentiate from amyotonia and myelodysplasia Diagnostic measures: Clinical, spinal radiographs, myelogram	Supportive
Peripheral Nerves	
Etiological considerations: Manipulation, fractures	Partial immobilization and appropriate positioning for 6 months intermittently

Diagnosis	Treatment
Clinical manifestations: Paralysis of upper arm or forearm with or without hand involvement Diagnostic measures: Differentiate from fractures	throughout day and night; use wrist splints if hand is involved; gentle range of exercises after 7 to 10 days of age; if persistent, perform neuroplasty

Peripheral Nerves: Brachial Palsy (Erb-Duchenne)

Etiological considerations: Fifth and sixth cervical nerves
Clinical manifestations: Cannot abduct, rotate externally, or supinate forearm

Peripheral Nerves: Brachial Palsy (Klumpke)

Etiological considerations: Seventh and eighth cervical nerves and first thoracic nerve
Clinical manifestations: Hand paralysis, ipsilateral ptosis and miosis

Peripheral Nerves: Phrenic Nerve

Etiological considerations: Traction Clinical manifestations: Respiratory distress, cyanosis Diagnostic measures: Chest radiograph with fluoroscopy; elevated diaphragm	Supportive; if no improvement, perform surgical application of the diaphragm

Peripheral Nerves: Facial Nerve

Etiological considerations: Pressure Clinical manifestations: Paralysis of one side of face, cannot close the eye Diagnostic measures: Clinical	Supportive; eye care; if persistent, perform neuroplasty

Liver or Spleen Rupture

Etiological considerations: Traumatic delivery, external chest compression (while resuscitating) Clinical manifestations: Poor feeding, pallor, tachypnea, tachycardia, shock, right and left upper quadrant mass Diagnostic measures: Isotope scan, surgical exploration	Treat shock and anemia Surgical intervention

Fractures: Clavicle, Humerus, Femur

Etiological considerations: Traumatic, iatrogenic Clinical manifestations: Inability to move the arm, absent Moro reflex Diagnostic measures: Radiograph of clavicle, humerus, or femur	Immobilization Strap arm to chest for 2 to 4 weeks with fractured humerus Traction suspension of both legs and spica cast with fractured femur

2. Vomiting

  a. Tracheoesophageal fistula

  b. Intestinal obstruction: Duodenal atresia, jejunoileal atresia, imperforate anus, meconium ileus, Hirschsprung's disease, malrotation and volvulus

3. Shock
    a. Ruptured abdominal viscus
    b. Necrotizing enterocolitis
    c. Intracranial bleeding
4. Externally apparent problems
    a. Fractures
    b. Omphalocele and gastroschisis
    c. Meningomyelocele
    d. Bladder extrophy

HYPOXIA

Signs and Symptoms

1. Prenatal
    a. Tachycardia
    b. Increased fetal movement followed by depression or bradycardia
2. Natal
    a. Meconium stained amniotic fluid
    b. Meconium aspiration
3. Neonatal
    a. Low Apgar score
    b. Hypotonia
    c. Cyanosis
    d. Respiratory depression

Pathophysiology

1. Redistribution of cardiac output
2. Tissue hypoxia
3. Respiratory and, later, metabolic acidosis
4. Anoxic brain damage

Clinical Manifestations

1. High-pitched cry
2. Hyperactive reflexes
3. Weak sucking reflex
4. Hypertonic and spastic
5. Pinpoint pupils, absent cough and gag reflexes, cranial nerve palsies, and disorders of muscle tone in severe anoxia

DISORDERS OF TEMPERATURE CONTROL AND BREATHING

Diagnosis

1. Lumbar puncture
2. CT scan
3. Ultrasound examination

Therapy

1. Ventilatory and circulatory support
2. Measures to prevent hemorrhage, hypocalcemia, hypoglycemia, aspiration pneumonia, seizures, further anoxia

Follow-Up

1. Gavage feeding (for difficulty in feeding)
2. Apneic spells
3. Seizure control
4. Prevent infection
5. Developmental assessment
6. Stimulation and exercise program

Neonatal Seizures

The evaluation of a newborn with seizures should follow a strict protocol because the etiologies are extremely varied and the implication of seizures in the neonatal period is severe.

GENERAL DIAGNOSTIC PROTOCOL

1. Monitor hematocrit, hemoglobin, blood glucose, serum calcium, phosphorus, magnesium, and electrolytes.

2. Obtain cultures of the blood, cerebrospinal fluid (CSF), urine, umbilicus, oropharynx, and nasopharynx.

3. Urine ferric chloride test and test for reducing substances.

4. Assure adequate ventilation and provide cardiovascular support; maintain the patient's temperature and administer intravenous fluids.

5. Until a systemic infection is ruled out, antibiotics (ampicillin, 200-250 mg/kg/24 hr, and gentamicin, 7.5 mg/kg/24 hr) should be given.

DIAGNOSTIC AND THERAPEUTIC PROTOCOLS

Table 1 gives diagnostic and therapeutic protocols for neonatal seizures of varied origins.

TABLE 1. *Diagnostic and treatment protocols*

Diagnosis	Treatment
Infection	
Etiological considerations: The most common organisms causing systemic infection in the newborn period are *E. coli* (and other enteric organisms), group B streptococci, and *S. aureus*	Antibiotic therapy should be guided by the organism obtained by culture and its sensitivity
Clinical manifestations: Irritability, tremors, lethargy, hypotonia, high-pitched cry, seizures, apnea, cyanosis, jaundice, hypertonia, vomiting, and diarrhea	Empirical therapy should begin with ampicillin, 200–250 mg/kg/24 hr, **and** gentamicin, 7.5 mg/kg/24 hr
Diagnostic measures: Cultures of blood, CSF and/or urine may be positive	

Diagnosis	Treatment

Hypocalcemia

Etiological considerations: Maternal parathyroid adenoma, bicarbonate therapy, high phosphorus level, acid citrated blood, low birth weight, diabetic mother, and traumatic delivery

Clinical manifestations: Irritability, tremors, high-pitched cry, seizures, apnea, cyanosis, hypotonia, hypertonia, and vomiting

Diagnostic measures: Serum calcium of ≤7.0 mg/100 ml, prolonged Q-T interval, tremors that disappear with intravenous calcium

10% Calcium gluconate, 1 to 3 mg/kg i.v. immediately, **then** 100 to 200 mg/kg i.v. four times a day, **then** oral therapy

Maintain treatment for 5 to 7 days, **then** monitor serum calcium levels

Hypoglycemia

Etiological considerations: Diabetic mother, placental dysfunction, anoxia, erythroblastosis, infection, leucine sensitivity, CNS hemorrhage, glycogen storage disease, galactose or fructose intolerance, islet-cell adenoma, Beckwith syndrome

Clinical manifestations: Tremors, cyanosis, seizures, apnea, irregular respirations, poor feeding, and hypotonia

Diagnostic measures: If blood glucose is ≤20 mg/100 ml in first 24 hr (≤30 mg/100 ml after first day of life) in premature infant; if blood glucose is ≤30 mg/100 ml in first 24 hr (≤40 mg/100 ml after first day of life) in full-term infant

50% Dextrose in water, 1 to 2 ml/kg i.v. immediately, **then** 10% dextrose in water, 75–100 ml/kg i.v., to keep blood glucose level >30 mg/100 ml

Raise to 15% dextrose in water, 75–100 ml/kg i.v., if no improvement

If seizures are persistent, give hydrocortisone, 5 mg/kg/day, **or** ACTH, 4 U i.m. twice a day, **or** glucagon, 100 to 300 μg/kg i.m. or i.v. (only in large infants)

Hypomagnesemia

Etiological considerations: Transient hypoparathyroidism, chronic diarrhea or vomiting, prolonged i.v. therapy, hyperaldosteronism, renal tubular disease, familial

Clinical manifestations: irritability, tremors, high-pitched cry, seizures, apnea, cyanosis, hypotonia, hypertonia, and vomiting

Diagnostic measures: Serum magnesium level <1.5 mEq/L

50% Magnesium sulfate: 0.1 to 0.2 ml/kg i.v.; repeat every 6 hr

Add 3 mEq/L of magnesium to i.v. fluid therapy

Hyponatremia

Etiological considerations: Iatrogenic (increased water ingestion); adrenogenital syndrome, syndrome of inappropriate secretion of antidiuretic hormone (SIADH), uncontrolled diarrhea, and gastrointestinal surgery

Clinical manifestations: Seizures, irritability, and lethargy

Diagnostic measures: Serum sodium <135 mEq/L

Replace sodium slowly: 5 to 10 mEq/L over 1- to 4-hr period

Restrict water intake

TABLE 1. *(continued)*

Diagnosis	Treatment

Narcotic and Alcohol Withdrawal

Etiological considerations: Maternal addiction to drugs

Clinical manifestations: Irritability, crying, tremors, sneezing, fever, vomiting, diarrhea, dyspnea, and cyanosis

Diagnostic measures: Specific drug levels; empirical response to narcotic antagonists

Place infant in quiet dark place
Intravenous fluids if needed
Tincture of paregoric, 1 to 4 drops/kg every 4 to 6 hr; taper over 1- to 6-week period, **or** chlorpromazine, 2 mg/kg/24 hr i.m. or p.o. in three doses **or** diazepam, 1 mg/kg i.m. or i.v. two or three times a day, **or** methadone, 0.5 to 1 mg i.m. every 8 hr; taper slowly over 1- to 6-week period

Thyrotoxicosis

Etiological considerations: Maternal thyrotoxicosis, maternal thyroidectomy

Clinical manifestations: Seizures, irritability, tremors, tachycardia, weight loss, goiter, jaundice, thrombocytopenia

Diagnostic measures: Elevated T_4 and long-acting thyroid stimulator

Lugol's solution, 1 drop 3 to 6 times a day, in mild cases, **or** propylthiouracil, 10 mg/kg/24 hr in three doses, **or** exchange transfusion, in very severe cases

Pyridoxine Deficiency

Etiological considerations: Maternal malnutrition, pyridoxine antagonists (isoniazid), inborn error of metabolism, maternal pyridoxine overdose

Clinical manifestations: Irritability and seizures

Diagnostic measures: Pyridoxine level or therapeutic-diagnostic intravenous pyridoxine

Pyridoxine hydrochloride, 50 mg i.m. or i.v.
Obtain electroencephalogram (EEG) while injecting pyridoxine (the EEG abnormalities will disappear)

CNS Hemorrhage

Etiological considerations: Mechanical injury, hypoxia, hemorrhagic disease, precipitous labor and delivery

Clinical manifestations: Lethargy, respiratory distress, apnea, cyanosis, pallor, decreased Moro reflex, decreased sucking, high-pitched cry, seizures, and bulging fontanelle

Diagnostic measures: Subdural tap, spinal tap (continuously hemorrhagic CSF and crenated red blood cells), ultrasound, CT scan

Phenobarbital, 5.0 mg/kg i.v. immediately; then 5 to 12 mg/kg/24 hr in three doses, **or** diazepam, 0.1 to 0.8 mg/kg i.m. or i.v. (do not use diazepam if jaundice is present)
Vitamin K; restrict fluids; mannitol and/or dexamethasone for cerebral edema

Nephrotic Syndrome

Nephrotic syndrome (NS) is a clinical condition representing multiple disorders, some of which are primary glomerulopathies and others part of a systemic disease process that secondarily involves the kidneys. Regardless of the etiology, the underlying renal defect is an increased permeability of the glomerular capillary membrane, which is manifested by massive proteinuria. The clinical condition of nephrotic syndrome requires the presence of four factors:

1. Hypoalbuminemia (below 2.5 g/dL)

2. Edema

3. Hyperlipidemia (usually based on cholesterol levels)

4. Massive proteinuria ($\geq$50 mg/kg/day)

The type of nephrotic syndrome seen in children most commonly is minimal change (nil) disease (MCD); it accounts for 80% to 85% of all nephrotic states in children. The name nil disease, a synonym for MCD disease, alludes to the absence of obvious histological changes in the kidneys (by light microscopy). MCD reaches its peak in preschool children (3 years of age) and is rare in the second decade. In children younger than 16 years of age, the incidence is 2 to 3 cases per 100,000 of population, with a male-to-female ratio of almost 3:1.

A familial incidence between 2% and 6% has been noted, and most recently a genetic predisposition (HL-A-DR7) has been described. This specific HL-A group association is the same one seen in individuals having allergic diatheses and elevated IgE levels. Because the immune system has been a prime target in the controversy over the etiology of nephrotic syndrome, the noted association with this HL-A group may ultimately provide us with a definitive understanding of the pathophysiological events in nephrotic syndrome. One plausible theory of the immune system's role is that individuals who develop nephrotic syndrome may be genetically predisposed and, following a specific antigenic insult, release a subpool of abnormal T lymphocytes that secrete lymphokines, causing changes in the glomerular capillary membrane. This insult to the glomerulus results in disruption of the membrane's barrier function (structural and electrostatic components) and permits massive efflux of proteins (Fig. 1).

SIGNS AND SYMPTOMS

The majority of patients who develop nephrotic syndrome report an antecedent nonspecific respiratory infection, but poison ivy, insect stings, medications (phenytoin), and immunizations (DPT) have all been observed to initiate the disease or participate in its relapse.

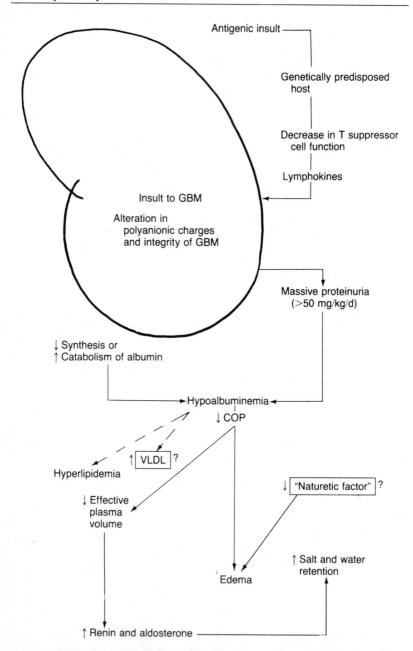

FIG. 1. Pathophysiology of nephrotic syndrome. GBM, glomerular basement membrane; COP, colloid osmotic pressure; VLDL, very low-density lipoprotein.

Edema is the most common presenting sign and varies from mild periorbital edema to anasarca. Remnants of the initiating illness may be present, but fever is distinctly unusual. The blood pressure tends to be normal, although mild elevations may occur transiently in up to 15% of affected children. Tachypnea and tachycardia are unusual, as the edema is not a result of vascular congestion but of interstitial fluid accumulation. Hepatomegaly without tenderness is common, and splenic enlargement occurs in less than 10% of affected children. Abdominal tenderness is usually absent, but fluid in the abdomen is frequent, as it is in other areas (e.g., pleura, scrotum).

In summary, although children with nephrotic syndrome may have a frightening appearance because of massive edema, they are not febrile or systemically ill unless infection has intervened or the nephrotic syndrome is the manifestation of a more serious systemic disease.

DIFFERENTIAL DIAGNOSIS

The differential diagnosis is related to entities causing massive proteinuria:

1. Minimal change disease

2. Focal sclerosing glomerulonephritis

3. Membranous glomerulopathy (primary versus secondary)

4. Membranoproliferative glomerulonephritis (primary versus secondary)

5. Congenital nephrotic syndrome

6. Crescentic glomerulonephritis

7. Focal proliferative glomerulonephritis

GENERAL DIAGNOSTIC PROTOCOL

There are general signs and symptoms that will be present to a greater or lesser degree in all types of nephrotic syndrome (Fig. 2).

1. Basic criteria

    a. Hypoalbuminemia

    b. Edema

    c. Hyperlipidemia (cholesterol levels)

    d. Massive proteinuria

2. Hematuria

    a. In 5% to 10% of children with MCD, but transient only

    b. Prevalent in other forms of NS

3. Complement

    a. Normal in MCD

    b. Decreased in membranous glomerulopathy (MGN) [systemic lupus erythematosis (SLE), malaria]

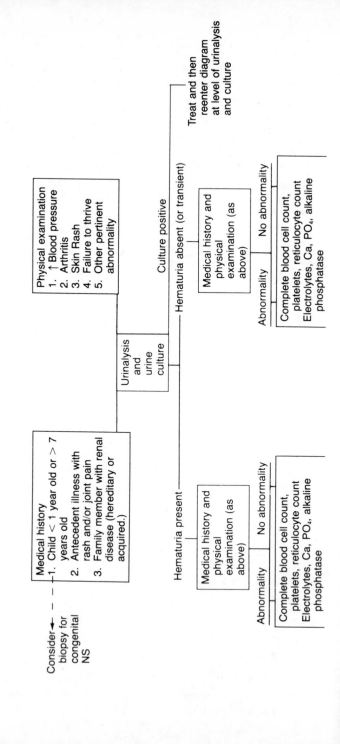

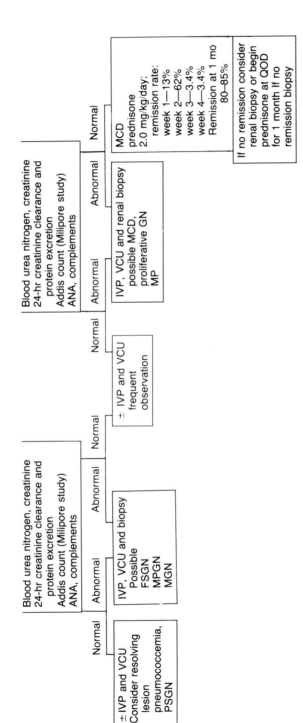

FIG. 2. General diagnostic and treatment protocols for nephrotic syndrome.

c. Decreased in type II membranoproliferative glomerulonephritis

4. Protein selectivity: In MCD, smaller molecules are usually allowed to pass through the membrane than in other forms of NS

5. Hypertension

   a. Evanescent if present in MCD

   b. Common in other forms of NS

GENERAL TREATMENT PROTOCOL

1. If incapacitating, edema may be temporarily decreased by use of agents to increase the colloid osmotic pressure and to clear excess fluid.

   a. Albumin, 1.0 to 1.5 g/kg i.v. over a period of 30 to 45 min.

   b. Furosemide (Lasix®), 1.0 mg/kg i.v., if hyponatremia is not a problem.

2. Albumin infusions should not be used routinely to raise serum albumin levels; infused albumin is lost quite rapidly (urine, interstitium, catabolism) and is expensive.

3. Salt restriction (2 g/day) is helpful while the patient is edematous, unless the patient is receiving diuretics or is a salt loser.

4. Definitive treatment includes prednisone (Fig. 3).

DIAGNOSTIC AND TREATMENT PROTOCOL

Table 1 gives diagnostic and treatment protocols for several nephrotic syndromes.

TABLE 1. *Nephrotic syndromes: Diagnostic and treatment protocols*

Diagnosis	Treatment
Focal Sclerosing Glomerulonephritis (FSGN)[a]	
There is some controversy as to whether this is both a nonspecific lesion accompanying a variety of renal diseases and a specific primary entity	Supportive
	Steroids, as in MCD, but relapses are frequent and resistance develops early
8% to 10% of childhood NS	
Presents as NS (66% of cases), asymptomatic proteinuria or acute nephritis	
Hypertension	

Diagnosis	Treatment

Microscopic hematuria in 70% of patients
with gross hematuria in 5%
Early evidence of reduced renal function

Membranoproliferative Glomerulonephritis (MPGN), Types I and II[a]

5% to 10% of childhood NS
Presents as NS, mild proteinuria and/or
hematuria, acute nephritis
Gross hematuria is not uncommon and may
be recurrent
Hypertension and edema are frequent
Early evidence of reduced renal function
Reduced C3 level
C3 nephritic factor (an autoantibody) is
detected frequently in type II
May be associated with partial lipodystrophy
and congenital hypocomplementemia

Supportive
Some success with intravenous pulse doses
of methylprednisolone or with alternate
day steroids

Membranous Glomerulopathy[a]

<1% to 2% of children with NS
Male-to-female ratio, 3:1
Presents as NS in two-thirds of children
Microscopic hematuria (50% of cases) with
gross hematuria occurring rarely
Hypertension (25% of cases) at time of
diagnosis
Renal function is normal until late in the
course of the disease

Supportive
Spontaneous remission in ≥25% of affected
children
Steroid treatment reserved for patients who
show a decline in renal function

Focal Proliferative Glomerulonephritis[a]

50% of cases occur with systemic disease,
especially anaphylactoid purpura
Presents with proteinuria and hematuria
after upper respiratory tract infection
Hematuria is often recurrent and
microscopic
NS is rare, transient, usually accompanied
by hematuria

Supportive

Mesangial Proliferative Glomerulonephritis[a]

Presents with two different patterns: Acute
nephritic hematuria (at times
NS), azotemia, and hypertension. Severe
NS, often associated with hematuria

Supportive
Steroid-resistant

Crescentic Proliferative Glomerulonephritis[a]

Clinical course is related to the percentage
of crescents
Presents commonly with NS and hematuria
Early renal insufficiency is prominent

Various methods have been attempted; the
most successful is early intervention with
antiplatelet or anticoagulant drugs

Congenital Nephrosis: Finnish Type[a]

Most common variety, which is autosomal
recessive
Associated with large placenta at birth

Prenatal diagnosis is possible by measuring
α-fetoprotein in amniotic fluid

TABLE 1. *(continued)*

Diagnosis	Treatment
Presents at several months of age with edema, failure to thrive Death in infancy due to infection and/or renal vein thrombosis	

Congenital Nephrosis: Idiopathic[a]

Not hereditary

Infectious Disease: Syphilis, CMV, Malaria[b]

The diagnosis in each is circumstantial unless a biopsy demonstrates a specific pattern or antigen Syphilis- and cytomegalovirus-induced are usually congenital Malaria is usually acquired	Supportive Directed against primary illness

Postinfectious Glomerulonephritis[b]

History of streptococcal glomerulonephritis or pneumococcemia
Shunt associated

Multisystem Diseases:
CTD (SLE), Neoplasia, Renal Vein Thrombosis, Hepatitis[b]

Manifestations of underlying illness by medical history, physical examination, and/or laboratory confirmation	Supportive Directed against primary disease

[a]Primary nephrotic syndrome.
[b]Secondary nephrotic syndrome.

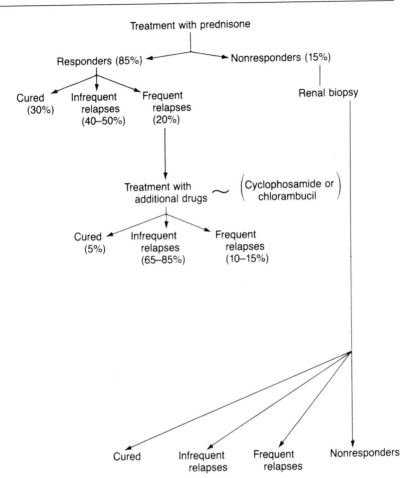

FIG. 3. Treatment of minimal change disease with prednisone. Responders: protein-free urine for 3 or more consecutive days; frequent relapses: more than 2 relapses in a given 6 month period; dependent: responds to steroids but relapses with decrease in dose; prednisone: 2 mg/kg/d for 28 days, if no response, then 2 mg/kg every other day for 28 days, if still no response, then renal biopsy.

Neuroblastoma

Neuroblastoma is the most common solid tumor of childhood and accounts for approximately half of all malignant tumors in neonates. Its incidence is reported to be about 1 per 10,000 live births. Seventy-five to eighty percent occur within the first 5 years of life. The tumor is slightly more common in males, but there is no significant racial or ethnic predisposition. A familial tendency may be present in conjunction with certain of the multiple endocrinopathies.

PATHOPHYSIOLOGY

This tumor originates from the pleuripotential neural crest cells (Fig. 1) and neuroblasts migrating from the developing spinal cord. Because of this origin, the tumor may be found in many diverse sites. However, more than 75% of neuroblastomas arise in the abdomen, at least half of these from the adrenal gland. The acute myoclonic encephalopathy may be immunologically based.

SIGNS AND SYMPTOMS

Approximately 25% of the patients with neuroblastoma are asymptomatic. Commonly occurring symptoms include abdominal or bone pain (37%), irritability (25%), and anorexia (12%). Usual signs include a palpable mass (54%), fever (37%), proptosis or orbital ecchymosis (23%), enlarged nodes (14%), weight loss, pallor, urinary problems, and vomiting. Hypertension occurs, but is uncommon (<1%). Symptoms from distant metastasis may occur.

Acute myoclonic encephalopathy may occur in patients with neuroblastoma. It consists of opsoclonus (rapid, multidirectional eye movements), truncal ataxia (in the presence of normal cerebrospinal fluid pressure), and myoclonus. The symptoms resolve after the tumor is removed, but it occasionally takes a long time.

DIFFERENTIAL DIAGNOSIS

Diagnostic considerations will, in part, depend on the location of the tumor. Neuroblastoma should be considered in any child who presents with unusual or atypical cerebellar findings.

1. Ganglioneuroma

2. Wilm's tumor

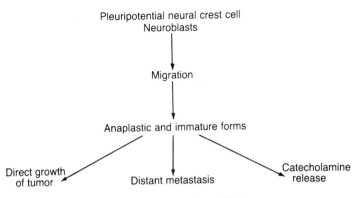

FIG. 1. Pathophysiology of neuroblastoma.

3. Pheochromocytoma

4. Lymphoma

5. Teratoma

STAGING OF NEUROBLASTOMA

Stage I: The mass is limited to the structure of origin.

Stage II: There is extension beyond the site of origin, but the tumor does not cross the midline; ipsilateral lymph node involvement may occur.

Stage III: There is direct extension of the tumor across the midline; regional lymph nodes may be involved bilaterally.

Stage IV: There is distant metastasis to other organs, nodes, skin, or bone.

Stage IVs: Includes patients in stage I or II who are <1 year of age with remote disease limited to the liver, skin, or bone marrow; there must be no evidence of bone metastasis on radiographic skeletal survey.

DIAGNOSTIC PROTOCOL

1. Obtain a complete history and perform a complete physical examination. Look for problems with bowel or bladder habits, difficulty in ambulation, swellings or masses, elevated blood pressure, ocular abnormalities, neurological abnormalities, or abnormal liver size.

2. Laboratory investigations

    a. Complete blood cell count, differential count, and platelet count

    b. 24-hr urinary vanillylmandelic acid (VMA) determination (15% to 20% of affected patients will have normal VMA) *c.* Liver function tests

    d. Coagulation profile

    e. Bone marrow aspiration or bone marrow biopsy

3. Radiographic investigations

    a. Chest radiograph

    b. Skeletal survey

    c. Intravenous pyelogram (will show downward displacement of a normal kidney if the adrenal gland is the point of origin; Wilm's tumor is intrarenal)

    d. Oblique spine radiographs and myelography if signs of cord compression or paravertebral involvement are present

    e. Brain, bone, liver nucleotide scans

    f. Arterial and venous contrast studies (for surgical approach to the tumor)

TREATMENT PROTOCOL

Diagnosis and treatment of neuroblastoma should be guided by an experienced pediatric oncologist and hematologist.

Therapy is guided by the staging of the disease.

Stage I: Surgery (<1 year old); surgery + radiation (>1 year old).

Stage II: Surgery + radiation + chemotherapy (vincristine and cyclophosphamide) (all ages).

Stage III: Surgery + radiation + chemotherapy (vincristine and cyclophosphamide) (<1 year old); surgery + radiation + chemotherapy (vincristine, cyclophosphamide, and doxorubicin) (>1 year old).

Stage IV: Palliative radiation + chemotherapy (all ages).

Stage IVs: Surgery + chemotherapy (vincristine and cyclophosphamide) (<1 year old).

Orbital Cellulitis

Orbital cellulitis is a severe, life-threatening infection within the ocular orbit (internal to the septum). A rapid diagnosis and early treatment are essential. Occasionally, surgical intervention is required. Differentiation between orbital cellulitis and preseptal cellulitis may be difficult on clinical grounds because of the significant swelling of the lids. However, every attempt should be made to examine the globe of the eye. Because of the involvement of retrobulbar structures, examination of the globe will yield clues to the diagnosis.

Meningitis, cavernous sinus thrombosis, and loss of vision are the major complications of orbital cellulitis (Fig. 1).

SIGNS AND SYMPTOMS

Fever, redness, pain, and periorbital swelling, along with an appearance of general toxicity, are characteristic but nonspecific findings. Proptosis, limitation of ocular motility, chemosis, and diminution of vision point toward infection posterior to the orbital septum.

DIFFERENTIAL DIAGNOSIS

1. Preseptal (periorbital) cellulitis
2. Conjunctivitis
3. Glaucoma
4. Trauma
5. Foreign body

DIAGNOSTIC PROTOCOL

1. Complete blood cell count: Frequently shows leukocytosis and a shift to the left.
2. Blood cultures: Multiple cultures should be obtained.
3. Culture of the ocular discharge.
4. Plain radiographs of the sinuses: To identify opacifications and/or other evidence of infection.
5. Plain radiographs of the orbits: If a penetrating injury or an orbital foreign body is suspected.

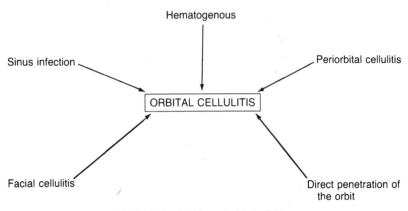

FIG. 1.   Pathophysiology of orbital cellulitis.

6. CT scan of the orbits: May reveal intraorbital abscess formation with displacement of the globe and retrobulbar structures.

7. Lumbar puncture: If meningeal extension is suspected.

TREATMENT PROTOCOL

---

1. Parenteral antibiotics are required. Staphylococci, streptococci, and pneumococci are the most common offending organisms. A semisynthetic penicillinase-resistant penicillin is an appropriate first choice: Nafcillin, 150 mg/kg/day i.v. in four equally divided doses for 14 days.

2. In younger children, *H. influenzae* may be the etiological agent and appropriate coverage should be added.

    a. Chloramphenicol, 100 mg/kg/day i.v. in four equally divided doses for 14 days.

    b. If the organism is susceptible, ampicillin, 200 mg/kg/day i.v. in four equally divided doses for 14 days, may be substituted.

3. Antibiotic therapy should be dictated by the results of culture and sensitivity testing.

4. If an intraorbital abscess or pyosinusitis is present, surgical intervention and drainage may be required.

5. Vision should be tested frequently.

Osteomyelitis

Osteomyelitis is an infection of bone and may be acute or chronic (Fig. 1). Virtually any organism may be the etiologic agent, but *Staphylococcus aureus* is the most common organism encountered in infants, and staphylococcus and streptococcus organisms are the most common in older children. *Hemophilus influenzae,* coliforms, and pneumococci also are responsible organisms. In patients with sickle-cell disease, osteomyelitis is not uncommon. Staphylococci, coliforms, and pneumococci are common agents in these patients. However, salmonella osteomyelitis occurs more often in patients with sickle-cell disease than in healthy patients. It should be considered in all sickle-cell disease patients with bone infections.

Osteomyelitis may exist alone or in conjunction with a septic arthritis. Differentiation is sometimes difficult, even with sophisticated radionucleotide techniques.

SIGNS AND SYMPTOMS

Fever is usually present and the patient may or may not appear to be ill. If an extremity is involved, there will be voluntary and involuntary splinting and limitation of motion secondary to pain. Pain, swelling, and "point" tenderness are characteristic. Redness and induration may also be present. Fistulization to the skin may occur, along with discharge of the purulent exudate.

DIFFERENTIAL DIAGNOSIS
---

1. Suppurative arthritis
2. Soft-tissue cellulitis
3. Subcutaneous abscess
4. Osseous tumor
5. Periostitis
6. Bone infarction (especially in patients with sickle-cell disease)
7. Nonsuppurative arthritis
8. Aseptic necrosis (e.g., Köhler's disease)

415

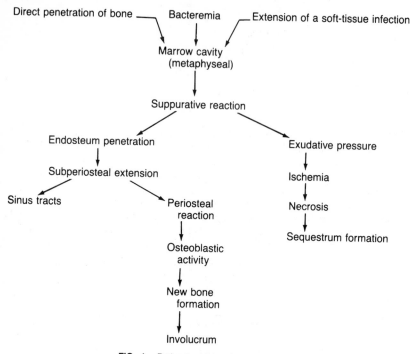

FIG. 1. Pathophysiology of osteomyelitis.

DIAGNOSTIC PROTOCOL

1. Osteomyelitis should be first suspected by clinical findings.

2. Complete blood cell count: May show leukocytosis and a shift to the left.

3. Erythrocyte sedimentation rate (ESR): Elevated.

4. Multiple blood cultures.

5. Culture and sensitivity of exudate: From the sinus tract (if present) or from aspiration of an identified bony focus; bone aspiration is indicated if there is a positive nucleotide scan plus clinical correlation.

6. Radiographs: May show bony destruction or periosteal reaction; however, radiographic changes do not occur early in the disease process, and clinical symptoms precede radiographic evidence by 5 days to 1 week.

7. Radionucleotide scan: False positives may result from significant contiguous arthritis or ischemic injury without infection.

TREATMENT PROTOCOL

1. Immobilization of the limb helps to decrease pain.

2. Intravenous antibiotics

   a. Nafcillin, 150 mg/kg/day in four divided doses; an appropriate empirical drug of choice, which may be started after appropriate cultures are obtained.

   b. If the patient is allergic to penicillin: Cephamandol, 100 mg/kg/day in four divided doses.

   c. If coliforms are suspected, add: Gentamicin, 5 to 7.5 mg/kg/day i.m. in two divided doses, **or** kanamycin, 15 to 30 mg/kg/day i.m. in two divided doses.

   d. If the patient has sickle-cell disease, add: Ampicillin, 200 mg/kg/day in four divided doses.

   e. If *H. influenzae* is suspected, add: Chloramphenicol, 100 mg/kg/day in four divided doses, **or** ampicillin, 200 mg/kg/day in four divided doses (if the organism is sensitive).

3. If pus is obtained from a needle aspiration, surgical drainage (or excision of the sequestrum) is indicated.

4. Parenteral antibiotics should be continued for 3 to 6 weeks; however, some authorities recommend 10 to 14 days of parenteral antibiotics (or until there is a significant decrease in symptoms and a decrease in the ESR) followed by oral antibiotics for 3 to 6 weeks. In order for oral therapy to be used, several requirements must be met: Compliance must be assured (most often the child must remain in the hospital); the exact organism must be known; and, the organism must be sensitive to the antibiotic (serum bactericidal concentrations must be monitored).

Otitis Media

Otitis media is the most frequent diagnosis made by physicians caring for children. The overall prevalence rate has been estimated as 15% to 20%, with at least one study showing that during the first 3 years of life, only 30% of children fail to develop an episode of otitis media. This disease can affect children of any age, including neonates, but its highest frequency is in children between the ages of 6 and 24 months. There is a marked decline about the time of school entrance. Boys tend to be affected more often than girls. Hispanics, American Indians, Eskimos, children from lower socioeconomic areas, and children who have been bottle fed also are more often affected.

The bacteriological focus of acute otitis media is strikingly consistent, except in neonates, in whom gram-negative organisms play a significant role. The pneumococcus is the most common organism found in cultures of middle ear fluids, followed closely by *H. influenzae*, group A streptococcus, and *S. aureus*. Cultures of middle ear fluid for viruses and *Mycoplasma* have shown a very low yield (only respiratory syncytial virus has been recovered with any notable frequency).

Although many investigators are convinced of the role of the immune system in the cause of otitis media, involvement of the eustacian tube appears to be the primary cause of otitis media. The eustacian tube is anatomically able to act as a conduit between the middle ear and the pharynx. Otitis media may develop in patients in whom the eustacian tube is unable to ventilate the middle ear cleft, equalizing pressure and replenishing oxygen; protect against sound pressures and contaminated secretions; and clear secretions produced by the middle ear via the nasopharynx. The eustacian tube in children is predisposed to functional obstruction due to its small amount of cartilage, short straight course, and poorly efficient muscle responsible for compliance in opening and closing. Any edema or nasopharyngeal mass at the opening of the tube can easily compress the orifice and result in mechanical obstruction (Fig. 1).

SIGNS AND SYMPTOMS

Classically, otitis media is preceded by an upper respiratory tract infection. There is sudden onset of otalgia and fever. Headache and other nonspecific symptoms may occur. Visualization of the tympanic membrane very often shows a distended erythematous structure with many of the landmarks poorly delineated. There is often significant fluid behind the membrane and pneumo-otoscopy will demonstrate poor compliance of the drum. During the acute phase of otitis media, there is often some decrease in hearing, which may correlate with decreased compliance secondary to the middle ear fluid. The effusion may remain for up to 10 to 12 weeks after successful treatment of the infection.

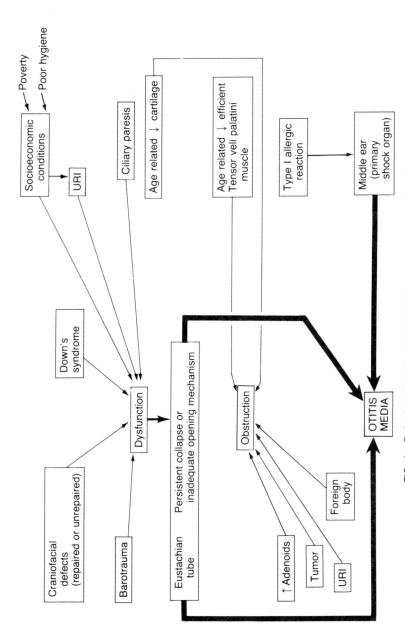

FIG. 1. Pathophysiology of otitis media. URI, upper respiratory tract infection.

DIFFERENTIAL DIAGNOSIS

1. Acute otitis media
2. Immune deficiency state
   (local ciliary defect, goblet-cell defect)
3. Neoplasia
4. Sinusitis

5. Foreign body
6. Active chronic otitis media
7. Recurrent purulent otitis media
8. Allergic diathesis (local)
9. Otitis externa

DIAGNOSTIC PROTOCOL

Acute Purulent Otitis Media (APOM)

Neonates

1. May occur as an isolated purulent or suppurative infection or may be associated with sepsis, pneumonia, or meningitis.
2. May occur as a silent infection and require careful otoscopy (with 2 mm speculum), noting immobility of the drum.
3. Newborns with low birth weight, jaundice, urinary tract infections, and infants whose mothers had preeclampsia or amnionitis are considered high risk for developing otitis media.
4. Proper evaluation, whether the infection is silent or occurs in a child with diarrhea, low grade fever, feeding problems, irritability, or failure to thrive, may require a myringotomy for the selection of an appropriate antibiotic.
5. Twenty percent of the organisms may be expected to be gram-negative *(E. coli* and *Klebsiella pneumoniae).*

Older Children

1. Isolated organisms in order of decreasing frequency at <3 years of age: *S. pneumonia, H. influenzae*, group A streptococcus, *S. aureus, N.* catarrhalis.
2. Often occurs in winter (January) and is preceded by several days of upper respiratory tract infection symptoms.
3. A mild antecedent prodrome abruptly develops into fever, otalgia, ear pulling, head shaking and/or systemic symptoms of diarrhea, vomiting and, occasionally, convulsions; some children complain of decreased hearing and/or vertigo.
4. Otoscopy will often reveal an erythematous, bulging or retracted tympanic membrane, which may show a fluid level or be translucent; be suspicious of foreign anatomical landmarks (i.e., foreign bodies).
5. There may be a purulent otorrhea, reflecting a perforated tympanic membrane (in this case the otalgia should have abated).
6. Pneumatic otoscopy is imperative and should show limited mobility of the tympanic membrane.

7. Unless an underlying disease or anatomical abnormality is present, otitis media is usually not a systemic infection.

Recurrent Purulent Otitis Media (RPOM)

1. Sixty-seven percent of all otitis media recurs within the first year, 19% within the second year, and 4% within the third year.

2. *S. pneumoniae* and *H. influenzae* should be suspected in recurrences.

3. Symptoms may recur within days or weeks of stopping therapy; some children may suffer a recurrence with almost every upper respiratory tract infection.

4. *S. aureus* and gram-negative organisms may become more prevalent with RPOM.

5. Signs and symptoms may be minimal or each episode may be similar to the original encounter with APOM.

6. Chronic otitis media with middle ear effusion developing into RPOM should be treated as multiple acute otitis media episodes superimposed on chronic otitis media.

Serous Otitis Media (SOM)

1. Most frequently the initiating event will be APOM; also the presence of SOM predisposes the patient to the development of APOM.

2. In the absence of a triggering event, attempt to exclude any underlying conditions (e.g., cleft palate, craniofacial abnormality, a genetic defect, impaired cilia motility syndromes, nasopharyngeal masses, sinusitis).

3. Complaints of impaired hearing, otalgia, disturbance of balance, and fullness in the ear are common; younger patients may show only irritability and restlessness; a popping sound on swallowing is not uncommon.

4. The tympanic membrane may range from amber to yellow (blue if blood is present) and air bubbles may be noted behind the drum.

5. In older children in whom the condition has persisted for more than several months, scarring and retraction of the drum may be noted.

6. Pneumatic otoscopy will provide some information regarding the degree of fluid present or tympanic membrane alteration.

Chronic Otitis Media (COM)

1. Isolated organisms: *Proteus* species, *Pseudomonas* species, *S. aureus*, *S. epidermidis*, mixed species, anaerobic organisms, *S. pneumoniae*, *H. influenzae*.

2. **Tissue destruction is irreversible**. Chronic otitis media may be active (infection, with drainage) or inactive (sequelae from prior infection and often without otorrhea).

   a. If active, a foul-smelling and bloody suppurative discharge may be present, with exuberant granulation tissue.

b. Cholesteotomas (six different types) must be sought for and referred for appropriate therapy.

TREATMENT PROTOCOL

Acute Purulent Otitis Media

Neonates

Antibiotics should be initiated expeditiously and in doses for sepsis after evaluation is completed.

Older Children

1. Following a thorough evaluation with limited laboratory investigations (as indicated) treat with a 7 to 10 day course of antibiotics: Amoxicillin, 40 mg/kg/24 hr p.o.in three divided doses, **or** Ceclor®., 40 mg/kg/24 hr p.o in three divided doses. Other antibiotics to consider are: Erythromycin/sulfisoxazole, 50 mg/kg/24 hr (erythromycin), p.o. in four divided doses; **or** trimethoprim/sulfamethoxazole, 8–10 mg/kg/24 hr (trimethoprim), p.o. in two divided doses.

2. Use of antihistamines and decongestants is controversial; they may delay the absorption of fluid from the middle ear.

3. Analgesia and antipyretics will usually make the child more comfortable and are an important part of the treatment regimen.

4. If the patient is in intolerable pain and/or if after 24 to 48 hr pain and fever are still considerable, a myringotomy should be performed for diagnostic and therapeutic reasons; the possibility of either an incorrect diagnosis or a resistant organism should be considered (e.g., ampicillin-resistant *H. influenzae*) and antibiotics altered appropriately.

5. The patient should be reevaluated after 2 weeks of therapy to determine the general state of health and the state of any middle ear effusion; in ≤10% of children this fluid may last 3 months or longer.

6. If middle ear effusion is present >3 months and/or the tympanic membrane appears to be abnormal, the patient should be referred to an otolaryngologist for further evaluation to prevent ongoing mild hearing loss.

7. Children with cleft palates or other craniofacial abnormalities should have otolaryngology evaluation within the first 3 months of life because of the high incidence of asymptomatic middle ear effusion and its correlation with conductive hearing loss and delays in language development; these problems are somewhat preventable by the use of tympanostomy tubes and should be considered in any child with prolonged middle ear effusion.

8. Severe complications (listed in order of frequency of fatal outcome; many are relatively rare since the introduction of antibiotics).

    a. Meningitis: Organisms from the middle ear can invade the dura.

    b. Brain abscess: Most often associated with cholesteotomas in chronic otitis media but may occur in APOM and usually involves the temporal lobe; if secondary to POM is usually mixed organisms.

c. Thrombosis of the sigmoid sinus.

d. Suppurative labyrinthitis: Onset is usually insidius until meningitis supervenes.

e. Facial nerve paralysis.

9. Minor complications

a. RPOM

b. Chronic otitis media.

c. Perforation of tympanic membrane (will usually close within 2 weeks spontaneously, otherwise consultation is indicated to prevent further morbidity).

Recurrent Purulent Otitis Media

1. Treat as in APOM, except when three or more acute episodes have occurred; in those cases, use prophylactic sulfisoxazole, 500 mg twice a day.

2. Myringotomy may be indicated.

3. Tympanometry and audiometry may be useful baseline and tracking information.

4. Otolaryngological consultation tympanostomy (PE tubes) may or may not be indicated and is related to the number of recurrences and the degree of impairment.

5. Initiate a screening evaluation for anatomical defects, allergic diathesis, and/or immunocompetence after second bout with RPOM.

6. Pneumococcal vaccine has been helpful in reducing the number of RPOM due to *S. pneumoniae*.

Serous Otitis Media

1. If no treatable cause is discovered a qualitative and quantitative assessment must be made regarding the degree of hearing impairment (typanometry and/or audiometry).

2. The use of antihistamines and/or decongestants is controversial.

3. Because of the high frequency of bacteria obtained in tympanocentesis from patients with SOM a short course of antibiotic treatment should be provided.

4. Autoinflation or self-ventilation of the middle ear space, whether physiologically (Valsalva) or with an inflator (e.g., Mathes inflator), should be suggested, with an appropriate explanation.

5. Consider otolaryngological consultation if hearing impairment is >25db, atelectasis of the tympanic membrane is present, the fluid persists, and/or for routine PE tubes.

Chronic Otitis Media

1. This diagnosis necessitates otolarynogological consultation from the outset.

2. Local instillation of antibiotics.

Pericarditis

Inflammatory and infectious diseases of the pericardium usually occur in association with other diseases, such as pharyngitis, pneumonia, skin infections, or sepsis. Pericarditis may also be a concurrent manifestation of a systemic disease, such as rheumatoid arthritis, uremia, or systemic lupus erythematosus. Occasionally, pericarditis occurs as an isolated disease with no identifiable etiology (benign idiopathic).

PATHOPHYSIOLOGY

The principal effect of pericarditis is determined by the amount and consistency of accumulated fluid and whether or not cardiac compression-tamponade is present. The hemodynamic alterations are the principal cause of mortality and morbidity and should be corrected on an emergency basis (Fig. 1).

SIGNS AND SYMPTOMS

Clinically, the manifestations of pericarditis are those of the primary pathological process. In addition, the patient will have the following specific manifestations.

1. Fever: Usually low-grade, except in infectious pericarditis, where it follows a septic pattern.

2. Chest pain: Variable, but most often mid–chest, stabbing, referred to the neck and shoulder, increases with inspiration, and relieved partially by sitting and leaning forward.

3. Respiratory distress: The degree of respiratory difficulty is directly related to the degree of cardiac dysfunction caused by effusion, tamponade, and constriction; constrictive pericarditis can occur concomitantly with the acute process or as a late complication (seen most commonly with tuberculous pericarditis and only rarely in pericarditis of other etiologies).

There is always some evidence of myocarditis in patients with pericarditis and myocardial disease must be ruled out.

ETIOLOGICAL CONSIDERATIONS

1. Rheumatic pericarditis: The most common cause of pericarditis in the pediatric age group; it is usually serofibrinous and the accumulated fluid is seldom large enough to cause tamponade; it does not result in constrictive pericarditis.

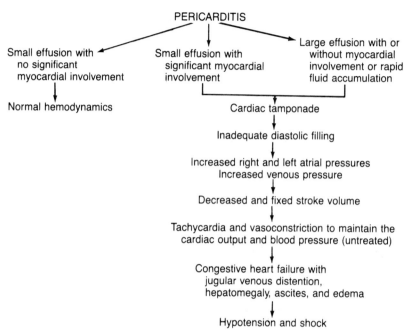

PERICARDITIS

Small effusion with no significant myocardial involvement

Small effusion with significant myocardial involvement

Large effusion with or without myocardial involvement or rapid fluid accumulation

Normal hemodynamics

Cardiac tamponade

Inadequate diastolic filling

Increased right and left atrial pressures
Increased venous pressure

Decreased and fixed stroke volume

Tachycardia and vasoconstriction to maintain the cardiac output and blood pressure (untreated)

Congestive heart failure with jugular venous distention, hepatomegaly, ascites, and edema

Hypotension and shock

FIG. 1.   Pathophysiology of pericarditis.

2. Purulent pericarditis: Produced most commonly by *H. influenzae* and *S. aureus,* but also caused by pneumococci, streptococci, and gram-negative organisms in newborn infants; it is almost always associated with a significant effusion of purulent exudate, clotted fibrin, and pus, which are difficult to aspirate; tamponade is a common complication.

3. Viral pericarditis: Caused most commonly by Coxsackie B_1 virus, but also caused by other viruses; it usually follows symptoms of an upper respiratory tract infection; pericardial fluid may accumulate, but it seldom causes any significant compression; the disease is self-limited, but it may be recurrent and result in constrictive pericarditis.

4. Tuberculous pericarditis: Associated with pulmonary tuberculosis and usually causes a significant effusion that often results in chronic constrictive pericarditis.

5. Uremic pericarditis: Occurs in chronic renal failure and is associated with significant effusions.

6. Postcardiotomy syndrome: May occur 1 to 4 weeks postoperatively and is associated with fever, but there is no evidence of infection; pericardial fluid may accumulate; the condition is almost always benign.

7. Pericarditis of juvenile rheumatoid arthritis: Rare in cases of pauciarticular juvenile rheumatoid arthritis, but present in about 35% of patients with the systemic

onset form; although it is usually benign, there may be significant effusion and cardiac dysfunction.

8. Pericarditis of the mucocutaneous lymph node syndrome: Occurs concomitantly with myocarditis, arthralgias, arthritis, hepatitis, and the erythema multiforme-like rash; pericarditis usually does not cause any complications and cardiac dysfunction is directly related to the coronary vasculitis and obstruction caused by the primary disorder.

9. Pericarditis associated with other diseases:

   a. Pericarditis due to *Listeria monocytogenes,* which causes widespread disease such as meningitis and pneumonia; it may be transmitted transplacentally to the fetus and newborn or by inhalation or ingestion after exposure to animals.

   b. Pericarditis associated with collagen-vascular disease, especially systemic lupus erythematosus.

   c. Pericarditis associated with a variety of other bacterial, viral, and mycotic organisms, such as *Mycoplasma,* meningococci, varicella, and *Candida.*

   d. Pericarditis associated with thalassemia and congenital hypoplastic anemia.

   e. Pericarditis associated with primary or secondary neoplastic disease and leukemia.

   f. Pericarditis associated with ulcerative colitis.

   g. Pericarditis of hypothyroidism.

   h. Pericarditis of Friedreich's ataxia.

   i. Pericarditis of storage diseases.

   j. Traumatic pericarditis.

10. Chronic constrictive pericarditis: Rare and usually idiopathic, but may be a sequala of recurrent viral pericarditis, tuberculous pericarditis and, occasionally, purulent pericarditis; it also may be the result of radiation therapy to the chest (especially in adults); the clinical picture is that of hemodynamic dysfunction secondary to cardiac compression that may be complicated by a variety of atrial arrhythmias. Occasionally, chronic pericarditis is associated with intestinal lymphangiectasia and growth failure, which must be differentiated from restrictive or obstructive myopathy and cor pulmonale.

DIAGNOSTIC PROTOCOL

Pericarditis should be suspected in any child who presents with chest pain. It should be ruled out in any infant or child who presents with any of the aforementioned disorders.

Medical History and Physical Examination

1. No significant effusion

   a. Quiet precordium.

b. No shift in the apical impulse.

c. Muffled heart sounds.

d. No significant heart murmurs, except with significant concomitant myocarditis or pancarditis, as in rheumatic fever.

e. Friction rub early in the process, which disappears if significant amounts of fluid accumulate.

2. Significant effusion

a. All of the above signs may be present except friction rub; however, friction rub may occur even with large effusions.

b. Small pulse volume, but normal heart rate; pulse volume may decrease further in inspiration.

c. Distended jugular veins.

3. Effusion with tamponade

a. All of the above signs may be present, including a small pulse volume in the presence of tachycardia; the pulse disappears in inspiration (pulsus paradoxus).

b. A paradoxical pulse can be confirmed by measurement of the blood pressure in inspiration and expiration; normally, in inspiration, the systolic pressure decreases by about 5 to 10 mm Hg; in tamponade, the systolic pressure decreases by more than 10 mm Hg.

c. Hepatomegaly, ascites, and edema may occur.

d. Hypotension and poor peripheral perfusion are often present (significant effusion can compress the left main bronchus, causing collapse of the lung).

4. Pericarditis may be differentiated from myocardial disease by the presence of the following physical and laboratory findings in patients with myopathic disease (hypertrophic or restricted).

a. Displaced apical impulse.

b. Presence of regurgitant murmurs.

c. Presence of gallop rhythm.

d. Prominent T-wave changes and ventricular arrhythmias.

e. Left atrial and left ventricular hypertrophy.

f. Left atrial pressure higher than right atrial pressure (equal in pericarditis).

g. Pulmonary artery pressure >45 mm Hg.

Laboratory Evaluations

1. To confirm pericarditis and effusion:

a. Chest radiograph: Normal if no effusion; if there is effusion, the cardiac shadow is enlarged, globular, and assumes the shape of a flask.

b. Electrocardiogram: S-T segment elevation early in the disease; later, the S-T segment becomes normal and the T wave becomes inverted; unlike myocardial infarction and ischemia, the T-wave inversion does not have reciprocal relations in leads I and III and the right and left precordial leads; the inverted T wave may persist for months; occasionally, the QRS voltages may be low.

   c. Echocardiography: The most reliable noninvasive method to demonstrate the fluid.

   d. Cardiac isotope scans: Used to demonstrate the pericardial border.

   e. Cardiac catheterization: Rarely necessary; elevated right atrial and pulmonary capillary pressures are demonstrated; poor myocardial contractibility is seen under fluoroscopy.

2. Other laboratory evaluations to determine etiology:

   a. Complete blood cell count.

   b. Urinalysis.

   c. Blood cultures.

   d. Throat cultures.

   e. Erythrocyte sedimentation rate (ESR), C-reactive protein (CRP), purified protein derivative (PPD) test.

   f. Antistreptolysin-O titer, streptococcal titer (Streptozyme), and anti-DNAase titer.

   g. Blood urea nitrogen (BUN), serum electrolytes.

   h. Liver function tests.

   i. Pericardiocentesis in suspected purulent pericarditis or if significant effusion is present (diagnostic and therapeutic).

   j. Viral titers (acute and convalescent).

   k. Rheumatoid factor.

   l. Antinuclear antibodies, including anti-DNA.

   m. Bone marrow.

   n. Endocrine and metabolic function tests.

TREATMENT PROTOCOL

1. If a significant effusion with tamponade is present (medical emergency) or if purulent pericarditis is present:

   a. Immediate therapeutic (as well as diagnostic) pericardiocentesis; needle aspiration is often not very effective when the fluid is purulent, thick, and contains fibrin clots.

   b. Pericardiectomy and continuous tube drainage may be necessary.

   c. Appropriate support of the cardiovascular dynamics and treatment of hypotension and shock; digoxin is contraindicated since it may cause further cardiac compromise and it may not be needed if the fluid can be evacuated immediately.

2. Treatment of the underlying condition

   a. Purulent pericarditis: Ampicillin (chloramphenicol if resistance to ampicillin is suspected) in children or gentamicin (in infants and newborns) **plus** a penicillinase-resistant antibiotic; antibiotics are given intravenously in appropriate doses until culture results are available and then treatment is modified accordingly; treatment is continued for 3 to 6 weeks, depending on the clinical response. A third generation cephalosporin may be the best choice if a single drug regimen is preferred.

   b. Rheumatic pericarditis: Treatment is same as that of rheumatic fever (i.e., eradication of streptococci, and anti-inflammatory agents).

   c. Viral pericarditis: Usually benign and requires no specific therapy; aspirin is often enough to control the symptoms; in recurrent or very severe pericarditis, steroids may be used.

   d. Tuberculous pericarditis: Patients should receive the standard antituberculous therapy plus steroids.

   e. Uremic pericarditis: Will improve with repeated dialysis and renal transplantation.

   f. Pericarditis of the postcardiotomy syndrome: Usually benign and requires no specific therapy; if severe, symptoms will improve with aspirin or indomethacin; if there is no response, steroids may be used.

   g. Pericarditis associated with juvenile rheumatoid arthritis: Responds to the anti-inflammatory agents used to treat the arthritis.

   h. Pericarditis of the mucocutaneous lymph node syndrome: Responds favorably to aspirin therapy, although coronary vasculitis may not.

   i. Constrictive pericarditis: Pericardiectomy.

Pertussis

Pertussis, an acute respiratory tract infection caused by *Bordetella pertussis*, is a serious disease of infancy and can be associated with significant morbidity and mortality (Fig. 1). Its incidence has decreased since the advent of a preventive vaccine. However, the associated immunity is not complete for all patients. This incomplete immunity, coupled with inadequate immunization, keeps pertussis active in many communities.

The major causes of morbidity and/or mortality from pertussis are bacterial bronchopneumonia and cerebrovascular accidents. Seizures may signify encephalopathy.

In older children and adults, pertussis is usually a mild illness. Low-grade fever, pharyngitis, rhinorrhea and a mild cough are most often the only symptoms. Adolescents and young adults have become the leading reservoir for the disease.

SIGNS AND SYMPTOMS

The incubation period of pertussis is 6 to 20 days, with an average of 1 week. Low-grade fever, profuse rhinorrhea, and a mild cough are characteristic of the catarrhal phase and last for 7 to 14 days. This phase is followed by a paroxysmal phase, which lasts 2 to 4 weeks. Rapid staccato series of coughs occur during a single expiration. A forceful inspiration occurs, causing the characteristic whoop. During the paroxysms, cyanosis, bulging neck veins, bulging eyes, protruding tongue, and drooling may occur. Facial petechiae and subconjunctival hemorrhage are not uncommon. Each paroxysm is frequently followed by vomiting. A whoop is not necessary for the diagnosis to be made, and pertussis should be considered in any infant or child who has lymphocytosis and a cough followed by vomiting. The paroxysmal phase is followed by a convalescent phase of 1 to 2 weeks in which the cough decreases in frequency and intensity.

DIFFERENTIAL DIAGNOSIS

1. Viral upper respiratory tract infection

2. Pneumonia

3. Foreign body aspiration

4. Cystic fibrosis

5. Cardiovascular disease

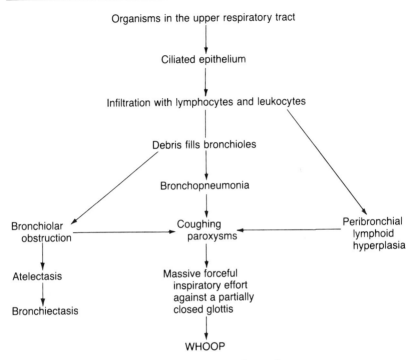

FIG. 1. Pathophysiology of pertussis.

DIAGNOSTIC PROTOCOL

1. Complete blood cell count: Usually shows a high white blood cell count and an absolute lymphocytosis; frequently, the lymphocytes account for more than 80% of the white blood cells.

2. Chest radiograph: May be normal or may show evidence of bronchopneumonia or atelectasis; a shaggy heart border is a normal finding in pertussis, even in the absence of bronchopneumonia; may rule out foreign body aspiration.

3. Blood cultures.

4. Viral cultures of the nasopharynx: Optional, since a negative culture does not rule out pertussis.

5. Fluorescent antibody staining: Frequently provides a rapid diagnosis; nasopharyngeal secretions are used.

6. *B. pertussis* culture: A negative culture on a cough plate does not rule out pertussis.

TREATMENT PROTOCOL

1. Hospitalization is required if the patient is younger than 1 year of age.

2. Allow nothing by mouth if the paroxysms are frequent; there is a high risk of food aspiration during a paroxysm.

3. Adequate fluids and electrolytes should be provided.

4. Small frequent feedings may be attempted if they are tolerated.

5. Erythromycin: 40 mg/kg/day p.o. in four divided doses for 5 to 7 days; may be preventive in the catarrhal (prodromal) phase but not in the paroxysmal phase: however, the organism will be eradicated from the nasopharynx.

6. Treatment of contacts

   a. Immunized children under 4 years of age: Booster DPT **plus** erythromycin, 40 mg/kg/day p.o. in four divided doses for 7 to 10 days (immunity is not absolute).

   b. Unimmunized contacts: Erythromycin, 40 mg/kg/day p.o. in four divided doses for 7 to 10 days.

$\mathbf{P}$hakomatosis

Phakomatosis is a term for a group of inherited familial diseases characterized by the presence of lens-like masses (Gr. *phakos* lens). A more descriptive term is neurocutaneous syndromes, implying clinical manifestations referable to the central nervous system and the skin. Several identifiable syndromes exist that exhibit characteristic cutaneous and central nervous system disturbances. Fourteen discrete syndromes have been described, but only the most common are discussed in this chapter.

The diagnosis of phakomatosis is usually based on the presence of characteristic clinical signs and symtoms.

PATHOPHYSIOLOGY

The diseases are genetically transmitted, most often in an autosomal dominant pattern (except ataxia-telangiectasia, which is autosomal recessive). The basic defect is usually the presence of multiple diffuse tumors (e.g., angiomas, fibromas) that have a systemic distribution (cutaneous and visceral) with a predilection for the central nervous system. There may or may not be other systemic manifestations. Most often, systemic symptoms are due to the extrinsic or intrinsic presence of the tumors.

DIAGNOSTIC AND TREATMENT PROTOCOLS

Table 1 gives diagnostic and treatment protocols for the most common syndromes of phakomatosis.

TABLE 1. *Phakomatosis: Diagnostic and treatment protocols*

Diagnosis	Treatment
Ataxia-Telangiectasia	
Skin: Café au lait spots, telangiectasia of the skin and conjunctivae CNS: Cerebellar ataxia Other: Immune deficiencies, bronchiectasis	Supportive and symptomatic
Neurofibromatosis: Recklinghausen's Disease	
Skin: Café au lait spots (six or more >1.5 cm in diameter), axillary freckles, neurofibromas (soft pedunculated masses) CNS: Neurofibromas (cranial nerves, spinal	Genetic counseling (though the transmission is autosomal dominant, approximately half of the cases result from spontaneous mutation)

TABLE 1. *(continued)*

Diagnosis	Treatment
roots, intracerebral), leading to various neurological symptoms, seizures, mild intellectual dysfunction Other: Multiple associated anomalies (e.g., bone cysts, megalencephaly, pseudoarthrosis of the tibia)	Anticonvulsant therapy if seizures are present Surgical removal of tumors if there is pain, functional impairments, or danger of malignant transformation

Sturge-Weber Disease: Encephalotrigeminal Angiomatosis

Skin: Nevus flammeus, or port-wine stain (a cutaneous angioma of the face that occurs most commonly in the ophthalmic division of the trigeminal nerve), congenital capillary hemangioma of the mucous membranes and the meninges CNS: Angiomata of the meninges and abnormal pial vessels (causes cortical anoxia, resulting in double contoured, curvilinear calcifications), seizures, mental retardation, hemiparesis, hemianopsia Other: Angioma of the choroid plexus of the eye, resulting in glaucoma	Seizures should be treated with appropriate anticonvulsants Physical therapy Special education, if required Frequent ocular examinations for glaucoma Surgical excision of cortical lesions, if seizures are intractable

Tuberous Sclerosis

Skin: Adenoma sebaceum (reddish brown nodules with a malar distribution appearing between 2 and 5 years of age and consisting of fibrous tissue and blood vessels), hypopigmented macules on the arms, legs, and trunk, shagreen patches (indurated areas over the back) CNS: Calcified "tubers" scattered through the gray matter (may bulge into the ventricle), seizures (in 90% of the patients, myoclonic seizures in the first year of life, progressing to grand mal and psychomotor seizures), mild to severe mental deficiency (in 60 to 70% of the patients), hyperactivity Other: Renal tubers (in 80% of the patients, causing compression symptoms)	Seizures should be treated with appropriate anticonvulsants Assess intellectual function and provide appropriate educational experiences Treat hyperkinesis (methylphenidate) Genetic counseling Evaluate parents for stigmata Surgical removal of tubers is indicated only if symptoms occur (e.g., obstructive nephropathy)

Lindau-Von Hippel Disease

Skin: None CNS: Cerebellar and spinal cord abnormalities secondary to hemangioma of the cerebellum and spinal cord, syringomyelia Other: Retinal angiomas (causing blindness), hypernephromas, cystic adenomas of other organs, arteriovenous aneurysms	Supportive and symptomatic Symptoms do not usually appear until late adolescence or young adulthood

Pneumonia

Respiratory tract infections are common during childhood and are responsible for significant morbidity and school absence. Because of the ubiquitousness of the organisms and ease of transmission in nursery and school situations, eradication and/or prevention of the infections is almost impossible. Early recognition and management of lower respiratory tract infections can effectively reduce resultant morbidity and mortality.

Certain forms of pneumonia occur in epidemics (e.g., *H. influenzae*). Appropriate prevention or epidemic control is possible, and routine prophylaxis is recommended for specified segments of the population.

Aspiration of foreign substances or of gastric contents can produce an intense inflammatory reaction. Sequelae are common and secondary bacterial infections occur.

PATHOPHYSIOLOGY

The exact pathophysiology of pneumonia varies with the offending organism. In general, there is infection and/or inflammation of the lower respiratory tract, alveolar exudation and transudation, edema of the mucosa and/or interstitium, diffusion and ventilation perfusion abnormalities. Occasionally, there is mucosal invasion, necrosis, and/or abscess formation.

SIGNS AND SYMPTOMS

The symptoms vary according to the type of pneumonia present and the extent of pulmonary involvement. Mild cough and coryza may be the only clinical findings. Fever may or may not be present. Rales secondary to alveolar exudation are frequently auscultated. Ronchi and upper airway sounds occur since there may be inflammation or infection along most of the pulmonary tree. Wheezing, dullness to percussion, diminished breath sounds, cyanosis, and asymmetrical auscultatory findings may also occur.

Patients present with various degrees of respiratory distress, which depend on the degree of pulmonary ventilatory dysfunction caused by obstruction to the diffusion of oxygen by alveolar fluid or exudate and/or interstitial inflammation and edema.

DIAGNOSTIC PROTOCOL

---

1. **Clinical findings:** The diagnosis of pneumonia is usually made on clinical grounds by the presence of rales, wheezing, asymmetrical breath sounds, diminished breath sounds, and/or respiratory distress.

2. **Chest radiograph:** Usually negative early in the course of the illness, radiographic evidence of pneumonia lags approximately 2 to 4 days behind the appearance of clinical symptoms.

3. **Cultures:** An accurate culture diagnosis is difficult and is frequently not obtained in patients with mild to moderate disease; blood cultures may yield the organism; patients with moderate to severe pneumonia, those not responding to empirical therapy, and those whose condition is deteriorating require culture diagnosis; the reliability of the culture is inversely proportional to the invasiveness of the procedure (e.g., Luken's aspiration, direct tracheal aspiration, transtracheal needle aspiration, bronchial washings, needle biopsy, thoracentesis, and open biopsy.

4. **Viral titers:** Require acute and convalescent serum and may not provide immediate information needed.

5. **Cold agglutinins:** Commonly elevated with mycoplasma pneumonia.

GENERAL TREATMENT PROTOCOL

---

1. The treatment of pneumonia is generally supportive and symptomatic: Adequate fluids, calories, humidity, and hydration; oxygen supplementation, if necessary; chest physical therapy and postural drainage; and occasionally assisted ventilation.

2. Antibiotic therapy

   a. Pneumonia in children is often viral in origin and, therefore, not amenable to antibiotic therapy; during epidemics of influenza pneumonia, adenine arabinoside may be used in patients with moderate to severe illness.

   b. When bacterial pneumonia is suspected, the initial choice of antibiotics is empirical and guided by the clinical findings, severity of the illness, and the presence of pathogens in the community; the pneumococcus organism is the most common cause of bacterial pneumonia in childhood; however, *H. influenzae* and *Mycoplasma* are not uncommon etiologies.

   c. Initial treatment is usually parenteral; if the clinical course improves significantly and the patient's condition is stable, medication may be given orally.

MANIFESTATIONS AND TREATMENT

Table 1 describes the manifestations and gives the corresponding treatment protocols for several types of pneumonia.

TABLE 1. *Pneumonia: Manifestations and treatment*

Clinical manifestations	Laboratory findings	Radiographic findings	Treatment
Pneumococcal			
Infants may manifest mild upper respiratory tract symptoms followed by an abrupt onset of fever and respiratory distress; signs of lobar consolidation may be present; abdominal distension may occur; Meningismus may occur, especially if the pneumonia is located in the right upper lobe. Older children and adolescents manifest symptoms similar to adults: Abrupt onset of shaking chill, fever, prostration, cough, cyanosis, and respiratory distress; signs of lobar consolidation may be present; chest pain and pleural effusions may occur	There is usually leukocytosis and a shift to the left on the complete blood cell count Blood cultures are positive in approximately 30% of the patients	Lobular or lobar consolidation Pleural reaction with effusion is common A diffuse infiltrate may be seen in younger patients	Parenteral penicillin G, 50,000 units/ kg/day in 4 divided doses for 10 days If the patient is ambulatory: procaine penicillin G, 600,000 units followed by 50,000 units/kg/day p.o. in 4 divided doses for 10 days If the patient is allergic to penicillin: cefazolin, 50 mg/ kg/day in 4 divided doses for 10 days
Mycoplasma			
The onset is slow; cephalgia, malaise, sore throat, and cough are commonly seen; moist rales are often auscultated diffusely throughout all lung fields	*M. pneumoniae* can be isolated from upper respiratory tract secretions, but significant time is required for the procedure Cold agglutinins are present in a titer greater than 1:64 Complete blood cell count is usually normal	Bronchopneumonia pattern to interstitial infiltration; lower lobes are commonly involved Pleural effusion with the above picture suggests another diagnosis; it is uncommon with mycoplasma pneumonia	Supportive and symptomatic Erythromycin, 50 to 100 mg/kg/day p.o. in 4 divided doses for 7 to 10 days

TABLE 1. *(continued)*

Clinical manifestations	Laboratory findings	Radiographic findings	Treatment
Viral			
The onset is variable, but it is usually preceeded by 1 to 2 weeks of upper respiratory tract symptoms, fever and cough may occur, rales are often heard, along with ronchi and wheezing, respiratory distress is variable and is usually worse in the young child (or otherwise compromised child) Secondary bacterial infections may occur	White blood cell counts are variable and may show a leukocytosis early in the course of the illness, and a lymphocytosis later Cultures are negative Viral titers yield only a retrospective diagnosis	Infiltrates are usually diffuse and/or interstitial; there may be a perihilar distribution Pleural effusions may occur Lobar consolidation may occur	Supportive and symptomatic In young or debilitated patients, adenine arabinoside may be used to treat significant influenzae pneumonia
Streptococcal			
Symptoms are similar to pneumococcal pneumonia but can be insidious in onset as in *H. influenzae* Radiograph often looks worse than the clinical condition appears Pleuritic pain is common and pleural fluid is often present	Leukocytosis and a left shift on the CBC is common Blood cultures are positive in approximately 10% of the patients There is an elevated serum antistreptolysin O titer	Disseminated interstitial infiltration	Parenteral penicillin G, 100,000 units/kg/day in 4 divided doses for 10 to 14 days
H. Influenzae			
The onset is usually insidious and may be preceeded by 1 to 3 weeks of upper respiratory tract complaints; fever, tachypnea and varying degrees of respiratory distress occur; rales, ronchi, dullness and increased	Leukocytosis and a left shift on the CBC may occur Blood cultures may yield the organism Counterimmunoelectrophoresis of pleural fluid, urine, bronchial washings, or tracheal aspirate may be positive for the organism	There is usually a lobar infiltrate in one or more lobes May appear as bronchopneumonia	Chloramphenicol, 100 mg/kg/day i.v. in 4 divided doses for 10 to 14 days If the organism is proven sensitive: *ampicillin*, 200 mg/kg/day i.v. in 4 divided doses for 10 to 14 days

Clinical manifestations	Laboratory findings	Radiographic findings	Treatment
fremitus, asymmetrical breath sounds may be present; the major difference from pneumococcal disease is the insidiousness of onset			

Staphylococcal

Clinical manifestations	Laboratory findings	Radiographic findings	Treatment
The patients are usually <1 year old or immunologically compromised Skin lesions are often present; there is an acute onset of fever, cough, tachypnea, and respiratory distress The patients appear to be quite ill; shock may be present Physical examination reveals rales, ronchi, dullness, and asymmetrical breath sounds	The white blood cell count is usually elevated with a left shift. Leukopenia is a poor prognostic sign Pleural fluid or tracheal aspiration reveals leukocytosis (>300/cm), decreased glucose concentration, and elevated protein concentration Gram stain will commonly reveal the organism	Rapidly progressive infiltrate, begins as a patchy bronchopneumonia and progresses to empyema and pyopneumothorax within a few hours. Pneumatoceles may or may not be present (they are not pathognomonic)	Nafcillin, 150 mg/kg/day i.v. in four divided doses for 2 to 4 weeks (depending on the clinical response), **or** other penicillinase-resistant penicillins If the organism is sensitive to penicillin: Aqueous penicillin G, 100,000 units/kg/day If the patient is allergic to penicillin: Cefazolin, 50 mg/kg/day for 3 to 4 weeks (depending on the clinical response) Drain any empyema Provide oxygen and chest physical therapy Treat shock

Pneumocystis carinii

Clinical manifestations	Laboratory findings	Radiographic findings	Treatment
Usually occurs in neonates or immunologically compromised patients The onset is insidious with cough, fever, and progressive respiratory distress, which is usually severe with relatively few pulmonary findings	Staining of the tracheal aspirate, bronchial washings, or biopsy specimen may reveal the organism	Bilateral infiltrates spread out from the hilum Diffuse granularity Hyperexpansion is usually present	Trimethoprim/sulfamethoxazole (trimethoprim, 20 mg/kg/day, **or** sulfamethoxazole, 100 mg/kg/day in 4 divided doses for 14 days)

Pneumothorax

Spontaneous pneumothorax is not common in children. It should be suspected whenever there is an acute onset of respiratory distress, particularly in infants and children who have underlying respiratory illnesses, those who have been resuscitated, those who are being ventilated or those who have received trauma to the chest (Fig. 1).

SIGNS AND SYMPTOMS

The signs and symptoms of pneumothorax vary, depending on the degree of pneumothorax. Most often there is an acute onset of respiratory distress manifested by tachypnea, intercostal retractions, subcostal retractions, and/or suprasternal retractions. There may be asymmetrical excursion of the thorax during the respiratory cycle. The breath sounds are most often asymmetrical, being diminished or absent on the side of the pneumothorax. Signs of cardiovascular compromise may occur. Cyanosis may or may not be present.

DIAGNOSTIC PROTOCOL

Suspect pneumothorax on clinical grounds if:

1. Respiratory distress in newborn
2. Acute onset of respiratory distress
3. Acute onset of chest pain
4. Decreased breath sounds
5. Muffled heart sounds or shifts in the cardiac apical impulse
6. Subcutaneous emphysema
7. Primary respiratory disorder with suddenly deteriorating condition, hypoxia, acidosis, or shock

If there is no time for a chest radiograph, the patient is in **acute distress, respiratory and/or cardiac arrest, or severe shock.**

1. Direct needle aspiration in the sitting position, using a 25-gauge needle (for infants) attached to a 50-cc syringe through a 3-way stopcock. Insert the needle through the second intercostal space in the anterior axillary line, lateral to the pectoralis major muscle **over the top** of the rib. In children, use the second

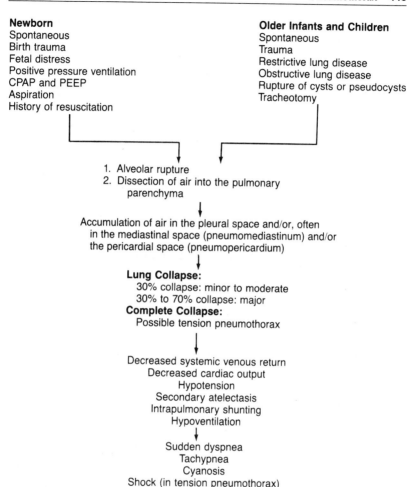

Newborn
Spontaneous
Birth trauma
Fetal distress
Positive pressure ventilation
CPAP and PEEP
Aspiration
History of resuscitation

Older Infants and Children
Spontaneous
Trauma
Restrictive lung disease
Obstructive lung disease
Rupture of cysts or pseudocysts
Tracheotomy

1. Alveolar rupture
2. Dissection of air into the pulmonary
   parenchyma

Accumulation of air in the pleural space and/or, often
in the mediastinal space (pneumomediastinum) and/or
the pericardial space (pneumopericardium)

Lung Collapse:
30% collapse: minor to moderate
30% to 70% collapse: major
Complete Collapse:
Possible tension pneumothorax

Decreased systemic venous return
Decreased cardiac output
Hypotension
Secondary atelectasis
Intrapulmonary shunting
Hypoventilation

Sudden dyspnea
Tachypnea
Cyanosis
Shock (in tension pneumothorax)
Cardiac tamponade (in severe pneumomediastinum or pneumopericardium)

FIG. 1.   Pathophysiology of pneumothorax. CPAP, continuous positive airway pressure; PEEP, positive end expiratory pressure.

intercostal space midclavicular line. Air will be aspirated. If air continues to leak, place chest tubes. Both sides of the chest must be tapped.

2. If no improvement, insert a needle into the pericardial space subcostally (subxyphoid).

3. Resuscitate, as necessary.

In the **absence of acute distress:**

1. Fiberoptic transillumination: May give false negative results.

2. Chest radiographs: Posteroanterior (in expiration) and lateral decubitus views (with affected side up).

   a. Extrapulmonary air with lung collapse (pneumothorax).

   b. Radiolucent rim following the contour of the mediastinum (pneumomediastinum).

   c. Radiolucent rim following the contour of the mediastinum but continuous over the diaphragmatic border of the heart (pneumopericardium).

   d. Small linear, reticular, or cystic radiolucencies wider in the periphery (pulmonary interstitial emphysema).

   e. Findings must be differentiated from diaphragmatic hernia, lung cysts, lobar emphysema, and artifacts (e.g., skin folds or clothing).

3. Arterial blood gases and pH.

4. Renal malformation studies should be performed in unexplained pneumothorax.

TREATMENT PROTOCOL

1. Emergency treatment and adequate resuscitation (acute distress)

   a. Needle aspiration.

   b. Chest tube placement.

   c. Correct acidosis.

   d. Ventilator therapy (can aggravate visceral pleural leaks but improves parietal pleural leaks, or flail chest; if needed, use the lowest possible inflation pressures).

2. If there is no underlying disease, no respirator therapy, no distress, no evidence of continuing air leak (stable condition), and pneumothorax < 30% of hemithorax:

   a. Observation and bed rest.

   b. 100% oxygen is contraindicated in newborn infants but may be used in older infants or children.

   c. Follow-up by monitoring vital signs, chest radiographs, arterial blood gas (ABG), and pH.

   d. The pneumothorax resolves within 24 to 48 hr.

3. If there is distress with no underlying pulmonary disease and no continuous air leak:

   a. Needle aspiration, as previously described.

   b. Observation and follow-up.

4. If there is continuous air leak: Insert a chest tube through a closed thoracotomy into the third intercostal space at the anterior axillary line (avoid the nipple area); place the tube under water seal, suction at 15 cm H_2O pressure.

5. If pneumothorax occurred with respiratory therapy or PEEP: Begin chest tube drainage, as described above.

6. Chronic small and asymptomatic pneumothorax: Evacuate with a chest tube.

7. Pneumopericardium with clinical evidence of compromised cardiac output (weak pulses, poor perfusion and shock): Needle aspiration through the subxyphoidal area; may require tube placement.

8. Pneumomediastinum: No treatment; usually asymptomatic; air is loculated and difficult to aspirate.

9. Recurrent pneumothorax (more than twice in the same hemithorax, especially with absence of underlying pulmonary disease): Pleural stripping or quinacrine instillation may be necessary if surgical intervention is contraindicated.

10. Bronchopleural fistula: Surgical therapy

11. Removal of chest tube.

  a. When no air leaks for 48 hr and chest radiograph is negative for 48 hr.

  b. Resolved underlying disease: Discontinue suction and put the tube under water seal; if no air leaks are observed, clamp the tube; if no reaccumulation of air is observed on chest radiograph 2 hr and 24 hr later, remove the chest tube.

Poisoning

Intentional ingestion of substances other than food is a common occurrence in infancy and childhood. The ingestion may be of a solid object, a toxic or potentially toxic substance, or a corrosive liquid or solid. Ingested substances vary in their toxicity, some requiring only the ingestion of a few drops and others the ingestion of more than a quart.

In general, children in the high-risk age group (1 year to 4 years) usually ingest 1 teaspoonful of liquid per swallow (4–5 ml) or approximately 0.27 ml/kg (Jones and Work, 1961). This may be helpful in estimating the volume of substance ingested and, ultimately, in the prognosis.

Of extreme importance to the practitioner is a knowledge of local resources available to assist in the management of acute intoxications. Perhaps most important is the provision of anticipatory guidance for parents and patients to prevent unintentional ingestions. Discussion of poisoning prevention should be part of routine health maintenance. Physicians may provide parents with information regarding Mr. Yuk programs, emergency telephone numbers, a supply of ipecac, and advice on how to childproof a home (e.g., installation of cabinet locks; placing detergents, cleaning fluids, and insecticides out of the reach of children; utilization of childproof caps; keeping medications and toxic substances in their original containers with their original labels in place).

SIGNS AND SYMPTOMS

The presenting signs and symptoms of poisoning depend on the substance and the amount ingested. Too often the offending agent is not known, and an accurate approximation must be made from a description of the substance or an accurate evaluation of the presenting signs and symptoms.

Most signs and symptoms of acute intoxications are nonspecific and can be mistaken for other disorders (e.g., infection, acute abdomen, epilepsy). However, the practitioner must have a high index of suspicion and consider poisoning whenever faced with a patient with unexplained cyanosis, seizures, cardiovascular collapse, coma, or other such conditions.

GENERAL DIAGNOSTIC PROTOCOL

1. The parents should be instructed to bring the bottle or contents of the agent ingested for evaluation.

2. Vomitus (or gastric aspirate) may be sent for drug, substance, and pH analysis.

3. Drug screening may be obtained, and analysis for heavy metals should be ordered. Lead should be included on the screening examination, since ingestion of a foreign substance may be a manifestation of pica.

4. The local poison control center should be notified for possible identification of the substance by its description and a description of the presenting signs and symptoms.

5. Complete blood cell count, urinalysis, chest radiograph, blood gases, electrolytes, blood urea nitrogen, creatinine, and liver function testing may be indicated.

GENERAL TREATMENT PROTOCOL

Treatment at Home

1. **Induce vomiting** (unless the ingested substance is a corrosive or volatile hydro-carbon, the patient is comatose, or seizures occur); **Do not waste time in transporting the patient to the hospital to attempt to induce vomiting**.

   a. Pharyngeal stimulation, **or**

   b. One teaspoonful of dry mustard in one glass of warm water, **or**

   c. Syrup of ipecac, 15 cc p.o., followed by copious amounts of water; repeat in 20 min if vomiting has not occurred.

2. **Dilute poison with milk** (or water if no milk is available).

3. Suggest that the parent bring the substance container, or the remainder of the contents of the container, to the hospital for analysis.

Treatment in the Hospital

1. **Induce vomiting** (unless a corrosive or volatile hydrocarbon was ingested, the patient is comatose, or seizures occur).

   a. Vomiting may be induced up to 12 hr after substance ingestion.

   b. If a volatile hydrocarbon was ingested, emesis may be induced, but it is best done with a cuffed endotracheal tube in place.

   c. Syrup of ipecac: 15 cc p.o., followed by copious amounts of fluids; repeat in 20 min if vomiting has not occurred.

2. Gastric lavage: If induction of emesis is unsuccessful, there is impending coma, or if the patient is comatose (**contraindicated if the ingested substance is corrosive**).

3. Activated charcoal: 1 to 3 teaspoonsful of activated charcoal in a slurry, either orally or by gastric lavage (**activated charcoal should not be given along with ipecac since the ipecac will be absorbed and will not function to induce emesis**).

4. Supportive and symptomatic care

   a. Intravenous fluids to maintain good urine output.

    b. Oxygen, if necessary.

    c. Anticonvulsants, if seizures are present.

    d. Cardiorespiratory support, if required.

5. Specific antidotes or regimens for specific toxins (see Table 1).

6. Dialysis (if the poison is dialyzable).

    a. Peritoneal dialysis.

    b. Hemodialysis.

TABLE 1. *Manifestations and treatment of poisoning*

Signs and symptoms	Antidote/treatment[a]
Acetone	
Similar to ethyl alcohol, but more potent anesthetic properties; upper respiratory tract and gastrointestinal tract irritant; may cause stupor and narcosis	Emesis Lavage with normal saline Supportive and symptomatic care
Adhesive Cement	
Rare if small quantities are ingested; inhalation causes symptoms similar to those of alcohol ingestion	Emesis Lavage with normal saline Supportive and symptomatic care Epinephrine may cause arrhythmias
Alkali	
Burning in the mouth, nausea, vomiting, hematemesis, cardiorespiratory collapse, gastrointestinal perforation and stricture, especially of the esophagus	**Do not induce emesis** Dilute with water and milk Cardiorespiratory support Steroids Esophagoscopy
Amphetamines	
Dilated pupils, sweating, nausea, vomiting, dry mouth, pallor, arrhythmias, tachycardia, hypertension, shock, lassitude, restlessness, psychosis, spasms, seizures, and coma	Emesis Activated charcoal Hydration Chlorpromazine
Analgesic Rubs (Methyl Salicylate)	
Gastritis, acid-base abnormalities, seizures and coma; symptoms may be similar to those of other salicylates ingestion	Emesis Dilute with milk or water Lavage with normal saline Activated charcoal
Barbiturates	
Miosis followed by dilatation of the pupil, hypotension, shock, respiratory depression, Cheyne-Stokes respirations, cyanosis, respiratory failure, drowsiness, decreased sensory abilities, ataxia, vertigo, stupor, coma, decreased deep tendon reflexes, and positive Babinski tests	Emesis Lavage with normal saline Activated charcoal Diuresis Dialysis Supportive and symptomatic care

Signs and symptoms	Antidote/treatment[a]

Chlorine Gas

Burning of the nose and throat, cough, irritation of the respiratory tract mucosa, cyanosis, dyspnea, and restlessness	Often no treatment is required Oxygen Respiratory support Sedation Cough suppressant

Clorox®

There may be no symptoms; burning and irritation of the mucous membranes may occur, but is usually mild; sodium hypochlorite in concentrations >5% may cause significant burns and should be handled as an alkali burn	Dilute with milk or water Demulcents may be utilized Cautious lavage if large quantities have been ingested Supportive and symptomatic care

Colognes

CNS depression and gastrointestinal tract irritation; toxic ingredient is usually ethanol	Emesis Lavage with normal saline Supportive and symptomatic care

Detergents

Mouth, throat, and esophageal irritation and edema; tetany can occur	**Do not induce vomiting** Dilute with water Calcium gluconate, if necessary

Diazepam

CNS depression, coma, respiratory depression, decreased blood pressure, stupor, and vertigo	Emesis Lavage with normal saline Activated charcoal Supportive and symptomatic care

Diphenhydramine

CNS stimulation, dilatation and fixation of the pupils, hyperthermia, central nervous system depression, coma, cardiorespiratory failure, and seizures	Emesis Lavage with normal saline Supportive and symptomatic care Physostigmine Diazepam Exchange transfusion

Diphenoxylate and Atropine

Signs of atropine toxicity and respiratory depression up to 24 hr after ingestion, possible ileus	Emesis Lavage with normal saline Naloxone (for respiratory depression)

Ethyl Alcohol

Exhiliration, incoordination, ataxia, vertigo, nausea, vomiting, stupor, coma, respiratory depression, hypoglycemia, and seizures	Emesis Lavage with sodium bicarbonate Supportive and symptomatic care Avoid using depressants Dialysis may be indicated

Ethylene Glycol

Exhiliration, incoordination, nausea, vomiting, depression, convulsions, cyanosis, pulmonary edema, respiratory failure, and renal failure	Emesis Lavage with normal saline Treat seizures with diazepam Respiratory support Provide adequate fluids and electrolytes Ethanol may be used to inhibit oxidation

TABLE 1. *(continued)*

Signs and symptoms	Antidote/treatment[a]

Hydrogen Peroxide

Mild gastrointestinal irritation (3–6% solution); more highly concentrated solutions are corrosive	Dilute with milk or water Supportive and symptomatic care

Iron Salts

Gastrointestinal irritation and hemorrhage, cardiovascular collapse, shock, and hepatic damage; usually an initial symptom-free interval	Emesis Lavage with 5% sodium bicarbonate Supportive and symptomatic care Deferoxamine

Isopropyl Alcohol

CNS depression, vertigo, incoordination, stupor, coma, cephalgia, nausea, vomiting, gastroenteritis, and hypoglycemia; pulmonary damage may occur; more irritating than ethanol and symptoms last 2 to 4 times longer	Ingestion of >5cc: Emesis Lavage with normal saline and 3% or 5% sodium bicarbonate Avoid depressants Do not use apomorphine to induce vomiting Supportive and symptomatic care Dialysis

Meperidine HCl

Euphoria, agitation, weakness, hallucinations, stupor, coma, respiratory depression, dry mouth, flushed face, tachycardia, shock, urinary retention, and variable pupillary responses	Respiratory support Supportive and symptomatic care Naloxone (antidote)

Meprobamate

CNS depression, ataxia, deep sleep, coma, shock, respiratory collapse, and seizures	Emesis Lavage with normal saline Activated charcoal Supportive and symptomatic care Osmotic diuresis Hemodialysis

Multivitamins

Rare unless there are large amounts of iron, vitamin A, or vitamin D in the preparation, which may cause central nervous system symptoms and symptoms of increased intracranial pressure	Emesis Lavage with normal saline Activated charcoal Mannitol Dexamethasone

Naphthalene

Gastric irritation and central nervous system irritation, seizures, coma, brown urine, dysuria, and hemolysis with glucose 6-phosphatase deficiencies	Emesis Lavage with normal saline Cathartic (magnesium sulfate but not mineral oil) Supportive and symptomatic care

Organophosphorous Compounds

Anorexia, nausea, sweating, salivation, lacrimation, abdominal pain, pallor, dyspnea, incontinence, muscle twitching, fasciculations, cephalgia, drowsiness, confusion, seizures, and respiratory arrest	Atropine Respiratory support Pralidoxime chloride (PAM)

Signs and symptoms	Antidote/treatment[a]

Petroleum Distillates

Burning of upper gastrointestinal tract, vomiting, euphoria, cephalgia, tinnitus, weakness, restlessness, incoordination, confusion, central nervous system depression, seizures, respiratory arrest, chemical pneumonia, and pulmonary edema	Do not induce emesis if a small amount was taken, if vomiting has already occurred, or if the patient is comatose If a large volume is ingested or the petroleum distillate is in combination with another significant toxin induce vomiting with ipecac with the patient in an upright position or with a cuffed endotracheal tube in place Supportive and symptomatic care Epinephrine may induce arrhythmias

Phenothiazines

Potentiation of CNS depressants, extrapyramidal symptoms, seizures, coma, dysphagia, hypothermia, opisthotonus, respiratory failure, cardiovascular collapse, bone marrow depression, and liver damage	Emesis Lavage with normal saline Diphenhydramine Supportive and symptomatic care Exchange transfusion

Phenytoin

Ataxia, drowsiness, vertigo, nystagmus, pupillary dilatation, cardiac arrhythmias, somnolence, hyperglycemia, and ketosis	Emesis Activated charcoal Insulin may be required for hyperglycemia Diuresis is not indicated Hemodialysis if the overdose is large

Propoxyphene

CNS depression, nausea, vomiting, respiratory depression, seizures, coma, and cardiac arrest	Emesis Lavage with normal saline Activated charcoal Respiratory support Naloxone (antidote) Supportive and symptomatic care

Warfarin

Hemorrhagic diathesis, vomiting, abdominal pain, prolonged prothrombin time; onset of symptoms may be delayed 24 to 36 hr after the ingestion	Emesis Vitamin K if the prothrombin time is abnormal

[a]Consult pertinent literature for specific dosages.

Precocious Puberty

Puberty is influenced by a variety of factors, the most crucial of which is the interaction between the hypothalamus, pituitary, and gonads. Before puberty, gonadal steroids suppress the hypothalamus and pituitary. At the onset of puberty, the hypothalamus becomes less sensitive to the suppressive effects of gonadal steroids, allowing the levels of luteinizing hormone (LH) and follicle-stimulating hormone (FSH) to increase and stimulate the gonads. This event occurs at about 11 to 12 years of age in girls and 12 to 13 years of age in boys. Because the age at onset of these changes is variable and covers a wide range, it is difficult to determine when puberty is precocious.

SIGNS AND SYMPTOMS

The onset of puberty before 8½ years of age in girls and 10 years of age in boys is considered precocious. Precocious puberty is divided into two groups.

1. True precocious puberty
   a. Always isosexual
   b. Precocity of the secondary sex characteristics
   c. Increased size and activity of the gonads
2. Pseudo precocious puberty
   a. Appearance of some secondary sex characteristics
   b. Sex characteristics may be isosexual or heterosexual
   c. Gonads do not mature
   d. No activation of normal pituitary-hypothalamic-gonadal interplay

DIFFERENTIAL DIAGNOSIS

True (Complete) Precocious Puberty

1. Idiopathic (constitutional, functional)
   a. Sporadic
   b. Familial (in the male)
2. Cerebral lesions
   a. Tumors destroying the pineal body

b. Brain tumors near the third ventricle

c. Hypothalamic hamartomas and congenital malformations

d. Hydrocephalus

e. Tuberous sclerosis and degenerative disease

f. Postinfection lesions (encephalitis, meningitis)

g. Cystic arachnoiditis

3. McCune-Albright syndrome (polyostotic fibrous dysplasia and abnormal pigmentation)

4. Associated with hypothyroidism

5. Silver's syndrome (syndrome of congenital asymmetry, short stature and elevated gonadotropins)

6. Gonadotropin-producing tumors

a. Hepatoma and hepatoblastoma

b. Chorionepithelioma

c. Teratoma

7. Drugs (gonadotropins and treatment of adrenal hyperplasia)

8. Exogenous obesity

Pseudo (Incomplete) Precocious Puberty in Girls

1. Isosexual (feminization)

a. Ovarian disorders: Granulosa cell tumor, theca-cell tumor, ovarian teratoma, functional ovarian cysts, choriocarcinoma, dysgerminoma, luteoma

b. Adrenal disorders: Adrenocortical tumors, Cushing's syndrome

c. Estrogen administration

2. Heterosexual (virilization)

a. Congenital adrenal hyperplasia

b. Testosterone-secreting tumors (adrenal)

c. Androgen-producing teratomas

d. Androgen administration

Pseudo (Incomplete) Precocious Puberty in Boys

1. Isosexual (virilization)

a. Congenital adrenal hyperplasia

b. Adrenocortical tumors

c. Leydig cell (interstitial) testicular tumors

d. Androgen administration

e. Teratomas containing adrenal tissue

2. Heterosexual (feminization)

   a. Adrenocortical tumors

   b. Estrogen administration

3. Other

   a. Hyperinsulinism

   b. Primordial dwarfism

   c. Excess of thyrotropin-releasing hormone

   d. Premature pubarche

   e. Premature thelarche

DIAGNOSTIC PROTOCOL

1. Complete medical history

   a. Drug intake.

   b. Use of hormone containing creams.

   c. Familial incidence.

   d. Multiple fractures (suggests McCune-Albright syndrome).

   e. Infections suggestive of CNS involvement.

   f. Symptoms and signs of CNS disease.

   g. Absence of vaginal bleeding (menstruation).

2. Complete physical examination

   a. General physical examination.

   b. Delineate secondary sex characteristics and determine if the patient has isosexual or heterosexual precocity.

   c. Compare the size of both testes to the penis and to each other (in adrenal hyperplasia there is enlargement of the penis but not the testes).

   d. Neurological examination (in precocity due to intracranial lesions, neurological symptoms are present before signs of sexual development).

   e. Pelvic examination with patient (if necessary, under general anesthesia) if a pelvic mass is suspected.

3. If the medical history and the physical examination do not reveal enough clues to suggest a diagnostic plan, the protocol in Table 1 may be followed.

4. Other tests

   a. Electroencephalogram: May be abnormal in true sexual precocity of functional origin.

   b. Urinary estrogens: May be elevated in ovarian granulosa cell tumor.

   c. Urinary pregnanediol: May be elevated in ovarian luteoma.

TABLE 1. *Precocious puberty: Diagnostic protocol*

Bone age	Urinary 17-ketosteroids	Urinary gonadotropins	Radioimmunoassay		Possible diagnosis and further investigation
			FSH	LSH	
Advanced	Normal or slightly increased	Increased	Increased	Increased	Constitutional precocious puberty; increased testosterone (boys) or estradiol (girls) if LH is greatly increased; rule out a possible gonadotropin-secreting tumor
			Decreased	Decreased	Rule out a possible functional ovarian lesion if estradiol and esterone levels are increased
Normal	Normal	Normal			Possible premature thelarche in absence of urinary estrogen level
Advanced	Slightly increased	Normal			Possible premature adrenarche (increased serum dehydroepiandrosterone); monitor plasma androgen level to rule out possible adrenal tumor
Normal or slightly advanced	Normal or slightly increased	Normal or increased			Rule out possible intracranial lesions, especially in boys, if there is no explanation for precocious puberty; further suggested tests: skull radiograph, electroencephalogram, CT scan, arteriographs
	Increased	Highly increased			Gonadotropin-secreting tumor (chorioepithelioma, teratoma, or hepatoma); monitor α-fetoprotein level; perform dexamethasone suppression test (17-ketosteroids do not suppress in hepatoma); perform testicular biopsy (Leydig cell hyperplasia with underdeveloped or degenerated seminiferous tubules)
	Slightly increased				Premature pubarche; true sexual precocity due to intracranial lesion
	Moderately or highly increased				Adrenogenital syndrome; adrenal tumor (increased dehydroepiandrosterone); testicular tumor; hepatoma (increased gonadotropins and α-fetoproteins); perform dexamethasone suppression test (possible virilizing adrenal hyperplasia if 17-ketosteroids suppress—testicular biopsy shows no spermatogenesis; possible interstitial cell testicular tumor, virilizing adrenal tumor, or hepatoma if 17-ketosteroids do not suppress)
Delayed			Increased	Increased	Hypothyroidism; monitor TSH, T_3 and T_4 levels
Delayed		Increased			Silver's syndrome

d. Skull radiographs: Enlarged sella turcica may be seen with hypothyroidism.

e. Radiographs of the long bones: Fractures in McCune-Albright syndrome.

f. Retroperitoneal pneumogram: To demonstrate ovarian or adrenal tumors.

TREATMENT PROTOCOL

1. Treat primary cause of precocious puberty, if demonstrable.

2. If there is no immediately demonstrable cause: Careful follow-up for several years to rule out a possible primary cause (e.g., intracranial lesion).

3. Psychological support of patient and family.

4. Prevention of sexual abuse.

5. Medroxyprogesterone (Provera®): Arrests the process, causes regression in breast development, and suppresses testosterone, but has numerous side effects, such as suppression of adrenal and pituitary axis; advanced skeletal maturation is not affected.

6. Danazol and cyproterone have been used for the same purpose.

Proteinuria

Isolated proteinuria refers to the presence of significant amounts of protein in the urine without other abnormalities of the urine sediment. Most nephrologists accept excessive (significant) proteinuria as 50 mg/dL or >200 mg/24 hr. A small amount of protein (usually albumin) in the urine is neither unusual nor abnormal. Thus, the distinction between normal and pathological proteinuria is quantitative rather than qualitative.

Proteinuria may also be defined in terms of its presentation (asymptomatic, symptomatic, intermittent, persistent) as well as its mechanism of appearance in the urine (increased glomerular permeability, overflow from elevated serum protein levels, renal tubular epithelial secretion, inadequate tubular reabsorption).

The incidence of significant proteinuria in a single urine test in preschool children is 2% to 5% and tends to increase with age, reaching 10% to 12% at puberty. It then gradually decreases in the early twenties. If multiple samples are obtained from those children with a positive single sample, the incidence of significant proteinuria decreases dramatically. Screening for proteinuria has been made simple through the use of albumin sensitive "dip sticks," which can detect proteinuria at a level of 15 mg/dL. Although there are false positives when a urine is markedly alkaline and false negatives at very high urine flow rates, there is a good correlation between the reading and the albumin concentration. Once a positive screening test is identified, verification with another laboratory test is in order. Precipitation tests for proteinuria using sulfosalicylic acid are sensitive, convenient, do not require heating, and are easily interpreted. Ultimately, the rate of excretion of protein is the most important indicator of the presence or absence of renal disease. In conjunction with quantitation of the protein found in the urine over a 24-hr period, the selectivity of the protein excreted may be useful in determining the significance, as well as the prognosis, of certain forms of proteinuria. As the permeability of the glomerular basement membrane increases, proteins of larger molecular weight pass through this filter and may imply a worse prognosis (Fig. 1).

SIGNS AND SYMPTOMS

Clinical manifestations of proteinuria depend on the disease state represented. A small amount of protein may be present in the urine of healthy people, but larger amounts may occur with no clinical manifestations. In nonselective and/or massive proteinuria, the signs and symptoms may be those of protein depletion and/or specific renal disease or dysfunction.

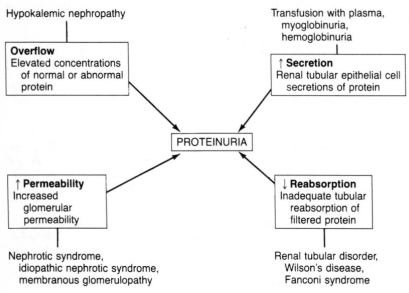

FIG. 1. Pathophysiology of proteinuria.

DIFFERENTIAL DIAGNOSIS

Symptomatic proteinuria, whether primary or secondary, has multiple etiologies. The evaluation in these categories is similar to the evaluation of isolated proteinuria, but more extensive and expeditious evaluation may be warranted and should include any tests specific for the disease entity suspected.

1. Primary renal disease
2. Secondary renal disease (kidneys affected by a systemic disorder)
3. Renal dysplasia
4. Chronic pyelonephritis
5. Hydronephrosis
6. Nephrotic syndrome
7. Renal vein thrombosis
8. Diabetes mellitus
9. Collagen-vascular disease
10. Hemoglobinuria
11. Constrictive pericarditis

Asymptomatic, isolated proteinuria may be secondary to exercise, fever, or orthostasis.

GENERAL DIAGNOSTIC PROTOCOL

1. When isolated proteinuria is discovered in an asymptomatic child, first repeat the test several times. If there is any doubt about the accuracy of the test, another method should be substituted, i.e., dip sticks versus sulfosalicylic acid.

2. If the protein is present in two or three consecutive daytime samples, then a test for orthostatic proteinuria should be performed. If the test shows inconsistent or questionable positive results, no further tests should be undertaken. The investigation for orthostatic proteinuria is simple and merely involves having the child urinate at bedtime and then collecting the first sample of urine in the morning prior to being up and about. It is helpful also to collect a second sample of urine on that day after the child has been out of bed and active for several hours. If the first sample is negative for protein, but the second sample is positive, then a diagnosis of orthostatic proteinuria is confirmed. If more quantitative information is required, after the child voids at bedtime, all urine passed is collected up to and including the first voided morning sample, and quantitatively measured.

3. If the test for orthostatic protein is negative (protein is present in an orthostatic pattern and/or an upright position), then further investigation is warranted and will depend on the quantity of protein excreted as well as any symptoms present.

   a. Initially, 24-hr urine protein excretion, as well as creatinine clearance, serum albumin, globulin, and cholesterol should be evaluated in conjunction with a complete blood cell count, blood urea nitrogen, electrolytes, and screening tests for possible collagen disease (C3 complement, antinuclear antibodies test).

   b. If urinalysis is suggestive of bacterial infection and/or the patient is symptomatic, a urine culture should be obtained and the patient treated appropriately.

   c. An intravenous pyelogram (IVP) may be obtained for anatomical delineation when quantitative protein measurements and urine cultures are performed but, regardless of sequence, urological consultation should be obtained for genitourinary studies.

4. If urine cultures are negative and no anatomical abnormality is detected on the IVP, a diagnostic percutaneous renal biopsy should be considered. Other indications for consideration of a biopsy include significant and persistent proteinuria, massive proteinuria ($>40/mg/m^2/hr$, or >2 g/24 hr), associated hematuria, any abnormal immune system studies, associated hypertension, or ongoing and untoward parental anxieties.

DIAGNOSTIC EVALUATION

Figure 2 outlines the procedure for the diagnostic evaluation of proteinuria.

DIAGNOSTIC AND TREATMENT PROTOCOLS

Table 1 gives the diagnostic and therapeutic protocols for several types of proteinuria.

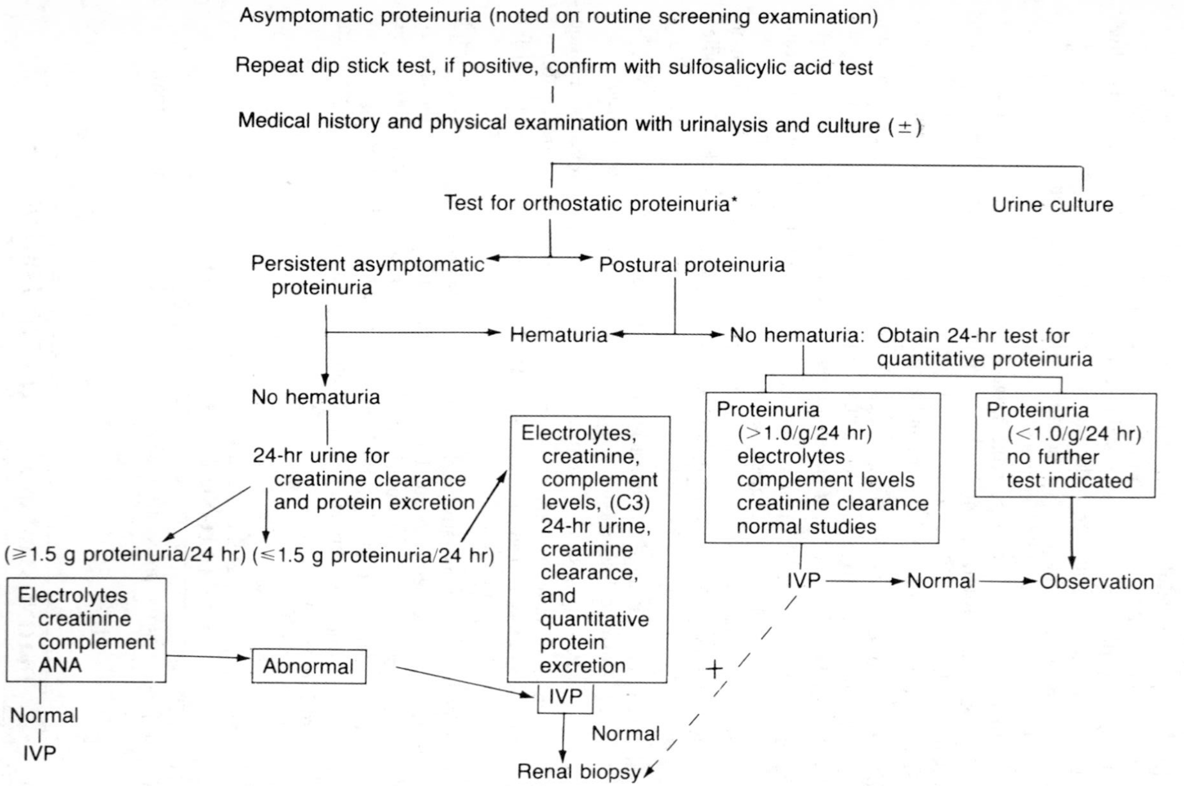

FIG. 2. Diagnostic evaluation of proteinuria. *, split urine × 3 (first morning urine, i.e., supine as well as an up-and-about urine) repeated 3 times.

TABLE 1. *Proteinuria: Diagnostic and treatment protocols*

Diagnosis	Treatment
Febrile	
Associated with febrile illness in 3% to 5% of children	Supportive and directed at the cause of the fever
Examination is directed toward determining the etiology of the fever	
Proteinuria is transient (2–3 days post-illness) and low grade (<500 mg/L)	
Test for proteinuria should be repeated during convalescent period	
Orthostatic	
Occasional history of healed glomerulonephritis	No treatment indicated
Proteinuria is usually discovered accidentally	Excellent prognosis
Physical examination is usually not remarkable	
Simple and definitive tests (see General Diagnostic Protocol)	
Exercise	
Mechanism: Alteration in renal hemodynamics, resulting in an exaggeration of the normal rates of protein filtration	No treatment indicated
Most often affects a healthy child who has undergone vigorous exercise	Excellent prognosis
Physical examination is not significant	
Repeat urine tests for protein three times; they should show significant proteinuria only after very vigorous exercise has occurred	
Proteinuria Associated with Acute or Chronic Pyelonephritis	
Mechanism: Probably tubular, but with severe renal disease, or may involve glomerular mechanism	
Medical history and symptoms may point to an acute urinary tract infection; proteinuria should be low grade and transient, reflecting probable tubular dysfunction	
Persistent or heavy proteinuria or proteinuria associated with other signs of renal disease	
Proteinuria Associated with Systemic Illness Without Primary Renal Pathology	
Pertinent information should be illicited regarding the specific illness, e.g., congestive heart failure	
Proteinuria Associated with Renal Parenchymal Disease[a]	
Information regarding the parenchymal disease will dictate evaluation and treatment	

[a]Nephrotic syndrome, glomerular disease, membrane proliferative, focal sclerosing tubular diseases, Wilson's disease, Fanconi syndrome, congenital galactosemia.

Respiratory Care

Respiratory care directed toward the maintenance of adequate oxygenation and preventing aspiration, accumulation of secretions, and infection is indicated in most infants and children who are admitted to the hospital for any reason. It is particularly important postoperatively and in all infants and children who are admitted with respiratory diseases, cardiac diseases, CNS and neuromuscular diseases, trauma, accidents, poisoning, severe fluid and electrolyte disturbances, shock, or burns, especially those of the face, neck, and chest.

To achieve the stated objectives of respiratory care, the following measures should be instituted.

1. Initial evaluation of the respiratory status
   a. Examine patient for signs of cyanosis.
   b. Obtain resting respiratory and heart rates.
   c. Examine lung fields for adequacy of air entry and exhalation.
   d. Observe patient for the presence of suprasternal retractions (upper airway obstruction), intercostal and subcostal retractions, and abdominal respiration.
   e. Monitor arterial blood gases and pH.
   f. Obtain a chest radiograph.
2. Respiratory care (individualized, depending on the initial evaluation)
   a. Allow nothing by mouth for moderate to severe respiratory distress.
   b. Intravenous [keep vein open (KVO) or therapy] if respiratory problems are present or anticipated.
   c. Frequently monitor vital signs until stable; continuous monitoring of respiration and heart rate for distressed patients or if problems are anticipated.
   d. Adequately humidified air (except in asthma, where humidity causes severe irritation and further airway obstruction).
   e. Respiratory and chest therapy by a qualified and experienced respiratory therapist.
      (1) Chest physiotherapy and mobilization of secretions.
      (2) Removal of secretions by gentle, nontraumatic suctioning.
      (3) Aerosol or intermittent positive pressure breathing (IPPB) therapy.
   f. Oxygen (tent or mask–nasal prongs may be used but are irritating) should be humidified and warm. Oxygen is used only if there is evidence of anoxia

($Pa_{O_2} < 65$ mm Hg); use the lowest concentration and flow rates to keep $Pa_{O_2} > 70$ mm Hg.

g. Frequent position changes, adequate ambulation, and encouragement of coughing.

3. Frequent reevaluation and assessment of respiratory status: Capillary blood gases or cutaneous measurements are adequate for follow-up if the Pa_{CO_2} is not very elevated or significant cyanotic heart disease is not suspected.

RESPIRATORY FAILURE

Despite adequate respiratory care, respiratory failure may develop and will lead, if not treated, to cardiac or respiratory arrest. Respiratory failure is the most common medical emergency in infants and children; its usual causes in the first two years of life are respiratory distress syndrome, pneumonia, asthma, upper airway obstruction, and accidents and poisoning.

Respiratory failure should be anticipated and early evidence recognized to ensure prompt and effective therapy. Signs of impending failure include any degree of hypoxemia, hypercapnea, tachycardia, drowsiness and fatigue, diaphoresis, and $Pa_{CO_2} \geqslant 60$ Torr.

Respiratory failure is diagnosed if three or more of the following conditions are present: cyanosis in 30% to 40% oxygen, absent air entry sounds, severe retractions and abdominal respiration, drowsiness, weakness, and fatigue, and/or agitation (air hunger).

INTUBATION AND MECHANICAL VENTILATION

Intubation and mechanical ventilation are indicated in the following conditions: arterial P_{O_2} that cannot be maintained above 50 Torr despite increasing the inspired oxygen concentration, arterial $P_{CO_2} > 65$ mm Hg, apnea, chest muscle paralysis, and/or inability to maintain a normal heart rate and adequate oxygenation despite the use of an ambu bag and adequate chest inflation.

Intubation (Team Effort Required)

1. Obtain adequate help.

2. Prepare adequate equipment and emergency drugs.

  a. Select endotracheal tube size according to patient's age

   (1) 2.5-3.0 mm: Premature to 3 months

   (2) 3.5-4.0 mm: 4 to 18 months

   (3) 4.0-5.0 mm: 2 to 5 years

   (4) 5.0-6.5 mm: 6 to 12 years

   (5) 6.5-8.0 mm: >13 years

  b. Adequate laryngoscope, straight and curved blades.

c. Drugs should include sodium bicarbonate, epinephrine, atropine, calcium gluconate; emergency cart with all the other emergency and resuscitation drugs should be available; other drugs for sedation and/or myoneural blockade should also be available.

d. Adequate suction machine and suction catheters.

e. Adequate nasogastric tubes.

3. Establish intravenous line if not already in place, preferably a CVP line.

   a. Umbilical vein catheter in newborns, positioned in the superior vena cava above the diaphragm (normal = 4-7 cm H_2O).

   b. Silastic catheters in external jugular in infants and small children.

   c. Silastic catheters inserted into the antecubital median basilic vein and advanced into the superior vena cava in older children (normal = 6-14 cm H_2O).

4. Attach patient to cardiac monitor.

5. Establish an arterial line

   a. Percutaneous plastic cannula into the radial artery or into the umbilical artery in newborns.

   b. Connect the cannula to a T-connector.

   c. Connect the T-connector to a continuous infusion pump of normal saline and heparin (1 unit/ml) at 3 ml/hr.

   d. The line can be used to withdraw arterial samples and in direct transducing of systemic pressures.

6. Aspirate the stomach with nasogastric tube.

7. Suction the oropharynx.

8. If intubation is to be carried out in an awake, resisting infant or child, it is desirable to use myoneural blockade (e.g., tubocurarine, 0.2 to 0.6 mg/kg **or** succinylcholine, 10 to 50 mg, by slow infusion).

9. Hyperventilate, using an ambu bag, mask and 100% oxygen.

10. Intubate under direct laryngoscopy, using nasotracheal tube (in emergencies, use orotracheal tube, size 14 and 16 in small infants and size 18 in full-term infants); do not hyperextend the neck during intubation; use Magill forceps to guide the nasotracheal tube into the trachea.

11. Atropine, 0.01 mg/kg s.c. (maximum dose, 0.4 mg) in case of bradycardia due to vagal reflex.

12. Aspirate secretions.

13. Ventilate with 100% oxygen.

14. Listen to both lungs and make sure that there is adequate air entry to both sides.

15. Fix the tube in place, using tincture of benzoin and waterproof adhesive tape.

16. Obtain a chest radiograph; ensure that the tube is in the trachea (not in the right main bronchus).

17. Attach patient to a respirator.

Mechanical Ventilation

1. Definitions

   a. Continuous distending airway pressure (CDAP) refers to all methods that attempt to maintain alveolar distention, including continuous negative airway pressure (CNAP) and continuous positive air pressure (CPAP).

   b. Intermittent positive pressure ventilation (IPPV).

   c. Intermittent positive pressure breathing (IPPB) refers to the use of mask and bag as opposed to ventilator.

   d. Positive end expiratory pressure (PEEP) must be set on the ventilator in the treatment of newborns; in older children, it may not be necessary to include it in the settings.

   e. Intermittent mandatory ventilation (IMV).

2. Ventilators

   a. Positive pressure flow: Determine the pattern of flow; the volume delivered and the pressure required to deliver it are determined by the pulmonary compliance.

   b. Pressure generators: Determine the pressure; the patterns of flow and volume are determined by the lung characteristics.

   c. The controlling cycles of the ventilator are time-cycled, pressure-cycled, volume-cycled, flow-cycled, or a combination of these.

   d. For infants and children <3 years of age, the machine should have variable inspiratory flow rate (50-200 ml/sec) and should be volume-cycled or time-cycled and pressure limited (e.g., Bourns pediatric ventilator).

   e. For older children, the machine should have variable flow rates (10-100 L/min), maximum pressure of 80 cm H_2O, adjustable cycling rate (6-100 breaths/min), and adjustable tidal volumes (10-200 ml/breath) (e.g., Bennett MA-1 ventilator).

3. Supportive care while on ventilator

   a. Frequent checks to ensure that the endotracheal tube is well fixed.

   b. Continuous monitoring of vital signs and clinical condition.

   c. FIO_2 and respirator settings should be checked frequently.

   d. Arterial blood gas (ABG) every 6 hr (more often if unstable) and 15 min after any change in settings.

   e. Airway care (sterile technique): Suction secretions, and perform tracheal toilet every 2 hr, including suction, ventilation with bag and mask and FIO_2 1.0 for 2 min, instill 0.5 to 5.0 ml of normal saline, suction, ventilation with bag and mask and FIO_2 for 2 min.

   f. Decompress stomach with nasogastric tube.

   g. Daily sputum cultures.

   h. Daily chest radiographs.

4. Weaning from the ventilator (attempted when primary disorder is under control and infant has improved and condition is stable)

   a. Start by lowering pressure: In pressure ventilators, 2 cm H_2O at a time (e.g., from 30 to 20 cm H_2O); repeat ABG if stable.

   b. Reduce FIO_2 0.05 at a time (e.g., from 0.6 to 0.4); repeat ABG if stable.

   c. Decrease the rate 2 to 4/min to the minimum as the infant increases spontaneous breathing.

   d. Intermittent use of CPAP to increase the periods of spontaneous respiration.

   e. When spontaneous respiration is tolerated for 1 hr, repeat ABG if stable; attempt extubation.

   f. Weaning may be attempted with the use of a T-adapter for 15 min; repeat ABG if stable; put patient back on the respirator for 1 hr, then place back on T-adapter for 15 min; repeat ABG if stable; attempt extubation.

   g. Weaning can be attempted by using IMV and gradually reducing the number of assisted breaths delivered.

   h. Weaning from PEEP: Decrease pressure gradually over a period of several hours until pressure is 2 cm H_2O; repeat ABG; if patient is breathing adequately but continues to need PEEP, wean using a T-adapter and CPAP; patient is ready to be extubated at PEEP 0 and normal ABG.

5. Extubation

   a. Tracheal toilet.

   b. Dexamethasone, 0.5 mg/kg i.v. or i.m.

   c. Deflate the endotracheal tube cuff, if inflated.

   d. Extubate.

   e. Racemic epinephrine (2.25%), 1 ml with 5 ml of saline, delivered by IPPB for 5 min; repeat every 1 to 2 hr.

   f. Maintain on dexamethasone, 0.25 mg/kg/day i.v. or i.m. in four divided doses, if necessary.

6. Failure to wean from the ventilator

   a. Chronic lung disease.

   b. Cardiac problems.

   c. CNS problems.

   d. One or more complications of mechanical ventilation.

7. Complications of mechanical ventilation

   a. Dehydration.

   b. Pneumothorax, pneumomediastinum, interstitial emphysema.

   c. Pneumonia and/or sepsis.

d. CNS disorders (e.g., seizures or hemorrhage).

e. Interference of the ventilator settings with normal hemodynamics.

For management of assisted ventilation problems see Table 1.

TABLE 1. *Management of problems encountered in assisted ventilation*

Problem	Treatment

Adequate heart rate, spontaneous breathing, Pao_2 <50 Torr **or** $Paco_2$ >55 Torr but <70 Torr	Oxygen mask and bag: Ventilate for 5 to 10 min every 30 min
	Select mask size according to child's weight:
	  Size 1: <1,000 g
	  Size 2: 1.0 to 1.7 kg
	  Size 3: 1.7 to 2.5 kg
	  Size 4: >2.5 kg
	Bag: 500 ml, 40 mm Hg safety valve

Oxygen mask and bag fail to keep Pao_2 >50 Torr **or** FIO_2 >0.6 is required to keep Pao_2 between 50 and 70 Torr	Infant very ill or <1,300 g: Start CDAP as CPAP via endotracheal tube
	Infant not very ill or >1,300 g: Start CDAP as CPAP via nasopharyngeal tube
	Use continuous flow respirator:
	  Pressure: 5 cm H_2O
	  FIO_2: 0.6
	  Flow: 5 to 10 L/min
	Reevaluate ABG in 15 min
	Increase pressure by increments of 2 cm H_2O until Pao_2 is appropriate
	Note: Gas inflow should be more than twice the infant's respiratory minute volume (RMV); RMV = RR × tidal volume; tidal volume = 10 to 15 ml/kg

Infant on CPAP and Pao_2 continues to be <50 Torr and $Paco_2$ <65 Torr **or** Pao_2 is normal but $Paco_2$ is rising	Replace nasopharyngeal tube by an endotracheal tube Decrease the CPAP (high CPAP can cause decreased venous return, decreased cardiac output, increased pulmonary vascular resistance, and R-L shunting

Infant on CPAP and Pao_2 continues to be <50 Torr and $Paco_2$ is normal and increasing despite FIO_2 of 0.6 to 1.0	Baby Bird ventilator:
	  Peak inspiratory pressure: 20 to 25 cm H_2O
	  PEEP: 3 to 5 cm H_2O
	  Respiratory rate: 20 to 25/min
	  Inspiratory duration: 1 to 1.5 sec
	  FIO_2: 0.6 to 1.0
	If Pao_2 does not improve, increase peak inspiratory pressure **or** increase PEEP **or** increase inspiratory time
	If $Paco_2$ is high, increase peak inspiratory pressure **or** decrease PEEP **or** decrease inspiratory time **or** increase expiratory time
	Bourns ventilator:
	  Flow rate: 3 to 5 L/min
	  Tidal volume: 10 to 15 ml/kg
	  Respiratory rate: 40 to 60/min
	  PEEP: 3 to 5 cm H_2O
	  FIO_2: 0.6
	If PEEP of 12 cm H_2O is reached and $Paco_2$ is still <50 Torr, make FIO_2 1.0

TABLE 1. *(continued)*

Problem	Treatment
	Bennett MA-1 ventilator: Respiratory rate: 15 to 30/min FIO_2: 0.4 to 0.6 Tidal volume: 10 to 15 ml/kg Dead space gas: 2 ml/kg Reduce FIO_2 until Pao_2 is between 70 and 100 Torr If $Paco_2$ is <30 Torr, decrease tidal volume **or** add dead space gas, 5 to 10 ml at a time, **or** decrease the rate.
Mechanical ventilation and Pao_2 is <50 Torr, FIO_2 is 1.0, and CPAP is 10 to 12 cm H_2O **or** Pco_2 is >70 to 80 Torr from any cause **or** apnea and bradycardia are not responsive to other therapy	IPPV Initial pressure: 15 to 20 cm H_2O Respiratory rate: 50 to 60/min Increase pressure by 2 or 3 cm H_2O until Pao_2 starts to fall Maintain Pao_2 between 50 and 80 mm Hg
Condition does not improve or improves and then suddenly deteriorates	Check blocked or dislodged tube Malfunctioning respirator Pneumothorax Extrapulmonary disease (e.g., CNS hemorrhage, cardiac disease)
Fighting the respirator	Check Pao_2, $Paco_2$, and pH Adjust the settings
Respirator settings are adequate, ABG and pH are acceptable, but patient continues to fight the respirator	Sedate with morphine, 0.1 to 1.0 mg/kg i.v. **or** curare, 0.3 to 0.5 mg/kg i.v., initially and then 0.1 mg/kg i.v., as needed
Evidence of injury to pulmonary capillaries (e.g., increased pulmonary venous pressure, prolonged open heart surgery, massive transfusions) **or** ABG suggestive of intrapulmonary shunts (e.g., Pao_2 <60 Torr with FIO_2 1.0 and $Paco_2$ normal or low) **or** multiple areas of collapse	PEEP with gradually increasing pressures until Pao_2 is between 60 and 80 Torr (maximum safe pressure, 10 to 12 cm H_2O)

Respiratory Distress in the Newborn

Respiratory distress in newborn infants may be produced by many pathological conditions. It differs from respiratory distress in older children in the frequency of particular etiologies and the presence of considerations unique to neonates.

SIGNS AND SYMPTOMS

Respiratory distress in newborn infants is manifested by retractions, tachypnea, and/or cyanosis, which are similar to the clinical findings in older children. Prolonged apnea ($>$20 sec), short apnea with bradycardia, excessive periodic breathing, shallow breathing with bradycardia, stridor, and/or grunting may also occur.

DIFFERENTIAL DIAGNOSIS

1. Pulmonary
   a. Transient upper airway obstruction (mucus)
   b. Respiratory distress syndrome
   c. Apnea
   d. Infection
   e. Transient tachypnea of the newborn
   f. Aspiration pneumonia
   g. Pneumothorax or pneumomediastinum
   h. Emphysema
   i. Bronchopulmonary dysplasia
   j. Esophageal atresia with fistula
   k. Diaphragmatic hernia
   l. Phrenic nerve palsy
   m. Congenital upper airway obstruction

2. Cardiac
   a. Congenital heart disease
   b. Congestive heart failure

3. Metabolic
   a. Acidosis
   b. Hypoglycemia
   c. Hypocalcemia
   d. Hypothermia
   e. Hyperthermia
   f. Septicemia

4. Hematological
   a. Anemia
   b. Polycythemia

5. Central nervous system
   a. Hemorrhage
   b. Meningitis or encephalitis
   c. Drug-induced
   d. Cerebral edema

GENERAL DIAGNOSTIC PROTOCOL

1. Clear the upper airway by gentle suctioning.

2. If cardiovascular compromise is present, resuscitate appropriately.

3. Obtain medical history and perform physical examination, paying close attention to the cardiovascular system, pulmonary system, and central nervous system.

4. Carefully pass a catheter through the external nares and nasopharynx and into the stomach to ensure a patency of the choanal passages and esophagus.

5. Monitor arterial blood gases (right radial, temporal, or umbilical artery sample).

6. Monitor blood glucose (Dextrostix®).

7. Determine hematocrit and hemoglobin.

8. Monitor serum calcium.

9. Obtain cultures of the blood, nose, trachea, gastric aspirate, and umbilicus.

10. Obtain cerebrospinal fluid for microsopic examination and culture.

11. Chest radiographs (posteroanterior and lateral views).

GENERAL TREATMENT PROTOCOL

General Measures

1. Suction, resuscitate.

2. Place infant in supine position.

3. Maintain abdominal temperature at 97°F (rectal at 98.5°F).

4. Monitor vital signs.

5. Allow nothing by mouth.

6. Administer i.v. fluids.

7. Administer oxygen as needed; monitor Pa_{O_2} and/or Tc_{PO_2}.

8. Correct respiratory acidosis (increased Pa_{CO_2}) by assisted ventilation.

9. Correct metabolic acidosis with sodium bicarbonate, according to base deficit.

10. Improve basic perfusion shock by administration of colloids and oxygen, which will improve acid-base balance.

11. Assisted ventilation if Pa_{CO_2} is >50 Torr or if there is apnea.

12. Correct anemia and shock.

13. Administer antibiotics.

14. Oral feeding, if no respiratory distress.

Oxygen Therapy

1. Use only if Pa_{O_2} is <50 Torr or if there is cyanosis.

2. Aim to keep Pao_2 between 60 and 80 Torr and not more than 100 Torr.

3. Oxygen should be warm (88°–93°F) and humidified.

4. Standardize the oxygen analyzer against room air (21%) and a known source of oxygen.

5. Observe infant for complications of oxygen therapy (pulmonary hemorrhage, bronchopulmonary dysplasia, and retrolental firbroplasia).

Assisted Ventilation Therapy

1. Intermittent positive pressure breathing (IPPB) using oxygen mask and bag.

   a. Indication: Pao_2 <50 Torr or $Paco_2$ >50 Torr.

   b. Mask size (according to infant's weight):
   Size 1: <1.0 kg
   Size 2: 1.0 to 1.7 kg
   Size 3: 1.8 to 2.5 kg
   Size 4: >2.5 kg

   c. Bag: 500 ml with 40 mm Hg safety valve (different ambu bags deliver different concentration of oxygen; hence, use appropriate ambu bag).

   d. Ventilate for 5 to 10 min every 30 min to 1 hr.

2. Continuous positive airway pressure (CPAP).

   a. Indication: To keep alveoli expanded in expiration if Po_2 is <50 Torr in 60% oxygen or if mask and bag therapy fails.

   b. Intubate.

   c. Administer desired concentration of oxygen at a minimum of 2 L/min.

   d. Gas inflow should be more than twice the infant's respiratory minute volume (RMV); RMV = RR × tidal volume; tidal volume = 4 ml/lb.

   e. Adjust screw clamp so that end expiratory pressure is 5 to 6 mm Hg.

   f. Increase end expiratory pressure by 2 mm Hg until Pao_2 is >50 Torr (maximum safe pressure, 12 mm Hg).

   g. Extubate if Pao_2 is normal at zero end expiratory pressure for at least 4 hr.

3. Intermittent positive pressure breathing, using mechanical ventilator.

   a. Indication: Apnea with bradycardia; failure of CPAP and IPPB by oxygen mask and bag.

   b. Intubate.

   c. Initial pressure of 15 to 20 cm H_2O (infants ≤1,000 g) up to 25 to 30 cm H_2O (infants >1,000 g).

   d. Decrease pressure by 2 to 3 cm H_2O if Pco_2 is normal.

   e. Intermittent mandatory ventilation respiratory rate of 30/min.

   f. If infant fights the respirator, sedate or curarize.

   g. Maintain airway patency by tracheal toilet.

h. Maintain Po_2 at 60 to 80 Torr and continuously monitor with Pao_2 transducer or $TcPo_2$.

i. Deep stomach decompressed by using a nasogastric tube.

4. Continuous positive pressure breathing (CPPB).

a. Indication: Positive end expiratory pressure (PEEP) can be maintained by CPPB to prevent alveolar collapse; use if Pao_2 is <50 Torr while on assisted ventilation and 80 to 100% oxygen.

DIAGNOSTIC AND TREATMENT PROTOCOLS

Table 1 gives the diagnostic and treatment protocols for a variety of respiratory distress syndromes as they affect the neonate.

TABLE 1. *Respiratory distress in the newborn: Diagnostic and treatment protocols*

Diagnosis	Treatment
Apnea	
Etiological considerations: Prematurity, CNS hemorrhage, infections, electrolyte imbalance, gastroesophageal reflux Manifestations: Prolonged apnea (>20 sec), periodic breathing with bradycardia, short apnea with bradycardia, shallow breathing with bradycardia, abnormal pneumogram Diagnostic measures: Abnormal pneumogram; exclude other factors such as CNS hemorrhage and upper airway obstruction	Feed slowly, decompress the stomach Remove nasogastric tube; treat hypoglycemia and hypocalcemia; prevent oropharyngeal obstruction; do not overflex or overextend the neck Theophylline, up to 8 mg/kg/day p.o.; serum level, 8 to 12 mg/100 ml
Bronchopulmonary Dysplasia	
Etiological considerations: Oxygen therapy with or without ventilator, poor bronchial drainage Manifestations: Chronic respiratory distress and cyanosis; prolonged need for respiratory support; diffuse rales Diagnostic measures: Chest radiograph in acute phase is similar to respiratory distress syndrome; later, it reveals cystic spaces (proliferative phase)	Supportive; no specific therapy
Congenital Heart Disease	
Etiological considerations: Positive family history, maternal diabetes, maternal alcoholism, congenital infection (rubella and Coxsackie virus), trisomies 21, 13-15, and 17-18, Turner's syndrome, large infant Manifestations: Respiratory distress, tachypnea without dyspnea, cyanosis not responsive to oxygen, heart murmur, arrhythmias	Congestive heart failure; digoxin and furosemide; restrict fluids Decreased pulmonary blood flow (pulmonary atresia); immediate surgery for Blalock-Taussig shunt (keep ductus arteriosus patent temporarily by using prostaglandins) Transposition: Rashkind septostomy Cardiac catheterization Surgical intervention

Diagnosis	Treatment

Diagnostic measures: Chest radiograph shows large heart, decreased or increased pulmonary vascular marking, abnormal electrocardiogram, abnormal echocardiogram, no response to inhaled oxygen

Meconium Aspiration

Etiological considerations: Prolonged labor, prolapsed cord, breech extraction, maternal hemorrhage, postmaturity, asphyxia, hypotension

Manifestations: Respiratory distress with tachypnea, rales, meconium upon tracheal aspiration

Diagnostic measures: Chest radiograph shows coarse, streaky infiltrates with areas of atelectasis and hyperinflation; flat diaphragm

Suction oropharynx and trachea before infant establishes respiration; do not use IPPB until clear from meconium; ultrasonic nebulization cultures; antibiotics (penicillin, gentamicin, 5 mg/kg/day); observe for pneumothorax; monitor CNS; use of steroids questionable

Patent Ductus Arteriosus

Etiological considerations: Prematurity and hypoxia, congenital heart disease, intrauterine infection

Manifestations: Ventilatory dependence, increasing oxygen requirement, lung edema, enlarging heart and symptoms of heart failure, heart murmur (may be absent), CO_2 retention

Diagnostic measures: Chest radiograph shows cardiomegaly and lung edema; abnormal electrocardiogram; echocardiogram shows left-atrial-to-aortic ratio of more than 1:2; aortogram shows L-R shunt at the ductal level

Restrict fluids; furosemide; treat hypoxia, indomethacin p.o. or i.v. if no contraindications (e.g., liver disease, bleeding, abnormal renal function); dose: experimental; if no response, use digoxin and furosemide; surgical ligation

Pneumonia

Etiological considerations: Premature rupture of membranes, prolonged labor, maternal infection, obstetrical manipulation, aspiration, *E. coli, Staphylococcus*, group B Streptococcus, *Candida, Listeria, Toxoplasma, Cytomegalovirus, Coxsackie virus, Pseudomonas, Klebsiella*

Manifestations: Respiratory distress, tachycardia

Diagnostic measures: Chest radiograph shows patchy densities with linear streaking toward the periphery

Sepsis evaluation; penicillin, 50,000 to 100,000 units/kg/day in two doses; kanamycin, 15 to 20 mg/kg/day in two doses **or** gentamicin, 7.5 mg/kg/day in two doses

Pneumothorax and Pneumomediastinum

Etiological considerations: Aspiration, uneven ventilation, vigorous resuscitation

Manifestations: Respiratory distress, shift of apical impulse, decreased breath sounds

Diagnostic measures: Chest radiograph shows air outside lung tissue and around the heart; use transillumination (diaphane light) for diagnosis

100% oxygen; needle thoracocentesis; closed intercostal drainage for reaccumulation with negative pressure of -10 to -15 cm H_2O; prevent vigorous crying

TABLE 1. *(continued)*

Diagnosis	Treatment

Pulmonary Hemorrhage

Etiological considerations: Prenatal and perinatal asphyxia, low birth weight, respiratory distress syndrome, chilling, infection, oxygen therapy, breech extraction
Manifestations: Bleeding from upper airway; frothy, bloody sputum; respiratory distress
Diagnostic measures: Chest radiograph suggests pulmonary edema

Vitamin K, 2 mg i.m., immediately
Replace lost blood with fresh whole blood
Supportive and high ventability settings of PEEP

Respiratory Distress Syndrome

Etiological considerations: maternal diabetes, hemorrhage, cesarean section, prematurity, asphyxia at birth, second born twin
Manifestations: Progressive symptoms of respiratory distress within 8 hr of birth; fixed heart rate, hypotension, hypothermia, harsh breath sounds, respiratory acidosis, low Po_2, increased Pco_2, increased bilirubin, right ventricular hypertrophy (RVH)
Diagnostic measures: Chest radiographs show reticulogranular pattern with or without bronchogram; decreased lung volume

Supportive oxygen therapy
Assisted ventilation with PEEP or CPAP

Tracheoesophageal Fistula

Etiological considerations: Polyhydramnios
Manifestations: Sudden deterioration of Apgar score, increased oral secretions, choking, flat abdomen
Diagnostic measures: Inability to pass nasogastric tube; radiopaque catheter or contrast study reveals the obstruction

Immediate surgical intervention
Levin tube in proximal oropharynx to prevent aspiration
Maintain nutrition

Transient Tachypnea of the Newborn

Etiological considerations: Normal delivery or pre- or postterm delivery caused by slow absorption of fetal lung field
Manifestations: Tachypnea, retractions and cyanosis relieved by oxygen
Diagnostic measures: Chest radiograph shows clear lungs, increased pulmonary vascular markings, fluid in tissues, usually no hypoxia and no acidosis

Oxygen

R esuscitation

The most successful way of preserving organ function is to **prevent** respiratory and cardiac arrest. Prevention is best achieved by careful monitoring of all patients with potential problems that might result in cardiorespiratory arrest. Monitoring is done best in the pediatric intensive care unit. Potential problems include patients with anoxia and respiratory distress, electrolyte disturbances, arrhythmias, acute CNS disease, hypo- or hyperglycemia, impending shock, and endotracheal tubes or tracheotomies that might be blocked by secretions (one of the most common and unacceptable causes of cardiorespiratory arrest), and patients who have been resuscitated (see Table 1).

MANAGEMENT PROTOCOL

1. Begin resuscitation if pulses cannot be felt or if the heart rate drops below 40 beats per minute.

    a. Suction.

    b. Mouth-to-mouth or bag-to-mouth ventilation at a rate of 40/min.

    c. Attach oxygen tube to ambu bag.

2. If heart rate does not increase and pulses do not become palpable in 30 to 45 sec

    a. Intubate (select tube size according to child's age)
       12–14 F (2.5–3.0 mm):   Premature to 3 months
       14–18 F (3.5–4.0 mm):   4 months to 2 years
       18–22 F (4.0–5.0 mm):   2 to 5 years
       22–28 F (5.0–6.5 mm):   5 to 13 years
       28–34 F (6.5–8.0 mm):   >14 years

    b. Continue ventilation and oxygen administration.

    c. Start cardiac massage by sternal compression at a rate of 80 to 120/min.

    d. Alternate ventilation and chest compression.

    e. Attach to cardiac monitor.

    f. Attach to ECG machine and run a continuous strip.

    g. Keep patient warm by warming lamps or blankets.

    h. Have someone not involved in ventilation and chest compression start intravenous infusion of 5% dextrose in normal saline (preferably a central line).

    i. Check adequacy of chest compression by palpation of the peripheral pulsations.

473

TABLE 1. *Management of problems encountered during resuscitation*

Problem	Treatment
Adequate QRS complex but poor pulses (inadequate cardiac output)	10% Calcium gluconate, 10 mg/kg (0.1 ml/kg) i.v. push
Cardiac arrhythmia	
Bradycardia (heart rate <60/min)	Atropine (may be repeated every 20 min) Neonate: 0.1 mg i.v. push Child: 0.01 mg/kg i.v. push (maximum dose, 0.6 mg) Adolescent: 0.6 mg i.v. push
Occasional premature atrial contractions	No treatment necessary
Multifocal, frequent premature ventricular contractions	2% Lidocaine, 20 to 50 μg/kg/min (maximum dose, 5 mg/kg)
Supraventricular tachycardia (atrial tachycardia)	Digoxin, 0.015 mg/kg i.v. push (maximum dose, 0.125 mg)
Ventricular fibrillation or tachycardia	DC shock Infant: 25 to 50 watt/sec Child: 50 to 100 watt/sec Large child: 100 to 200 watt/sec 2% Lidocaine, 1 mg/kg i.v. push; repeat every 5 to 10 min (maintenance dose, 20 to 50 μg/kg/min)
Asystole	Calcium gluconate, 30 mg/kg (0.3 ml/kg) i.v. push; repeat every 15 min Epinephrine (repeat every 5 to 10 min) Infant: 1:10,000—0.01 mg/kg (0.1 ml/kg) i.v. push Child: 1:1,000—0.01 mg/kg (0.1 ml/kg) i.v. push DC shock (see above)
Adequate QRS complex but poor peripheral perfusion and (normal or high CVP but hypotensive or normotensive) normal CVP as follows: Infant: 4 to 7 cm H_2O Child: 6 to 15 cm H_2O	Dopamine, 50 mg/500 ml of 5% dextrose in water (1.0 to 2.5 ml/kg/hr) **or** isoproterenol (Isuprel®), 1.0 mg/100 ml of 5% dextrose in water (5 ml/hr) Albumin, Plasmanate®, **or** blood, 10 ml/kg i.v.; repeat every 30 min if CVP is still decreased; 5% dextrose in normal saline or lactated Ringer's solution, 10 to 20 ml/kg i.v.
Shock, no response to volume expansion, and impending cardiac arrest	Methoxamine (Vasoxyl®), 0.25 mg/kg i.m. (maximum dose, 15 mg) **or** phenylephrine HCl (Neo-Synephrine®), 0.1 mg/kg i.m. (maximum dose, 7 mg) Hydrocortisone (Solu-Cortef®), 25 mg/kg i.v. push, immediately Continue fluid expansion Insert arterial line Monitor CVP, arterial pressure, urine output and specific gravity
Prolonged resuscitation (>5 min) and suspected cerebral hypoxic insult (CNS resuscitation and preservation)	Hyperventilate; keep Pco_2 at 20 to 25 Torr Restrict fluids Cooling blankets; keep core temperature at 90°F Chlorpromazine, 0.1 to 0.2 mg/kg, to prevent shivering and central pooling Hydrocortisone Infant: 1 mg/kg i.v. push Small child: 4 mg/kg i.v. push

Problem	Treatment
Seizures	Large child: 6 mg/kg i.v. push Adolescent: 8 mg/kg i.v. push Maintenance dose, 0.25 to 0.50 mg/kg/24 hr (maximum, four doses) Mannitol, 1 g/kg i.v. over a 15-min period Avoid excessive stimulation Diazepam (Valium®), 0.3 to 0.7 mg/kg i.v. push over a 1-min period (maximum dose: infants, 5 mg; children, 10 mg) **or** 2 mg i.v. push every 3 min until seizure stops (maximum dose, 10 mg) **or** phenytoin (Dilantin®), 8 to 10 mg/kg i.v. in normal saline (25 mg/min) **plus** 3 mg/kg i.m., if successful (maintenance dose, 5 to 8 mg/kg/day i.m. or p.o. in three divided doses)

3. If spontaneous heartbeat does not occur and asystole is persistent after 1 min of external cardiac compression: Sodium bicarbonate, 2 mEq/kg iv. push, **and** epinephrine 1:10,000 (infants) or 1:1,000 (children) 1 ml iv. or intracardiac injection

4. If asystole is persistent 30 sec after epinephrine administration

   a. Calcium gluconate, 30 mg/kg (0.3 ml/kg) iv. or intracardiac injection.

   b. Special medications and procedures:

     (1) 50% Dextrose, 1 ml/kg i.v. push.

     (2) Naloxone, 0.01 mg//kg i.m. or i.v. push; repeat every 2 to 3 min as needed (maximum, three doses).

     (3) Mannitol, 1 g/kg iv. over a 15-min period.

     (4) Hyperventilate.

5. If asystole is persistent 30 sec after the above procedures

   a. Administer a single DC shock (2 watt/sec/kg):
   Infants: 15–30 watt/sec
   Children: 30–60 watt/sec
   Adolescents: 60–100 watt/sec
   Adults: 150–300 watt/sec

   b. If single shocks are ineffective, use paired shocks.

6. If asystole is persistent

   a. Repeat bicarbonate epinephrine and calcium gluconate administration.

   b. Wait 1 min and administer DC shock again.

7. Indications of successful resuscitation

   a. Normal heart rate.

   b. Normal QRS complexes on the ECG.

    c. Normal color.

    d. Palpable peripheral pulses, indicating adequate peripheral tissue perfusion.

8. If spontaneous respirations are still absent, place on mechanical ventilation. After condition is stable, perform the following procedures:

    a. Monitor arterial blood gases and pH.

    b. Control ventilation and oxygen administration to keep P_{O_2} between 70 and 100 Torr and P_{CO_2} <45 Torr (in case of severe anoxia and possible anoxic effects on the CNS, it is desirable to keep P_{CO_2} <30 Torr).

    c. Evaluate the blood pressure and status of peripheral perfusion; if inadequate, administer dopamine, 50 mg/500 cc of 5% dextrose in water at a rate of 1.0 to 2.5 cc/kg/hr **or** isoproterenol (Isuprel®), 1.0 mg/100 ml of 5% dextrose in water i.v. at a rate of 5 cc/hr **or** fluid replacement (dopamine or Isuprel®) should be used only if the patient is **not** volume depleted and the central venous pressure (CVP) is normal or high; if the CVP is low and the patient is in shock, fluid replacement is the most essential therapy.

9. Determine the primary cause as well as possible complications of the event and treat accordingly

    a. Anoxic brain damage.

    b. Pneumothorax or pneumomediastinum.

    c. Cardiac tamponade.

    d. Liver (or other organ) lacerations.

10. Obtain chest radiograph to check endotracheal tube placement and to rule out complications.

11. Continue monitoring.

12. Make certain that the endotracheal tube is properly placed and fixed and that it stays patent.

Reye's Syndrome

Reye's syndrome is a clinicopathological entity manifested by encephalopathy and fatty degeneration of the viscera. It affects children of all ages (peaking at ages 4 and 11 years) and, in rare instances, adults. There are no definite sexual or racial predilections, although preliminary data indicate a general preponderance of the disease in white middle class children. There is also a higher incidence in black infants in the inner city's lower socioeconomic high density areas, which may indicate exposure to communicable diseases at an earlier age than their counterparts in less crowded areas. Reye's syndrome occurs in both epidemic and sporadic forms with an overall annual incidence of 1.3 to 2.7 cases per 100,000 population in children under 17 years of age.

In some patients, there is a suggestion of a genetic predisposition. The syndrome has been shown to follow viral infections, especially influenza type B and varicella infections, and may be one of the most common causes of death in viral-related central nervous system diseases (Fig. 1).

SIGNS AND SYMPTOMS

The clinical features of Reye's syndrome are remarkably similar in children from 1 through 16 years of age. The disease is ushered in by a viral infection which, in the prodromal phase, consists of upper respiratory tract or gastrointestinal symptoms. After a period of several days, during which the child appears to be recovering, repetitive vomiting occurs. Within 1 to 2 days, behavioral changes become obvious and range from combativeness to coma. Hyperventilation, seizures, gastrointestinal bleeding, hepatomegaly, and liver dysfunction are concomitant features.

In infants under 1 year of age, diarrhea, instead of vomiting, and/or respiratory distress are the main symptoms. In this age group, seizures and sudden apnea, suggesting other diseases, may be prominent and thus delay the appropriate diagnosis.

The prognosis for survival, both quantitatively and qualitatively, has made quantum leaps over the past few years. Better supportive therapy and intracranial pressure monitoring appear to have significantly decreased some of the severe neurological sequelae. Children over the age of 2 years who survive Reye's syndrome apparently function at a grossly normal level. However, there may be specific deficits in school achievement, visual motor functioning, and concept formation, which correlate to some degree with the severity of the disease and the length of coma.

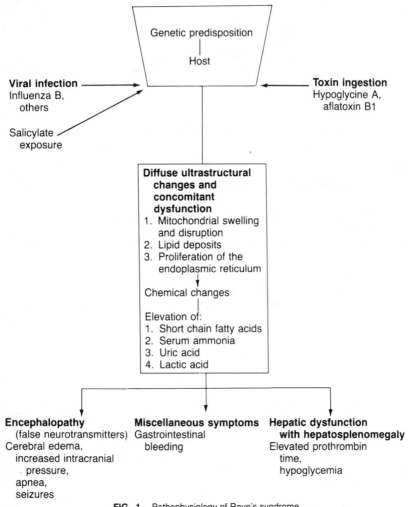

FIG. 1. Pathophysiology of Reye's syndrome.

The symptoms and signs of Reye's syndrome may be classified into the following stages:

Stage 1: Vomiting and lethargy.
Stage 2: Disorientation, delerium and combativeness, appropriate response to noxious stimuli.
Stage 3: Obtundation, coma, decorticate posturing, preserved pupillary reflexes.
Stage 4: Coma, decerebrate rigidity, loss of oculocephalic reflexes, dilated and fixed pupils.
Stage 5: Absent deep tendon reflexes, respiratory arrest, and flaccidity.

DIFFERENTIAL DIAGNOSIS

1. Urea cycle defects

2. Organic acid abnormalities

3. Drugs or toxins (e.g., salicylates, valproic acid, lead, methylbromide, isopropyl alcohol)

4. Systemic carnitine deficiency

5. CNS infection (bacterial or viral)

6. Jamaican vomiting sickness

7. Hepatic encephalopathy

DIAGNOSTIC PROTOCOL

1. The diagnosis of Reye's syndrome rests primarily on the medical history. The disorder is strongly suggested by a history of viral illness with upper respiratory tract or gastrointestinal symptoms, followed by vomiting and/or diarrhea with rapid progression to central nervous system obtundation.

2. Evidence of hepatic dysfunction (elevation of SGOT, SGPT, clotting factors), an elevated ammonia level, and absence of central nervous system infection point to the possibility of Reye's syndrome.

3. The differential diagnostic entities that mimic Reye's syndrome are somewhat limited; with hyperammonemia, elevated transaminase levels, abnormal coagulation factors, and a normal bilirubin level, only the following should be suspected: ingestion of toxins, inborn errors of metabolism, CNS infection, postinfectious encephalopathy, and hepatic coma; a thorough medical history and physical examination, along with the above tests and neurological consultation, will allow a diagnosis with a reasonable degree of certainty.

4. In the patient with atypical disease (e.g., <1 year old), a liver biopsy may be required.

TREATMENT PROTOCOL

1. Admit all children with a tentative diagnosis of Reye's syndrome to a pediatric intensive care unit; clinical staging and appropriate concomitant treatment must be carried out as soon as possible.

2. Insert arterial and venous lines for medication and fluid infusion and monitoring of pressures, along with a nasogastric tube and Foley catheter, as needed.

3. Monitor fluid intake and output carefully.

4. Intravenously infuse appropriate electrolyte solutions and 15% to 20% hypertonic glucose at less than normal rates (two-thirds of maintenance) to minimize exacerbating cerebral edema.

5. Any patient showing even mild central nervous system symptomatology should be intubated and mechanically ventilated, as required.

6. Hyperthermic episodes should be avoided; keep the temperature at a normal level through the use of a cooling mattress.

7. Avoid all extraneous, irritating stimuli.

8. Nonspecific, supportive measures include control of electrolytes and glucose at normal levels, chest physiotherapy, antiseizure medication, and electroencephalographic monitoring of seizure activity.

9. Continuously monitor intracranial pressure; treat episodes of increased intracranial pressure rapidly and vigorously.

R heumatic Fever

Rheumatic fever is an inflammatory multisystem disease that is a sequela of pharyngeal infection with a group A streptococcus (e.g., tonsillitis, tonsillopharyngitis, scarlet fever, or otitis media). It does not follow streptococcal infections of the skin. Rheumatic fever derives its importance from the fact that it can cause carditis and result in chronic heart disease.

PATHOPHYSIOLOGY

1. Not all patients with rheumatic fever give a history of a definitive antecedent tonsillitis.

2. Not all patients with suspected acquired rheumatic heart disease give a history of rheumatic fever.

3. Although streptococcal infections are common, only few children acquire rheumatic fever (host factors).

4. The tendency to develop the disease may be familial (genetic factors).

5. The clinical manifestations resemble those of a hypersensitivity reaction (immunological factors); it is now thought that rheumatic fever may be an autoimmune reaction.

6. Rheumatic fever occurs most commonly between the ages of 5 and 15 years (peak age, 6–8 years).

7. Crowding appears to play a significant role in the spread of streptococcal infection and the incidence of rheumatic fever.

8. Although there has been a decline in the morbidity and recurrent attacks of rheumatic fever, the decline in the frequency of first attacks is less striking.

9. Aggressive therapy with anti-inflammatory agents suppresses the signs and symptoms of rheumatic fever, but there is no definite evidence that these agents modify the outcome and lessen the chances of acquiring permanent heart disease, even if they are used early. **Hence, an accurate diagnosis should be sought before the initiation of therapy**.

10. The best approach to the disease continues to be adequate treatment of streptococcal infections and prevention of recurrent attacks.

SIGNS AND SYMPTOMS

Symptoms of rheumatic fever develop 1 to 5 weeks following the streptococcal infection (chorea occurs after 2 to 6 months). Fever is almost always present in the early stages. It becomes low grade after the first week and may persist 2 to 4 weeks after its onset.

The major manifestations include arthritis, carditis, erythema marginatum, chorea, and subcutaneous nodules. The arthritis is migratory and usually involves the large joints. Carditis is present if the patient develops congestive heart failure, cardiomegaly, and the appearance of significant murmurs (mitral and/or aortic insufficiency). Supportive evidence of carditis may appear as persistent tachycardia, ST and T wave changes on the electrocardiogram and atrioventricular (A-V) blocks or friction rub. Erythema marginatum appears as a serpiginous rash over the chest and trunk; it may disappear in a few hours or days and may be recurrent. Chorea, characterized by involuntary purposeless movements, may precede or follow other manifestations. Subcutaneous nodules range from 0.1 to 1.0 cm in diameter and occur most commonly over the extensor surfaces of the joints. They are nontender and occur most commonly after multiple attacks of carditis.

The minor manifestations include arthralgia, fever, prolonged P-R interval, elevated erythrocyte sedimentation rate (ESR) and positive C-reactive protein, previous history of rheumatic fever or rheumatic heart disease, epistaxis, abdominal pain, and pneumonitis. The tissue response is manifested by inflammation and dilatation of the valvular ring, valvular damage, and leaflet scarring, initially causing regurgitation (stenosis requires months to years to develop, most commonly involving the mitral and aortic valves). The Aschoff body, unique to rheumatic fever, is found in myocardial tissue as a result of either myocardial damage or blockage of cardiac lymphatic channels and may be present years after the clinical evidence of rheumatic activity.

DIFFERENTIAL DIAGNOSIS

1. Rheumatoid arthritis
2. Bacterial arthritis (septic joint)
3. Serum sickness
4. Hypersensitivity reactions
5. Systemic lupus erythematosus
6. Infective endocarditis
7. Sickle-cell anemia
8. Henoch-Schönlein purpura
9. Leukemia
10. Osteomyelitis
11. Local joint injury
12. Viral or bacterial pericarditis or myocarditis

LABORATORY PROCEDURES

1. Complete blood cell count (CBC): Leukocytosis and possibly anemia.
2. Urinalysis: Usually negative.

3. Erythrocyte sedimentation rate (ESR): Elevated if the disease is active; may be elevated in anemia and other inflammatory disorders.

4. C-reactive protein (CRP): Positive early in the disease.

5. Throat culture: Usually negative.

6. Blood culture: Negative.

7. Serological tests: Antistreptolysin O (ASO) **and**: Streptozyme® screening test (anti-DNase B, anti-NADase); the ASO titer starts rising about 10 days to 2 weeks following a streptococcal infection and may persist for 3 months; levels of 250 to 320 TU: borderline elevated; levels >500 TU: clear evidence of a recent infection (two serial determinations showing a rise in the titer are clear evidence of infection, irrespective of the level).

8. Chest radiograph: Normal, except in congestive heart failure, cardiomegaly or pneumonitis.

9. Electrocardiogram: Normal, except if there is pericarditis or arrhythmias.

10. Liver function tests: Prior to aspirin therapy.

11. Tests for other diseases (if serological evidence of an antecedent streptococcal infection cannot be shown in two or more serial determinations; may be difficult to obtain in chorea):

    a. Latex fixation test for rheumatoid arthritis.

    b. Radiographs of the involved joint.

    c. Aspiration of the joint.

    d. Immune profile.

    e. Antinuclear antibodies test, including anti-DNA.

    f. Hemoglobin electrophoresis.

    g. Echocardiography.

    h. Bone scan.

DIAGNOSTIC PROTOCOL

The diagnosis of rheumatic fever is made on clinical grounds and is based on a combination of the different manifestations (the Jones criteria). The diagnosis depends on the following essential factors:

1. The presence of two major manifestations.

2. The presence of one major and two minor manifestations.

3. Evidence of an antecedent streptococcal infection.

4. No evidence of other diseases that may mimic rheumatic fever.

If the patient has arthritis, arthralgia cannot be used as a minor manifestation. If the patient has carditis, prolonged P-R interval cannot be used as a minor manifestation.

TREATMENT PROTOCOL

1. Bed rest
   a. Bed rest during the acute and active stage of the disease.
   b. Complete and strict bed rest if the patient has carditis with heart failure.
   c. No strenuous activity as long as the ESR is elevated.
   d. No competitive activities until 1 to 2 months following normalization of the ESR.

2. Eradication of streptococci
   a. Pharyngitis, otitis media: Penicillin G, 25,000 units/kg/day p.o. or i.m.
   b. Cellulitis: Penicillin G, 50,000 to 100,000 units/kg/day p.o., i.m., or i.v.
   c. Pneumonia, empyema, bacteremia: Penicillin G, 100,000 to 200,000 units/kg/day i.v. or i.m.
   d. Meningitis: Penicillin G, 300,000 units/kg/day i.v.
   e. Alternative drugs: Erythromycin, cephalosporin, clindamycin.

3. Anti-inflammatory agents
   a. Arthritis without carditis or with mild carditis: Aspirin, 100 mg/kg/day in four to six doses for 3 to 4 weeks (maximum dosage, 130 mg/kg/day); maintain blood level of 20 to 35 mg/100 ml; follow liver function tests.
   b. Carditis without heart failure: Steroids (prednisone), 2 mg/kg/day for 4 weeks; while tapering, start the patient on aspirin and continue aspirin for 2 weeks after steroids are discontinued.
   c. Carditis with heart failure: Steroids (prednisone), 2 mg/kg/day for 4 to 6 weeks, tapering over the next 2 weeks (aspirin may or may not be used during the tapering period).
   d. Anticongestive measures: Digoxin and diuretics should be used if heart failure is present, despite the increased sensitivity of the myocardium to digitalis.
   e. Chorea
      (1) Bed rest.
      (2) Quiet surroundings.
      (3) Medications such as chlorpromazine, phenobarbital, diazepam, and haloperidol may be helpful.
      (4) Psychological support and psychiatric evaluation.
   f. Prevention of recurrences: **Lifetime prophylaxis is indicated in all patients whether there is residual heart disease or not:**
      (1) Benzathine penicillin, 600,000 units (<60 lb) **or** 1.2 million units (>60 lb) every 28 days i.m.
      (2) Penicillin G, 125 to 250 mg p.o. twice a day.
      (3) Sulfisoxazole (Gantrisin®), 0.5 to 1.0 g/day p.o.

Rickets

Rickets is a disease of growing children. It consists of several subgroupings characterized by bony lesions that fail to undergo calcium salt deposition in their matrix and preosseous cartilage.

Normally, tropocollagen, a disorganized precursor of collagen, develops into collagen as it organizes into long cellular strands. Osteoid material is laid down on these strands and then undergoes a process of calcification, resulting in calcified cartilage. In a very smooth and predetermined sequence (Fig. 1), the calcified cartilage is invaded by capillaries, which causes dissolution of the area and leeching of the calcium. The calcified cartilage cells die and are replaced by osteoblasts, which subsequently form bone. In all the subsets of rickets, the osteoid material is not appropriately calcified, thus allowing the osteoblasts to proliferate in a disorganized, uncontrolled fashion (radiographically shown as flaring).

Defective mineralization in rickets is a function of several factors and one of the most important is the calcium-phosphorus product ($Ca^{2+} \times PO_4^{3-}$). In simple (vitamin D deficiency) rickets, the correction of either serum calcium or serum phosphorus in such a way that the calcium-phosphorus product is normalized results in correction of the bony changes. Unfortunately, correction of this factor has little effect on the rickets of renal osteodystrophy and renal tubular acidosis. Other variables, such as the presence of sufficient alkaline phosphatase in an alkaline medium (in the fluid surface of the bone) permit cleavage of the pyrophosphonate bond, allowing precipitation of the phosphorus in the bone. This reaction and others appear pivotal, along with equally important roles for magnesium and citrate in the processes of bone mineralization and/or reabsorption.

SIGNS AND SYMPTOMS

There are at least five distinct categories included in the definition of rickets. These range from simple vitamin D deficiency rickets to primary matrix defects. Despite the broad scope of etiologies, they all share similar signs and symptoms based on the common lack of bone salt in their matrices. Children with rickets tend to have short stature with proportionate or disproportionate limbs. They suffer from friability of their bones. Certain subtypes of rickets cause severe acidosis, irritability, and a propensity toward tetany and amino acidurias. In subsets associated with renal and/or gastrointestinal variants, the symptoms may be overshadowed by the complexities and complications of the underlying disease process.

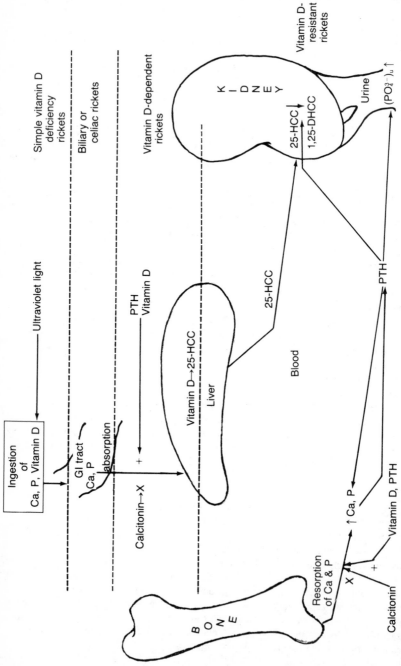

FIG. 1. Pathophysiology of rickets. X, interferes with or blocks process; +, catalyzes process; 25-HCC, 25-hydroxycholecalciferol; 1,25-DHCC, 1,25-dihydroxycholecalciferol; PTH, parathyroid hormone; $PO_4^{3-}{}_u$, urine phosphate concentration.

DIFFERENTIAL DIAGNOSIS

1. Rickets
   a. Rickets due to a deficiency of biologically active vitamin D
      (1) Simple rickets (vitamin D deficiency)
      (2) Biliary and cellular rickets
      (3) Vitamin D-dependent rickets
   b. Vitamin D-resistant rickets
      (1) X-linked familial hypophosphatemic rickets
      (2) Fanconi syndrome (tyrosinosis)
      (3) Vitamin D-refractory rickets with hyperglycinuria and/or glucosuria
      (4) Rickets secondary to a primary form of renal tubular acidosis
   c. Renal osteodystrophy
   d. Primary matrix defects
      (1) Metaphyseal dysostosis
      (2) Hypophosphatasia
      (3) Pseudohypophosphatasia
   e. Miscellaneous: Anticonvulsant drug-induced (phenytoin and phenobarbital may induce enzymes that inactivate 25-HCC)
2. Osteoporosis: Defined not as a qualitative problem of bone but as an absolute decrease in total mass and is an acquired form of osteopenia, implying loss of bone density.
3. Osteomalacia: Rickets occurring after linear growth of the skeleton has stopped.

DIAGNOSTIC AND TREATMENT PROTOCOLS

Table 1 gives the diagnostic and treatment protocols for the various forms of rickets.

TABLE 1. *Rickets: Diagnostic and treatment protocols*

Type	Genetics	Aminoaciduria	Characteristics	Serum calcium/phosphate	Serum alkaline phosphatase	PTH	Treatment
Deficiency rickets							
Simple rickets	–	–	Irritability, weakness, failure to thrive, rachitic rosary, craniotabes, fraying, and cupping of metaphyses	↓/↓	↑	↑	Dietary calcium; sunlight (ultraviolet radiation), vitamin D, 1.5 to 2.0 ml/day (15,000 units)
Vitamin D-dependent	r	+	As above; failure of 1-hydroxylation of 25-hydroxy vitamin D	↓/↓ or N	↑	↑	1,25-dihydroxy-cholecalciferol (1,25-DHCC), 0.5 to 1.0 µg/d or 1000–2000 units/day of vitamin D
Secondary (e.g., biliary obstruction, celiac disease)	–	±	Signs associated with specific disease entity; inability to absorb and/or failure of 25-hydroxylation of vitamin D	↓/↓	↑	↑	1,25-DHCC 0.5 µg/d or vitamin D_2 (Drisdol) 4000–8000 units (0.2–0.4 mg)/d
Vitamin D-resistant							
Vitamin D-resistant	X-linked r	–	Short stature, especially lower extremities	N/↓	↑	↓ ↑	Vitamin D, 30,000 to 50,000 units/day; phosphate (long-term)
Fanconi syndrome	r/R	+	Failure to thrive, metabolic acidosis, pyrexia, dehydration	±/↓	↑	± ↑	Depends on lesion, but HCO_3^-, potassium, and phosphorus supplements are indicated
Hypophosphatemic with hyperglycinuria and/or glucosuria	r	+	Normal plasma glycine and glucose, but significant urine spillage	N/↓	↑	↑ ±	Same as in vitamin D-resistant rickets

Condition			Clinical features				Treatment
Secondary to renal tubular acidosis (distal form)	?/R	+	Nephrocalcinosis, lithiasis	N/↓	↑	↑ ±	Same as in vitamin D-resistant but buffer (HCO₃⁻) is needed
Renal osteodystrophy	—	+/−	Renal failure, acidosis, magnesium abnormalities, radiographic evidence of hyperparathyroidism	↑/↓	↑	↑/↓	Treat renal failure, plus phosphate binders, activated vitamin D, and calcium supplements
Primary matrix defect Metaphyseal dysostosis (4 varieties)	r/R	+/−	Peculiar facies (±) short bowed limbs, short stature, joint contractures, recurrent infections (thymic abnormality)	±/±	↑	?	Treatment is supportive
Hypophosphatasia	r	+	Anemia, short ribs, small rib cage, hypoplastic bones, failure to thrive. Elevated serum phosphoethanolamine	↑ ±/−	↓↓→	?	Treatment is supportive
Pseudohypophosphatasia (possible allele of hypophosphatasia)	r	+	Similar to hypophosphatasia	↑/↓	N	↑	Treatment is supportive
Miscellaneous Anticonvulsant drug-induced	—	−	Associated with use of phenobarbital or phenytoin	↓/↑	↑	↑	Activated vitamin D
Osteoporosis (nutritional, idiopathic, immobilization, medication induced, homocystinuria)	r/−	±	Distinction from rickets is usually made by medical history and physical examination, but radiographs show osteopenia, not fraying and cupping. Laboratory results will be dependent on the etiology				Disease specific

TABLE 1. *(continued)*

Type	Genetics	Aminoaciduria	Characteristics	Serum calcium/ phosphate	Serum alkaline phosphatase	PTH	Treatment
Osteomalacia			Rickets occurring after linear growth has stopped, but the histological changes are similar. Therefore, parameters will parallel entities previously discussed in this chapter				Disease specific

r: Recessive
R: Dominant
+ : Present
– : Absent
+/– : Present or absent
r/R: May be recessive or dominant depending on variant
r/– : Either a genetic pattern of inheritance or sporadic

Salicylate Intoxication

Salicylate intoxication was responsible for accidental poisoning and death of many children before safety caps came into use in the early 1970s. Since then, the number of accidental deaths secondary to salicylism has decreased, but ingestions still occur. Insufficient anticipatory guidance and the inclusion of salicylates in many combination over-the-counter medications keep salicylate intoxication an important consideration in discussions of poisonings.

Salicylates are variably absorbed from the gastrointestinal tract. The level in the blood may increase significantly up to 6 hr after the ingestion. Blood salicylate levels after 6 hr are used to evaluate the severity of the intoxication.

SIGNS AND SYMPTOMS

Salicylates directly stimulate the central nervous system respiratory center and cause increased ventilation and a profound respiratory alkalosis (Fig. 1). When they are present in high concentrations, oxidation phosphorylation is uncoupled, resulting in metabolic acidosis, which usually supervenes in younger children. Fever, tinnitus, and vomiting are also common. Irritability, restlessness, delerium, hallucinations, seizures, and coma may occur. These represent symptoms of central nervous system toxicity of acidosis and/or dehydration. Respiratory failure and cardiovascular collapse are the common causes of death.

DIAGNOSTIC PROTOCOL

1. Complete blood cell count: Symptoms of salicylism frequently appear to be similar to those of acute respiratory tract infections.

2. Urinalysis: Utilized for screening for infections and monitoring urine pH; specific gravity is helpful in monitoring the state of hydration.

3. Electrolytes, blood urea nitrogen, and creatinine: The primary abnormalities noted with salicylism are related to the acid-base status of the patient, and the kidney is the organ of excretion.

4. Blood glucose: Hypoglycemia occurs with salicylism.

5. Blood salicylate level: Plot on the Done nomogram (see Fig. 2).

6. Blood lead level: Ingestion of a foreign substance may be a symptom of pica.

7. Blood pH and blood gases: Abnormalities in the acid-base status are the primary pathophysiological events.

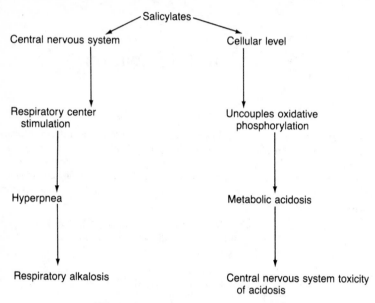

FIG. 1.   Pathophysiology of salicylate poisoning.

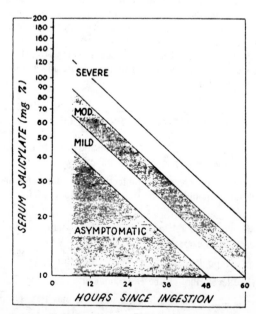

FIG. 2.   Done nomogram for assessment of the severity of salicylate intoxication in children. (From Done, A.K. 1960, *Pediatrics*, 26:800, with permission.)

TREATMENT PROTOCOL

1. Induce vomiting or perform gastric lavage with normal saline.

2. Administer activated charcoal.

3. Provide enough fluids to maintain adequate urinary output and treat dehydration.

4. Hypoglycemia should be corrected with intravenous infusions of glucose.

5. Sodium bicarbonate, 3 to 5 mEq/kg over a 2- to 4-hr period; repeat as needed; functions to normalize the pH and protect the CNS against the effects of acidosis; also keeps the pH of the urine >7.5 and facilitates excretion of the salicylate.

6. In severe cases, dialysis or exchange transfusions may be required.

7. The remainder of the treatment is supportive and symptomatic.

Seizure Disorders

Seizures are the clinical manifestation of abnormal central nervous system neuronal activity. They are paroxysmal, stereotypic, and associated with altered states of consciousness. The presentation varies with the type of seizure and the location of the abnormal activity in the nervous system. Some seizures may remain localized in a particular area, causing focal motor manifestations; others may spread to involve many areas, resulting in generalized seizures.

The etiologies are as varied as the types. Neuronal damage secondary to hypoxia, hypoglycemia, trauma, infections, or toxins are possible causes. Damage from space-occupying lesions, glial scarring, embolism, hemorrhage, or increased pressure may result in seizures. It is important, however, to note that damaged neurons may seize, but dead neurons cannot.

Seizures tend to be familial, but no specific genetic transmission has been found. Fever, fatigue, emotions, and other factors are known to precipitate convulsive episodes in patients predisposed to seizures. The majority of episodes (and etiologies) are idiopathic (Fig. 1).

SIGNS AND SYMPTOMS

The signs and symptoms of seizures vary according to the type of seizure disorder and the location of the abnormality within the central nervous system. The manifestations may vary from subclinical effects to major motor convulsions. However, with most seizures, there are concurrent perceptual abnormalities and changes in levels of consciousness.

Many patients with seizure disorders present with mixed manifestations, are complicated diagnostically, and require multiple medications.

DIFFERENTIAL DIAGNOSIS

1. Febrile seizures
   a. Simple febrile convulsion
   b. CNS infection
   c. Seizure with fever (may be a manifestation of an afebrile seizure disorder)
   d. Toxic ingestion
2. Afebrile seizures

   a. Grand mal
   b. Petit mal
   c. Psychomotor
   d. Focal seizures
   e. Myoclonic
   f. Infantile spasms
   g. Akinetic
   h. Toxic

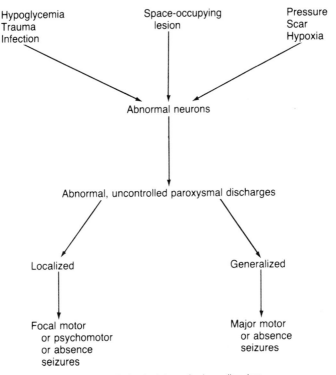

FIG. 1. Pathophysiology of seizure disorders.

GENERAL DIAGNOSTIC PROTOCOL

1. The diagnosis frequently rests on the medical history and manifestations of the seizure. Therefore, a complete history, including family history, gestational and natal history, previous seizures, illnesses prior to the seizure, medications, onset, description, and duration of the seizure, must be obtained. A complete and detailed neurological examination, both postictally and interictally and including an electroencephalogram (EEG), is essential.

2. Complete blood cell count and urinalysis.

3. Electrolytes.

4. Blood urea nitrogen and creatinine.

5. Calcium and phosphorus.

6. Blood gases.

7. Blood glucose.

8. Toxicology screening.

9. Blood lead level.

10. Cerebrospinal fluid examination.

11. Other tests may be indicated, according to the presentation (e.g., amino acid screening if an amino acid abnormality is suspected, skull radiographs if tuberous sclerosis or Sturge-Weber syndrome is suspected).

DIAGNOSTIC AND TREATMENT PROTOCOLS

Table 1 gives the diganostic and treatment protocols for various seizure disorders.

STATUS EPILEPTICUS: TREATMENT PROTOCOL

1. Ensure an adequate airway: Clear the airway of obstruction, insert an airway (if necessary), or intubate (if control of ventilation is required).

2. Administer oxygen.

3. Monitor vital signs, obtain the medical history and perform a physical examination.

4. Establish an intravenous line and administer 5% dextrose in 0.25% saline.

5. Obtain initial laboratory evaluations.

6. Medications

    a. Diazepam, 0.3 mg/kg to 1.0 mg/kg i.v. every 3 to 5 min (maximum dose, 10 mg). **There is danger of respiratory depression or respiratory arrest; assisted ventilation and cardiac support must be** *immediately* **available**; the seizures are usually rapidly controlled.

    b. Phenytoin, 5 to 8 mg/kg i.v. slowly (no more rapidly than 25 mg/min); monitor the electrocardiogram during the infusion; if the seizures are controlled, maintenance dose is 5 to 8 mg/kg/day i.m. or p.o. in two or three divided doses.

7. **Extreme care must be taken using intravenous anticonvulsant therapy.** The most common cause of death in children with seizure disorders is the injudicious use of medications and failure to closely monitor the patient during their administration.

TABLE 1. *Seizure disorders: Diagnostic and treatment protocols*

Diagnosis	Treatment
Akinetic	
Clinical characteristics: Paroxysmal complete loss of tone and posture, frequently resulting in a fall; episode lasts for approximately 10 to 15 sec and is usually not preceded by an aura; usually no	A multidrug regimen is usually required: Phenobarbital, 3 to 5 mg/kg/day **and** ethosuximide, 5 to 25 mg/kg/day, **or** valproic acid, 15 to 30 mg/kg/day, **or** trimethadione, 15 to 40 mg/kg/day

Diagnosis	Treatment

postictal state; seizures may cluster throughout the day

EEG: Atypical spike-and-wave discharges, which may temporarily disappear after the intravenous administration of diazepam

Focal

Clinical characteristics: Motor or sensory, or both, depending on the location of the lesion in the CNS; convulsive activity may begin in an isolated portion of the body and remain isolated or may progress and result in a generalized seizure (classical Jacksonian epilepsy)

EEG: May show focal epileptiform activity

Angiography: May be required if a space-occupying lesion is considered

Phenobarbital, 5 mg/kg/day, **or** phenytoin, 5 to 8 mg/kg/day, **or** primidone, 5 to 25 mg/kg/day

Surgery may be required if a space-occupying lesion is present

Grand Mal

Clinical characteristics: Most common form of epilepsy; classically an aura (olfactory, ocular, or auditory) occurs, followed shortly by a generalized tonic or clonic seizure, which lasts for several minutes; it is usually self-limited; postictal depression usually occurs; transient focal neurological abnormalities may occur (Todd's paralysis)

EEG: Abnormal spike discharges may be seen

Phenobarbital, 5 mg/kg/day, **or** phenytoin, 5 to 8 mg/kg/day

Infantile Spasms

Clinical characteristics: Seizures occur in children between the ages of 3 and 9 months; appear as sudden clusters of exaggerated Moro reflexes; often a developmental delay and mental retardation; spasms are usually replaced by major motor or akinetic seizures as the child grows older

EEG: Frequently shows the pattern of hypsarrhythmia

ACTH, 150 units/m^2/day for 6 weeks

Hydrocortisone, 60 mg/day for 3 to 4 months, after cessation of ACTH

Diazepam, up to 30 mg/day, has been used in patients with refractory seizures

The seizures are usually extremely difficult to control and multiple drug regimens are usually required

Myoclonic

Clinical characteristics: Usually a massive contraction of a single muscle or group of muscles; may appear as a generalized startle type of posturing; seizures often associated with CNS infection or CNS degenerative diseases and metabolic diseases

EEG: Usually consistent with the underlying disorder

Same as for infantile spasms

Petit Mal

Clinical characteristics: Attacks occasionally difficult to recognize; "absence" attacks lasting 5 to 15 sec; no motor activity, no aura, and no postictal depression; child

Ethosuximide, 5 to 25 mg/kg/day, is the drug of choice

Other agents: Valproic acid or trimethadione

Some authorities believe phenobarbital or

TABLE 1. *(continued)*

Diagnosis	Treatment
may appear to be daydreaming; often school failure EEG: Diagnostic pattern of 3-Hz spike-and-wave discharges	phenytoin should be given because of the liklihood of development of major motor seizures as the child grows older

Psychomotor

Clinical characteristics: Usually purposeless, paroxysmal, stereotypic behaviors; an aura, followed by subjective experiences, automatisms, or postural changes; attack ends with postictal depression; usually alterations in consciousness EEG: Abnormal spikes usually isolated to the temporal lobe	Primidone, 5 to 25 mg/kg/day Other agents: Carbamazepine, phenobarbital, or phenytoin

Simple Febrile Convulsions

Clinical characteristics: Usually a brief generalized convulsion, which occurs in the presence of fever (usually >102°F) in children 6 months to 6 years old, who were previously neurologically normal; convulsions are self-limited and usually benign; diagnosis is usually made by exclusion of other etiologies EEG: Usually shows no abnormalities	Most authorities do not recommend chronic treatment for the first simple febrile convulsion; treatment is usually recommended if the initial seizure is prolonged, if there are multiple seizures in the same febrile episode, if there is a history of more than two seizures, or if there is a likelihood of the development of afebrile seizures (e.g., a strong family history of seizures, first seizure before 12 months of age) Phenobarbital, 5 mg/kg/day, chronically

Septicemia

Septicemia refers to active multiplication of bacteria within the bloodstream beyond the amount the body can normally clear. It differs from the commonly occurring bacteremia, in which there is no active multiplication and host defenses have not been breached. Septicemia results when the normal defense mechanisms are overwhelmed by a massive inoculum or compromised extrinsically or intrinsically. The immunologically compromised host is prone to develop systemic infections because of a decreased ability to localize infections. The effect may occur normally in the neonatal period or may be induced by concurrent infection or disease or by drugs (e.g., corticosteroids, cancer chemotherapeutic agents).

PATHOPHYSIOLOGY

There is a breach of the external defenses, inadequate immune function or phagocytic function, and/or an overwhelming inoculum of bacteria. There is a dynamic balance between multiplication, filtration, and killing of the organisms (Fig. 1).

SIGNS AND SYMPTOMS

The presentation of septicemia varies with the age of the patient. Usually, the signs and symptoms of septicemia are nonspecific. Hyperthermia or hypothermia may be present (hypothermia is more common in the neonate or premature infant). The patients usually appear to be quite ill and no localizing source of infection can be readily found. Lethargy, irritability, changes in feeding habits, vomiting, diarrhea, abdominal distention, seizures, and/or cardiovascular collapse may occur. In certain patients (e.g., those undergoing chemotherapy, those with sickle-cell disease, and neonates) localized infections cannot be adequately walled-off or limited, and metastatic infection is common. Since the organisms commonly causing local infections also are common systemic or CNS pathogens, disseminated infection should be sought and treated until it is proved to be absent. The most common organisms cultured are *Streptococcus pneumoniae*, and *Hemophilus influenzae*. *E. coli*, *Pseudomonas*, and *Klebsiella* are three common gram-negative organisms isolated from the immunocompromised host. Patients with compromised splenic function (e.g., sickle-cell anemia, splenectomy) have specific problems handling encapsulated organisms, primarily pneumococcus.

Septic shock may occur. It is characterized by cardiovascular compromise and decreased peripheral perfusion. Metabolic acidosis is severe. Complement is activated,

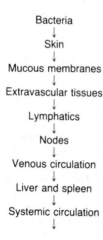

Bacteria
↓
Skin
↓
Mucous membranes
↓
Extravascular tissues
↓
Lymphatics
↓
Nodes
↓
Venous circulation
↓
Liver and spleen
↓
Systemic circulation
↓

FIG. 1. Pathophysiology of septicemia.

causing peripheral vascular abnormalities, and disseminated intravascular coagulation may occur. Vigorous treatment is required and, in addition to antibiotics, corticosteroids and heparin therapy may be indicated.

DIAGNOSTIC PROTOCOL

1. Complete blood cell count: The white blood count is usually elevated; leukopenia is not uncommon and reflects an overwhelming infection or inadequate host defense mechanisms.

2. Urinalysis and urine culture: The urinary tract may be the source of infection.

3. Chest radiograph: The respiratory tract may be the source of infection.

4. Culture of any exudate and Gram stain: These may reveal the offending organism.

5. Cerebrospinal fluid examination: A disseminated infection may seed the meninges, especially in younger children, neonates, and immunologically compromised hosts.

6. Blood cultures: Multiple cultures are usually required.

7. Buffy coat smear.

8. Counterimmunoelectrophoresis and *Limulus* lysate testing: Usually, they are rewarding when done on cerebrospinal fluid, joint fluid, pleural fluid, or urine, but not as rewarding when done on blood.

TREATMENT PROTOCOL

1. Supportive and symptomatic care: Intravenous fluids and provision of adequate calories to maintain a positive nitrogen balance.

2. Antibiotic therapy: This is usually done with the suspicion of septicemia. The choice of drug is empirical (treat the organism that carries the highest index of suspicion), but multiple drug regimens are most often employed to provide broader spectrum of coverage.

   a. Suspected *N. meningitidis* or *S. pneumoniae*: Penicillin, 100,000 to 200,000 units/kg/day i.v. in four divided doses

   b. Suspected *H. influenzae*: Chloramphenicol, 100 mg/kg/day i.v. in four divided doses

   c. Suspected gram-negative organisms: Gentamicin, 3 to 5 mg/kg/day i.m. or i.v. in two or three divided doses.

3. If septic shock is suspected, support circulation with fluids and pressor agents, and provide ventilation assistance and oxygen; corticosteroids may be required; heparin may be required if disseminated intravascular coagulation is present.

Sexually Transmitted Diseases

Sexually transmitted diseases (STD) are problems not only for our patients who contract them, but also for public health (epidemiological) reasons. There appears to be a rapidly escalating number of infected individuals along with the presence of previously unknown varieties and presentations of these diseases. STD infects not only the patient, but also, if pregnancy ensues, possibly the fetus and newborn.

Several factors play a major role in the increasing prevalence of venereal disease: improved laboratory recognition, greater public awareness and earlier treatment, increasing incidence of premarital sex, multiple sexual partners, and use of nonbarrier contraceptives.

Alterations in immunity of the population plays a significant role in the patterns of sexually transmitted diseases (Fig. 1). Improvements in socioeconomic status, suburban growth, decreased population densities, and better public health conditions change sequences of exposure to various organisms. Contact that occurred during infancy is now often delayed until young adulthood (e.g., primary herpes 1 infection in young children, resulting in partial immunity against herpes type 2 infections in adults). Reduced contact between the young infant and mother, decreasing the transmission of passive immunity to the child, may also be involved.

DIFFERENTIAL DIAGNOSIS

1. Bacterial disease
   a. *Neisseria gonorrheae*
   b. *Chlamydia trachomatis*
   c. *Treponema pallidum*
   d. *Hemophilus ducreyi*
   e. *Mycoplasma hominis*
2. Viral disease
   a. Herpes simplex virus, type 2 (occasionally)
   b. Cytomegalic inclusion virus
   c. Genital warts
   d. Molluscum contagiosum
   e. Hepatitis virus, type B (sexual transmission among homosexuals)
3. Protozoal disease
   a. *Trichomonas vaginalis*
   b. *Giardia lamblia*
   c. *Entamoeba histolytica* (sexual transmission among homosexuals)
4. Ectoparasitic disease
   a. *Phthirus pubis* (crab louse)
   b. *Sarcoptes scabiei* (scabies mite)

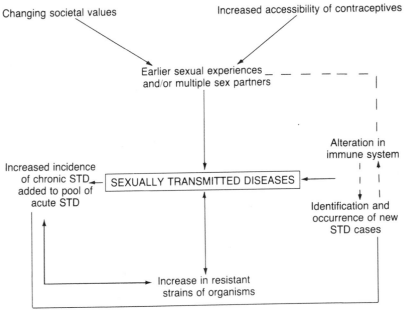

FIG. 1. Pathophysiology of sexually transmitted diseases.

DIFFERENTIAL DIAGNOSIS BY SYMPTOM

1. Vaginitis (vaginosis)

    a. Herpes simplex virus, type 2 (HSV-2)

    b. Gonococcal

    c. Trichomoniasis

    d. Candidiasis

    e. Nonspecific vaginitis (*Gardnerella vaginalis* and vaginal anaerobes)

2. Urethritis (male or female)

    a. Gonococcal

    b. Nonspecific urethritis (chlamydial, ureaplasma)

    c. Candidiasis

    d. Cytomegalic inclusion virus (CMV)

    e. Trichomoniasis

3. Acute pelvic inflammatory disease (endometritis, salpingitis, parametritis, and/or peritonitis)

    a. Gonococcal

    b. Chlamydial

    c. Mixed (anaerobic and aerobic bacteria as well as *M. hominis*)

4. Female lower genital tract infection (cervicitis, vulvovaginitis, urethritis)

    a. Gonococcal

    b. Chlamydial

    c. Trichomoniasis

    d. Herpes simplex virus

    e. *Gardnerella vaginalis*

5. Proctitis

   a. Gonococcal

   b. Herpetic

   c. Chlamydial

   d. Treponematosis

   e. Lymphogranuloma venereum (LGV)

6. Pharyngitis

   a. Gonococcal

   b. Herpetic

7. Ulcer-inguinal adenopathy syndrome

   a. HSV-2

   b. Syphilis

   c. LGV

   d. Chancroid

   e. Granuloma inguinale

TABLE 1. *Sexually transmitted diseases: Diagnostic and therapeutic protocols*

Diagnosis	Treatment
Scabies *(Sarcoptes scabiei)*	

Scabies *(Sarcoptes scabiei)*

Diagnosis	Treatment
Medical history: Male predominance (3:1); frequency in adults, 0.4% to 1.39% Most frequent in teenagers but infants are also infected (symptomatology is less specific) Spread by close intimate contact with an infected person, rarely from clothing or bedding Pruritis, the most common complaint and disabling feature, does not develop until about 4 to 6 weeks after the initial infection, and occurs with the greatest intensity at night when the individual is covered with blankets, thereby warming the skin and causing increased activity of the mite Physical examination: Skin lesions are diffuse and may involve any part of the body, but classically are located in the intertrigenous areas, and tend to be papular or papulovesicular, unless they have been present for a long time (in which case they may become eczematoid) or the patient has been scratching them Skin burrows are evidence that the female has dug a hole through the layer of skin and has burrowed her way to lay her eggs; these are rarely found in infants Laboratory confirmation: Rapid diagnosis can be made by microscopic examination of a skin scraping from a burrow or a new, nonexcoriated lesion. Except in infants, it is very unusual to find scabies above the neck, as compared with lesions involving pubic lice Infestation can occur from dogs or other domestic animals, but the dog mite cannot reproduce in humans; moreover, it spares the genitals and interdigital webs; treatment of the dog mite is not indicated	Nonspecific: Since the mite cannot survive more than 2 days away from the human host, personal bedding and bathroom articles of treated persons should be stored for 48 hr or laundered in a washing machine and dryer (the organism is very sensitive to temperatures above 120°F) Specific: Topical application of lindane cream or lotion (Kwell®) left in place for 8 to 12 hr; repeat application 1 week later In older children, Kwell® should be applied from the neck down, not just in the place of the obvious lesions. Crotamiton cream is an alternative therapy Infectivity is lost 24 hr after the treatment Secondary infections are common and present as pustules, bullae, or diffuse crusting lesions. Impetigo is the most common of these pyodermas and requires prompt treatment with penicillin to avoid the nonsuppurative streptococcal infections

Diagnosis	Treatment

Pediculosis Pubis[a] (Crab lice)

Medical history: Intimate body contact 2 to 3 weeks previously (rarely spread by infested clothing or bedding)

Pruritus occurs following the 2 to 3 week incubation period, as well as complaints by the affected individual regarding the unesthetic appearance of the lice in the body hair

Physical examination: The lice are attached to the hair in the area of the pubis, lower abdomen, thighs, and buttocks

Following orogenital sex, the lice may be found on the eyelashes and eyebrows

Laboratory confirmation: There are no specific laboratory tests other than identification of the crab lice, which can be seen with the naked eye

Nonspecific: Wash and dry clean clothing and bedding or sequester them for a month or more. Bathe and dry thoroughly

Specific: Apply 1% gamma benzene hexachloride (Kwell®) from the neck to the feet and do not remove for 12 hr; thereafter bath vigorously to remove lotion; repeat application 1 week later

Kwell® shampoo may also be indicated but should be removed after 5 min; repeat in 1 week

Gonorrhea[b] (Neisseria gonorrheae)

Epidemic in the U.S.

The oldest of the five classic venereal diseases; known to the Hebrews (depicted in the biblical reference to the necessity for sanitary controls)

Uncomplicated (urethritis, cervicitis, vaginitis)

Medical history: Most frequent in young adults with teenagers as the second most commonly affected group

Gonorrheal organisms in the genital tract, anal canal, oropharynx, or other areas, except for the conjunctiva, strongly imply sexual contact

Transmission of this disease from toilet seats, bath towels, drinking glasses, etc., although an interesting theoretical consideration has not been shown to have any practical importance

75% of females and 10% of males may be asymptomatic

The gonorrheal organism has fastidious growth and survival requirements; it must have moisture, and dies immediately upon drying

The pathogenic forms of the gonococcus have pili, which is true of most gram-negative organisms infecting the urinary tract. The pili allow the organisms to stick to each other, to the mucosal cell of the genitals, and to crypts of the anus, thereby allowing them to propagate and survive

When the gonococcal organism dies, it liberates an endotoxin, an irritant, which accounts for the purulent discharge and erosive balanitis and cervicitis

Symptoms may occur as early as 1 day or as late as 2 weeks following sexual contact, with an average incubation period in males

Adolescents and children who weigh more than 45 kg

Uncomplicated gonorrheal infection:
Aqueous procaine penicillin G, 4.8 million units, in two sites, **plus** probenecid, 1 g p.o. **or** Tetracycline, 0.5 g p.o., four times a day for 7 days **or** Ampicillin, 3.5 g p.o., **plus** probenecid, 1 g p.o.

Children who weigh less than 45 kg

Uncomplicated gonorrheal infection:
Aqueous procaine penicillin G, 100,000 units/kg i.m. combined with probenecid 25 mg/kg p.o. **or** amoxicillin 50 mg/kg p.o. **plus** probenecid 1 g p.o.

TABLE 1. *(continued)*

Diagnosis	Treatment

of 3 to 5 days. In females, because the cases are often asymptomatic, it is difficult to know the incubation period exactly
Laboratory confirmation: Gram-negative intracellular *Diplococcus* is seen in the smears. There is some controversy as to the efficacy of a positive endocervical smear; such smears were previously thought to be helpful only in the male, but since only 80% to 90% of women with endocervical gonorrhea will have positive cultures for *N. gonorrheae*, the smear is probably a reliable index of infection when it is classically positive in the presence of a negative culture in a child

Pelvic Inflammatory Disease (PID) and Epididymitis

The most serious complication of gonorrhea, occurring in 10% to 15% of all infected females
Results in a high percentage of sterility in females (15%), in ectopic pregnancies, and possibly in increased perinatal morbidity and mortality
Medical history: Sexual exposure 1 to 2 months previously
Patient is often sexually active with complaints of lower abdominal pain and/or penile or vaginal discharge; acute salpingitis in the female is the counterpart of epididymitis in the male
Subjective symptoms may be very mild and go unnoticed (numerous studies from infertility clinics show bilateral tubal scarring and occlusion without a history of PID)
Physical examination: Lower abdominal tenderness and spasm
Pelvic examination reveals marked pain on moving the cervix (Chandelier sign) and adnexal tenderness
Occasionally, an adnexal mass may be palpable and tender
Purulent cervical discharge is often present
Laboratory confirmation: Leukocytosis may be present in up to 50% of affected females
Increased erythrocyte sedimentation rate (sometimes considered useful to help differentiate PID from appendicitis)
Positive Gram stain (controversial)

For confirmed gonococcal PID: The patient should be hospitalized for acute salpingitis if there is any question of appendicitis, ectopic pregnancy, pelvic abscess, or if pregnant. Other indications for hospital admission: possible noncompliance, markedly severe symptoms, or outpatient treatment is impractical
Inpatients: Aqueous crystalline penicillin 20 million units i.v. for 72 to 96 hr and followed by ampicillin, 0.5 g p.o. every 6 hr for 10 days **or** doxycycline 100 mg i.v. every 12 hr, **plus** metronidazole 1 g i.v. every 12 hr for at least 4 days **and then** both drugs at the same dose p.o. for a total of 10–14 days; if response is not adequate within 48 to 72 hr laparoscopy or culdocentesis should be performed
Outpatients: In females, procaine penicillin G, 4.8 million units i.m. followed by doxycycline 100 mg p.o. every 12 hr for 10–14 days. In males, tetracycline, 500 mg p.o. four times a day for 10 to 14 days
For penicillin-allergic patients or penicillin-resistant gonorrhea (e.g., exposure took place in the Far East): Spectinomycin, 2.0 g i.m. or tetracycline, 0.5 g p.o. every 6 hr for 10 days

Disseminated Gonococcal Infection[b]

Infection within previous 2 months in 1 to 3% of patients
Arthritis develops in 1–3% of affected patients
Medical history: Sexually active female, usually just premenstrual, but may occur in pregnancy

Septicemia: Aqueous crystalline penicillin, 10 million units i.v. daily for 10 days
Meningitis and/or bacterial endocarditis may occur as complications

Diagnosis	Treatment

Abrupt onset with chills, fever, headaches, malaise, accompanied by joint or synovial pain

Physical examination: Skin lesions tend to occur early in the course, at the same time joint pain is occurring; lesions are usually acral macules which develop a target vesicle

The initial lesion progresses to a pustule and then a purpuric lesion

Meningeal or cardiac manifestations, although rare, may occur and reflect seeding of these organs

Arthritis and/or tenosynovitis, especially of the wrist or dorsum of the hands, may occur as (1) an acute hot, painful joint with purulent fluid and a positive Gram stain and culture or (2) as a painful joint with few objective signs and negative cultures on joint aspirations

Laboratory confirmation: Blood cultures are usually positive if obtained when chills are occurring

Identification of the organism from scrapings of a skin lesion (Gram stain and/or culture)

Positive endocervical or urethral culture

Lumbar puncture, if indicated

Aspiration of involved joint

Gonococcal Pharyngitis[b]

Less than 5% of gonorrhea cases

May be the only culture-positive site, even in asymptomatic child

Medical history: Oral-penile exposure is a must; cunnilingus does not usually cause this syndrome

No age group is immune (we have just documented this involvement in a 3-year-old child)

Physical examination: affected patients may have an (1) erythematous pharynx with micropustules on the tonsils, (2) an erythematous and mildly edematous pharynx with diffuse minute pustules, or (3) a normal appearing throat (gonococcal carrier)

Laboratory confirmation: Positive throat culture or a positive fluorescent test

Initiate treatment as in cervicitis or urethritis: Aqueous procaine penicillin G, 4.8 million units i.m.

Does not respond to ampicillin or spectinomycin

Gonococcal Proctitis

Medical history: Penile-rectal exposure (also possible to aspirate the organism from the vagina into the rectum at time of defecation, by incorrect wiping, and/or with very tight fitting jeans)

Physical examination: Asymptomatic carrier

Pain and swelling with increased pain on defecation

Procaine penicillin G, 4.8 million units i.m. followed by ampicillin, 0.5 g p.o. four times a day for 4 or more days

Penicillin-sensitive patient: Spectinomycin, 4 g i.m.

TABLE 1. *(continued)*

Diagnosis	Treatment
Pain on defecation with blood and pus on underwear Laboratory confirmation: Positive culture	

Syphilis[b] *(Treponema pallidum)*

Syphilis is an acute and chronic infection, spread principally by sexual exposure (95% of all syphilis is transmitted sexually):
Kissing (kissing a person who has lesions of primary or secondary syphilis on the lips or oral cavity)
Transplacentally to the fetus
Digital sex play
Transfusion
Accidental inoculation by contaminated needles
The disease appears in four stages: Stage 1: Chancre
Stage 2 (secondary stage): Generalized eruption with systemic symptoms
Stage 3 (latent stage): Reactive blood test but no symptoms
Stage 4 (late or tertiary stage): a slowly destructive stage, appearing >4 years after the initial infection and involving one or more body systems
Male to female predominance (2.9:1)
Forty cases of gonorrhea occur to each single case of syphilis
There appears to be no natural immunity to syphilis, and no way of introducing immunity short of an actual infection

Primary Syphilis[b]

Diagnosis	Treatment
Medical history: Sexual contact occurs an average of 3 weeks prior to the appearance of single or multiple genital chancres; the chancre is initially painless Physical examination: The chancre begins as a papule which then erodes and becomes ulcerative; it is painless, "punched out" with yellowish discharge There is contiguous large, hard lymphadenopathy In female patients, primary chancres appear most often on the labia, but may also occur in the cervix, fornix, or urethra (as a result of preliminary sex play, chancres may occur anywhere) Chancres of the lips are the most common extragenital lesions Any indolent painless lesion that does not heal within 2 weeks, regardless of location, should be considered as a possible syphlitic lesion Laboratory confirmation: Identification of the spirochete on dark-field examination	Aqueous procaine penicillin G, 4.8 million units i.m. daily for 8 to 10 days (total 600,000 units), **or** benzathine penicillin G, 2.4 million units i.m. (1.2 million units in each buttock), **or** tetracycline, 500 mg p.o. four times a day for 12 days

Diagnosis	Treatment

A positive blood test, such as the rapid plasma reagin (RPR) test; it is usually positive by the time the patient presents a week or so after the initial lesion occurs

Serological conversion shows that by the second week, 50% of the patients are zero converters, which increases to 75% at three weeks, and almost 100% at the end of the fourth week

The fluorescent treponemal antibody-absorption (FTA-ABS) test is the most sensitive of the treponemal tests; it tends to be more sensitive than the reagin tests in both early and late syphilis

The FTA-ABS test is most useful to distinguish between biologically false positive and true positive tests and to help establish a diagnosis of syphilis in patients who have clinical evidence of the disease, in patients who have clinical evidence but negative blood and cerebrospinal fluid serology tests, and in patients with epidemiological evidence but negative clinical and serological findings

Secondary Syphilis[b]

The secondary stage follows the onset of the chancre by 90 to 100 days (average, 3 weeks)

A chancre is frequently present at the beginning of the secondary stage, but healing usually appears within 6 to 8 weeks after its exposure

The manifestations are myriad, but early in the course a flulike syndrome with nasal discharge, lacrimation, sore throat and arthralgia is prevalent, with a mildly elevated temperature; Generalized lymphadenopathy, along with hepatosplenomegaly, may be present

A generalized rash completes the picture of secondary syphilis and is darkfield positive; the nonpruritic rash involves the mucous membranes, the hands and feet

The earliest rash shows a macular and/or papular eruption, appearing 6 to 8 weeks after the infectious exposure; the macular rash very rapidly becomes a macular-papular eruption, which rapidly evolves into the papular eruption of secondary syphilis (the papular eruptions in a moist area are called condylomalata and are filled with spirochetes)

The third type of rash in the sequence of these skin lesions are the pustular lesions, which may be accompanied by symptoms similar to those of chickenpox (headache and arthralgia); these lesions are especially frequent around the fingernails and toenails and are filled with treponemes

Benzathine penicillin G, 2.4 million units i.m., repeat in 7 days; **or** crystalline procaine penicillin G, 600,000 units i.m. daily for 10 days

If patient is penicillin-sensitive: Tetracycline, 500 mg p.o. four times a day for 12 days

Syphilis will develop in 5% to 30% of untreated sexual partners, so it would seem worthwhile to prophylactically treat the known contacts

A Herxheimer reaction may be expected when the patient is treated at this stage of secondary syphilis

TABLE 1. *(continued)*

Diagnosis	Treatment

Latent Syphilis[b]

Diagnosis	Treatment
Latent syphilis is a laboratory diagnosis Latent syphilis is classified as early latent or late latent Early latent: Patient within the past year has had untreated primary or secondary syphilis, a history of primary or secondary lesions, or a negative reagin test or is <30 years of age Late latent: Patient for more than one year has had untreated primary or secondary syphilis, a history of primary or secondary lesions, or a negative reagin test within the past 4 years, or is >30 years of age	Same as treatment of primary or secondary syphilis

Late Syphilis[b,d]

Diagnosis	Treatment
Late mucocutaneous syphilis Nodular syphilis Noduloulcerative syphilis Gummatous Osseous Visceral (lungs, abdomen, liver, spleen, gallbladder, intestines, kidneys, and bladder) Cardiovascular Neurosyphilis See Bibliography for additional reading on late syphilis Medical history, physical examination, laboratory confirmation Painless, asymptomatic, sharply demarcated ulcers The surface of the long bones, especially the tibia, are similar to a saber; far more frequently involved are the flat bones, such as the skull; the syphilitic process may penetrate the skull and directly involve the meninges The joints may be involved and arthralgia may be present, but radiographic examination is usually negative; In late syphilis, there may be a painless, hydroanthrosis, especially of the knees, Clutton's joints, and Charcot's disease of neurogenic origin Manifestations of neurosyphilis are myriad, ranging from deep tendon reflex abnormalities to paresis in meningal vascular syphilis; none of these changes are unusual	Benzathine penicillin G, 7.2 million units i.m. daily for 7 days, repeat three times, **or** tetracycline, 500 mg p.o. four times a day for 30 days Evaluation for neurosyphilis requires analysis of cerebrospinal fluid (e.g. cell count, protein level) and specific types of reagin tests

Early Congenital Syphilis[b,e]

Diagnosis	Treatment
Include a blood test for syphilis at the first prenatal visit; it should detect all infected pregnant women and ensure adequate treatment to prevent fetal infection or cure any infection of the fetus	Treatment depends on the cerebrospinal fluid findings: If abnormalities are found, then treatment should begin immediately (rather than a watchful waiting period to determine whether the positive reagin test was

Diagnosis	Treatment

Abnormal findings may be seen at birth, but more often are not seen until the first 2 to 4 weeks of life, they parallel the findings seen in secondary syphilis in adults

A flulike syndrome with lacrimation and nasal discharge, numerous mucous patches on the nasal mucosa (showing numerous spirochetes); the child may also have a hoarse cry and eroded/denuded areas in the oropharynx, arthralgia, and osteochondritis

Generalized hard adenopathy

A maculopapular or bullous eruption accompanied by hepatosplenomegaly

Early syphilitic lesions in the mother (i.e., primary or secondary stages) almost always have a negative effect on the fetus, ranging from abortion to congenital syphilis. However, the longer the mother has had the disease, the less chance there is of significant fetal infection

A reagin test should be performed on the child and the mother. If the mother has been treated early in the pregnancy, over the next few months the infant's quantitative levels will continue to drop and should be negative at the end of 3 months

The IGM-FTA-ABS test has been used, but very few centers are still performing this test

A positive darkfield examination is diagnostic as is a positive FTA-ABS test (in the post neonatal period)

An examination of the spinal fluid is imperative

passive transfer); the regimen is that of intramuscular or intravenous injections every day

Infants with normal CSF should receive banzathine penicillin G, 50,000 units/kg i.m. for 1 dose, **or** penicillin G procaine, 50,000 units/kg i.m. for 10 days

Infants with abnormal CSF should receive aqueous crystalline penicillin G, 50,000 units/kg i.m. or i.v. daily in 2 divided doses for 10 days, **or** aqueous procaine penicillin G, 50,000 units/kg i.m. for 10 days (in children with abnormal CSF a 10 day course of treatment is the minimum duration)

Late Congenital Syphilis[b,f]

Manifestations include frontal bossing, short maxilla, high arched palate (Hutchinson's triade), Hutchinson's teeth, interstitial keratitis, eighth nerve deafness, saddle nose, mulberry molars, clavicular abnormalities, protuberant mandible rhagades, saber skin, scaphoid scapula and Clutton's joint

See treatment schedule for early congenital syphilis

Lymphogranuloma Venereum (LGV) *(Chlamydia trachomatis)*

Medical history: Spread principally by sexual exposure, either genital, oral, or rectal, and is infectious as long as the skin lesion is present

Incubation period is 7 to 12 days, with a delayed presentation or onset of adenitis at 10 to 15 days

Complaints of headache, nausea, myalgias and/or arthralgias, as well as inguinal adenopathy (much more frequent in males)

Complement fixation test with a rising titer and a positive Frei test (hypersensitivity test following an injection of LGV antigen)

Sulfadiazine or sulfisoxazole, l g p.o. four times a day for 3 weeks **or**

Tetracycline, 0.5 g p.o. four times a day for 7 days, followed by 1 g four times a day for 2 weeks

TABLE 1. *(continued)*

Diagnosis	Treatment
Physical examination: Female patients present with vulvovaginal or rectal lesions, or both	
Chronic indolent weeping ulcers of the female genital tract may destroy significant amount of tissue, but may heal completely or leave tunnels and fistuls	
Male genital lesions are comparable, but are more often edematous and associated with ulcers of the scrotum and perineum	
LGV proctitis may reveal blood, mucus, and pus in the rectum along with tenderness and pain. Anoscopy may reveal an erythematous, friable rectal mucosa with punctate hemorrhages, superficial ulcers, and polypoid-type granulations. Mucosal sloughing is common with resultant strictures, especially at the anorectal ring	

Chancroid *(Hemophilus ducreyi)*

Diagnosis	Treatment
Medical history: Almost always sexual transmission and most frequent in persons with poor habits of personal hygiene	Sulphisoxazole 1 g p.o. four times a day for 2 to 4 weeks
The most common of the minor venereal diseases	
Attacks skin, not mucous membranes, but, rarely, may cause chancroidal ulceration in oral cavities	
Male predominance (20:1)	
Incubation period is 12 hr to 3 days	
Physical examination: Penile lesion is a small macule, progressively developing into a pustule, which ruptures and leaves a small ulcer on a red base; the ulcer increases in size and is rapidly joined by other ulcers	
Inguinal adenopathy follows within the week and is usually unilateral with swollen, tender nodes which rapidly become soft and fluctuate but without the sinuses of LGV	
Female patients may have labial, cervical or anal involvement (may also be an asymptomatic carrier)	
Constitutional signs are minimal, if present at all	
Laboratory confirmation: Smears from the lesion or aspirate from the lymph may be examined by Gram, Wright, or Pappenheim stain	
Fluorescent antibody test is available but not widely done	

Granuloma Inguinale

Diagnosis	Treatment
Chronic ulcerative disease involving the genitals, groin, peritoneum, or thighs	Tetracycline, 500 mg p.o. four times a day for 7 days, followed by 250 mg four times a day for 2 weeks
Medical history: Mainly a tropical disease, rarely seen the United States	It may be necessary to repeat a course of treatment
Physical examination: Irregular, red, friable, nontender ulcer	Erythromycin, in a similar dosage, may be

Diagnosis	Treatment
Adenopathy is a frequent concomitant Laboratory confirmation: Donovan bodies stained with Wright or Giemsa stain Histopathological diagnosis is possible Biological confirmation by culture can be performed within 48 hr of infection	substituted for tetracycline Long-term follow-up is needed because of the possibility of squamous cell carcinoma in the area of the ulceration

Cytomegalic Inclusion Virus (CMV)

Depending on circumstances, may be a STD Semen and cervical secretions have a high frequency of CMV Cervical CMV in women at STD clinics is 20 times more frequent than in other settings Medical history: Among 15 to 35 year-olds, sexual transmission may be the most common mode of infection, with an increased incidence of CMV in sex partners of infected people Significance lies in its relationship to malignancies (Kaposi sarcoma) and to congenital malformations following *in utero* infection Physical examination: Cervical discharge (10% to 25% of females attending STD clinics relative to <2% of the general population) Laboratory confirmation: Culture from semen and cervical cultures Serological proof	None

Condyloma Acuminata[c] (Genital Warts)

Medical history: Sexually transmitted and usually not noted in the absence of discharge when the papova-papilloma virus has infected the genital area Physical examination: May be single or in clusters Distribution is universal, from fingers to the bucal mucosa	Small lesions may be destroyed with 20% podophyllin in alcohol Larger lesions should be removed surgically

Herpes Progenitalis[c]

Medical history: about 70 to 90% of herpes type 2 occurs below the belt line, whereas the reverse is true with herpes type 1 A distinction must be made between primary and secondary herpes type 2; primary type 2 has an incubation period of about 36 hr and then large, discreet vesicles on an erythematous base with tender, enlarged lymph nodes and several weeks of a very uncomfortable state Physical examination: In recurrent herpes, there are clusters of small vesicles on an erythemotous base which are pruritic rather than painful; lymphadenopathy is not prominent and the evolution is usually about 10 days (recurrent herpes type 2 is not a reinfection, but a reactivation)	Supportive: Emollient creams are usually sufficient to decrease the pruritus and discomfort Specific: Intravenous acyclovir (Zovirax®) has been shown to be effective in the treatment of serious initial genital herpes infections 5% Acyclovir ointment has been shown to be helpful in the initial attacks of genital herpes; it reduces healing time and, in some cases, decreases the duration of viral shedding and pain Recurrent infection: Recurrent genital herpes, unfortunately, is not amenable to benefits from acyclovir or any other currently available medication

TABLE 1. *(continued)*

Diagnosis	Treatment
The genital ulceration inguinal adenopathy syndrome in the United States is most frequently caused by a herpes type 2 infection, with syphilis being a close second	
Anoscopy should be routine for patients who have rectal discharge, pain, or diarrhea; primary herpetic proctitis may show multiple rectal ulcers associated with systemic symptoms such as fever and malaise	
Laboratory confirmation: Culture of the lesion for herpes virus	
Papanicolaou stain of scrapings from the base of the lesion	

[a]Ectoparasitic disease.
[b]Bacterial disease.
[c]Viral disease.
[d]Latent syphilis is usually a slow progressive inflammatory disease of adults.
[e]Early congenital syphilis clinical manifestations occur before age 2.
[f]Late congenital syphilis clinical manifestations occur after age 2.

Shock

Shock is defined as circulatory collapse resulting in poor tissue perfusion. Poor tissue perfusion causes cellular hypoxia and metabolic acidosis. If the sequence of events leading to tissue hypoxia is not interrupted, shock becomes irreversible (Fig. 1).

The successful treatment of shock depends on its early recognition and aggressive management aimed at restoring adequate blood flow to the peripheral vascular beds (not only raising the blood pressure).

SIGNS AND SYMPTOMS

In general, states of shock are characterized by hypotension, decreased intravascular volume, and decreased central venous pressure. Shock is usually characterized by pallor (manifestation of decreased peripheral perfusion), diaphoresis (sympathetic response), tachycardia, and tachypnea. In cardiogenic shock, however, the hypotension is associated with severely decreased cardiac output and increased central venous pressure, which complicates the standard treatment of shock (i.e., volume expansion).

ETIOLOGICAL CONSIDERATIONS

Neonates

1. Signs and symptoms of shock
   a. Hypotonia
   b. Weakness
   c. Lethargy
   d. Mottled, gray, or cyanotic cold skin
   e. Hypothermia
   f. Shallow, rapid breathing
2. Predisposing conditions

   a. Birth injury (e.g., cord injury, intracranial hemorrhage)
   b. Hypothermia
   c. Sepsis
   d. Respiratory distress syndrome, pneumonia
   e. Congenital heart disease
   f. Hemorrhage
   g. Pneumothorax

515

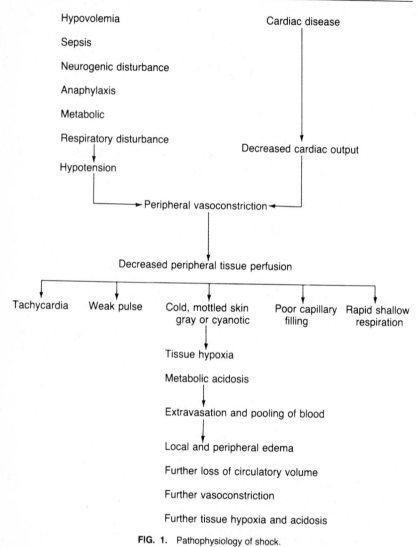

FIG. 1. Pathophysiology of shock.

Older Infants and Children

1. Signs and symptoms of shock

   a. Disorientation

   b. Weakness

   c. Lethargy and unresponsiveness

   d. Cold, clammy skin

   e. Poor capillary filling

   f. Rapid, weak pulse

2. Predisposing conditions

a. Gastroenteritis and dehydration

b. Hemorrhage

c. Burns

d. Abdominal trauma (e.g., splenic rupture)

e. Myocarditis, pericarditis, cardiac tamponade

f. Cardiac arrhythmias

g. Intractable congestive heart failure

h. Sepsis

i. Anaphylactic reactions

j. Diabetes

k. Adrenocortical disorders

l. Upper airway obstruction

m. Spinal injuries

n. Electrocution

o. Poisoning and drowning

p. Pulmonary embolism

q. Disseminated intravascular coagulopathy

DIAGNOSTIC PROTOCOL

1. **Shock should be recognized immediately and therapy started before any other diagnostic or investigative studies are done.**

2. The diagnosis is established if physical examination shows the following evidence of poor peripheral perfusion:

    a. Cold, clammy, gray or cyanotic skin

    b. Poor capillary filling

    c. Weak, thready, and rapid pulse

    d. Nonpalpable pulse

    e. Low blood pressure

3. Hypotension probably exists with the following systolic blood pressures (serial measurement of the blood pressure to establish a trend is more important than just one measurement):

    a. <45 mm Hg at 1 week of age

    b. <65 mm Hg at 1 year of age

    c. <75 mm Hg at 1 to 6 years of age

    d. <85 mm Hg after 6 years of age

TREATMENT PROTOCOL

Immediate Management

1. Oxygen by mask.

2. Intravenous fluids, using lactated Ringer's solution or normal saline, 20 ml/kg, given as rapidly as possible (over a 30-min to 1-hr period).

3. Obtain blood for typing and crossmatching.

4. Monitor vital signs as soon as condition permits (e.g., electrocardiogram, chest radiograph).

5. Continue intravenous fluid administration until an appropriate volume expander (5% albumin, Plasmanate®, or blood) is available.

6. Sodium bicarbonate, 1 mEq/kg i.v., immediately.

7. Specific therapy if predisposing condition is evident.

   a. Sepsis: Intravenous antibiotics.

   b. Hemorrhage: Blood replacement.

   c. Anaphylaxis: Epinephrine.

   d. Pneumothorax: Chest tube.

   e. Tamponade: Pericardiocentesis.

   f. Poisoning: Antidotes.

   g. Upper airway obstruction or trauma with continuous bleeding: Surgical intervention.

Irreversible Shock

1. Administer 5% albumin, Plasmanate®, or blood (10 ml/kg) as rapidly as possible.

2. Establish a central venous pressure (CVP) line.

3. Consider placement of an arterial line (useful for accurate blood pressure determinations and monitoring of blood gases).

4. Keep the patient warm.

Irreversible Shock and Impending Cardiac Arrest

1. Repeat sodium bicarbonate, 1 mEq/kg i.v.

2. Levarterenol bitartrate (Levophed® Bitartrate), 0.05 mg/kg/min, and titrate rate by blood pressure (should not be used routinely; causes further vasoconstriction).

3. Hydrocortisone (Solu-Cortef®), 25 mg/kg i.v. push (maintenance dose, 12 mg/kg/24 hr in four doses).

4. Continue aggressive volume expansion monitored by the CVP.

Irreversible Shock and CVP 7 to 14 cm H_2O

Isoproterenol (Isuprel®), 0.1 mg/ml i.v. drip (0.05 to 4.0 mg/min) **or** dopamine, 2 to 5 mg/kg/min i.v. drip (maximum, 20 mg/kg/min).

Postshock Management

1. Appropriate investigative studies.

2. Continuous monitoring of vital signs.

3. Electrocardiogram and chest radiograph, if not previously obtained.

4. Monitor urine output and specific gravity; if output is less than optimal, the CVP is normal, and the blood pressure is stable, administer mannitol, 1 g/kg i.v. (25% sol, 250 mg/ml) **or** furosemide (Lasix®), 2 mg/kg i.v. (do not use mannitol in presence of hyperosmolarity).

Specific Shock Syndromes

1. Hypovolemic shock

  a. Volume expansion, using saline and 5% albumin (or blood in case of hemorrhage) until the CVP is normal (6 to 15 cm H_2O in children, 4 to 7 cm H_2O in newborns).

  b. In burns, give packed red blood cells to keep the hematocrit above 30% and maintain the oxygen carrying capacity.

2. Anaphylactic shock

  a. Volume expansion.

  b. Epinephrine 1:10,000 aqueous solution, 0.01 ml/kg i.m., followed by 0.01 ml/kg i.v.; repeat every 20 min, if needed.

  c. Diphenhydramine (Benadryl®), 5 mg/kg in four doses p.o. i.v. or d.m. (maximum dose 150 mg/day).

  d. Hydrocortisone (Solu-Cortef®), 25 mg/kg i.v. push (maintenance dose, 12 mg/kg/24 hr in four doses).

  e. Aminophylline, 12 mg/kg/day i.v. in four doses (for respiratory distress or wheezing).

3. Neurogenic shock

  a. Volume expansion.

  b. Methoxamine, 0.25 mg/kg i.m. or 0.08 mg/kg i.v. over a 15-min period.

4. Cardiogenic shock

  a. Fluid therapy should be guided by LA pressures (not the CVP); a Swan-Ganz catheter passed into the pulmonary wedge position reflects the left atrial (LA) pressure.

  b. Relieve tamponade, if present.

  c. For bradycardia, use atropine, 0.01 mg/kg i.m. (maximum dose, 0.6 mg or 0.15 mg for newborns).

  d. Solu-Cortef® for postoperative atrioventricular (A-V) blocks.

  e. Treat cardiac arrhythmias, if present.

  f. Digitalize and use diuretics, if necessary.

  g. Isuprel® or dopamine (most effective if the CVP is normal; volume expansion is essential prior to their use).

  h. Phlebotomy may be necessary if the CVP is dangerously high.

5. Septic shock
   a. Volume expansion.
   b. Intravenous antibiotics.
   c. Solu-Cortef®.
   d. Heparin for disseminated intravascular coagulopathy.

S hort Stature

Short stature may be the most common complaint of patients seen by endocrinologists. It is estimated that 10 million children are evaluated for growth disturbances each year. Only a fraction of the investigations uncover significant abnormalities (Fig. 1). Most of the children evaluated reflect the normal continuum of growth patterns.

Discrepancies and variations in growth are poorly tolerated by both the parents and the patients. Their anxieties are related to the public's growing awareness of the role of preventive health care and the need for early diagnosis of disease to allow optimal and successful treatment. Consequently, parents seek advice earlier and for milder degrees of disease.

The significance of growth retardation should not be minimized. In children, any change in growth patterns or velocity may be the first sign of a significant medical problem. Health professionals are able to track growth on standard growth charts and, since linear growth often reflects basic health, both the static height and the growth velocity may provide sensitive and early recognition of disease.

SIGNS AND SYMPTOMS

The most rapid period of extrauterine somatic growth occurs during the first 3 years of life. The normal high velocity of growth during that period of development may obscure all but the most significant problems. From the fourth year of life through early puberty, growth occurs at a more consistent rate.

Along with somatic growth, there is also a change in body proportions. The infantile proportion (trunk and head account for the majority of the child's height) moves toward adolescent proportions (where the crown-rump height is equal to the heel-pubis height). The upper segment-to-lower segment ratio (US:LS) provides information that the measurement of linear somatic growth cannot. Arm span must also be measured. Patients with bone or cartilage disorders tend to have short extremities relative to both their trunks and their height.

Normal growth must be interpreted in association with secondary sexual development that the child may be undergoing. Pubertal development causes a more rapid rate of skeletal maturation, thereby resulting in epiphyseal fusion and minimizing further growth.

DIFFERENTIAL DIAGNOSIS

1. Familial short stature (racial or genetic).
2. Constitutional retarded growth and delayed adolescence.

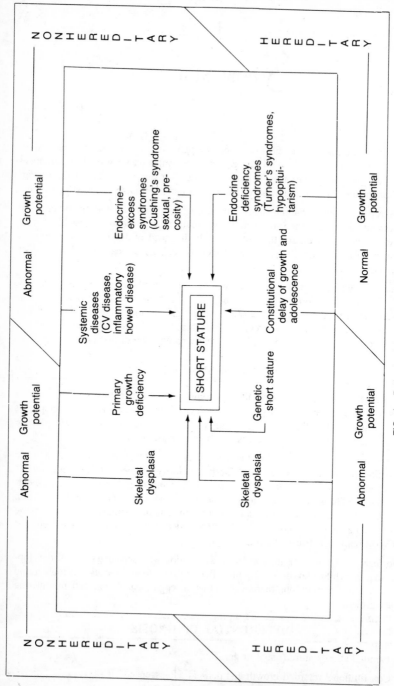

FIG. 1. Pathophysiology of short stature.

3. Endocrine disturbances (e.g., growth hormone deficiency, somatotropin, hypothyroidism, adrenal insufficiency, Cushing's syndrome, or androgen excess).

4. Primordial short stature: Infants noted to have small stature at birth with a subsequent pattern of growth that runs parallel to but below the third percentile (with appropriate body proportions).

5. Metabolic disorders.

6. Constitutional diseases of bone (e.g., chondrodysplasia and dysostosis).

7. Chromosomal defects: Autosomal or X-linked (although the genetic abnormality may result in short stature, the familial background of growth development and height potential may still exert a significant influence in concert with the genetic chromosomal abnormality).

8. Malignancies and chronic systemic diseases (e.g., inflammatory bowel diseases, cardiovascular diseases, central nervous system diseases, renal diseases, and pulmonary diseases).

9. Psychosocial dwarfism (maternal deprivation). See Failure to Thrive chapter.

10. Miscellaneous syndromes.

DIAGNOSTIC PROTOCOL

Figure 2 outlines diagnostic and therapeutic protocols for short stature.

TREATMENT PROTOCOL

1. Disorders with normal growth potential.

   a. Specific hormonal replacement for the deficiency syndromes.

   b. Medical management of any underlying systemic disease.

   c. Surgical intervention, as needed.

2. Disorders with decreased growth potential.

   a. Growth hormone will increase velocity but ultimate height will not be changed. (An exception is Turner's syndrome wherein treatment will result in actual increase in stature.)

   b. A short course of testosterone in boys with constitutional growth delay may be helpful if the delay is causing increased emotional stress.

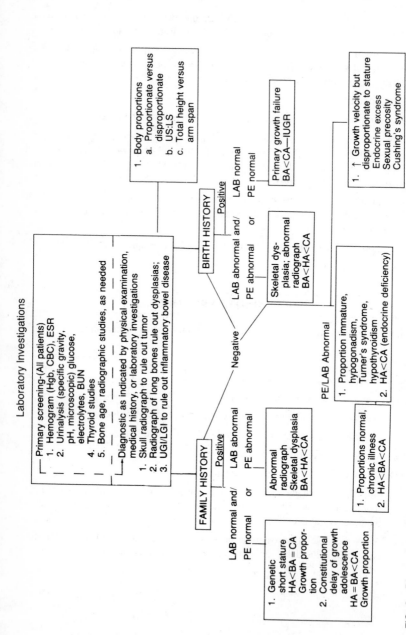

FIG. 2. Diagnostic protocol of short stature. Hgb, hemoglobin; CBC, complete blood cell count; ESR, erythrocyte sedimentation rate; BUN, blood urea nitrogen; UGI, upper gastrointestinal; LGI, lower gastrointestinal; PE, physical examination; HA, height age; BA, bone age; CA, chronologic age; LAB, laboratory studies; IUGR, intrauterine growth retardation; US, upper segment; LS, lower segment.

Spinal Dysraphism

Spinal dysraphism refers to a complex of disorders that have in common the failure of complete closure of the neural tube in the embryo. The disorder ranges from the mild spina bifida occulta to the severe meningomyelocele.

Spina bifida occulta is characterized by failure of fusion of the posterior vertebral arch. A meningocele is a cystic lesion in which the meninges and spinal fluid protrude through the posterior bony defect. The most severe form consists of a cystic protrusion of the meninges and the spinal cord.

PATHOPHYSIOLOGY

The exact pathophysiological mechanism of failure of fusion of the neural tube is not known. There tends to be a familial distribution, but the exact genetic transmission has not been established.

SIGNS AND SYMPTOMS

Patients with spina bifida occulta are usually asymptomatic. The lesion is most often discovered coincidently when a radiograph is taken for another reason. It is estimated that the lesion occurs in approximately 10% of children. There may be an associated presacral or lumbar sinus or dimple. Occasionally, urinary incontinence, gait abnormalities, lumbar lipoma, or lumbar teratoma may occur. In such cases, further diagnostic procedures should be performed.

Cystic lesions occur with meningoceles, but because they do not contain spinal cord components, there are usually no neurological abnormalities and the patients lead normal lives.

Meningomyelocele is a serious lesion. Neurological deficits, consisting of bladder and bowel incontinence and paralysis of the lower extremities, are common. The level of the lesion determines the extent of the paralysis. Hydrocephalus is usually present secondary to Arnold-Chiari malformation, abnormal development of the cerebellum and brainstem. Intelligence is usually normal.

DIAGNOSTIC PROTOCOL

---

1. The diagnosis is usually made on physical examination.

2. α-Fetoprotein is elevated in the amniotic fluid of mothers whose fetuses have

meningomyelocele. Since there is a familial incidence, prenatal diagnosis may be useful.

3. Early neurosurgical consultation is essential in the initial evaluation and management of spinal dysraphism.

4. Spinal radiographs, including the sacrum, may give information regarding the extent of the lesion.

5. Myelogram may be indicated to identify the extent of the lesion (it is usually not performed in patients with meningomyelocele).

6. The extent of the lesion is usually determined by the level and extent of the paralysis.

TREATMENT PROTOCOL

1. Early closure of the defect.

2. Treat meningitis, if present.

3. Ventriculoperitoneal shunting and monitoring to identify or prevent intracranial infections.

4. Counseling and support for the patient and family.

5. Control of bowel and bladder incontinence and prevention of urinary tract infections.

6. Orthopedic procedures, if necessary, and bracing. Physical therapy and rehabilitation are usually required to aid the patient in ambulation.

7. Close follow-up and monitoring; coordination of care should be the responsibility of the general practitioner.

Substance Abuse

The physician who cares for children must constantly be aware of the many who are substance abusers. Substances of abuse are readily available and easily acquired, increasing the risk of a child or adolescent presenting with adverse effects from their use (Fig. 1). The substances chosen for abuse tend to vary according to their immediate availability. Because of the sense of omnipotence among adolescents and the psychological and emotional variability of the adolescent period of development, experimentation with central nervous system altering substances by adolescents is common, but the age of the abusers is **constantly decreasing**. Of great concern is the large number of preadolescents and adolescents who are turning from drug abuse to the most commonly abused substance, alcohol.

Substance abuse must be considered in two ways: its short-term consequences and its long-term management. The recognition and differential diagnosis of the patient who presents with acute symptoms from an abused substance are of utmost importance. Rapid diagnosis and management may have a significantly positive effect on outcome. The following discussions are concerned with the short-term consequences of the most commonly abused substances. Long-term consequences are related to addiction, both physiological and psychological. Detoxification is a long and painstaking process, requiring a multidisciplinary effort. It is highly specialized and is not considered in this volume.

SIGNS AND SYMPTOMS

The signs and symptoms of the abuse of various substances are shown in Table 1.

DIAGNOSTIC PROTOCOL

Known Substance Abuse

1. Medical history
    a. Low expectations of academic performance.
    b. Greater value placed on independence than on academic performance.
    c. Greater tolerance of less conventional methods of performance.
    d. Little susceptibility to parental influence.
    e. Greater involvement in other problem behavior (e.g., delinquency, truancy).

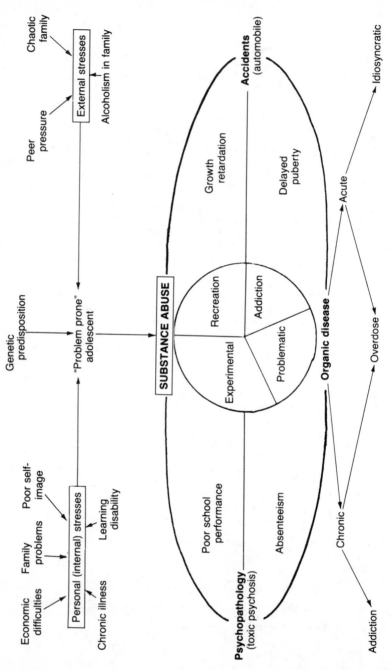

FIG. 1. Pathophysiology of substance abuse.

TABLE 1. *Symptoms and signs of substance abuse*

Symptoms and signs	Barbiturates[a]	Opiates (heroin)[a]	PCP	Amphetamines	Alcohol[a]
Coma/agitation	+/+(w)	+/−	−/+	−/+	+/+
Pupils	−	Pinpoint	Pinpoint	Dilated	−
Muscle twitching/ convulsions	+(w)/+(w)	−/−	+/+	+/+	+/+
Respiratory rate	Increased early, decreased late	Decreased	Increased	Increased	−
Pulse rate	−	Decreased	Increased	Increased	−
Dry mouth	−	+	+	+	−

[a]Naloxone (Narcan®) responsive.
+, Present; +(w), present in acute drug withdrawal; −, absent, not characteristic, or not diagnostic.

    f. Minimal participation in conventional activities (e.g., sports, school activities).

    g. Unusual amounts of friction with parents and friends.

    h. Family history of alcoholism, chaotic behavior patterns.

2. Clinical assessment

    a. Accelerated maturity (e.g., appearance, heterosexual versus isosexual relationships).

    b. Behavioral instability (e.g., mood swings, depression, poor sleeping and eating patterns, sadness, suicidal ideation, hopelessness).

    c. Mental status.

Acute Drug Ingestion

1. Medical history and clinical assessment

    a. Drugs ingested in decreasing order of frequency: Salicylates, diaxepam (Valium®), acetaminophen.

    b. Current or previous episodes of drug or substance abuse, with possible treatment by family or friends.

    c. Identify substance ingested, quantity ingested, route of ingestion, and time of ingestion (symptoms usually begin within 2 to 3 hr of ingestion).

    d. Recent trauma or medical illnesses.

    e. Travels, hobbies, exposure to illness.

2. Physical examination

    a. Determine level of consciousness.

    b. Potential grouping of signs and symptoms.

    c. Specific, well-known signs and symptoms.

    d. Determine presence of any unrelated diseases.

  e. Ecchymosis, track marks, or other signs of drug abuse.

  f. Vital signs.

  g. Pupils (mydriatic versus miotic).

  h. Diaphoresis.

  i. Salivation.

  j. Hyperthermia versus hypothermia.

3. Laboratory investigations

  a. Skull radiographs (if trauma is suspected).

  b. Abdominal radiographs (if radiopaque material such as iron, phenothiazine, chloral hydrate, or lead is suspected).

  c. Complete blood cell count, platelet count, electrolytes, blood urea nitrogen, creatinine.

  d. Toxicology studies (obtain quantitative level if therapy will be specifically altered).

   (1) Blood barbiturate, alcohol, PCP levels.

   (2) Urine narcotics, amphetamines, PCP levels.

TREATMENT PROTOCOL

Known Substance Abuse

Age and pattern of substance use or abuse will dictate treatment.

1. Experimentation or recreational use (marijuana or alcohol): Counseling regarding untoward possibilities (e.g., accidents, poor school performance, growth retardation, delayed puberty).

2. Problem use

  a. Counseling, as above.

  b. Psychotherapy or counseling directed toward special problems.

  c. Family therapy.

3. Addiction: Hospitalization and detoxification.

Acute Drug Ingestion

1. Intravenous infusion of fluids and medications.

2. Naloxone (Narcan®), 0.01 mg/kg i.v. or i.m. (neonates) or 0.01 to 0.03 mg/kg i.v. or i.m. (children) or 0.4 mg/kg/dose i.v. or i.m. (adolescents); repeat as necessary at 3- to 4-min intervals up to three times; the greater the amount of narcotic ingested the more rapidly the symptoms will return; alcohol ingestion will show a nonspecific response or no response.

3. 50% Glucose, 1 ml/kg i.v.

4. For amphetamine, barbiturate, or alcohol ingestion: If not comatose, syrup of ipecac, 30 ml (adult dose) p.o.; repeat in 20 min if necessary.

5. For PCP ingestion: Nasogastric lavage with activated charcoal.

6. For phenobarbital ingestion: Sodium bicarbonate, 1 or 2 mEq/kg every 4 hr (alkalinizes the urine).

7. For PCP or amphetamine ingestion: Ammonium chloride, 2 or 3 mEq/kg every 6 hr, **and** ascorbic acid, 1 or 2 g (acidifies the urine).

8. For barbiturate, amphetamine, or ethanol ingestion: Dialysis may rarely be indicated.

Sudden Infant Death Syndrome

Sudden infant death syndrome (SIDS) is the unexpected death of an infant who is not seriously ill and whose death remains unexplained by pathologist's examination of the circumstances surrounding the death (i.e., complete autopsy, including toxicology studies, blood cultures, and radiographic examination, as indicated). The mortality rate ranges from 10,000 to 13,000 deaths per year in the United States, which makes SIDS the largest single cause of postneonatal infant mortality and responsible for the deaths of one-third of all infants between 1 week and 1 year of age.

The incidence rates vary by geographic location, race, season, maternal age, level of parental education, number of antenatal physician visits, and other well-defined risk factors (see Fig. 1). These unexplained infant deaths leave a series of intense psychological reactions. Possibly one of the most prevalent is guilt. The physician who cared for the child may share in this guilt reaction by questioning, in the same introspective manner as the parents, what he or she might have done differently. A postmortem examination is essential. Ten to fifteen percent of these cases will be unexplained after the examination, but it may indirectly provide an indication for monitoring other children at risk.

SIGNS AND SYMPTOMS

The manifestations of SIDS are only available in retrospect and are obviously nonscientific and extremely subjective when related by the grief-stricken parents. Nonetheless, retrospective questioning of parents has yielded significant information. Some SIDS children seem to be less responsive to their external environment than their siblings. In addition, many are less active, have shortness of breath when feeding, and an "abnormal" cry. Only rarely is this information thought to be significant and conveyed to the physician before the child's death.

Other groups of children, possibly physiologically related to SIDS children, must act as models to provide further data on the signs and symptoms of SIDS. The first group consists of those who have suffered "near-miss" SIDS. These children have suffered apneic episodes that were witnessed and interrupted by resuscitation. The resuscitative efforts were not always successful and occasionally resulted in neurological damage. No definitive conclusions can be drawn as to the children's neurological and physiological responses before the near-miss episode. However, it is recognized that there is significant risk of the occurrence of another near-miss episode. Certain events are statistically related to a repetition of a near-miss episode: immunizations, colds, and a period of 1 month after a previous episode.

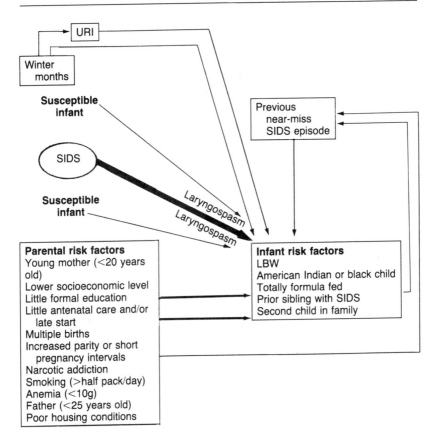

FIG. 1. Pathophysiology of sudden infant death syndrome (SIDS). LBW, low birth weight.

The second group of models consists of the siblings of SIDS children. The risk of apnea and SIDS in this group is thought to be five to ten times that of other children. Monitoring studies performed on these children have shown both neurological and physiological abnormalities in their respiratory sensitivity to P_{CO_2} (findings similar to those in the near-miss SIDS group).

A third group that may correlate with SIDS children are children with primary infantile apnea.

DIFFERENTIAL DIAGNOSIS

1. Primary infantile apnea
2. Abnormal ventilatory response to carbon dioxide
3. Aspiration
4. Gastroesophageal reflux with bronchospasm

5. Choanal atresia and/or other anatomical obstructive airway abnormality

6. Cardiac conduction abnormalities (prolongation of the Q-T interval)

   a. Idiopathic

   b. Electrolyte-induced

7. Atlantooccipital instability

8. Toxic ingestion

9. Anaphylactic reaction

10. Child abuse

11. Intracerebral bleeding

12. Sepsis

13. Endocrinopathy (thyroid, adrenal insufficiency)

14. Genetic and/or inborn error of metabolism

15. Neonatal narcotic withdrawal

16. Foreign body

DIAGNOSTIC AND TREATMENT PROTOCOLS

Near-Miss SIDS Children

1. There is some evidence that near-miss SIDS children who require significant resuscitative intervention have almost a 60% chance of repeating the episode, with less flexibility in the amount of time available for intervention.

2. Near-miss SIDS children who ultimately die may show an increased incidence of various abnormal anatomical features (e.g., muscularized arterioles).

3. Physiological abnormalities concerned with respiratory controls, manifested by increased P_{CO_2} at rest and decreased responsiveness to rising P_{CO_2}, may exist before the resuscitation episode.

4. Sleep apnea (>20 sec) and excessive short apnea (12–20 sec) are also more common in children with near-miss SIDS.

Siblings of SIDS Children

1. Siblings of children who have died of SIDS have a fivefold to tenfold increase in the risk of developing SIDS episodes.

2. SIDS children and slightly more than 10% of their siblings share similar P_{CO_2} problems (e.g., retention and decreased sensitivity to change).

3. Siblings of SIDS children may have detectable and measurable physiological and neurological abnormalities.

Monitoring Near-Miss SIDS Children and Siblings

1. Monitoring raises the issues of expense, availability of equipment and service, and stress and anxiety on the parents, who will be responsible for the child after leaving the hospital with monitoring equipment.

2. The monitor costs $1,000 to $2,000, and the average duration of the infant's hospital stay for evaluation averages four days, with few subsequent readmissions.

3. Monitoring is recommended for 6 months and the average age of discontinuance of monitoring is 8.3 months.

4. The pathologist is the ultimate source of information and advises the clinician as to the probability of a SIDS episode in a near-miss SIDS child or a sibling of a SIDS child; the physician must then collaborate with the parents in determining the advisability and necessity of a home monitoring and alarm system for other children; the parents' thoughts regarding their ability to handle the monitoring and resuscitation procedures msut be fully expressed.

Syncope

Syncope is defined as a sudden episode of loss of consciousness, usually lasting less than 1 min. Syncope may be precipitated by a variety of disorders, but the basic pathophysiological disturbance is a sudden decrease in cerebral blood flow. Previously present CNS disorders may facilitate the onset of a syncopal episode.

Because cerebral dysfunction in syncope is reversible and because treatment is oriented toward therapy of the primary and underlying cause, syncope must be differentiated from a seizure disorder, which is also manifested by a sudden episode that may result in unconsciousness. Seizures are followed by a postictal state; syncopal episodes are not.

ETIOLOGICAL CONSIDERATIONS

1. Vasovagal syncope
2. Cardiac syncope
   a. Tachycardia
   b. Bradycardia
   c. Heart block (Stokes-Adams syndrome)
   d. Sick sinus syndrome
   e. Asystole
   f. Congenital heart disease
      (1) Critical aortic stenosis
      (2) Idiopathic hypertrophic subaortic stenosis
      (3) Tetralogy of Fallot with critical right ventricular outflow obstruction
      (4) Prolonged Q-T interval and mitral click syndrome
3. Orthostatic hypotension
   a. Physiological or idiopathic syncope
   b. Sudden decrease in systemic venous return (venous pooling)
   c. Volume depletion
      (1) Hemorrhage
      (2) Dehydration
      (3) Hyponatremia
   d. Sympathetic dysfunction
4. Cerebral occlusive disease
   a. Basilar artery insufficiency
   b. Subclavian steal syndrome
   c. Aortic arch syndrome
5. Carotid sinus syndrome
6. Hypoxia
7. Anemia
8. Hyperventilation and decreased P_{CO_2}
9. Hypoglycemia
10. Others
    a. Glossopharyngeal neuralgia
    b. Cough syncope
    c. Hysterical fainting
    d. Micturition syncope

DIFFERENTIAL DIAGNOSIS

1. Coma
2. Seizure disorders
3. Breath-holding spells
4. Hypoventilation syndromes
5. Labyrinthitis episodes and vertigo
6. Basal migraine
7. Apneic spells
8. Inguinal hernia (affected children may sweat and feel faint after exercise)

DIAGNOSTIC PROTOCOL

If the infant or child is unconscious, the approach should be the same as that used for coma (see Coma chapter). Significant life-threatening disease must be ruled out and treated immediately.

Medical History

Medical history is **crucial** to an accurate diagnosis (see Table 1).

Physical Examination

1. Rule out possible neurological disease or diabetes.
2. Symptoms and diagnosis on examination immediately following the syncopal attack.

    a. Decreased blood pressure, slow heart rate: Vasovagal syncope.

    b. Normal blood pressure, slow heart rate: Bradyarrhythmia.

    c. Decreased blood pressure, normal or slightly increased heart rate: Orthostatic syncope.

    d. Decreased blood pressure, markedly increased heart rate: Tachyarrhythmia.

Investigative Procedures

1. Admit patient to pediatric intensive care unit for continuous monitoring.
2. Document blood pressure and heart rate in the upright (after 5 min of standing still) and recumbent positions; normally there is no difference.
3. Electrocardiogram.
4. Chest radiograph.
5. Echocardiogram.
6. Holter monitoring for 24 hr (Holter monitoring and/or cardiac catheterization with intracardiac electrophysiological studies may be needed to document significant cardiac arrhythmias).
7. Exercise test.
8. Fasting blood glucose and glucose tolerance test.

TABLE 1. *Causes of syncope*

Syncopal episode	Etiology	Possible diagnosis
Following pain, fear, anxiety, excessive food or alcohol intake, closed quarters (e.g., school, church); only if sitting or standing; always preceded by nausea and uncomfortably warm feeling	Hypotension	Vasovagal syncope
Following palpitation	Tachyarrhythmia, causing decreased cardiac output	Tachyarrhythmia (severe sinus tachycardia, paroxysmal atrial tachycardia)
Following open heart surgery	Decreased cardiac output	Sick sinus syndrome
On exertion	Decreased cardiac output	Aortic stenosis, pulmonary hypertension
Preceded by cyanosis	Anoxia	Tetralogy of Fallot, breath-holding spell, apneic spell
After prolonged squatting or sitting; standing abruptly; no prodromal symptoms (e.g., nausea or warmth)	Orthostatic hypotension	Hypotension
Following bleeding, water loss (severe diarrhea), diuretic therapy	Orthostatic syncope	Volume depletion and decreased cardiac output
Induced		
Neck turning, wearing a tight necktie	Carotid sinus syndrome	Hypotension
Throat pain and bradycardia	Glossopharyngeal neuralgia	Hypotension
Cough	Cough syncope	Hypoventilation, reflexive
Micturition	Micturition syncope	Reflexive
Hyperventilation, numbness, paresthesias	Hyperventilation syncope	Decreased P_{CO_2}
Occurs only when people are present, no prodromal symptoms, no change in vital signs	Hysterical syncope	Involuntary, but may be induced
Following food ingestion; accompanied by prodromal signs (e.g., sweating)	Hypoglycemic syncope	Hypoglycemia
Sudden, with no prodromal history, especially on arising from recumbent position	Cardiac	Sudden decrease in cardiac output
With unconsciousness lasting longer than 1 to 4 min	Cardiac, hypoglycemic, or hysterical syncope; postictal states	Decreased cardiac output, hypoglycemia, seizures

9. Complete blood cell count and urinalysis.

10. Blood urea nitrogen serum and electrolytes.

11. Hyperventilation and cautious unilateral carotid massage.

12. Electroencephalogram.

13. Brain scan (blood flow studies and/or cerebral arteriography when indicated).

14. Apnea monitoring in infants.

15. Arterial blood gases and pH.

TREATMENT PROTOCOL

1. The regimen must be guided by the etiology of the syncopal episode.

2. Treat the underlying disorder.

T etanus

Tetanus is the clinical syndrome resulting from the disseminated toxin produced by an infection with *Clostridium tetani*. The organism multiplies locally and produces exotoxin, which has a predilection for the central nervous system (Fig. 1).

The organism is a gram-positive rod which resembles a drumstick because of the production of a terminal spore. It is found most commonly in soil and in manure of sheep, cattle, and horses.

The prognosis of tetanus is variable, being fatal in approximately 60% of affected patients. Age, length of incubation period, height of fever, extent of involvement, and treatment measures will, to some extent, affect the prognosis.

SIGNS AND SYMPTOMS

Progressive neurological symptoms appear after a variable incubation period of approximately 5 to 14 days. There is stiffness of the voluntary musculature, which usually begins in the muscles of the jaw (lockjaw) and neck. The stiffness progressively increases in severity and spreads to involve the muscles of the rest of the body. Risus sardonicus, opisthotonus, stiff extremities, and abdominal rigidity are characteristic of tetanus. External stimuli may provoke or exacerbate the spasms. Involvement of respiratory musculature and the larynx may cause compromise of the airway, resulting in respiratory failure, hypoxia, coma, and/or death.

The patient's temperature is usually normal. A fever during the course of the illness is a poor prognostic sign. Resolution of symptoms is gradual, with muscles of the jaw being last to remit.

During the course of the illness, there is no alteration of consciousness. The patient is alert and responsive.

Tetanus neonatorum occurs in newborns approximately 1 week of age and is characterized by difficulty sucking (secondary to jaw involvement), excessive crying, continuous or intermittent generalized spasms (frequently precipitated by external stimuli), opisthotonus, respiratory distress, cyanosis, and/or shock. The presentation in the newborn is variable, and any or all of the symptoms may be present.

DIFFERENTIAL DIAGNOSIS

1. Bacterial or aseptic meningitis
2. Poliomyelitis
3. Encephalitis
4. Rabies
5. Tetany, hypocalcemia
6. Strychnine poisoning
7. Peritonitis

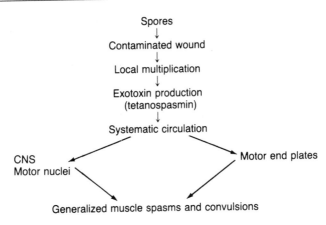

FIG. 1. Pathophysiology of tetanus.

DIAGNOSTIC PROTOCOL

1. Complete blood cell count: May show signs of viral or bacterial infection.

2. Urinalysis.

3. Calcium and blood glucose: Hypocalcemia and hypoglycemia can cause seizures.

4. Cerebrospinal fluid evaluation: To rule out meningitis and/or encephalitis.

5. Culture and Gram stain of wound exudate.

6. History of trauma and inadequate or questionable immunization status suggests the diagnosis.

7. Blood gases.

8. Toxic screening for other poisons.

9. Chest radiograph and flat plate radiograph of the abdomen.

TREATMENT PROTOCOL

1. Supportive and symptomatic care: Adequate hydration and oxygen, mobilization of secretions, airway management (intubation or tracheostomy, if necessary), minimal external stimuli.

2. Antibiotic therapy: Aqueous penicillin G, 100,000 units i.v. every 4 hr (300,000 units/kg/day i.v. in six divided doses for 10 to 14 days).

3. Passive immunization: Human tetanus immune globulin (TIG), 3,000 to 6,000 units i.m. **or** bovine tetanus antitoxin (TAT), 50,000 to 100,000 units (one half i.m. and one half i.v.); **used only if the patient is not sensitive to bovine serum**.

4. Sedation: Diazepam (Valium®), 8 mg/kg (<2 years old) or 10 to 40 mg/kg (>2 years old) in eight divided doses, **or** phenobarbital, 2 to 3 mg/kg/day in four divided doses, **or** chlorpromazine, 2 mg/kg/day i.m. or p.o. in four divided doses (not recommended for use in infants; may be used in combination with phenobarbital) **or** D-tubocurarine (ventilation must be controlled).

Thyroid Disease

Management of problems of the thyroid gland in infants and children requires a detailed understanding of the physiology of the thyroid gland, which is beyond the scope of this chapter. The main emphasis is on an explanation of when to suspect a thyroid disorder and how to investigate it. Mass screening programs of newborns allows for the early detection and treatment of hypothyroidism, which, in the past, was a leading cause of psychomotor retardation.

PATHOPHYSIOLOGY

Figure 1 outlines the pathophysiology of thyroid disease.

SIGNS AND SYMPTOMS

Patients may present with manifestations of either hypothyroidism or hyperthyroidism, or they may be euthyroid. The thyroid gland should be investigated and thyroid function tests (thyroid hormone studies) should be performed when any of the following symptoms or signs are present:

1. Newborn infants
   a. Hypotonia and sluggishness
   b. Poor peripheral circulation
   c. Myxedema
   d. Macroglossia and umbilical hernia
   e. Hypothermia and bradycardia
   f. Persistent unexplained jaundice
   g. Suspected Down's syndrome
   h. Large posterior fontanelle
2. Older infants and children
   a. Dry, thick skin
   b. Coarse, brittle hair
   c. Unexplained constipation
   d. Hypertrophy of the calf muscles (Debré-Sémélaigne syndrome)
   e. Psychomotor and/or physical retardation
   f. Unusual sexual development
   g. Evidence of other endocrine disorders (e.g., diabetes)
   h. Weakness, emotional instability, anxiety, excessive sweating, and tachycardia
   i. Diffuse thyroid enlargement (goiter)
   j. Nodular and/or tender thyroid gland
   k. Unusually coarse features

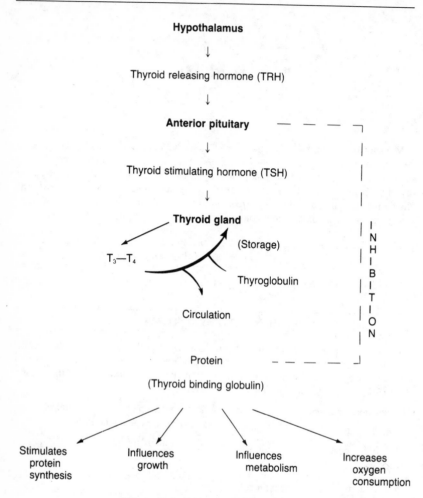

FIG. 1.   Pathophysiology of thyroid disease.

ETIOLOGICAL CONSIDERATIONS

Hypothyroidism

1. Congenital

   a. Aplasia or hypoplasia of the thyroid gland (most common causes).

   b. Radioiodine administered to the mother during pregnancy for treatment of tumors or hyperthyroidism.

c. Developmental defects of the pituitary and/or hypothalamus with deficiencies of thyroid releasing hormone (TRH) and thyroid stimulating hormone (TSH).

d. Defective synthesis of thyroxine, resulting in goiter (cretinism).

2. Acquired

  a. Congenital hypothyroidism not detected earlier in life.

  b. Thyroidectomy (iatrogenic or as treatment for hyperthyroidism).

  c. Chronic infections.

  d. Chemically induced by such agents as iodides, cobalt, lithium, or para-aminosalicylic acid (PAS).

  e. Lymphocytic thyroiditis (most common cause).

  f. Radiographic destruction.

Hypothyroid patients must be differentiated from infants and children with Down's syndrome, chondrodystrophy, gangliosidosis, Hurler's syndrome, or exogenous obesity.

Hyperthyroidism

1. Graves' disease (diffuse toxic goiter, thought to be an autoimmune disease).

2. Toxic uninodular goiter (Plummer's disease).

3. Functional thyroid carcinoma.

4. Acute suppurative thyroiditis.

5. TSH pituitary secreting tumors.

6. McCune-Albright syndrome.

7. Congenital (in newborns).

Hyperthyroid patients must be differentiated from infants and children with chorea, anxiety states, emotional disorders, pheochromocytoma, or hyperactive states (CNS dysfunction with hyperactivity).

Goiter

Patients may be hypothyroid, hyperthyroid, or euthyroid.

1. Congenital (may be due to antithyroid drugs given to the mother during pregnancy, defective thyroxine synthesis, or teratoma).

2. Endemic goiter (actual or relative iodine deficiencies, as in periods of rapid growth).

3. Sporadic goiter (due to lymphocytic thyroiditis, defective thyroxine synthesis, treatment with iodides, and idiopathic).

4. Thyroid adenoma.

5. Goiter and congenital deafness (Pendred's syndrome).

DIAGNOSTIC PROTOCOL

Thyroid Function Tests

1. Serum levels of T_3 and T_4 (for adequate interpretation of the value of T_4, the level of thyroid binding globulin should be known since it may be increased or decreased in a variety of conditions and, hence, change the measured level of T_4, although the patient may be euthyroid).

2. Serum thyroxine-binding globulin (TBG) as determined by the resin-T_3 uptake (RT_3U) test: TBG is increased in pregnancy, newborn period, oral contraceptives use, intermittent porphyrias, and as a genetic defect (X-linked dominant disorder); TBG is decreased in patients receiving steroids, in nephrotic syndrome, in major stress, and as a congenital deficiency.

3. The product of serum T_4 and RT_3U (T_4-RT_3 index); used to interpret the T_4 (not as an independent test of thyroid function); phenytoin interferes with thyroid function tests; normal values of serum hormones change with age and the methods used (normal values should be established for the specific laboratory doing the determinations).

4. Serum TSH by radioimmunoassay.

5. TRH stimulation test.

6. Radioisotope studies (sodium pertechnetate ^{99m}Tc accumulation).

Obtain Serum Level of T_4

1. Low or borderline T_4

    a. Obtain T_4-RT_3 index: If normal, the patient has TBG abnormalities; if decreased, the patient may have hypothyroidism.

    b. Obtain serum level of TSH: Elevated TSH indicates hypothyroidism; normal TSH indicates hypothalamic or pituitary dysfunction.

    c. Administer TRH, 7 mg/kg i.v., and measure TSH: In normal response, TSH is increased by 5–40 M units/ml within 30 min; normal response localizes the defect to the hypothalamus; no response (and low T_4) localizes the defect to the pituitary.

2. Elevated T_4

    a. Obtain T_4-RT_3 index: If increased, the patient may have hyperthyroidism.

    b. Obtain serum level of TSH: Depressed TSH indicates hyperthyroidism; normal TSH indicates thyrotoxicosis (rarely, T_4 is normal and only T_3 is elevated, indicating T_3 thyrotoxicosis).

3. Normal T_4 with no goiter and no symptoms

    a. Obtain serum level of T_3: If normal, the patient has no thyroid abnormalities; if elevated, suspect T_3 thyrotoxicosis.

    b. Obtain serum level of TSH: Normal or low.

4. Normal T_4 with goiter, but no symptoms

a. Obtain serum level of T_3: Elevated T_3 indicates endemic goiter; normal or borderline low T_3 indicates colloid goiter or Hashimoto's thyroiditis.

b. Obtain serum level of TSH: Normal or slightly elevated in endemic or colloid goiter and moderately elevated in thyroiditis.

c. Thyroid isotope scan: Abnormal in thyroiditis; normal in colloid goiter.

d. Perchlorate discharge test results in more than 10% iodide discharge in thyroiditis.

e. Agglutination test for thyroid antibodies: >1:16 is diagnostic of thyroiditis.

f. Open biopsy might be indicated.

Other Tests

1. Bone age: Decreased in hypothyroidism; normal or slightly advanced in hyperthyroidism.

2. Serum cholesterol and carotene: Elevated in hypothyroidism and decreased in hyperthyroidism (not reliable in infants <1 year old).

3. Red blood cell glucose-6-phosphate dehydrogenase (G6PD) activity is decreased in hypothyroidism and normal or increased in hyperthyroidism.

4. Circulating antibodies to thyroglobulin are found in most patients with hyperthyroidism.

5. Skull radiographs may reveal some abnormalities in patients with pituitary disease.

6. Radioisotope studies (^{99m}Tc) are performed to detect ectopic thyroid, evaluate thyroid nodules, assess presence or absence of thyroid tissue in suspected agenesis.

7. Radioiodine studies, perchlorate tests, and studies of thyroid tissue may be used to determine the biochemical nature of the defect in congenital goiterous hypothyroidism.

TREATMENT PROTOCOL

Hypothyroidism

1. Levothyroxine

   a. Newborns and infants: 0.25 mg initially, then increase by 0.025 to 0.05 mg every 2 weeks until required level is reached.

   b. Children: 0.05 mg initially for 2 weeks (total dose, 100 mg/m^2), then increase by 0.025 to 0.05 mg every 2 weeks until desired level is reached; usual requirement, 0.1 mg/m^2; monitor by serum T_4 and TSH determinations.

2. Triiodothyronine: More rapid but short-lived effect; should not be used for maintenance therapy.

3. Levothyroxine or iodine (in iodine deficiency): For hypothyroidism in goiter.

Hyperthyroidism

1. General measures: Bed rest; adequate diet high in calories, carbohydrates, and vitamins; propranolol to control tachycardia and thyroid storm and preoperatively in doses of 20 to 100 mg every 6 hr.

2. Medical therapy

   a. Propylthiouracil, 75 to 300 mg/day in four doses until patient is asymptomatic and thyroid tests are normal; maintenance dose, 50 to 100 mg/day in three doses.

   b. Methimazole and iodide are less desirable forms of therapy.

   c. Congenital hyperthyroidism is treated by iodide; propranolol is given in case of arrhythmias.

3. Surgical therapy (if medical therapy is unsuccessful). Subtotal thyroidectomy (preoperative preparation): Bed rest, diet, propranolol, propylthiouracil for 2 to 4 weeks, iodide-saturated solution of potassium iodide, 1 to 10 drops daily for 21 days before surgery and 1 week after surgery.

Thyroiditis

1. Suppurative thyroiditis: Antibiotics.

2. Chronic lymphocytic thyroiditis (Hashimoto's disease): Levothyroxine, 100 mg/m^2; steroids may be needed to reduce the size of the thyroid gland.

Thyroid Nodules (^{99m}Tc Scan)

1. Hard and growing rapidly with tracheal and vocal cord involvement: Surgical exploration for possible thyroidectomy.

2. Questionable: Give suppressive L-thyroxin therapy, 0.2 mg/day; surgical exploration if growth continues over a period of 2 to 4 months or nodule does not decrease by at least 50% in 6 months. (Surgical exploration is preferable to suppressive trials. Postoperatively replacement therapy and/or radiotherapy may be necessary.)

Total Parenteral Nutrition

The purpose of total parenteral nutrition (TPN) is to provide intravascularly all the nutritional requirements for normal metabolism and growth when they cannot be provided orally or enterally.

If all the nutritional caloric requirements are to be met, a hyperosmolar solution (800–900 mOsm/L) is usually necessary, since the volume of infusate is limited. Infusing a hyperosmolar solution requires the use of a large vessel with rapid flow. Peripheral veins may be used when the infusate is less concentrated and additional calories are either not needed or are provided by a fat emulsion (Intralipid®). Nutritional requirements and TPN problems differ according to the patient's age, the primary disorder, and the objectives. Therefore, recommendations for premature infants, full-term newborns, infants, and older children are different.

Because infants and children cannot be subjected to acute changes in composition or concentration of hyperosmolar solutions, the institution and termination of therapy must be done gradually. The patient must also be carefully monitored during the entire course of infusion.

INDICATIONS

Premature Infants or Full-Term Newborns

1. At 72 hr of age if infant cannot be fed, using peripheral vein TPN.

2. Whenever the caloric intake cannot be provided by the enteral route.

Infants and Children

1. After 4 to 6 days of intravenous fluids and inability to feed or provide adequate caloric intake.

2. Loss of 6% or more of body weight while on intravenous fluids.

   a. If expected to be fed within a week, use peripheral vein TPN.

   b. If expected not to be fed before 2 or more weeks, use central vein TPN.

   c. If expected to be fed within 10 to 14 days (most infants, such as those with necrotizing enterocolitis and chronic diarrhea), use peripheral vein TPN if infant is not in a depleted or unstable condition and use central vein TPN if infant is very ill and in a depleted or unstable condition.

Consider TPN in infants and children with intractable and chronic diarrhea, Crohn's disease, ulcerative colitis, anorexia nervosa, chronic pancreatitis, esophageal disease, severe malnutrition and wasting, as well as postoperatively and in children in prolonged comatose states.

CONTRAINDICATIONS (RELATIVE AND ABSOLUTE)

1. If the infant can be provided with adequate nutrition enterally, either orally or nasogastrically.

2. Total bilirubin of $\geqslant 5$ mg/100 ml in premature infants and $\geqslant 8$ mg/100 ml in full-term and older infants.

3. Liver disease.

4. Severe respiratory distress.

5. Serious bleeding disorders.

6. Fat emulsions should not be used in cases of liver disease and hyperlipidemia.

TPN SOLUTIONS

TPN solutions should provide a source of nitrogen (amino acids), calories (glucose, with or without the use of fat emulsions), electrolytes, minerals, and vitamins (Table 1). The use of free amino acids is preferable to the use of casein or fibrin hydrolyzates. The TPN solution should be prepared daily in the hospital's pharmacy (Table 2). Fat emulsions are needed to prevent deficiencies of essential fatty acids; they are administered via a separate intravenous line.

TECHNICAL ASPECTS OF TPN

1. TPN should be performed in a pediatric intensive care unit.

2. A solution with 10 or more grams of dextrose and providing more than 80 cal/kg/day must be infused in a central vein. Less hyperosmolar solutions and fat emulsion may be infused in a peripheral vein.

3. Use silicone catheters; if not available, Teflon or polyvinyl catheters may be used.

4. Perform a jugular vein cut-down in infants or insert the catheter percutaneously in the antecubital basilar vein; advance to the superior vena cava.

5. Change the dressing and reapply an antiseptic ointment every 3 days, following strict aseptic techniques.

6. Attach a 0.22 M membrane filter between the catheter and fluid column.

7. Use a constant infusion pump.

8. The fat emulsion is infused separately through a peripheral vein or through a T or Y connector and separate infusion pump; if the T or Y connector is used, hang the lipid bottle higher than that of the amino acid-glucose solution to prevent backflow.

TABLE 1. *Recommended nutritional requirements for TPN*

	Daily amount	
	Newborn infants	Older infants and children
Dextrose	10–20 g/kg	15–30 g/kg
Protein	2.0–2.5 g/kg	2.5–3.0 g/kg
Lipid	0.5–1.0 g/kg	2.0–3.0 g/kg
Sodium chloride	2–3 mEq/kg	3–4 mEq/kg
Potassium		
Phosphate	2 mEq/kg	
Chloride		2–4 mEq/kg[a]
Calcium gluconate[b]	1–2 mEq/kg	2–4 mEq/kg
Magnesium sulfate	0.1–0.2 mEq/kg	0.25 mEq/kg
Zinc sulfate	150 micrograms/kg	150–300 micrograms/kg
Copper sulfate	20 micrograms/kg	20–40 micrograms/kg
Manganese	2 micrograms/kg	5–10 micrograms/kg
Iodine	10 micrograms/kg	maximum 130 micrograms/kg
Chromium	0.15 micrograms/kg	0.20 micrograms/kg
Vitamins[b]	0.5 ml/100 ml	1–3 ml/100 ml
Volume	125–135 ml/kg (maximum, 200 ml/kg)	120–150 ml/kg
Calories	100–120/kg	75–125/kg

[a]2 mEq/kg as phosphate.
[b]Administer calcium gluconate and vitamins D and E enterally (not in the solution) as soon as the patient's condition permits.
Additional requirements: Vitamin K, 1 mg i.m. every 1 to 2 weeks; vitamin B_{12}, 50 mg i.m. every month; folic acid, 2 mg i.m. every 2 weeks.

9. Do not use the lines for any other purposes.

10. If infection is suspected, remove the catheter over a wire, insert a new one on the wire, and culture the used catheter.

11. Check the site frequently for evidence of phlebitis, thrombosis, or subcutaneous infiltration and tissue necrosis.

12. The infusion may be administered constantly or every 12 hr to allow mobility.

13. Start gradually.

   a. 10% Dextrose solution with electrolytes at one and one half times maintenance rate for 24 hr.

   b. 20% Dextrose solution with amino acids at three quarters maintenance rate for 12 hr.

   c. Increase the intravenous rate by 10% every 12 hr until 135 ml/kg/24 hr is reached.

   d. The fat emulsion should be started at no more than 15 ml/kg/day over a 12-hr period.

   e. If there are no complications, increase the lipid by 5 ml/kg/day until 30 to 40 ml/kg/day is reached.

TABLE 2. *Daily total parenteral nutrition (central or peripheral) order form*

A. Amino acids/dextrose solution suggested formulae (check one)
☐ 1. For adult patients
    Crystalline amino acids .... 4.25 ⎫
    Dextrose .... 25.0 ⎬ g in 100 ml
☐ 2. For neonatal, pediatric or adult patients
    Crystalline amino acids .... ____ ⎫ in 24 hr **or** ____ ⎫ g in 100 ml
    Dextrose .... ____ ⎬
☐ 3. For renal patients
    Essential amino acids 5.4% .... 250 ml ⎫ **or** ____ ⎫ g in 100 ml
    Dextrose 70% .... 500 ml ⎬

B. Electrolytes and other additives: (to be added in 24 hour supply)

☐ Sodium chloride .... ____ mEq   ☐ *Sodium (as phosphate) ...... ____ mEq
    or   or
☐ Sodium acetate .... ____ mEq   ☐ *Potassium (as phosphate) .... ____ mEq
☐ Calcium gluconate .... ____ mEq   ☐ *Trace elements (ped.)........ ____ ml
☐ Magnesium sulfate .... ____ mEq   ☐ Zinc chloride 1,000 mcg/ml ... ____ ml
☐ Hyperlyte .... ____ ml   ☐ Ascorbic acid .... ____ mg
☐ Insulin regular .... ____ U   ☐ Folic acid.................... ____ mcg
☐ Potassium chloride .... ____ mEq   ☐ Vitamin B_{12} .... ____ mcg
    or   ☐ MVI Conc .... ____ ml
☐ Potassium acetate .... ____ mEq   ☐ Berocca C .... ____ ml
                                       ☐ _____ .... ____

    *Refer to the electrolyte and incompatability notes

C. Intralipids 10%   Rate of administration: ____ml/hr for 24 hr
                     Number of hours if prescribed for less than 24 hr: ____hr

---

MD Signature: _____   Level: _____

Date: _____   Room no./bed no. _____

Time: _____   Weight of the patient: _____

Bottle sequence: _____   Patient Addressograph

TPN#_____

Electrolyte notes
1. **Amino acid:** Each 100 ml contains 1 ml of sodium and 1 μM of phosphate ions, which will always be in addition to the electrolytes ordered.
2. **Calcium gluconate:** 1 g = 4.8mEq of Ca^{++}
3. **Magnesium sulfate:** 1 g = 8.12 mEq of Mg^{++}
4. **Hyperlyte vial:** Each 25 ml contains Na^+ = 25 mEq, K^+ = 40.5 mEq, Ca^{++} = 5 mEq, Cl = 33.5 mEq, acetate 40.6 mEq, and gluconate = 5 mEq.
5. **Sodium phosphate:** 1 ml contains 4 mEq of Na^+ and 3 mM of P.
6. **Potassium phosphate:** 1 ml contains 4.4 mEq of K^+ add 3 mM of P.
7. **Pediatric trace elements:** Each 0.5 ml contains, zinc 100 mcg, copper 20 mcg, chromium 0.17 mcg, manganese 6 mcg (recommended dose up to 5 years of age: 0.5 ml/kg/d). **Note:** Since zinc requirement for neonates (recommended dose) is 300 mcg/kg/day, and extra 200 mcg/kg/day may be ordered separately for neonatal patients.
Incompatibility note:
Calcium and phosphate/ions: (conditional compatability) Calcium up to conc. of mEq is compatible with phosphate up to conc. of 20 mM/liter when present in the same TPN bottle. Calcium ion may be increased to 12 mEq if phosphate ion is decreased to 15 mM/liter.

Monitoring

1. Continuously monitor vital signs and catheter site.
2. Weigh infant daily.

3. Measure head circumference and height weekly.

4. Monitor hemotocrit, white blood cell count, blood urea nitrogen, blood glucose, electrolytes, and pH every day for 4 days and then every week.

5. Monitor serum magnesium, calcium, phosphorus, and protein levels initially and then every week.

6. Monitor SGOT, SGPT, lactic dehydrogenase, alkaline phosphatase, total and direct bilirubin, and creatinine levels initially and then every week.

7. Monitor copper, zinc, and iron levels initially and then every month.

8. Urinalysis daily.

9. Serum evaluation for hyperlipemia daily.

10. Cultures, as indicated.

11. Sunflower seed oil applications to the skin.

Complications

1. Catheter-related

    a. Infection (sepsis, shock, endocarditis).

    b. Phlebitis, thrombosis, embolism.

    c. Cardiac arrhythmias.

2. Metabolic

    a. Hyperglycemia.

    b. Hypoglycemia.

    c. Electrolyte disturbances.

    d. Hypophosphatemia.

    e. Hyperammonemia (treated by arginine and/or ornithine infusion; could be prevented by adding arginine, 0.5 to 1 mm/kg/day; to avoid coma, the amino acid concentration in the infusate may have to be increased gradually over a 2-day period).

    f. Acidosis (treated by decreasing glucose infusion rate by 50% plus sodium bicarbonate or sodium acetate).

    g. Zinc deficiency causing acrodermatitis (first evidence may be decreased alkaline phosphatase).

    h. Hypomagnesemia.

3. Lipid (do not use lipids in very low birth weight infants)

    a. Hyperlipidemia.

    b. Deposition in the lungs and the reticuloendothelial system.

    c. Aggravate hyperbilirubinemia.

    d. Acute syndrome of fever, respiratory distress, cyanosis, vomiting, and local skin irritation (discontinue TPN).

4. Other complications

   a. Hepatocellular damage.

   b. CO_2 production secondary to glucose oxidation, and aggravating respiratory distress and ventilator therapy.

WEANING

1. Start with oral fluids (90–150 ml/day).

2. Decrease the intravenous infusion rate and volume and increase the enteral intake and volume.

3. Use a lactose-free formula.

4. Once the enteral intake includes 2 to 2.5 mg/kg/day of protein and 100 cal/kg/day, discontinue TPN.

5. Use 10% dextrose i.v. for 12 hr.

6. Use 5% dextrose i.v. for 12 hr and then discontinue.

Tuberculosis

Tuberculosis is an infectious disease caused by *Mycobacterium tuberculosis*. The incidence and significance of the disease has changed markedly over the years since the discovery of its etiology and effective treatment. Diagnostic techniques and mass screening programs permit early diagnosis of primary infections and early treatment, decreasing the prevalence of active disease, although it is still present. Accurate diagnosis and management of children with tuberculosis is essential to maintain a good prognosis.

PATHOPHYSIOLOGY

The pathophysiology of tuberculosis is outlined in Fig. 1.

SIGNS AND SYMPTOMS

In adults and older children, it is common for patients with tuberculosis to be asymptomatic. However, more than half of the infants with tuberculosis have symptoms. Cough, pulmonary findings and infiltrates, pleural effusions, and/or hilar adenopathy are several findings that suggest pulmonary involvement. Nonspecific findings of failure to thrive, fever of unknown origin, and/or hepatosplenomegaly may also be present. Patients with miliary tuberculosis present signs and symptoms of either diffuse pulmonary and/or systemic involvement. Hepatosplenomegaly is common and the patients appear to be significantly ill.

Cervical adenopathy may occur in the presence or absence of systemic involvement. Abacteruric pyuria may occur in patients with miliary involvement.

Tuberculous meningitis is manifested as part of systemic disease or as an isolated phenomenon. There are three distinct stages: The first stage is characterized by nonspecific findings of fever, malaise, lethargy, vomiting, and a generally ill appearance; following, in stage 2, are neurological signs and symptoms, especially those of meningeal irritation (e.g., stiff neck, Kernig's and Brudzinski's signs), although the younger the patient, the less consistent the findings; stage three is characterized by sensorial changes in addition to the symptoms associated with the other stages.

DIFFERENTIAL DIAGNOSIS

1. Pneumonia: Bacterial, viral, mycoplasma, fungal
2. Aspiration

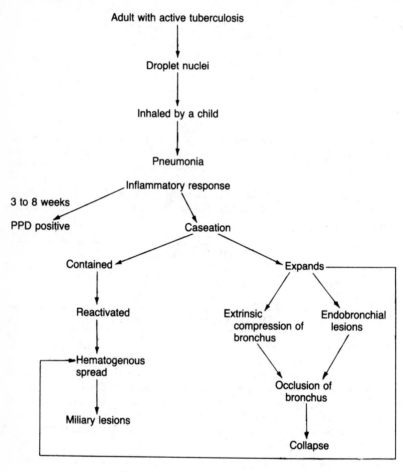

FIG. 1.   Pathophysiology of tuberculosis.

3. Tumor

4. Meningitis: Septic, aseptic

5. Septicemia

6. Urinary tract infection

DIAGNOSTIC PROTOCOL

1. Purified protein derivative (PPD) skin test.

2. Chest radiograph.

3. Early morning gastric aspirates (three) for acid-fast staining and culture for the tubercle bacillus.

4. Liver function tests to identify miliary lesions.

5. Urinalysis and urine culture (acid-fast staining of the first morning void may also be helpful).

6. Pleural biopsy, lymph node biopsy, and/or liver biopsy.

7. Blood cultures.

8. Cerebrospinal fluid examinations.

TREATMENT PROTOCOL

1. Recent PPD conversion with a normal chest radiograph: Isoniazid (INH), 5 to 10 mg/kg/24 hr p.o. for 12 months (complete blood cell count and liver function testing before and several times during the course of treatment).

2. Mild active pulmonary disease (two-drug regimen): INH, 10 mg/kg/24 hr, plus para-amino salicylic acid (PAS), 0.2 to 0.3 g/24 hr, **or** ethambutol (ETH), 15 mg/kg/24 hr (>13 years old), **or** rifampin (RIF), 10 to 20 mg/kg/24 hr.

3. Extensive pulmonary disease, miliary disease, and/or meningitis

   a. Supportive and symptomatic care, especially cardiovascular and respiratory support.

   b. Adequate hydration and calories.

   c. Control seizures, if present.

   d. Antituberculous therapy (triple therapy): INH, 15 mg/kg/24 hr, **plus** RIF, 10 to 20 mg/kg/24 hr, **plus** streptomycin, 20 to 40 mg/kg/24 hr (maximum dose of 1 g/day); continue regimen for 12 weeks, then switch to INH **plus** PAS or INH **plus** ETH for 24 months.

4. Pyridoxine, 25 to 50 mg/day, is usually given to children >8 years of age who are taking INH.

5. Corticosteroids have been used in patients with tuberculous meningitis and those with disseminated disease.

Ulcerative Colitis

Ulcerative colitis is a major chronic inflammatory disease of the bowel. The etiology of the disease is unknown. Acute exacerbations and remissions of symptoms occur and are characteristic. Successful diagnosis and management of the disease requires that the practitioner have a high index of suspicion. There is no cure, but affected patients may live a relatively normal life with few modifications and/or restrictions.

PATHOPHYSIOLOGY

The etiology and pathophysiological mechanisms of ulcerative colitis are unknown. There is diffuse inflammation of the rectum and descending colon, although the entire colon may be involved. More than 30% of the patients with ulcerative colitis have involvement of the terminal ileum. The inflammation is limited to the mucosa and submucosal regions, although crypt abscesses can occur. The mucosa is friable and, occasionally, ulcers are present.

SIGNS AND SYMPTOMS

Diarrhea, often mucopurulent or bloody, and abdominal pain are common. Fever is often present. The most common extraintestinal manifestation of ulcerative colitis is arthritis. Ninety percent of the patients exhibit involvement of the rectum early in the disease. However, perianal involvement is unusual. Physical findings are less striking than in Crohn's disease and primarily consist of nonspecific, diffuse abdominal tenderness. Failure to thrive, weight loss, anorexia, and developmental (maturational) delay are more commonly seen in patients with Crohn's disease than with ulcerative colitis, but these findings do occur in the latter disease. Abdominal cramps prior to defecation, tenesmus, waking at night to defecate, pallor, anemia, erythema multiforme, liver disease, and iritis may occur.

DIFFERENTIAL DIAGNOSIS

1. Crohn's disease
2. Acute gastroenteritis: Viral, bacterial *(Salmonella, shigella)*, parasitic
3. Hirschsprung's disease (with enterocolitis)
4. Malabsorption syndromes

5. Gastrointestinal tract tumors

6. Atopic disorders

DIAGNOSTIC PROTOCOL

1. Complete blood cell count.

2. Urinalysis.

3. Stool cultures.

4. Stool smear for polymorphonuclear leukocytes, ova, and parasites.

5. Electrolytes, blood urea nitrogen, and creatinine.

6. Liver function tests and clotting studies.

7. Proctoscopy and/or sigmoidoscopy.

8. Barium enema with postevacuation radiographs: Shaggy, barium-filled ulcers, loss of haustral markings, and shortening of the colon are seen.

9. Upper gastrointestinal series and a small bowel radiograph.

10. Rectal biopsy.

TREATMENT PROTOCOL

Dietary Considerations

1. Avoid high fiber foods, fresh fruits, milk products, and any food that causes exacerbation of symptoms; these foods should be eliminated for 2 to 3 weeks; intake may be resumed after adequate control is achieved, but specific foods that cause exacerbations should be avoided and not resumed.

2. Ferrous sulfate (6 mg/kg/24 hr p.o. in three divided doses), if iron deficiency anemia is present.

3. Diarrhea may be controlled by diphenoxylate hydrochloride, 2.5 to 5 mg/dose; use depends on the age of the child; toxic megacolon may occur with the use of antidiarrheal drugs and the medication should be immediately discontinued if the patient experiences abdominal distention.

4. Nutrition must be adequate to maintain a positive nitrogen balance; total parenteral nutrition may be required in some patients.

Medications

1. Sulfasalazine

    a. Used in patients with mild symptoms and those initially controlled with prednisone.

    b. Begin with 250 to 500 mg four times a day for 2 or 3 days; if there are no side effects or reactions, the dosage may be increased to 2 to 8 g/24 hr for 3 months.

    c. After there is adequate control of symptoms, the dosage may be decreased to 1 to 2 g/day for long-term administration.

2. Prednisone

    a. Begin with 2 mg/kg/day p.o. for 2 to 3 weeks (maximum dose, 60 mg); taper the dose by 5 mg every other week.

    b. If chronic prednisone administration is required, an every-other-day regimen should be employed.

    c. Acute exacerbations may be treated with ACTH or hydrocortisone.

3. Arthritis and/or ankylosing spondylitis may be treated with salicylates

Surgery

Indications for surgery are: Poor response to medical therapy, toxic megacolon, increased chance of developing malignancy (adenocarcinoma), severe maturational and growth retardation.

Urinary Tract Infections

Urinary tract infections often occur in children and are a relatively common cause of their hospitalization. The incidence of uncomplicated urinary tract infection ranges from 0.03% in schoolboys to a high of 3% in preterm infants. In almost all age groups, other than neonates, girls have a significantly higher rate of infection than boys. In neonates, this ratio may be reversed due to a higher incidence of congenital renal malformations in boys. These deformities are often associated with ascending or hematogenously spread infections. Most uncomplicated urinary tract infections (i.e., not recurrent or unassociated with anatomical abnormalities) are caused by a single organism (*E. coli, Proteus,* or *Klebsiella*). Complicated infections are more often caused by *Pseudomonas, Staphylococcus,* or mixed organisms.

Urinary tract infections may result when bacteria infect the urinary tract through poor hygiene or poor toilet habits in girls and may be exacerbated by infrequent bladder emptying. In neonates, the usual route of seeding is hematogenous. Other causative factors, other than reflux, may be more idiosyncratic and relate to the individual immune response of the host (Fig. 1).

There is an ongoing controversy as to whether asymptomatic bacteriuria should be treated as urinary tract infection. Asymptomatic bacteriuria is defined as the growth of more than 10^5 colonies of a single organism per milliliter of urine in three consecutive urine samples, with no associated host symptoms. Many urologists tend to treat asymptomatic bacteriuria as recurrent urinary tract infection (see Treatment Protocol).

The basis for treatment of urinary tract infection centers on the differentiation between upper urinary tract infection (pyelonephritis) and lower urinary tract infection (cystitis). In theory, a lower urinary tract infection is one that is confined to the bladder, whether or not there is actual invasion of the bladder mucosa (as in hemorrhagic cystitis). Cystitis is not thought to be a harbinger of future renal insufficiency, unless it is chronic and involved with advanced degrees of reflux. Cystitis usually causes symptoms of dysuria, burning, frequency, and dribbling, but rarely a high spiking fever and chills. Upper urinary tract infections are classically associated with fevers and chills and the potential for pyelonephritic changes within the kidneys. The treatment of upper urinary tract infections is usually parenteral, whereas lower urinary tract infections require only oral antibiotic therapy (a short course of the antibiotic is usually sufficient).

SIGNS AND SYMPTOMS

Signs and symptoms of urinary tract infection vary according to the age of the child. Neonates may have a history of maternal antepartum infection, congenital

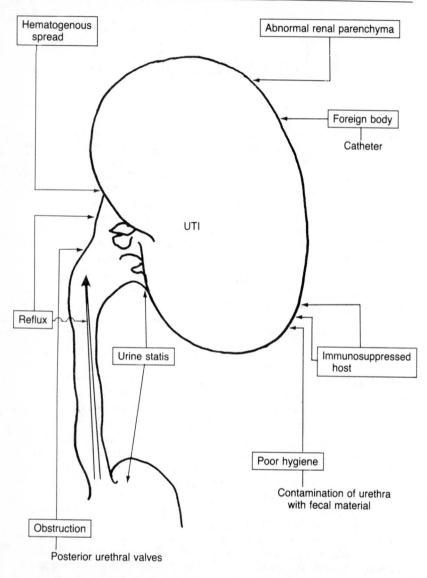

FIG. 1. Pathophysiology of urinary tract infection (UTI).

anomalies, anorexia, irritability, vomiting, diarrhea, or jaundice. Signs of septicemia, failure to thrive, meningitis, seizures, respiratory irregularities, cyanosis, fever, or hypothermia may be present. Older children may present with complaints of fever, chills, vomiting, incontinence, urgency, dysuria, anorexia, or backaches. Frequency, urgency, incontinence, fever, or hematuria may occur. As previously stated, chills, high fever, back pain, and abdominal pain are more common when the upper urinary tract is involved.

DIFFERENTIAL DIAGNOSIS

1. Upper urinary tract infection (pyelonephritis)
2. Lower urinary tract infection (cystitis)
3. Urethritis
4. Prostatitis
5. Meatitis
6. Foreign body
7. Chemical irritants
8. Nonspecific vaginitis

DIAGNOSTIC PROTOCOL

Indirect Detection Methods for Upper and Lower Urinary Tract Infections

1. Urine microscopy: Although not specifically diagnostic, this procedure can provide an accurate provisional diagnosis of a urinary tract infection.

   a. Pyuria: White blood cells (pus cells) in the urine, indicative of inflammation but not specific for urinary tract infection; significant pyuria is usually defined as >5 to 10 white blood cells per high power field in a centrifuged specimen; may occur with fever, glomerulonephritis, dehydration, or poor collection techniques. Riley (1975) showed that only 40% of patients with >10 white blood cells per high power field had significant bacteriuria. Dodge (1969) showed that only 50% of females with asymptomatic bacteriuria had pyuria. Quantitative leukocyte excretion rates showed that only 74% of the patients studied (over a 3-hr period) had urinary tract infections.

   b. Glitter cells: Glitter cells are pale-staining large white blood cells identified with a Sternheimer-Malbin stain and thought to be evidence of an upper urinary tract infection; the frequently cited motility of the cytoplasmic granules in these cells depends on the osmolality of the urinary solution; the significance of these cells is questionable.

   c. Leukocyte casts: Reflect inflammation but not necessarily infection, within the kidneys; must be differentiated from white blood cell clumps.

   d. Gram stain: Identification of one or more bacteria per high power or oil field in an **uncentrifuged** specimen correlates 70% to 85% with 100,000 colonies of bacteria per milliliter of urine obtained by culture of a clean voided midstream sample.

2. Urine culture

   a. Clean voided midstream urine specimens, are often contaminated with periurethral bacteria. The periuretheral area should be carefully cleaned with an iodine-based solution, followed by thorough rinsing of the antiseptic. In a symptomatic patient, the growth of 100,000 colonies of a single organism from a clean voided urine specimen represents an 80% to 85% probability of infection; in an asymptomatic patient, this growth would indicate a probability of less than 80%. For statistical accuracy an asymptomatic patient must have three consecutive urine cultures, each growing the same organism in significant numbers; a symptomatic patient will only require two similar cultures. Fulfillment of the above criteria will indicate 95% probability of a urinary tract infection.

b. Catheterized urine specimens are less often contaminated than clean voided specimens, but this procedure is looked upon negatively by many pediatricians for fear of introducing organisms through the urethra into the bladder. The probability of that event (6%) is more a question of the catheterization technique than of the procedure itself. Significant bacterial growth in a single catheterized urine specimen is statistically much more valid than in a single clean voided urine specimen and correlates strongly with a urinary tract infection.

c. Suprapubic aspiration, although more invasive than other procedures, can save the patient and parent repeated office or hospital visits, as well as the expense of having multiple urine tests. Growth of more than 200 colonies per milliliter of urine is significant. Misleading results were obtained 38% of the time when clean voided specimens were compared with the results obtained by suprapubic aspiration. The potential complications of suprapubic aspirations are minimal, consisting mainly of microscopic hematuria and minor discomfort for the patient.

Direct Detection Methods for Upper Urinary Tract Infections

1. Bladder wash-out: This test consists of catheterizing the child, instilling an antibiotic solution into the bladder, followed by rinsing of the solution from the bladder, and draining the bladder, thereupon collecting urine for a culture; a single positive test is statistically significant.

2. Ureteral catheterization: Although this procedure correlates well with urinary tract infections, it is too invasive for general clinical application.

3. Culture of renal biopsy material: Although infection may be documented in the course of renal biopsy, this procedure is usually done to determine the prognosis or treatment of other conditions.

Indirect Detection Methods for Upper Urinary Tract Infections

1. Determination of specific serum antibodies against the infecting organism: This test is designed to detect infections of the renal parenchyma with the production of antibodies against the invading organism; infections of the lower urinary tract theoretically do not result in antibody production; antibodies against the "0" antigen of *E. coli* (the most common organism causing simple urinary tract infection) are utilized.

a. The test appears to be invalid within the first 2 months of life.

b. The test is specific for the antibody tested and thus depends on the number of occurrences, i.e., in the first pyelonephritic episode IgM antibody might be expected to be produced; therefore, it is important to determine if a hemagglutination or precipitation test is needed.

2. Antibody-coated bacteria in the urine: This test is again based on the principle that bacterial infections of the renal parenchyma (not the lower urinary tract) will produce antibodies that coat the offending bacteria and can be detected by fluorescent methods; this test may be more sensitive than titrating serum antibodies, as above; it is not affected by proteinuria, but tends to be less sensitive in children than in adults.

3. Urinary lactic dehydrogenase isoenzymes: This test relies on two different isoenzyme patterns, reflecting upper versus lower urinary tract damage, with the former being reflected by slower moving isoenzymes (fourth and fifth components).

4. Erythrocyte sedimentation rate and c-reactive protein: These are both altered by acute phase reactants and thus may be nonspecific in their response. Some data show that quantitative CRP≥20 mg/100 ml may reflect upper urinary tract infection.

Office and/or Rapid Screening Techniques

1. The pour-plate culture technique is standard for the culturing of bacteria in most laboratories. This method has withstood the test of time and is both valid and reliable, but is usually too time consuming for office practice.

2. A thorough microscopic examination and Gram stain of an uncentrifuged urine specimen correlates with culture results approximately 80% to 90% of the time.

3. Chemical screening methods: These methods depend on viable bacteria in the urine to produce the required chemical change. Ideally, they require a clean voided morning urine specimen collected before fluid or food ingestion.

    a. Griess nitrite test: Most gram-negative bacteria convert nitrate to nitrite in urine, and the latter product results in this reagent turning red; false positive rates are low (0.3%); false negative rates tend to be slightly higher.

    b. Triphenyltetrazolium chloride test: This test is cumbersome and requires a 4-hr incubation period; a red precipitate indicates a positive test. False negative rates are variable, but may be in the range of 35%; false positive rates range from 8% to 10%.

    c. Glucose test method: This test depends on the catabolism of urine glucose to <1 mg/100 ml (2–20 mg/100 ml normally present) by viable bacteria. (It requires a hypersensitive reagent strip which can detect better than 1 mg/100 ml of glucose in the urine.) Obviously, this test cannot be used in diabetics and should not be used when the patient is undergoing water diuresis, which may result in a smaller number of bacteria per aliquot (dilution). The test has high false negative rates (*Pseudomonas* is also frequently not detected); the false positive rate is 2% to 10%.

4. Immediate cultures

  a. Dipstick (Testuria®): This test depends on the absorption and growth of bacteria on a piece of filter paper with agar. The presence of more than four colonies after incubation indicates a positive test; the error rate is <5%.

  b. Dip slide (Uricult®): This slide is impregnated with culture media. False negatives occur in <10% and false positives in <3%.

Medical History, Physical Examination, Laboratory Investigations

1. Assessment of the severity and significance of the infection.

2. Identification of microorganisms in subsequent sensitivity tests.

3. Identification of factors that may predispose the child to infection (e.g., steroids, immunosuppressive drugs, glycosuria).

4. Determine the presence or absence of sepsis associated with any potential structural abnormalities or underlying disease.

5. Determine the efficacy of therapy at 48 hr; a culture of the urine should be sterile if the therapy has been adequate.

6. Both boys and girls with urinary tract infections may have underlying anatomical abnormalities. Several authorities advocate delaying radiographic examinations of girls older than 3 years of age until a second infection has been documented, but we believe that every child with a urinary tract infection should have radiographic evaluation, including an IVP and a voiding cystourethrogram. Although many children who undergo these procedures will have no significant anatomical abnormalities, many others will benefit from early detection of significant obstructive disease or severely incompetent vesicoureteral junctions. The question of radiation to the child may become academic as more facilities are able to do the above studies using radionuclide cystourethrogram.

7. Delay anatomical studies after urinary tract infection to minimize the possibility of confusing mild reflux induced by infection with anatomic abnormality. Although <1% of randomly selected children are found to have reflux, nearly 50% of infants with urinary tract infections have at least mild reflux. Moreover, approximately 25% of them have associated anatomical abnormalities at the time of their first diagnosed urinary tract infection.

8. Radiographic studies may reveal multiple structural abnormalities consisting of defects in the upper and lower tracts (vesicoureteral reflux, ureteral pelvic junction obstruction, calyceal obstruction, bladder diverticuli, and intravesicle obstruction).

TREATMENT PROTOCOL

General

1. Provide symptomatic treatment of fever or vomiting, as needed.

2. Encourage fluid intake to ensure adequate diuresis.

3. Encourage complete and frequent bladder emptying if the child is capable.

4. A bladder analgesic such as phenazopyridine hydrochloride (Pyridium®) (7–10 mg/kg/day) is occasionally helpful for dysuria.

5. Acidification of the urine by ascorbic acid (250–500 mg three times a day) has proved to be helpful in some patients.

6. Hospitalization may be necessary in patients with systemic symptoms and is mandatory in neonates.

Acute Uncomplicated Urinary Tract Infection

1. Immediate treatment is age dependent.

   a. Neonates

   (1) In neonates, urinary tract infections can constitute one of the components of a gram-negative septicemia or can be the site of origin of bacteremia.

   (2) Suprapubic tap or bladder catheterization is mandatory when sepsis is suspected in neonates.

   (3) Neonates should receive parenteral antibiotic therapy (ampicillin and/or gentamicin) for 10 to 14 days.

   b. Older children

   (1) In older children, an orally absorbable, nontoxic antibiotic, such as a short-acting sulfonamide or ampicillin, is usually recommended for 10 days.

   (2) The urine should be recultured in 48 hr; if treatment has been successful, there should be no growth of bacteria.

   (3) Follow-up cultures are essential over a period of about 2 years because of the frequency of recurrence: One week after completion of therapy, monthly for 6 months, every second month for 6 months, and every third month for 1 year.

   (4) A single dose of an antibiotic orally or intramuscularly may be successful treatment for lower urinary tract infection.

Relapse or Reinfection

1. Patients with a subsequent relapse (same bacteria) or reinfection (different species of bacteria) who have no anatomical abnormality, should be given an additional course of antibiotics, often the same one used to treat the original infection.

   a. Although the organisms in recurrent infection are not usually the same as the original infecting agent, some authorities believe that they are usually from the same groups of bacteria causing uncomplicated infections *(E. coli, Klebsiella, Proteus).*

   b. An infection-free period of 1 year will often imply a long-term remission.

   c. Frequent recurrences, whether associated with structural abnormality or not, are best treated with low dose, once-daily suppressive therapy for 6 months to 1 year: Nitrofurantoin, 1 to 2 mg/kg/day, *or* trimethoprim, 2 mg/kg/day, *and* sulfamethoxazole, 10 mg/kg/day.

Structural Abnormality

The ultimate treatment must be a team approach and tailored to the patient's needs.

Vesicoureteral Reflux

Vesicoureteral reflux and its potential long-term consequences to the kidneys is an extremely controversial topic. In very young patients, who have marginal competence of the antireflux mechanisms, reflux may be merely a maturational component without sequelae in the healthy host. In the mature and properly functioning antireflux mechanism, the ureters pass obliquely through the bladder wall through submucosal tunnels to their termination, the ureteral orifices. Lengthening of the submucosal tunnels by dynamic mechanisms of the bladder and neurological control helps to close the ureteric openings and prevent the reflux of urine.

It is not known with certainty that persistent reflux of sterile urine causes progressive renal scarring. If it does, at what point is antireflux surgery indicated? It has been shown that in approximately 40% to 50% of patients with reflux there will be spontaneous resolution over a period of time. Unfortunately, in younger children (particularly in those younger than 3 years of age), the time required for lengthening of the ureters by growth may be unacceptable. It is in this group that the risk for renal damage is the highest.

PATHOPHYSIOLOGY

The pathophysiology of vesicoureteral reflux is indefinite (see Differential Diagnosis).

SIGNS AND SYMPTOMS

There are few specific symptoms that may be ascribed directly to reflux. Some patients complain of pain in the area of the kidneys during the initiation of urination (corresponding to the time refluxing urine strikes the kidneys). Most other symptoms appear to be related to complications associated with or caused by reflux (e.g., urinary tract infection and/or hypertension). Certain clinical or laboratory signs may be seen: abnormal urine sediment, decreased ability to concentrate urine (especially in cases with infected urine), signs of renal insufficiency, irregular or focal scarring of renal tissue, lack of growth in the affected kidney(s), abnormal renal anatomy, and/or decreased somatic growth.

DIFFERENTIAL DIAGNOSIS

The differential diagnosis of vesicoureteral reflux may be based on its manifestations, but more readily lends itself to an elaboration of the types of defects resulting in reflux, the anatomical configurations of the refluxing orifices, and the grading or staging of reflux. Reflux may be unilateral or bilateral and low pressure (appearing soon after the contrast is instilled into the bladder) or high pressure (appearing at voiding). Reflux may also show gradation in the degree of reflux:

Grade 1: Reflux into the ureters only.

Grade 2: Reflux into the calyces without ballooning.

Grade 3: Reflux into the calyces with ballooning.

Grade 4: Intrarenal (parenchymal) reflux.

In considering the causes of reflux, each of the grades should be considered in an attempt to determine the severity of the reflux.

Primary Reflux

Anatomical maldevelopment of the ureterovesical junction.

1. Abnormalities of the ureteral orifice involving position and/or shape, e.g., lateral placement of the ureteral orifice with an abnormal configuration (golf-hole, stadium, or horseshoe).

2. Ureteral duplication (complete) with ectopic placement and ureter usually going to lower pole; often associated with infection.

3. Paraureteral diverticulum.

4. Familial reflux nephropathy.

Secondary Reflux

1. Infection, inflammation, and/or irritation in the ureterovesical angle.

2. Neurogenic dysfunction (occasional resolution with maturation of the nerve).

3. Renal disorders (increased production or decreased concentrating ability may indirectly result in reflux by altering the anatomy of the ureters and bladder).

4. Obstructive uropathies (posterior and anterior urethral valves, bladder outlet obstruction, meatal stenosis).

5. Congenital anomalies of the kidney (shape or position).

6. Miscellaneous

   a. Prune belly syndrome.

   b. Exstrophy of the bladder.

7. Postsurgical procedure, especially of the ureterovesical angle.

DIAGNOSTIC PROTOCOL

1. Urinalysis and urine culture; if the culture is positive, treat with a short course of antibiotics.

2. If the culture is negative or 6 weeks after adequate treatment, obtain an intravenous pyelogram and a voiding cystourethrogram (VCU).

3. If the reflux is grade 3 or 4, a significant anatomical defect is present, and/or renal scarring is noted, refer the patient to a urologist for cystoscopy and surgical correction (ureteroneocystotomy).

4. If surgical intervention is delayed, obtain urine cultures every 6 weeks after treatment; if the infection recurs, suppressive therapy is indicated.

5. A VCU should be obtained every 6 months and reviewed with the urologist.

TREATMENT PROTOCOL

1. The regimen must be based on the age of the child at the time of diagnosis, the degree of reflux, the presence or absence of associated deformities, any changes in the kidneys secondary to reflux, and any secondary systemic changes ascribed to the reflux.

2. A very youthful child with a grade 3 or 4 reflux who has associated deformities and/or systemic changes requires surgical intervention.

3. Medical therapy is appropriate for a child with grade 2 reflux who has yet to undergo a growth spurt, is beyond the most sensitive age for developing atrophic pyelonephritis (4–5 years), and is not showing untoward kidney changes.

  a. Keep urine sterile with appropriate antibiotics.

  b. Routine urine cultures for early detection of infection.

  c. Tincture of time (wait for lengthening of the ureters with the child's growth).

Vomiting

Vomiting may be a symptom of gastrointestinal tract dysfunction, or it may be a nonspecific symptom of a systemic disease process. However, it may result in a secondary pathological disturbance because of fluid, electrolyte, and/or calorie loss.

GENERAL TREATMENT PROTOCOL

1. Hydrate: Provide fluids to account for deficits, ongoing losses, and maintenance.

2. Electrolytes and acid-base balance: Correct deficits, account for ongoing losses, and provide maintenance.

3. Treat the underlying cause.

DIAGNOSTIC AND TREATMENT PROTOCOLS

Table 1 gives diagnostic and treatment protocols for various vomiting disorders.

TABLE 1. *Vomiting: Diagnostic and treatment protocols*

Diagnosis	Treatment
Central Nervous System Related	
Tumor, increased intracranial pressure, infection, migraine Acute, insidious, or cyclical onset of symptoms Vomiting may or may not be projectile Often associated with neurological signs and symptoms	Treat the underlying cause
Drugs	
Chemotherapy, ipecac–intentional or unintentional, aminophylline, lead, others Onset of vomiting is usually acute and associated with ingestion or administration of a drug	Chemotherapy reactions may be pretreated with phenothiazines (e.g., Compazine®, Thorazine®) Tigan®
Extraintestinal Infection	
Septicemia, urinary tract infection, otitis media, pneumonia, meningitis Acute or indolent onset of symptoms Vomiting may or may not be associated with diarrhea Fever is often present Associated symptoms may occur	Treat the underlying cause

572

Diagnosis	Treatment

Gastrointestinal Tract Anatomical Abnormalities

Pyloric stenosis, volvulus, atresia, stenosis, intussusception, Hirschsprung's disease, others Acute or chronic symptoms Occasionally, vomiting is projectile (e.g., pyloric stenosis) Abdominal physical findings are usually remarkable and may show signs of obstruction	Surgical treatment of the underlying cause

Gastrointestinal Tract Infection

Bacterial, viral, parasitic Insidious or acute onset of symptoms Upper or lower gastrointestinal tract involvement Vomiting is usually nonprojectile Fever and/or diarrhea may be present	Clear liquids (if the patient cannot receive alimentation orally, intravenous fluids and electrolytes are required) Electrolyte solutions (Lytren®, Pedialyte®) may be given orally >10% Dehydration or large ongoing fluid losses necessitate intravenous therapy Advance the patient to a regular diet after 24 hr, or as tolerated

Labrynthine (Motion Sickness)

Acute onset of vomiting associated with travel and motion (e.g., air, car, sea)	Antihistamines are effective but must be utilized before travel

Metabolic Diseases

Diabetic ketoacidosis, uremia, Reye's syndrome, hypercalcemia, metabolic abnormalities Acute or chronic symptoms Vomiting is usually nonprojectile Frequently associated with other signs and/or symptoms (e.g., dehydration, polydispia, renal failure, seizures	Treat the underlying cause

Poor Feeding Techniques

Improper feeding technique, inadequate food storage or preparation Regurgitation to forceful emesis Patient is usually otherwise healthy (failure to thrive may occur)	Anticipatory guidance, health education, reassurance Failure to thrive may necessitate hospitalization

Pregnancy

Morning sickness Hyperemesis gravidarum Acute or insidious onset Usually occurs in the first trimester of pregnancy	Doxylamine succinate and pyridoxine (Bendectin®) Antihistamines and phenothiazines but their usefulness is limited

Radiation

Onset of vomiting is usually acute and associated with radiation therapy	Antihistamines, trimethobenzamide (Tigan®), pyridoxine Haloperidol is effective, but is not recommended because of the high incidence of extra-pyramidal symptoms

Wilm's Tumor

Wilm's tumor is the second most common abdominal malignancy in childhood and the most common malignant tumor of the genitourinary tract. It is relatively rare, with approximately 400 new cases being reported each year. It usually occurs in children younger than 5 years of age (78% of cases) with the peak incidence occurring in the third or fourth year of life.

There appears to be a familial tendency, but there is no predilection for either sex. The tumor is bilateral in approximately 10% to 15% of affected patients. Associated congenital anomalies occur in approximately 15% of patients with Wilm's tumor.

The prognosis of Wilm's tumor depends on the histological characteristics of the tumor (better differentiated cell types carry a better prognosis), the age at diagnosis (the younger the patient at diagnosis, the better the prognosis), and the stage of the tumor at diagnosis (the more limited the tumor, the better the prognosis). The stages are defined as follows (Fig. 1):

Stage 1: The tumor mass is limited to the kidney and is completely resectable

Stage 2: The tumor extends beyond the kidney, but is still completely resectable (local extension beyond the kidney only)

Stage 3: The tumor is not completely resectable; it is confined to the abdomen, with no hematogenous metastasis

Stage 4: Bilateral renal involvement is present (at the time of diagnosis or any time after the diagnosis is made)

SIGNS AND SYMPTOMS

Patients usually present with the complaint of abdominal swelling or an abdominal mass discovered by the parents. Pain is unusual, unless the tumor is exceptionally large, growing very rapidly, and/or hemorrhaging. Hypertension and/or hematuria (usually microscopic) occurs in 25% of affected patients.

Other less common clinical manifestations include fever, hypotension, dyspnea, anemia, anorexia, diarrhea, or symptoms related to metastasis to the lungs, liver, or lymph nodes.

Associated congenital anomalies include nonfamilial aniridia, hemihypertrophy, Beckwith's syndrome, sexual ambiguity, genitourinary abnormalities (e.g., horseshoe kidneys, duplications, aplasia, hypoplasia, cryptorchidism, hypospadius), chromosomal abnormalities, microcephaly, and recurved otic pinna.

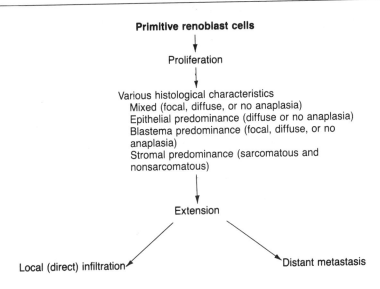

FIG. 1. Pathophysiology of Wilm's tumor.

DIFFERENTIAL DIAGNOSIS

1. Hydronephrosis
2. Polycystic kidney
3. Visceromegaly (organs other than kidneys)
   a. Hepatomegaly
   b. Splenomegaly
4. Other intra-abdominal tumors

DIAGNOSTIC PROTOCOL

1. Abdominal radiographs: Calcifications occur in approximately 10% of affected patients.
2. Chest radiograph: Pulmonary metastasis is the most common extra-abdominal site.
3. Abdominal ultrasonography: Reveals a solid tumor mass or enlarged kidney; the tumor is part of the kidney.
4. Intravenous pyelogram (IVP): Reveals an intrarenal mass with distortion of the

renal calyces (differentiated from neuroblastoma of adrenal origin by the fact that neuroblastoma is extrarenal and displaces a normal kidney downward).

5. Complete blood cell count.

6. Urinalysis: Microscopic hematuria occurs in approximately 25% of affected patients.

7. Angiography, aortography: May or may not be helpful; most useful when the kidney cannot be visualized on IVP.

8. Bone marrow aspiration: Rarely is there extension of the tumor to the bone or marrow.

TREATMENT PROTOCOL

1. The diagnosis and treatment of Wilm's tumor should be guided by an experienced pediatric oncologist and hematologist (oncologic therapeutics are extremely complicated and hazardous to the patient and must be performed by those experienced in tumor treatment).

2. Therapy is generally determined by the stage of the tumor:

Stage 1: Surgery + chemotherapy (actinomycin D and vincristine)

Stage 2: Surgery + radiation + chemotherapy (actinomycin D, vincristine, and adriamycin for 15 months)

Stage 3: Same as stage 2

Stage 4: (also patients with unfavorable histological findings at any stage): Surgery + radiation + chemotherapy (actinomycin D, vincristine, adriamycin, and ?cyclophosphamide for 15 months).

Appendixes

Acetaminophen Nomogram

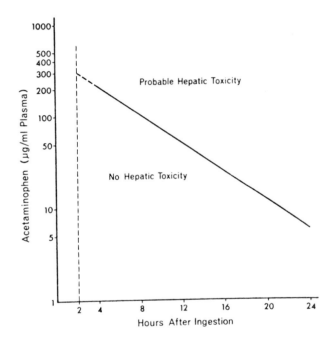

Semilogarithmic plot of plasma acetaminophen levels versus time. [Reproduced with permission from Rumack B.H., and Matthew, H. (1975): Acetaminophen poisoning and toxicity. *Pediatrics* 55:873. © American Academy of Pediatrics.]

Blood Transfusions

TRANSFUSIONS AND BLOOD COMPONENT THERAPY

Whole Blood Transfusion

1. Whole blood is usually used when larger volumes of blood are required (e.g., during surgery, to combat shock, in exchange transfusions).

2. In the absence of acute blood loss, the maximum transfusion volume should be 5 ml/lb of body weight (3 ml/lb if the hemoglobin is <5 g/100 ml).

3. Platelets in whole blood survive for approximately 6 hr at 0 to 6°C.

4. Blood must be warmed before infusion.

5. Clotting factors may not be present in adequate concentrations (factor VIII decreases after 8 hr, factor V after 3 days).

6. Certain biochemical abnormalities (e.g., acidosis, hyperkalemia, hypocalcemia) may result when large volumes of blood are transfused. These abnormalities are usually secondary to the type of anticoagulant used and the age of the blood transfused.

7. Do not use heparinized blood greater than 24-hr old, ACD solution (acid, citrate, dextrose) greater than 48-hr old, or CPD solution (citrate, phosphate, dextrose) greater than 5 days old.

8. A modified exchange transfusion should be performed if congestive heart failure is present.

9. In an emergency, use type-specific blood if available immediately, O negative packed cells, or whole blood (use AB negative plasma to resuspend the packed cells).

FACTOR VIII of 1 (see Bleeding Disorders chapter)

1. Use cryoprecipitate or fresh frozen plasma (the activity should be checked for each preparation used).

2. One unit of factor VIII/kg will raise the plasma factor VIII by approximately 2%.

3. The patient's partial thromboplastin time (PTT) is prolonged with factor VIII levels <40% of normal.

4. Factor VIII levels of 10% to 20% may stop soft-tissue bleeding, but higher levels are often required to stop other bleeding.

   a. Hemarthrosis: 20 units/kg initially, then 10 units/kg every 12 hr for 2 days.

b. Soft-tissue bleeding: 20 units/kg as a single infusion.

c. Serious soft-tissue bleeding: Same as for hemarthrosis.

d. Surgery: 50 units/kg initially, **then** 25 units/kg every 12 hr for 7 to 10 days, **and** 8 to 10 units/kg every 12 hr for the second week.

e. Severe surface bleeding: Same as for surgery.

Packed Red Blood Cells

1. Packed red blood cells (RBCs) are used primarily to raise the hemoglobin concentration in anemic and chronically ill patients when volume infusion is not a consideration or is contraindicated.

2. Calculation of transfusion requirements:

$$\text{Transfusion volume} = \frac{(\text{desired Hb level} - \text{patient's Hb level}) \times \text{body weight (kg)} \times \text{blood volume}}{\text{Hb concentration of packed RBCs}}$$

Blood volume = 80 to 85 cc/kg body weight in infants and 69cc/kg in adults. Hemoglobin (Hb) concentration of packed RBCs is usually 22 to 24 g/100 ml.

3. The volume transfused should generally not exceed 10 ml/kg.

4. Each gram of hemoglobin transfused contains approximately 3.4 mg of iron.

Platelets

Transfusion of platelet concentrate: 1 unit/10 lb of body weight should raise the platelet count by $50,000/mm^3$.

TRANSFUSION REACTIONS

Allergic Reaction

1. Signs and symptoms

    a. Urticaria.

    b. Pruritus.

    c. Periorbital edema.

    d. Laryngospasm.

    e. Cardiovascular collapse.

2. Treatment

    a. Stop the transfusion.

    b. Administer diphenhydramine, epinephrine, and/or steroids.

    c. A combination of antihistamines and steroids may be required.

Febrile Reaction

1. Signs and symptoms
   a. Variable degrees of fever and/or chills.
   b. Myalgia.
   c. Nausea and vomiting.
   d. Hemolysis and hemoglobinuria **do not** occur.

2. Treatment
   a. Stop the transfusion.
   b. Antipyretics and/or analgesics may be required.

Hemolytic Reaction

1. Signs and symptoms
   a. Same as for febrile reaction, but usually more marked.
   b. Acute hemolysis and hemoglobinuria.
   c. Hypotension and shock.

2. Treatment
   a. Stop the transfusion.
   b. Force diuresis with mannitol (50 to 100 ml of 20% solution); give fluids to keep the urine flow 1 to 3 ml/min.
   c. Give fluids containing 25 mEq of sodium bicarbonate after the initial mannitol infusion.

Body Surface Area Approximation from Weight

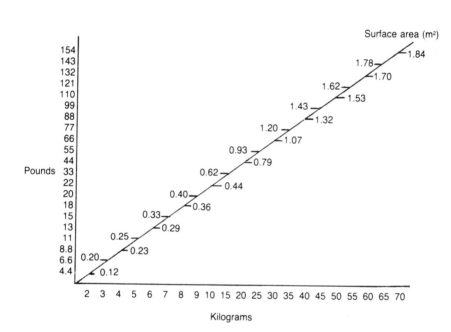

Calculations in Pediatrics

1. Anion gap

   = (sodium) − [(chloride + bicarbonate)]

2. Blood volume (total)

   Children and adolescents = 80 × weight (kg)
   Neonates and infants = 85 × weight (kg)

3. Creatinine clearance

$$= \frac{\text{urine creatinine (mg/dL)} \times \text{urine volume (ml/min)}}{\text{plasma creatinine (mg/dL)}} \times \frac{1.73}{\text{surface area (m}^2)}$$

4. Electrolytes, deficits

   mEq required = (desired − actual) × 0.6 × weight (kg)

5. Endotracheal tube size

   Internal diameter (mm) $= \dfrac{\text{age (years)} + 16}{4}$

6. Fat absorption coefficient

$$= \frac{\text{grams of fat ingested} - \text{grams of fat excreted}}{\text{grams of fat ingested}} \times 100$$

7. Fluids, deficits

   For each 5% of water loss, provide 50% over maintenance fluid requirement (e.g., 5% = maintenance plus 50% of maintenance; 10% = maintenance plus 100% of maintenance; 15% = maintenance plus 150% of maintenance)

8. Fluids, maintenance

   1,200 − 1,500 ml/m^2/24 hr, **or**
   100 ml/kg for the first 10 kg (0–10 kg)
    50 ml/kg for the next 10 kg (10–20 kg)
    20 ml/kg for each kg thereafter (>20 kg)

9. Hendersen-Hasselbach equation

$$\text{pH} = 6.1 + \frac{\log[\text{HCO}_3]}{0.3(\text{P}_{\text{CO}_2})}$$

10. Iron saturation

$$= \frac{\text{serum iron}}{\text{TIBC}} \times 100$$

11. Mean corpuscular hemoglobin (MCH)

$$= \frac{\text{hemoglobin (g/100 ml)}}{\text{RBC (million/mm}^3)} \times 10$$

12. Mean corpuscular hemoglobin concentration (MCHC)

$$= \frac{\text{hemoglobin (g/100 ml)}}{\text{hematocrit (\%)}} \times 100$$

13. Mean corpuscular volume (MCV)

$$= \frac{\text{hematocrit (\%)}}{\text{RBC (million/mm}^3)} \times 10$$

14. Mentzner formula

$$= \frac{\text{MCV}}{\text{RBC}}$$

(iron deficiency if >13.5; thalassemia if <11.5)

15. Metric conversions

1 in = 2.54 cm
1 kg = 2.2 lb

16. Osmolality, serum

$$= 2(\text{sodium}) + \frac{\text{glucose (mg/dL)}}{18} + \frac{\text{BUN (mg/dL)}}{2.8}$$

17. $Q-T$ interval correction

$$= \frac{\text{measured } Q-T}{\sqrt{R-R \text{ interval}}}$$

18. Temperature conversion

$$°F = (9/5 \times °C) + 32$$
$$°C = (°F - 32) \times 5/9$$

19. Transfusions, coagulation factors

See Bleeding Disorders chapter

20. Transfusions, packed red blood cells

$$= \frac{(\text{blood volume} \times \text{desired hemotocrit} - (\text{blood volume} \times \text{present hematocrit})}{\text{hematocrit of packed RBC (usually 60\% to 70\%)}}$$

21. Transfusions, partial exchange

$$\text{Vol (ml)} = \frac{\text{weight (kg)} \times 75 \text{ mg/kg} \times \text{desired rise in hemoglobin}}{22 \text{ g/100 ml} - [(\text{hemoglobin initial} + \text{hemoglobin desired})/2]}$$

22. Transfusions, platelets

1 unit increases the platelet concentration $12 \times 10^3/\text{mm}^3$

23. Tubular reabsorption of phosphate

$$= 1 - \frac{(\text{serum creatinine}) (\text{urine phosphate})}{(\text{serum phosphate}) (\text{urine creatinine})} \times 100 = 75\% \text{ to } 100\%$$

Common Pediatric Procedures

CAPILLARY BLOOD SAMPLING

1. Warm the extremity.
2. Use a sterile lancet (a #11 scalpel blade may be used, but take care to limit the depth of penetration beneath the skin).
3. Clean the area with alcohol **(let the alcohol dry before puncturing the skin).** The most convenient areas for obtaining the sample are the lateral aspect of the heel in neonates and small infants and the lateral aspect of the distal phalanx of the finger in older children. The heel pad and the palmar surface of the finger should be avoided.
4. Wipe away the first drop of blood with a dry sterile gauze pad, then begin the collection into capillary tubes. The tube is held at an angle within the drop of blood. It is drawn into the tube via capillary action. Aspiration is not necessary. Keep the tip of the tube away from the skin, since obstruction of the lumen may occur.
5. Seal one end of each tube with clay to avoid spillage.
6. Be sure not to squeeze the extremity; the blood must flow freely from the puncture site.

EVACUATION OF PLEURAL AIR

1. In an emergency situation, evacuation of air may be accomplished with a 22-gauge needle attached to a syringe and a 3-way stopcock. **This is a temporizing measure; chest tube insertion is the procedure of choice.**
    a. The area should be cleaned with iodine solution and alcohol and left to dry.
    b. The needle is inserted into the pleural cavity at the superior border of the third or fourth intercostal space in the midaxillary line.
    c. Air is evacuated with the syringe, the stopcock is adjusted to expel the air, and is then readjusted to again aspirate air from the pleural cavity.
2. Chest tube insertion
    a. The lateral chest wall should be cleaned with iodine solution and alcohol and left to dry.
    b. Sterile procedures are used throughout the insertion.
    c. An incision is made in the third or fourth intercostal space in the midaxillary line.
    d. A blunt dissection over the superior portion of the rib is performed in order to reach the pleural cavity.

e. The catheter is inserted into the pleural space and connected to a water seal and suction (15 to 20 cm H_2O pressure is used).

f. The catheter is secured with sutures and tape, then covered with a sterile dressing.

EXTERNAL JUGULAR PUNCTURE

1. Obtaining blood from the external jugular vein is a relatively simple and well-tolerated procedure. It should be used when children have small, inadequate, or unobtainable veins in the extremities.

2. The child should be appropriately and gently restrained on a bed or examination table.

3. The neck is gently extended and laterally flexed (this is easy to accomplish if the assistant will hold the child's head over the edge of the bed or table, supporting it from below).

4. The external jugular vein will distend when the child cries. The course of the vein can then be easily identified.

5. The area should be cleaned thoroughly with iodine solution and alcohol and left to dry.

6. When the vein is distended, a scalp vein needle is inserted and the blood withdrawn.

7. Upon removal of the needle, pressure is applied over the puncture site and the child is placed in an upright position.

LUMBAR PUNCTURE

1. The child should be gently and appropriately restrained (either lying laterally or in the sitting position); the neck and hips should be flexed.

2. Identify the second or third lumbar intercostal space.

3. The area should be cleaned with iodine solution and alcohol and left to dry (strictly adhere to aseptic technique).

4. A lumbar puncture needle (**a trocar is essential**) is inserted into the intercostal space and advanced until the dura is perforated (a subtle pop may be felt).

5. The trocar is carefully removed from the needle and cerebrospinal fluid pressure is measured. After the pressure is measured, the fluid is allowed to flow freely into the specimen containers (the fluid must not be aspirated; aseptic technique must be continued).

6. After the collection of fluid, the needle is removed and pressure is applied to the puncture area.

RADIAL ARTERY PUNCTURE

1. The radial artery should be identified by palpation.

2. The child's arm should be gently restrained with the palmar side up.

3. The area should be cleaned with iodine solution and alcohol and left to dry.

4. Two fingers are placed over the course of the artery (one proximal and one distal to the proposed puncture site) and the needle is inserted perpendicularly to the artery.

5. If possible, the arterial blood should be allowed to flow freely into the syringe. If the flow is slow, gentle suction may be applied.

6. If no blood is obtained and the needle has been inserted to the appropriate depth, gently withdraw the needle while looking for blood return (i.e., the artery may have been traversed with the needle).

7. After obtaining the appropriate sample, the needle is withdrawn and pressure is applied over the artery for 5 to 7 min. This assures hemostasis (significant hematoma formation may occur if inadequate pressure is applied).

SUPRAPUBIC TAP OF THE URINARY BLADDER

1. In preparation for a bladder tap, it is wise to place a urine collection bag over the patient's urethra; many children will urinate just prior to the aspiration.

2. The bladder should be full (it may or may not be palpable).

3. The area should be cleaned with iodine solution and alcohol and left to dry; aseptic technique must be employed throughout the procedure.

4. The child should be gently and appropriately restrained.

5. A 22-gauge (1½-inch) needle is aseptically attached to a sterile syringe.

6. Insert the needle 1 to 2 cm above the symphysis pubis with the syringe angled slightly toward the posterior. Be sure the needle is inserted into the abdomen in the midline.

7. After the bladder is entered, gently aspirate the urine.

8. Gross and/or microscopic blood may appear in the voided urine after a suprapubic aspiration.

PARACENTESIS

1. The child should be gently and appropriately restrained.

2. Clean the abdomen with iodine solution, as in surgical preparation.

3. Using sterile technique, insert the needle (an intravenous catheter is often more desirable in this procedure) into the abdominal cavity just lateral to the rectus abdominus muscle in the right or left lower quadrant.

4. Gently aspirate the fluid **(do not remove too much fluid too rapidly from the peritoneum; a dynamic equilibrium has been established and the removal of excessive fluid may precipitate massive fluid shifts and hypotension).**

5. If no fluid is obtained on aspiration, or if air is withdrawn, remove the needle and attempt the procedure with new sterile instruments. Aspiration of air usually signifies entrance into the bowel or bladder and bowel entrance contaminates the needle.

THORACENTESIS

1. The child should be gently and appropriately restrained (preferably in the sitting position).

2. The area should be cleaned with iodine solution and alcohol and left to dry.

3. The area to be tapped is identified by percussing the level of the fluid. The area should then be anesthetized.

4. A 22-gauge needle is attached to a sterile syringe and a 3-way stopcock.

5. The needle is inserted over the superior border of the lower rib and the fluid is gently aspirated from the pleural cavity.

6. Remove the needle and cover the puncture site with a sterile dressing.

7. Examine the chest by auscultation and percussion after the procedure is completed to assure expansion of the lung.

8. A chest radiograph may be required if pneumothorax is suspected.

UMBILICAL ARTERY CATHETERIZATION

1. Measure the shoulder to umbilicus length and calculate the length of insertion of the catheter.

2. Prepare the umbilicus for an aseptic procedure.

3. Place an umbilical tape around the base of the stump and tighten just enough to prevent bleeding.

4. Cut the umbilical stump 1 to 2 cm from the base.

5. Identify the umbilical vessels (there are two arteries and one vein; the arteries are thick walled and smaller than the vein).

6. Gently dilate the orifice of one of the arteries (with the tip of a small clamp) and insert the catheter. Advance the catheter to the predetermined length.

7. Secure the catheter to the stump with a silk suture.

8. Obtain an abdominal radiograph to determine the position of the tip of the catheter; it should be just above the level of the diaphragm and away from the juncture of the renal arteries.

VENOUS CUTDOWN

1. The long saphenous vein is the most common vein used for venous cutdown, but other superficial veins may be used; the procedure is similar for all.

2. The most suitable point of entry into the long saphenous vein is just anterior and slightly superior to the medial malleolus.

3. The area is prepared for an aseptic procedure.

4. An incision with a scalpel is made over and perpendicular to the course of the vein.

5. Dissect bluntly the soft tissue to expose and free the vein from the surrounding soft tissue.

6. Place two silk sutures around the vein. Tie the distal suture, leaving the proximal suture slack. It will be used later to secure the catheter.

7. Carefully incise the vein to make an aperture large enough to insert the catheter.

8. The catheter is gently advanced into the vein and blood return is ensured (a small amount of normal saline may be instilled to ensure that the catheter tip is in the lumen of the vessel).

9. The catheter is secured with the proximal suture.

10. The skin incision is closed with silk sutures and a sterile dressing is applied (an antibiotic ointment is usually recommended).

Diet and Nutrition

CALORIC REQUIREMENTS BY AGE

<1–1 year	100–120 cal/kg
1–3 years	100 cal/kg
4–6 years	90 cal/kg
7–9 years	80 cal/kg
10–12 years	70 cal/kg
13–15 years	60 cal/kg
16–19 years	50 cal/kg

FLUID REQUIREMENTS BY AGE

<1–6 months	2–3 oz/kg
3 months	140–160 ml/kg
6 months	130–155 ml/kg
9 months	125–145 ml/kg
1 year	120–135 ml/kg
2 years	115–125 ml/kg
4 years	100–110 ml/kg
6 years	90–100 ml/kg
10 years	70–85 ml/kg
14 years	50–60 ml/kg
18 years	40–50 ml/kg

FEEDING AMOUNT AND FREQUENCY

Amount

Age in months + 3 (<1–6 months of age) = oz/feeding

Frequency

Birth: Every 3 hours = 8 feedings/day

2–3 months: Every 4 hr = 6 feedings/day

4–6 months: Every 5 hr = 5 feedings/day

1 year: 4 feedings/day

Calories

Protein 15%

Carbohydrates 45%

Fat 40%

RECOMMENDED DAILY ALLOWANCES

Table 1 gives the recommended daily allowances for essential nutrients

FORMULA COMPOSITION

Table 2 gives the nutrient components of a variety of infant formulas

SPECIAL DIETS

Ketogenic Diet

1. General considerations
   a. May be of use in the treatment of intractable grand mal epilepsy or minor motor seizures.
   b. Best results in children 2 to 5 years of age, but may be tried up to 8 years of age.
   c. Supervision is essential.
2. Starting diet
   a. Initial period of starvation (3–7 days): 400 to 800 ml of water per day; diet is started when patient has lost 10% of body weight and has +4 acetone in urine (terminate diet if serum carbon dioxide is <10 mEq/liter or if untoward reactions occur).
   b. One-third of calculated diet is offered the first day, with increase to two-thirds and to full diet on successive days.
   c. Routine evaluations
      (1) Vital signs every 4 hr
      (2) Daily morning weight
      (3) Urinalysis twice daily
      (4) Fasting blood glucose, carbon dioxide, potassium and uric acid monitoring every 3 days and before discharge
   d. Eliminate drugs gradually over a 2-week period after starting the diet.

TABLE 1. *Recommended daily allowances*

Age (years)	Weight (kg)	Height (cm)	Calories	Proteins (g)	Calcium (g)	Vit. A (IU)	Thiamin (mg)	Riboflavin (mg)	Niacin (mg)	Vit. C (mg)	Vit. D (IU)	Iron (mg)
<0.5	7	63	kg × 115	kg × 2	0.5	1,500	0.4	0.4	6	35	400	kg × 1
0.5–1	9	72	kg × 100	kg × 1.8	0.6	1,500	0.5	0.5	8	35	400	15
1–3	13	87	1,200	25	0.8	2,000	0.6	0.8	8	40	400	15
3–6	18	107	1,500	30	0.8	2,500	0.8	0.8	11	40	400	10
6–9	26	126	2,100	40	1.0	3,500	1.1	1.3	15	40	400	10
Boys												
9–12	35	140	2,400	45	1.1	4,500	1.3	1.4	16	40	400	10
12–14	43	151	2,700	50	1.4	5,000	1.4	1.4	18	45	400	18
14–18	59	170	3,000	60	1.4	5,000	1.5	1.5	20	55	400	18
Girls												
9–12	35	140	2,200	50	1.1	4,500	1.1	1.3	15	40	400	18
12–14	44	154	2,300	50	1.3	5,000	1.2	1.5	15	45	400	18
14–18	53	158	2,300	55	1.3	5,000	1.2	1.5	15	50	400	18

TABLE 2. Formula composition

	Fat (% wt/vol)	Protein (% wt/vol)	Carbohydrate (% wt/vol)	Vit. A (IU/qt)	Vit. D (IU/qt)	Vit. C (mg/qt)	Iron (mg/qt)	Ca (mg/qt)	P (mg/qt)	Na (mEq/L)	K (mEq/L)	Ca (mEq/L)	P (mEq/L)
Standard formulas													
Cow's milk	4.1	3.5	5.0	940	38	17	—	1,300	1,004	25	36	61	53
Enfamil®	3.7	1.5	7.0	1,500	400	50	1.4	615	473	11	18	32	32
Human	3.8	1.25	7.0	1,400	95	40	—	320	146	7	14	17	9
Similac®	3.4	1.7	6.6	2,500	400	50	—	662	473	11	23	34	30
S-26®	3.6	1.5	7.2	2,500	400	50	7.5	400	310	7	14	21	21
Soy formulas													
Mull-Soy®	3.6	3.1	5.2	2,000	400	40	5	1,200	800	16	40	60	46
Sobee®	2.6	3.2	7.7	1,500	400	50	8	946	473	22	33	50	32
Special formulas													
Lofenalac®	2.7	2.2	8.5	1,500	400	50	15	897	690	25	37	47	47
Nutramigen®	2.6	2.2	8.5	1,500	400	30	9	887	683	17	26	50	45
Similac® + Iron	4.2	2.1	8.0	3,000	480	60	15	800	610	13	27	41	36
Cho-free + 12% D/W®	3.5	1.8	6.4	—	—	—	8	850	630	15	22	—	—
Lytren®	0	0	7.00	—	—	—	—	80	155	25	25	—	—
Pedialyte®	0	0	5.00	—	—	—	13	80	0	30	20	—	—
Portagen®	3.2	2.3	7.7	—	—	—	—	630	473	14	21	—	—
Skim milk	0.2	3.5	4.9	—	—	—	—	1,240	1,010	26	34	—	—

3. Calculating the diet

    a. Fat (4 g), protein (1g/kg), and carbohydrate (grams).

    b. The 4:1 ratio is a dietary unit and yields 40 calories.

    c. Calories: 60 to 75 cal/kg/day.

    d. Determine number of dietary units needed per day (i.e., calories divided by 40).

    e. Calculate grams of fat needed per day (i.e., dietary units divided by 4).

    f. Calculate grams of protein needed per day on the basis of 1 g/kg/day.

    g. Obtain grams of carbohydrate needed per day by the difference.

4. Discontinuing the diet: After 2 years on the diet, it is reduced to a 3:1 ratio over a 3-month to 1-year period and then to a 2:1 ratio over a 3-month period; a normal diet can then be resumed.

5. Complications

    a. Hypoglycemia.

    b. Uric acid nephropathy.

    c. Severe acidosis.

Gluten-Free Diet

1. For gluten-sensitive enteropathy (e.g., celiac disease).

2. Allowed foods (food should be well cooked)

    a. Rice, infant rice cereal, puffed rice.

    b. Corn.

    c. Potatoes, yam, turnip, carrots, beets.

    d. Squash, peas, green beans, asparagus, tomatoes, olives.

    e. Bananas, pears, peaches, apricots, berries, fruit juices.

    f. Chicken, beef, pork, lamb, fish (fresh).

    g. Eggs, milk, cheese, butter.

    h. Gelatin, desserts, custards.

    i. Honey, jelly, sugar, molasses.

3. Foods to avoid

    a. Bread, wheat products, cakes, doughnuts, and pancakes.

    b. All baby foods in jars.

    c. Frankfurters, sausages, luncheon meat, meat loaf.

    d. Meat, meat loaf.

    e. Chili, stews, fish or meat pastes, and ham.

f. All thick salad dressings.

g. Gravy and creamed vegetables.

h. Commercial ice creams.

i. Candy and chocolate.

j. Macaroni and noodles.

Low-Calorie Diet

1. For obesity.
2. Weight should not be abruptly reduced.
3. Allow a period of adjustment.
4. Teach self-esteem by encouraging activities.
5. Good nutrition, especially during adolescence, should be maintained by having adequate protein and calcium and less fat and carbohydrate.
6. During adolescence, the minimum requirement for adequate growth is 1,300 cal/day for girls and 1,400 cal/day for boys. Older children (adults) can have as low as 1,000 cal/day. At least 20% of calories should come from protein.
7. Spread the calories over three meals. Encourage intake of raw carrots, celery, and raw vegetables.
8. Fad diets result in loss of weight through loss of water and muscle and should be discouraged.

Athlete's Diet

1. Fat, not protein, is the prime fuel for muscle.
2. Under extreme efforts, all muscle energy comes from carbohydrates.
3. On the day of events, give liquid diet: 1,000 calories composed of 75% carbohydrates and 25% proteins.
4. Do not restrict water intake during exercise; allow intake of some distilled water and/or 0.2% saline solution.

Cystic Fibrosis Diet

1. 200 cal/kg/day given every 3 to 4 hr.
2. Limit total fat, but do not abolish it.
3. Use 1% fat milk.
4. Protein: 4 g/kg/day.
5. Vitamins: Twice the recommended dose, including vitamins K and E.
6. Pancreatic enzymes (VioKase®) should be used: ½ to 1 tsp of powder per feeding (infants) or 3 to 6 tablets per meal (older children).

7. Do not let enzyme stand on food and do not cook or heat food with enzyme on it.

Vegetarian Diet

1. A pure vegetarian diet (vegan) is not adequate.

2. Lactovegetarian, or lacto-ovo-vegetarian diets are adequate.

Lactose-Free Diet

1. For primary or secondary lactose intolerance from congenital lactase deficiency, acute gastroenteritis (viral, bacterial, protozoal, toxic), celiac disease, galactosemia, cystic fibrosis, Crohn's disease, giardiasis, ulcerative colitis, short bowel syndrome, neomycin administration.

2. Foods to avoid

   a. All milk and milk products (e.g., butter, cream, cheese, yogurt, prepared foods containing dry milk).

   b. Liver.

   c. Peas.

   d. Soybeans.

3. Provide a milk substitute (lactose-free formula) for affected infants; fruit juices are appropriate substitutes for older children.

4. In the temporary (transient) forms of lactose intolerance, lactose-containing products may be slowly reintroduced after 2 to 6 weeks.

Milk Protein-Free Diet

1. For milk protein intolerance

2. Foods to avoid

   a. All milk and milk by-products

   b. Prepared foods containing dry milk

3. Provide a milk substitute (soy protein or meat base formula) for affected infants.

VITAMIN, MINERAL, AND PROTEIN CONTENT OF FOOD ITEMS

Vitamin A

1. 10,000 units of vitamin A in 1 oz liver, ½ cup dark greens, or ½ cup cooked carrots.

2. 1,000 units of vitamin A in 1 tomato, 1 apricot, ½ cup peaches, ½ cup squash, or ½ cup lettuce.

3. 500 units of vitamin A in ½ cup green vegetables, 8 oz milk, 1 egg, 1 tbsp butter, or 1½ cups cheddar cheese.

Iron

1. 3 mg of iron in 3 tbsp cream of wheat, ½ cup beans, or 1 oz liver.

2. 1 mg of iron in 1 oz meat or fish, 1 egg, or 2 dried prunes.

3. 0.5 mg of iron in 2 apricots, 1 potato, or 1 fruit.

Calcium

1. 0.3 g of calcium in 8 oz milk, 1½ oz cheese, or 1½ cups ice cream.

Vitamin C

1. 50 mg of vitamin C in 1 orange, ½ cup orange juice, ½ cup any citrus juice, 1 large tomato, 1 cup cantaloupe, 10 large strawberries, or ⅓ raw pepper.

2. 10 to 20 mg of vitamin C in 1 potato or ½ cup tomato juice, raw fruit or vegetable.

Protein

1. 7 g of protein in 1 egg, 1 oz meat, 8 oz milk, or 2 tbsp peanut butter.

2. 3 g of protein in ½ cup cereal, ⅔ cup ice cream, ½ cup milk pudding, or 1 slice of bacon.

3. 2 g of protein in 1 slice of bread, 1 serving of cake, or 1 potato.

4. 1g of protein in 1 serving of fruit or vegetables.

CALORIC, SALT, AND CARBOHYDRATE CONTENTS OF FOOD ITEMS

Table 3 gives the amounts of calories, salt, and carbohydrates found in various food items.

Listed here are activities and the corresponding calories/kg/hr required to perform them.

Caloric Energy Requirements

Sleeping	1.10 (cal/kg/hr)
Sitting	1.32
Standing	1.54
Housework	2.20
Light exercise	2.75

Walking	3.30
Trade work (e.g., carpenter)	3.85
Active exercise	4.18
Walking fast	4.40
Descending stairs	4.95
Loading heavy objects	5.5
Heavy exercise	6.05
Active sports	7.15
Running	8.20
Ascending stairs	15.0

TABLE 3. *Caloric, salt, and carbohydrate content of food items*

Food	Amount	Calories	Salt[a]	Carbohydrate[b] (g)
Almonds (salted)	12	102	+	3
American cheese	1 slice	103	+	T
Apple	1 small	74		11
Apple pie	⅙	277	+	42
Apricots	5	103		22
Artichoke	1	53		10
Asparagus	12	25		4
Bacon	3 strips	104		T
Banana	1	103		23
Banana split	1	453	+	44
Beans (baked)	1 cup	204		48
Beans (string)	1 cup	25		5
Beef (chopped)	¼ lb	352		0
Beef (roast)	1 serving	304	+	0
Beef (corned)	1 serving	252	+	0
Beef (filet)	1 serving	253		0
Beef (steak)	1 serving	204		0
Beef (porter steak)	1 serving	402		0
Beef (ribs)	1 serving	204		0
Beets	½ cup	37	+	10
Biscuits	2 small	112	+	15
Blue cheese	1½ oz	152	+	T
Bread (white)	1 slice	87	+	30
Bread (French)	1 slice	52	+	10
Bread (rye)	1 slice	72	+	12
Brick cheese	1½ oz	156	+	T
Broccoli	1 cup	43		6
Brownies	1	152	+	16
Brussels sprouts	1 cup	62		12
Butter	1 tbsp	102		T
Cabbage	1 cup	41		7
Cake	1 piece	200–300		30–60
Candy	1 oz	110		28
Carrots	1 medium	25		5
Carrot juice	1 cup	52		13

Food	Amount	Calories	Salt[a]	Carbohydrate[b] (g)
Cauliflower	1 cup	34		5
Celery (cooked)	1 cup	25	+	3
Cottage cheese	½ cup	201	+	9
Cherries	1 cup	73		20
Chicken (broiled)	1 serving	202		0
Chicken (fried)	½ medium	324		0
Chicken (soup)	1 cup	174	+	34
Chocolate	1 bar (2 oz)	252		32
Clams	12 medium	104	+	3
Cocoa	1½ tbsp	51		13
Coffee (black)	1 cup	0		T
Corn-on-cob	1 avg	103		19
Crab	3 oz	93	+	T
Cream (20%)	3 tbsp	101	+	2
Cream (whipped)	1 tbsp	52		T
Cucumber	1 8-in	20		3
Custard	½ cup	127		24
Danish pastry	1 piece	252	+	24
Dates	4	101		23
Doughnut	1 piece	152	+	21
Dressing (French)	1 tbsp	102	+	4
Dressing (Italian)	1 tbsp	48		0
Duck	1 serving	301	+	0
Eggs	1 avg	73	+	T
Egg yolk	1	63		T
English muffin	1	152	+	21
Fig bars	2	102		22
Figs (fresh)	4 small	123		24
Fish (baked)	1 serving	204		0
Fish (fried)	1 serving	323		0
Fish (tuna)	½ cup	252	+	0
Flour	1 cup	402		84
Frankfurter	1 avg	126	+	0
Frosting	1 tbsp	53		6
Fruit cocktail	1 serving	104	+	19
Grapefruit	½ small	52		11
Grapes	1 cup	92		16
Halavah	1 oz	126		18
Ham (baked)	1 slice	355		1
Hamburger	2 oz	202		0
Honey	1 tbsp	63		17
Ice cream	1 scoop	153	+	14
Jam	1 tbsp	52		14
Juices				
Apple	1 cup	125		28
Grape	½ cup	75		18
Grapefruit	6 oz	73		15
Lemon	½ cup	30		9
Orange	4 oz	53		10
Pineapple	1 cup	124		30
Prune	½ cup	85	+	23
Tomato	1 cup	48		10
Lamb chop (broiled)	1	253	+	0
Lamb chop (fried)	1	325	+	0
Lamb roast	1 serving	177	+	0
Lemon	1 avg	23		5
Lemon meringue pie	1 piece	353	+	45

TABLE 3. *(continued)*

Food	Amount	Calories	Salt[a]	Carbohydrate[b] (g)
Lentils	1 cup	112		17
Lettuce	½ head	19		3
Liver	1 serving	154		4
Lobster (tail)	Avg serving	101	+	T
Macaroni	1 cup	200		39
Mango	1	101		19
Margarine	1 tbsp	101	+	0
Mayonnaise	1 tbsp	101	+	T
Milk	¾ cup	126		8
Milk (skimmed)	1 cup	84	+	13
Milk shake	1	352	+	30
Mints (after dinner)	5	52		14
Molasses	1 tbsp	52		13
Muffins	1	110		24
Mushrooms	½ cup	15		3
Mustard	1 tbsp	10	+	T
Nuts (cashew)	7	76		8
Nuts (pistachio)	16	51		2
Oil (vegetable)	1 tbsp	101		0
Olives	6 small	53	+	T
Onion (raw)	1 large	51		11
Orange	1	74		14
Oyster (baked)	12	85	+	8
Oyster (fried)	6	252	+	4
Pancakes with butter and syrup	3	473	+	37
Peach	1	50		18
Pear	1	73		18
Petits fours	1	102	+	25
Pineapple	1 cup	75		16
Pine nuts	1 tsp	25		1
Pizza	⅛ of 12-in	250	+	25
Plums	1	30		7
Popcorn	1 cup	52	+	11
Pork chop	1	224		0
Potato	1	127		28
Potato chips	½ cup	103		7
Potato (French fried)	6	102	+	12
Potato (mashed)	1 medium	183	+	28
Prunes	4	102		24
Pudding (rice)	½ cup	172		32
Rice (boiled)	¾ cup	104		22
Rice (fried)	1 cup	206		22
Salami (hard)	1 oz	126	+	T
Sardines	4	103	+	T
Shrimp (fried)	10	202	+	11
Soda pop	6 oz	76		19
Sole filet (fried)	1 serving	201		0
Sole (broiled)	1 serving	106		0
Soup (chicken)	1 cup	103	+	2
Soup (creamed)	1 cup	202	+	12
Soup (mushroom)	1 cup	201	+	13
Soup (tomato)	1 cup	103	+	13
Soup (onion)	1 cup	101	+	4
Soup (vegetable)	1 cup	103	+	11
Spinach	½ cup	26	+	3

Food	Amount	Calories	Salt[a]	Carbohydrate[b] (g)
Strawberries	1 cup	51		12
Sugar	1 tsp	18		4
Sundaes	1 avg	400		24
Tangerine	1 large	34		8
Tomato	1	25		4
Turkey	1 serving	176		0
Watermelon	1 piece	102		22
Yogurt	1 cup	165		13

[a] + indicates high salt content.
[b] T indicates trace amount.

Drugs Causing Hemolysis in Patients with Glucose 6-Phosphate Dehydrogenase Deficiency

Glucose 6-phosphate dehydrogenase deficiency is also known as primaquine-sensitive hemolytic disease. Patients with the deficiency of this enzyme experience acute hemolytic disease when exposed to certain foods or drugs. The definitive treatment is to avoid the substances that cause hemolysis. The following are the more common substances implicated:

1. Aniline dyes
2. Antipyrine
3. Aspirin
4. Chloramphenicol
5. Fava beans
6. Furazolidone
7. Methylene blue
8. Naphthalene
9. Nitrofurantoin
10. Para-aminosalicylic acid
11. Phenacetin
12. Primaquine
13. Probenecid
14. Sulfa drugs and sulfa-containing products
15. Vitamin C (in large doses)
16. Vitamin K (water soluble)

Drugs Excreted in Breast Milk

The following drugs are transferred in the breast milk to the nursing infant. Mothers who are breast feeding should use caution when taking any medication, and the baby should be observed closely for any adverse effects from the mother's medication. (Modified from Sheldon 1981.)

Acetazolamide

Amantadine HCl[a]

Aminoglycoside antibiotics

Aminophylline

Amitriptyline[b]

Amphetamines

Antineoplastic medications

Aspirin

Atropine

Azathioprine[a]

Barbiturates[b]

Carbamazepine

Cephalosporins

Chloral hydrate

Chloramphenicol[a]

Chlordiazepoxide

Chlorophenothane (DDT)[a]

Chlorothiazide

Chlorpromazine[b]

Chlorthalidone[b]

Cimetidine[b]

Clindamycin

Clonidine[b]

Coumarins

Dextropropoxyphene

Diazepam[b]

Diazoxide[a]

Dicumarol

Diethylstilbestrol[a]

Digoxin

Epinephrine

Estrogen

Ethacrynic acid

Ethanol

Ethosuximide

Furosemide

Heparin

Hexachlorophene

Imipramine[a]

Indomethacin

Insulin[c]

Iodines[a]

Isoniazid[a]

Laxatives

Levothyroxine[b]

Lithium carbonate[a]

Marijuana[a]

Meprobamate[b]

Methadone[b]

Methyl dopa

Methyltestosterone[a]

Metronidazole[b]

Morphine[b]

Nalidixic acid[b]

Nicotine

Nitrofurantoin[b]

Oral contraceptives

Penicillamine[a]

Penicillins

Pentazocine[b]

Phenobarbital

Phenylbutazone

Phenytoin

Potassium iodide[a]

Prednisone

Primidone[a]

Prochlorperazine

Promethazine

Propranolol

Propylthiouracil[a]

Pyridoxine

Quinine

Radioisotopes[a]

Reserpine

Sulfonamides[b]

Sulfonylureas[a]

Tetracyclines[a]

Trimethadione[b]

Trimethoprim/sulfa-methoxazole[b]

Valproic acid

Vitamin D

---

[a]Contraindicated.

[b]Avoid, if possible; otherwise, monitor baby closely.

Drugs Used in Pediatric Practice

Every effort has been made to provide accurate drug doses. Since information about doses, uses, and side effects of currently used drugs is continuously changing, and to avoid using incorrect doses, **the reader is *urged* to double-check all drug information provided and to review the manufacturer's description of action, indications, contraindications, and recommended doses before the use of *any* drug.**

Drugs	Indications	Dosage
Amino acid preparations		
Travasol® 5.5% or 8.5% injection (with or without electrolytes)	Parenteral nutrition	Variable, depending on protein and caloric requirements
L-amino acid	5.5 g/100 ml 8.5 g/100 ml	
Total nitrogen	924 mg/100 ml 1.42 g/100 ml	
pH	6.0 6.0	
Sodium acetate	431 mg/100 ml 594 mg/100 ml (70 mEq/L)	
Potassium phosphate	522 mg/100 ml 522 mg/100 ml (60 mEq/L)	
Magnesium chloride	102 mg/100 ml 102 mg/100 ml (10 mEq/L)	
Standard Vivonex® Diet	Enteral nutrition	Variable, depending on protein, caloric, and fluid requirements
Calories	300/80–g packet	
Amino acid	6.56 g/80 g	
Carbohydrate	69.2 g/80 g	
Fat (linoleic acid)	0.435 g/80 g (0.348 g/80 g)	
Sodium	20 mEq/L/300 ml	
Potassium	30 mEq/L/300 ml	
Vitamins A, B, C, D, E, iron, calcium, iodine, copper, zinc, magnesium	100% U.S. RDA supplied by six 80-g packets	
High Nitrogen Vivonex® Diet	Enteral nutrition	Variable, depending on protein, caloric and fluid requirements
Amino acid	13.3 g/80-g packet	
Carbohydrate	63 g/80 g	
Fat (linoleic acid)	0.26 g/80 g (0.2 g/80 g)	
Analgesics and antipyretics		
Acetaminophen (Tempra®, Tylenol®, Liquiprin®)		5 to 10 mg/kg every 4 hr (maximum dose, 0.3 to 0.6 g every 4 hr)
Aspirin	Antipyretic	60 mg/kg/day in four to six doses (maximum dose, 3.6 g/day)
	Antirheumatic	100 mg/kg/day in four to six doses

605

Drugs Used in Pediatric Practice *(continued)*

Drugs	Indications	Dosage
Codeine		0.5 to 1.0 mg/kg p.o. or s.c. every 4 hr
Meperidine (Demerol®)		6 mg/kg/day p.o., i.m., i.v., or s.c. in four to six doses (maximum dose, 100 mg)
Morphine		0.1 to 0.2 mg/kg s.c.; repeat every 4 hr as needed
Antacids		
Cimetidine (Tagamet®)	Do not use in children <16 years old	20 to 40 mg/kg/day p.o. in four doses (maximum dose/day 1,200 mg); for intravenous use, dilute in 100 ml 5% D/W and give over a 20-min period
Magaldrate (Riopan®)		Tablets (chew or swallow) or suspension (1 or 2 tsp) between meals and at bedtime
Aluminum hydroxide (Amphogel®)		2 to 8 ml p.o. with meals
Anticoagulants		
Warfarin sodium (Coumadin®)		Initial: 10 to 15 mg/day p.o. for 2 or 3 days **or** 20 to 60 mg p.o., i.v., or i.m. Maintenance: 2 to 10 mg/day p.o.; adjust dose according to prothrombin time
Heparin		Initial: 50 to 75 units/kg i.v. Maintenance: 10 to 25 units/kg/hr continuous i.v. **or** 100 units/kg i.v. every 4 hr
Anticonvulsants		
Diazepam (Valium®)	Status epilepticus	0.3 to 0.75 mg/kg i.v. over a 1- to 2-min period; repeat every 15 min no more than twice (maximum single dose, 10 mg)
	Sedative	0.1 to 0.8 mg/kg p.o. in three or four doses **or** 0.1 to 0.3 mg/kg i.m. or i.v.; repeat every 2 to 4 hr as needed
Paraldehyde	Status epilepticus	10 ml in 90 ml normal saline (5 to 40 drops/hr) i.v. **or** 0.3 mg/kg rectally (repeat every 4 to 6 hr) **or** 0.15 mg/kg deep i.m. every 4 to 6 hr (maximum dose, 4 to 10 ml)
Phenobarbital	Status epilepticus	15 mg/kg i.v. slowly (give half of dose first and repeat in 5 min) **or** 10 mg/kg i.m. **or** 4 to 6 mg/kg/day p.o. in two doses (as a chronic anticonvulsant)
Phenytoin (Dilantin®)	Status epilepticus	Initial: 15 mg/kg i.v. in normal saline (50 mg/min) Maintenance: 5 to 8 mg/kg/day p.o. in one dose (maximum dose, 0.3 to 0.5 g/day)

Drugs	Indications	Dosage
Bromides		25 to 75 mg/kg/day p.o. in three or four doses
Clonazepam (Clonopin®)		0.01 to 0.03 mg/kg/day p.o. in three doses; increase dose every 3 days up to 0.1 to 0.2 mg/kg in three doses. Maximum 20 mg/day
Valproic acid (Depakene®)		10 to 15 mg/kg/day p.o. in two doses; increase weekly by 5 to 10 mg/kg/day to a maximum dose of 60 to 80 mg/kg/day
Mephenytoin (Mesantoin®)		3 to 10 mg/kg/day p.o. (maximum dose, 0.1 to 0.3 g three times a day)
Primidone (Mysoline®)		Initial: 125 mg p.o. two times a day (<8 years old) **or** 250 mg p.o. two times a day (>8 years old); increase dose gradually. Maintenance: 12 to 24 mg/kg/day p.o.
Carbamazepine (Tegretol®)		15 to 25 mg/kg/day p.o. in two to four doses
Trimethadione (Tridione®)		20 to 50 mg/kg/day p.o. in three or four doses
Ethosuximide (Zarontin®)		10 to 25 mg/kg/day p.o. in one or two doses, with food
Haloperidol (Haldol®)	Not FDA approved for use in children <12 years old	1 to 2 mg p.o. two or three times a day (maximum dose, 15 mg/day)
Acetazolamide (Diamox®)		8 to 30 mg/kg/day p.o. in three or four doses (maximum dose, 1.5 g/day)
ACTH	Infantile spasms	40 to 60 units/day i.m. in two doses; taper after 4 weeks
Antidiabetic agents		
Rapid-acting insulin		
Crystalline zinc	Ketoacidosis	0.1 unit/kg i.v., **then** 0.1 unit/kg/hr continuous i.v. **or** 15 to 20 min before meals s.c.
Intermediate-acting insulin		
Equal parts of semilente and ultralente or one part of regular to three or four parts of NPH		Tentative starting dose: 0.3 to 0.5 unit/kg/day
Oral insulin		
Chlorpropamide (Diabinese®)		100 to 250 mg/day p.o.
Sulfonylurea (Tolbutamide®)		Initial: 0.5 to 2 g/day p.o. in divided doses; taper to 1 g/day over a 3-day period. Maintenance: 2 g/day (maximum)
Antidiarrheic agents		
Donnagel PG®		≤10 to 20 lb: ½ tsp every 6 hr; 20 to 30 lb: 1 tsp every 6 hr; ≥30 lb: 1 or 2 tsp every 6 hr

Drugs Used in Pediatric Practice *(continued)*

Drugs	Indications	Dosage
Diphenoxylate (Lomotil®)		Adults: 2 tsp initially, **then** 1 tsp four times a day Children: 2.5 mg two or three times a day Adults: 5 mg three or four times a day
Antidotes Acetylcysteine (Mucomyst®)	Acetaminophen poisoning	140 mg/kg p.o. (diluted to a 5% solution in juice or soft drink), **then** 70 mg/kg every 4 hr for 3 days
Disulfiram (Antabuse®)	Alcohol deterrent; discontinue alcohol use for 12 to 24 hr before use of drug	Initial: 500 mg/day p.o. for 2 weeks Maintenance: 125 to 250 mg/day
Physostigmine (Antilirium®)	Anticholinesterase	0.5 mg i.m. or i.v. slowly; repeat as needed (maximum dose, 2.0 mg)
Atropine	Organic phosphate or insecticide poisoning	0.01 mg/kg p.o. or s.c. every 4 hr as needed (maximum single dose, 0.4 mg)
BAL (Dimercaprol®)	Arsenic poisoning	2.5 mg/kg deep i.m. every 4 hr for 5 days; repeat in 10 days if needed
Activated charcoal	Universal antidote	0.5 g/kg mixed with water
Deferoxamine*a*	Iron poisoning Shock	15 mg/kg/hr i.v. for 8 hr; repeat every 8 hr if needed
	Stable	90 mg/kg i.m. every 8 hr
Edetate calcium disodium (Calcium Disodium Versenate®)	Lead poisoning	12.5 mg/kg i.v. or i.m. (maximum dose, 75 mg/kg/day)
1% Methylene blue	Methemoglobinemia	0.2 ml/kg i.v. over a 10-min period
Naloxone (Narcan®)	Narcotic antagonist	5 to 10 µg/kg i.m. or i.v.; repeat as needed (maximum dose, 0.4 mg)
Protamine sulfate	Heparin poisoning	1 mg/100 units of heparin in previous 3 to 4 hr
Pralidoxime chloride (Protopam Chloride®)	Organic phosphate poisoning (use with atropine)	Infants: 250 mg i.v. (500 mg/min) Children: 1 g i.v.
3% Sodium nitrite	Cyanide poisoning	Hemoglobin, 8 g/dL: 0.22 ml/kg i.v. 10 g/dL: 0.27 ml/kg i.v. 12 g/dL: 0.33 ml/kg i.v. 14 g/dL: 0.39 ml/kg i.v.
25% Sodium thiosulfate	Cyanide poisoning (use following sodium nitrite)	Hemoglobin, 8 g/dL: 1.10 ml/kg i.v. 10 g/dL: 1.35 ml/kg i.v. 12 g/dL: 1.65 ml/kg i.v. 14 g/dL: 1.95 ml/kg i.v. Repeat if needed, using half doses

*a***Test dose:** 2 g i.m. If urine is positive (pink) begin 20 mg/kg every 4 to 6 hr i.m. **or** 10–15 mg/kg/hr by continuous or intermittent i.v. infusion.

Drugs	Indications	Dosage
Methadone		0.7 mg/kg/day p.o. or s.c. in four doses
Antiemetics		
Bendectin®	Adult use only	2 tablets at bedtime
Prochlorperazine (Compazine®)		Children: 0.25 to 0.375 mg/kg/day p.o. or rectally in two or three doses Adults: 25 mg rectally two times a day **or** 5 mg p.o. three times a day **or** 0.25 mg/kg/day i.m. in three or four doses
Dimenhydrinate (Dramamine®)		5 mg/kg p.o., i.m., or i.v. in four doses (maximum dose, 300 mg/day)
Emetrol®		Infants and children: 1 or 2 tsp at 15-min intervals until vomiting stops Adults: 1 ot 2 tbsp
Chlorpromazine (Thorazine®)		2 mg/kg/day p.o., i.m., or i.v. in four doses **or** 4 mg/kg/day p.r. in four doses (maximum dose, 800 mg/day)
Trimethobenzamide (Tigan®)		15 mg/kg/day p.o. or i.m. in three or four doses
Antihistamines		
Hydroxyzine (Atarax®)		Children: 1 or 2 mg/kg/day p.o. in three doses; preoperatively, 1 mg/kg i.m. Adults: 25 to 50 mg p.o. three times a day
Diphenhydramine (Benadryl®)		Children: 4 to 6 mg/kg/day p.o. in four doses **or** 2 mg/kg i.v. over a 5-min period Adults: 100 to 200 mg/day p.o. in four doses
Antihypertensive agents		
Diazoxide (Hyperstat®)	Hypertensive crisis	3 to 5 mg/kg i.v. as bolus injected within 30 sec; repeat in 30 min and then every 2 hr as needed
Guanethidine (Ismelin®)		0.2 mg/kg/day p.o. in one dose; increase weekly by 0.2 mg/kg/day to maximum dose of 75 mg/day
Hydralazine (Apresoline®)		0.75 mg/kg/day p.o. in four doses (increase over a 4-week period to a maximum dose of 7 mg/kg/day) **or** 0.15 mg/kg i.m. or i.v. every 4 hr (maximum dose, 300 mg/day)
Magnesium sulfate		50% solution: 50 to 100 mg/kg i.m. every 4 hr 1% solution: 100 mg/kg i.v. slowly
Methyldopa (Aldomet®)		10 mg/kg/day p.o. in two or three doses; increase dose every 2 days to a maximum

Drugs Used in Pediatric Practice *(continued)*

Drugs	Indications	Dosage
		of 65 mg/kg **or** 3 g/day (whichever is less)
Nitroprusside (Nipride®)	Dilute with 5% D/W and wrap in aluminum foil	1.0 µg/kg/min i.v.; titrate dose to blood pressure
Propranolol (Inderal®)		0.5 to 1.0 mg/kg/day p.o. in four doses
Reserpine (Serpasil®)		0.02 mg/kg/day p.o. in two doses **or** 0.07 mg/kg i.m.; repeat every 8 to 24 hr as needed (maximum dose, 2.5 mg/day)
Antimicrobials Chloroquine (Aralen®)	Amebicide Malaria suppression: treat for 2 weeks before exposure and for 8 weeks after leaving endemic area	Adults: 5 mg/kg/day p.o. on same day of each week (maximum dose, 500 mg/day or 800 mg/dose)
	Acute illness	10 mg/kg/day p.o. (maximum dose, 600 mg), **then** 5 mg/kg/day p.o. (maximum dose, 300 mg) 6 hr after first dose, **then** 5 mg/kg/day p.o. 18 hr after second dose, **then** 5 mg/kg/day p.o. 24 hr after third dose
	Extraintestinal amebiasis	10 mg/kg/day p.o. for 2 days, **then** 5 mg/kg/day p.o. for 2 or 3 weeks
Metronidazole (Flagyl®)	Trichomoniasis, giardiasis, and amebiasis	35 to 50 mg/kg/day p.o. in three doses (maximum dose, 250 mg every 8 hr)
Antibiotics Amikacin (Amikin®)	Aminoglycoside; gram-negative organisms, including *Pseudomonas* and *serratia*	Neonates: 7.5 mg/kg i.m. every 12 hr Children: 7.5 mg/kg i.m. every 8 hr **or** 7.5 mg/kg i.v. over a 1-hr period Peak blood level: 15 to 30 mg/ml
Gentamicin	Aminoglycoside; gram-negative organisms; some activity against *Staphylococcus*; used orally for nursery outbreaks of diarrhea due to enteropathogenic *E. coli*	Premature infants: 2 mg/kg i.m. every 8 hr Neonates: 2.5 mg/kg i.m. every 8 hr Children: 2.5 to 3.0 mg/kg i.m. every 8 hr Adolescents: 1.7 mg/kg i.m. every 8 hr Intravenous dose: Same as intramuscular dose in all cases; give over a 1-hr period Peak blood level: 6 to 10 mg/ml
Kanamycin	Aminoglycoside; *E. coli*, *Proteus*, some *Pseudomonas*, *Staphylococcus*,	50 to 100 mg/kg/day p.o. in four doses **or** 7.5 mg/kg i.m. every 12 hr (premature infants or neonates <7 days

Drugs	Indications	Dosage
	mycobacteria	old) **or** 10 mg/kg i.m. every 8 hr (older infants and children) (maximum dose, 1 g/day i.m. in two doses) Intravenous dose: Same as intramuscular dose in all cases; give over a 20-min period Peak blood level: 15 to 30 mg/ml
Neomycin	Aminoglycoside; parenteral or oral use is not recommended	
Spectinomycin	Aminoglycoside; *N. gonorrheae*	Adults: 2 g i.m. in one dose
Streptomycin	Aminoglycoside; tuberculosis, *H. influenzae*, enterococci; should never be used as the only drug	20 mg/kg i.m. every 12 hr (maximum dose, 1 g every 12 hr)
Tobramycin	Aminoglycoside; *E. coli*, enterobacteria, *Klebsiella*, *Proteus*, *Pseudomonas*	Children: 2.5 to 3.0 mg/kg i.m. every 8 hr Adults: 1.0 to 5.0 mg/kg/day i.m. in three doses
Cephalothin (Keflin®)	Gram-positive cocci, penicillin-resistant *Staphylococcus*, *E. coli*, *Proteus*, and *Klebsiella*	Neonates: 50 mg/kg i.v. or i.m. every 6 hr Children: 80 to 160 mg/kg i.v. or i.m. in four to six doses (maximum dose, 12 g/day)
Cephalexin (Keflex®)	Same spectrum as cephalothin	25 mg/kg p.o. every 8 hr (maximum dose, 1 or 2 g/day)
Cefazolin (Ancef® or Kefzol®)	Same spectrum as cephalothin; do not use in neonates	25 mg/kg i.v. or i.m. every 6 hr
Cefaclor (Ceclor®)	Effective against *H. influenzae*	15 mg/kg p.o. every 8 hr (maximum dose, 1.5 g)
Cefamandole (Mandol®)	Same spectrum as cephalothin	Neonates: 32.5 mg/kg i.v. or i.m. every 8 hr Children: 50 mg/kg i.v. or i.m. every 6 hr (maximum dose, 12 g/day)
Cefoxitin (Mefoxin®)	Same spectrum as cephalothin, but extended to include *providencia*, *serratia*, and *B. fragilis*	50 to 100 mg/kg/day i.m. or i.v. in four doses (maximum dose, 12 g/day)
Chloramphenicol	Gram-positive and gram-negative organisms, *Salmonella*, *Rickettsia*, *Chlamydia*, *Bacteroides*, anaerobic *Streptococcus*, resistant *H. influenzae*; do not use in premature infants	Children: 50 to 100 mg/kg/day p.o. or i.v. in four doses Neonates: 25 to 50 mg/kg/day i.v. in four doses
Erythromycin	Gram-positive cocci, *Mycoplasma*, *Chlamydia*, *B. pertussis*, *Rickettsia*, *Brucella*	20 to 50 mg/kg/day p.o. in four doses **or** 10 to 20 mg/kg/day i.m. in four doses (maximum dose, 1 or 2 g/day) Intravenous dose: Same as oral or intramuscular dose;

Drugs Used in Pediatric Practice *(continued)*

Drugs	Indications	Dosage
Lincomycin (Lincocin®)	Most aerobic Gram-positive cocci and common anaerobic organisms	give over a 1-hr period 30 to 60 mg/kg/day p.o. in four doses (maximum dose, 5 g/day) **or** 20 to 100 mg/kg/day i.m. or i.v. in four doses
Clindamycin (Cleocin®)	Same spectrum as lincomycin	10 to 25 mg/kg/day p.o. in four doses **or** 10 to 40 mg/kg/day i.m. or i.v. in four doses
Nitrofurantoin (Furadantin®)	Treatment and prophylaxis of urinary tract infection	5 to 7 mg/kg/day p.o. in four doses (maximum dose, 400 mg/day): reduce dose to 2.5 mg/kg/day after 10 days
Penicillin G or penicillin V		50,000 to 100,000 units/kg/day p.o. in four doses
Aqueous penicillin G		25,000 to 400,000 units/kg/day i.v. in six to twelve doses (maximum dose, 24 million units)
Procaine penicillin G		25,000 to 50,000 units/kg/day i.m. in one or two doses (maximum dose, 4.8 million units)
Benzathine penicillin G		600,000 to 1.2 million units i.m. (maximum dose, 1.2 million units)
Methicillin, oxacillin, nafcillin	Penicillinase-resistant organisms	Neonates: 25 to 50 mg/kg/day i.m. or i.v. in two or three doses Children: 100 to 300 mg/kg/day i.m. or i.v. in four to six doses (maximum dose, 12 g/day)
Cloxacillin, dicloxacillin	Penicillinase-resistant organisms	25 to 100 mg/kg/day p.o. in four doses (maximum dose, 4 g/day)
Ampicillin	Broad spectrum; Gram-positive cocci, enterococci, *Listeria,* Gram-negative organisms such as *H. influenzae, Shigella, Salmonella, Proteus,* and *E. coli*	Neonates: 100 mg/kg/day i.m. or i.v. in two or three doses (maximum dose, 4 g/day) Children: 50 to 400 mg/kg/day i.m. or i.v. in six doses (maximum dose, 12 g/day)
Amoxicillin	Same spectrum as ampicillin	20 to 40 mg/kg/day p.o. in three doses (maximum dose, 3 g/day)
Carbenicillin	Same spectrum as ampicillin, but extended to include *Pseudomonas* and *Proteus*	50 to 100 mg/kg/day p.o. in four doses **or** 400 to 600 mg/kg/day i.m. or i.v. in six to twelve doses (maximum dose, 40 g/day)
Ticarcillin	Same spectrum as carbenicillin	200 to 300 mg/kg/day i.m. or i.v. in six doses (maximum dose, 30 g/day)
Sulfonamides (Sulfadiazine,	Gram-positive cocci and bacilli	150 mg/kg/day p.o. in four

Drugs	Indications	Dosage
triple sulfas, and sulfisoxazole)	(not enterococci) and gram-negative organisms, including *H. influenzae*, *Chlamydia*, *Actinomyces*, *Nocardia*, and *Protozoa*	doses **or** 100 mg/kg/day i.v. in four doses (maximum dose, 5 g/day)
Tetracyclines (Tetracycline, chlortetracycline, and oxy-tetrocycline)	*Rickettsia*, *Chlamydia*, and *Mycoplasma*; gram-positive organisms; do not use in children <8 years old	20 to 40 mg/day p.o. in four doses (maximum dose, 1 or 2 g/day)
Doxycycline		2 to 4 mg/kg/day p.o. in two doses (maximum dose, 300 mg/day)
Minocycline	Carriers of *N. meningitides*	4 mg/kg/day p.o. in two doses
Co-trimoxazole (Trimethoprim, sulfamethoxazole, TMP-SMX)	Most gram-positive and gram-negative organisms; *H. influenzae*, *P. carinii*	8 to 20 mg/kg/day of TMP **and** 40 to 100 mg/kg/day of SMX p.o. in two doses (maximum dose, 960 mg/day TMP and 4.8 g/day SMX)
Vancomycin	Resistant staphylococcal infections, staphylococcal and antibiotic-induced enterocolitis associated with toxin-producing *Clostridium*	2 to 4 g/day p.o. in four doses **or** 20 to 30 mg/kg/day i.v. in two doses (children) **or** 2 or 3 g/day i.v. in four doses (adults)
Colistin	*Pseudomonas*, *E. coli*, *Enterobacteria*, and *Klebsiella*	15 mg/kg/day p.o. in four doses **or** 1.5 to 2.5 mg/kg/day i.m. in two doses (neonates) **or** 2.5 to 5 mg/kg/day i.m. in two to four doses (older children)
Nalidixic acid	Gram-negative urinary tract infection	40 to 50 mg/kg/day p.o. in four doses (maximum dose, 4 g/day)
Polymyxin B	*Pseudomonas*	2.5 mg/kg/day i.m. or i.v. in four doses (maximum dose, 200 mg/day)
Antifungal agents Amphotericin B[b] (Fungizone®)	*Candida*, *Cryptococcus*, *Blastomyces*, *Coccidioides*, and histoplasmosis	1 mg/kg/day **or** 1.5 mg/kg i.v. every other day over a 4- to 6-hr period (starting dose, 0.25 mg/kg/day)
Clortrimazole	Topical use only for cutaneous and vaginal candidiasis	
Flucytosine (Ancobon®)	Cryptococcal meningitis (use with amphotericin B); do not use for *Candida*	150 mg/kg/day p.o. in four doses
Griseofulvin	Tinea, microsporum, and *Trichophyton*	
Grifulvin V® or Grisactin® Fulvicin P/G®		Children: 10 mg/kg/day p.o. in one dose (maximum dose, 500 mg/day) 5 mg/kg/day p.o. in one dose (maximum dose, 250 mg/day)
Nystatin (Mycostatin®)	*Candida*; not absorbed orally	Neonates: 200,000 to 400,000

[b]**Test dose: Daily dose:** 0.1 mg/kg i.v. on day one of therapy, infused over 6 hr. Given once per day; increase to 0.5–1.0 mg/kg/day by increments of 0.1 mg/kg. **Or, alternate day therapy**: used when infection controlled. Give 2 × daily dose every other dose. Maximum daily dose is 1.5 mg/kg/day.

Drugs Used in Pediatric Practice *(continued)*

Drugs	Indications	Dosage
		units/day p.o. in three or four doses Children <2 years old: 400,000 to 800,000 units/day p.o. in three or four doses Children >2 years old: 1 to 2 million units/day p.o. as above
Antihelminthics Mebendazole (Vermox®)	*Enterobius*	Single dose of a 100-mg tablet p.o.
	Trichuris, Ascaris, Ancylostoma, Necator; do not use in children <2 years old	100 mg (one tablet) p.o. morning and evening for 3 days
Piperazine (Antepar®)	*Enterobius, Oxyuriasis*	50 mg/kg/day p.o. in one dose for 7 days (maximum dose, 2 g/day)
Pyrvinium pamoate (Povan®)	*Ascaris, Enterobius*	5 mg/kg p.o. in one dose (maximum dose, 0.25 g)
Thiabendazole (Mintezol®)	Same spectrum as mebendazole, but extended to include cutaneous larva migrans and *Strongyloides*	25 mg/kg/day p.o. (maximum dose, 3 g/day) for 4 days (*Trichuris*) or for 2 days (*Ascaris, Ancylostoma, Necator, Strongyloides*, or larva migrans) or for 1 day and repeated once 7 days later (*Enterobius*)
Antiparasitics Chloroquine phosphate	*Plasmodium vivax,* nonresistant *P. falciparum*	10 mg/kg p.o. (maximum dose, 600 mg), **then** 5 mg/kg p.o. 6 hr later (maximum dose, 300 mg), **then** 5 mg/kg p.o. 18 hr after second dose, **then** 5 mg/kg p.o. 24 hr after third dose
Chloroquine hydrochloride		2 mg/kg/day i.m. or i.v. for 3 days
Quinine sulfate	Resistant *P. falciparum*	25 mg/kg/day p.o. in three doses for 3 days
Pyrimethamine	Use with quinine; also use in histoplasmosis	<10 kg: 6.25 mg/day p.o. two times a day 10–20 kg: 12.5 mg/day p.o. two times a day 21–40 kg: 50 mg/day p.o. two times a day >40 kg: 25 mg/day p.o. two times a day
Sulfadiazine	Use with quinine and pyrimethamine	100 to 200 mg/kg/day p.o. in four doses for 5 days (maximum dose, 2 g/day)
Quinine dihydrochloride	***Caution: Dangerous***; use for 1 day then use oral medications	8 mg/kg i.v. diluted in 100 ml of normal saline and given over a 1-hr period; repeat every 8 hr, if needed, for 1

Drugs	Indications	Dosage
Primaquine phosphate	Use with chloroquine for *P. vivax*; do not use within 5 days of quinacrine therapy	day (maximum dose, 25 mg/kg/day) <10 kg: 2 mg/day for 14 days 11–20 kg: 4 mg/day for 14 days 21–40 kg: 6 mg/day for 14 days 41–55 kg: 10 mg/day for 14 days >55 kg: 20 mg/day for 14 days
Fansidar (Pyrimethamine + sulfadoxine)	Use with quinine	Adult: Single dose of 1 tablet p.o./week
Dehydroemetine	Life-threatening dysentery	1.5 mg/kg/day i.m. in two doses for 5 days
Diloxanide furoate	Invasive amebiasis	20 mg/kg/day p.o. in three doses for 10 days
Diiodohydroxyquin	*Dientamoeba fragilis, Balantidium*	30 to 40 mg/kg/day p.o. in three doses for 21 days
Pentavalent antimony (Antimony sodium stibogluconate)	*Leishmania*	10 mg/kg/day i.v. slowly for 6 days
Pentamidine	Antimony-resistant leishmaniasis	3 mg/kg/day i.m. in one dose for 10 days
Suramin	*Trypanosoma*	10% fresh aqueous solution: 20 mg i.v. (test dose), **then** 20 mg/kg/day i.v. on days 1, 3, 7, 14, and 21
Tryparsamide	Trypanosomiasis with CNS involvement	20 to 40 mg/kg i.v. once a week for 10 weeks
Gamma benzene hexachloride (Kwell® or Gamene®)	Scabies, pediculosis, skin infestations; do not use in infants	Lotion or cream applied to body for 4 hr, to pubic area for 24 hr, or to hair and scalp for 5 min and then washed off; repeat in 10 days
Crotamiton (Eurax®)	Scabies or pediculosis in infants	External use
Antituberculous agents Ethambutol	Use in adults only	15 to 25 mg/kg/day p.o. in one dose
Isoniazid		10 to 20 mg/kg/day p.o., i.m., or i.v. in one or two doses (maximum dose, 600 mg/day)
Para-aminosalicylic acid		0.2 to 0.3 g/kg/day p.o. in three doses (maximum dose, 12 g/day)
Streptomycin		20 to 40 mg/kg/day i.m. in one or two doses (maximum dose, 1 g/day)
Rifampin	For tuberculosis	10 to 20 mg/kg/day p.o. in one dose (maximum dose, 600 mg/day)
	For meningococcus carriers	20 mg/kg/day p.o. in two doses for 2 to 4 days (maximum dose, 1,200 mg/day)

Drugs Used in Pediatric Practice *(continued)*

Drugs	Indications	Dosage
Antiviral agents		
Adenine arabinoside (Vidarabine, Vira-A®)	Herpes encephalitis and neonatal herpes	15 mg/kg/day continuous i.v. over a 12-hr period
Amantadine (Symmetrel®)	Prophylaxis during influenza A epidemics	Children 1 to 9 years old: 4 to 8 mg/kg/day p.o. in three doses (maximum dose, 150 mg/day)
		Older children: 200 mg/day p.o. in two doses
Idoxuridine (Stoxil®)	Topical ophthalmic use	0.1% solution **or** 0.5% ointment
Antimigraine agents		
Cafergot P-B®		½ or 1 tablet at first sign of attack, **then** ½ or 1 tablet every 30 min for a total of 2 to 4 tablets
Propranolol (Inderal®)		<35 kg: 10 to 20 mg p.o. three times a day
		>35 kg: 20 to 40 mg p.o. three times a day
Antineoplastics		
Actinomycin D (Dactinomycin)		0.015 mg/kg/day i.v. for 5 days
Amethopterin (Methotrexate)		0.12 mg/day p.o. or i.m. (maximum dose, 5 to 10 mg/day) **or** 0.25 to 5 mg/kg/week intrathecally **or** 3 to 5 mg/kg i.v. every other week
Azathioprine (Imuran®)		3 to 5 mg/kg/day p.o.or i.v.
Busulfan (Myerlan®)		Children: 0.06 mg/kg/day p.o.
		Adults: 2 mg p.o. one to three times a day
Chlorambucil (Leukeran®)		0.1 to 0.2 mg/kg/day
Cyclophosphamide (Cytoxan®)		2 to 8 mg/kg/day p.o. or i.v. for at least 7 days **or** 20 to 50 mg/kg once a week
Mechlorethamine (Nitrogen mustard)		0.1 mg/kg/day i.v. slowly for 4 days
Mercaptopurine (Purinethol®)		2.5 to 4 mg/kg/day p.o. in three doses
Vinblastine (Velban®)		Children: 0.1 to 0.2 mg/kg i.v. once a week
		Adults: 0.1 to 0.15 mg/kg i.v. once a week
Vincristine (Oncovin®)		1.5 mg/m^2 i.v. once a week for 4 to 6 weeks, then every 2 weeks (maximum dose, 2 mg)
Antispasmodics		
Donnatal®	Gastrointestinal distress	10 lb: 0.5 ml every 4 hr
		20 lb: 1 ml every 4 hr
		30 lb: 1.5 ml every 4 hr
		50 lb: ½ tsp every 4 hr
		75 lb: ¾ tsp every 4 hr
		100 lb: 1 tsp every 4 hr
		Adults: 1 or 2 tablets three times a day

Drugs	Indications	Dosage
Ditropan®	Urinary bladder distress	Children >5 years old: 1 tsp two times a day (5 mg/5 ml) Adults: 1 5-mg tablet two or three times a day (maximum dose, 20 mg/day)
Bethanechol (Urecholine®)	Gastroesophageal reflux	0.3 to 0.6 mg/kg/day p.o. in four doses; one-third or one-fourth of the oral dose may be given subcutaneously
Bronchodilators Epinephrine (Adrenaline®)		1:1,000 aqueous solution: 0.01 ml/kg s.c.; repeat every 15 min up to three times (maximum dose, 0.5 ml) 1:200 (Sus-Phrine®): 0.005 mg/kg s.c. in one dose (maximum dose, 0.15 ml) Racemic (2.25%): 0.05 mg/kg diluted to 3 ml with saline, via nebulizer every 2 hr as needed (maximum dose, 0.5 ml)
Metaproterenol (Alupent®)	Use only in children >6 years of age	6–9 yrs (under 60 lb): 10 mg (one tsp or one 10-mg tablet 3×/day p.o. > 9 yrs (over 60 lb): 20 mgs p.o. 3×/day
Aminophylline		5 to 7 mg/kg i.v. over a 15- to 20-min period, **then** 0.8 mg/kg/hr continuous i.v.; **or** 5 to 7 mg/kg p.o. every 6 hr
Terbutaline (Brethine®)		Children 12 to 15 years old: 2.5 mg p.o. three times a day Adults: 5 mg p.o. three times a day **or** 0.25 mg s.c.; if needed, repeat once after 20 min
1% Isoetharine (Bronkosol®)		0.5 ml diluted 1:3 with saline in oxygen aerosol every 4 hr as needed
Cromolyn (Intal® or Aarane®)	Not for acute attacks	20 mg by inhalation via Spinhaler® every 6 hr
Theophylline (Slo-Phyllin®)		5 to 8 mg/kg p.o. every 6 hr
Cardiovascular drugs Atropine	Bradyarrhythmias	0.01 to 0.03 mg/kg i.v.; repeat as needed (maximum dose, 1 mg)
Epinephrine (Adrenaline®)	Bradyarrhythmia, cardiac arrest	Intracardiac: 0.1 ml/kg of 1:10,000 solution Intravenous: 0.1 to 1.0 μg/kg/min of 1:50,000 solution
Digoxin	Congestive heart failure, paroxysmal atrial tachycardia (PAT), atrial fibrillation and flutter	Digitalizing dose: 0.02 to 0.04 mg/kg/day p.o.; one-half of dose is given immediately, one-fourth of dose is given 6 to 8 hr later, and one-fourth of dose is given 6 to 8

Drugs Used in Pediatric Practice *(continued)*

Drugs	Indications	Dosage
		hr after second dose (maximum dose, 2.0 mg/day) Maintenance dose: One-fourth of digitalizing dose is given in two doses 12 hr apart (maximum dose, 0.5 mg/day) Intravenous dose: Two-thirds of oral dose
Phenytoin (Dilantin®)	Ventricular arrhythmia, digoxin toxicity	1 to 5 mg/kg i.v. slowly; repeat as needed (maximum dose, 500 mg in 4 hr)
2% Lidocaine	Ventricular arrhythmia	0.5 to 1.0 mg/kg i.v.; repeat every 5 to 10 min as needed **or** 20 to 40 ug/kg/min continuous i.v. (maximum dose, 5 mg/kg)
Isoproterenol (Isuprel®)	Heart block, bradycardia, cardiogenic shock	1 to 4 mg/l of 5% D/W, continuous i.v. (0.5 to 4.0 μg/min)
Quinidine	Ventricular arrthymia, PAT, and other atrial arrthymias	2 to 10 mg/kg p.o. every 3 to 6 hr
Methoxamine (Vasoxyl®)	PAT	0.1 mg/kg i.v.
Dopamine (Intropin®)	Hypotension, cardiogenic shock	5 to 10 μg/kg/min continuous i.v. (maximum dose, 20 to 50 μg/kg/min)
Propranolol (Inderal®)	Avoid use if surgery is imminent	0.01 to 0.15 mg/kg i.v. slowly; repeat every 6 to 8 hr as needed (maximum single dose, 10 mg) **or** 0.5 to 1.0 mg/kg/day p.o. in three or four doses (maximum dose, 60 mg/day)
Procainamide (Pronestyl®)		40 to 60 mg/kg/day p.o. in four to six doses
Metaraminol (Aramine®)	Hypotension	0.1 mg/kg i.m. or s.c. immediately and as needed **or** 0.01 mg/kg i.v. as needed **or** 0.5 to 4.0 μg/kg/min continuous i.v.
Neo-Synephrine®	Hypotension, PAT	0.1 mg/kg s.c. or i.m. every 1 or 2 hr as needed **or** 10 mg/100 ml of saline; adjust rate to desired effect
Tolazoline (Priscoline®)	To keep the ductus arteriosus patient in cyanotic-ductus-dependant congenital heart disease	1 to 2 mg/kg i.v., **then** 1 or 2 mg/kg/hr continuous i.v.
Prostaglandin (PGE₁)		0.1 μ/kg/min continuous i.v. drip
Diuretics		
Spironolactone (Aldactone®)		1.7 to 3.3 mg/kg/day p.o. in three or four doses
Acetazolamide (Diamox®)		5 mg/kg/day p.o. or i.m. in one dose
Chlorothiazide (Diuril®)		20 mg/kg/day p.o. in two

Drugs	Indications	Dosage
		doses (maximum dose, 2.0 g/day)
Hydrochlorothiazide (Hydrodiuril®)		2 or 3 mg/kg/day p.o. in two doses (maximum dose, 200 mg/day)
Furosemide (Lasix®)		2 mg/kg/day p.o. in three or four doses **or** 1 mg/kg i.v. or i.m. every 2 hr as needed (maximum single dose, 6 mg/kg)
25% Mannitol		200 mg/kg i.v. over a 3- to 5-min period (test dose), **then** 0.5 to 2 g/kg i.v. over a 30- to 60-min period (diuresis) **or** 400 mg/kg continuous i.v. (loading dose) and 13 g/hr/1.73 m² (maintenance dose)
Electrolyte preparations Ammonium chloride		75 mg/kg/day p.o. in four doses (maximum dose, 2 to 6 g/day)
Calcium chloride (27% calcium)		250 to 300 mg/kg/day p.o. as 2% solution in four doses
Calcium gluconate		500 mg/kg/day p.o. in three to six doses **or** 100 mg/kg i.v. slowly as needed
Calcium lactate		500 mg/kg p.o. every 4 to 8 hr
Magnesium citrate		4 ml/kg p.o.
Magnesium sulfate		25 to 50 mg/kg i.v. or i.m. every 4 to 6 hr for three or four doses, **then** 12 to 15 mg/100 ml of intravenous fluids (maintenance dose)
Phosphorus supplements		1 or 2 g/day p.o. in four doses
Potassium supplements (Chloride, gluconate, or Triple X)		1 or 2 mEq/kg/day p.o.
Sodium polystyrene sulfonate (Kayexalate®)		Children: 1 mEqK/1 g of resin p.o. (practical exchange rate) of resin p.o. every 6 hr **or** rectally every 2 to 6 hr Adults: 15 g p.o. every 6 hr **or** 30 to 60 g rectally every 6 hr
Emetics Syrup of ipecac		9 to 12 months old: 10 ml p.o. 1 to 12 years old: 15 ml p.o. >12 years old: 30 ml p.o. followed by 100 to 500 ml of clear fluids p.o.; repeat once after 20 min, if needed
Laxatives Colace®		5 mg/kg/day p.o. in three or four doses
Dulcolax®		0.3 mg/kg p.o. 6 hr before desired effect; 5 to 10 mg rectally

Drugs Used in Pediatric Practice *(continued)*

Drugs	Indications	Dosage
Milk of magnesia (Magnesium hydroxide)		0.5 ml/kg/dose p.o.
Psychotropic drugs		
Dextroamphetamine (Dexedrine®)	Anorexic agent, hyperactivity	2.5 to 40 mg/day p.o. in two or three doses; increase daily dose by 2.5 mg as needed to a maximum dose of 1 mg/kg/day
Imipramine (Tofranil®)	Sedation	1.5 mg/kg/day p.o. or i.m. in three or four doses
	Enuresis	25 mg p.o. at bedtime; increase to 50 to 75 mg (maximum dose, 300 mg/day)
Methylphenidate (Ritalin®)	Hyperactivity, attention deficit disorders (ADD); use for children <6 years old	5 mg p.o. two times a day; increase weekly by 5 to 10 mg to a maximum dose of 60 mg/day
Pemoline (Cylert®)	Hyperactivity, ADD; not recommended for use in children <6 years old	37.5 mg/day p.o.; increase weekly by 18.75 mg to a maximum dose of 112.5 mg/day
Thioridazine (Mellaril®)	Use for children 2 to 12 years old	0.5 to 3.0 mg/kg/day p.o. in two to four doses (maximum dose, 20 to 800 mg/day)
Sedatives		
Chloral hydrate		1 to 30 mg/kg p.o. or rectally every 6 hr as needed (maximum dose, 50 mg/kg/day or 2.0 g)
Diazepam (Valium®)		0.1 to 0.8 mg/kg/day p.o. in three or four doses **or** 0.1 to 0.3 mg/kg i.m. or i.v. slowly; repeat every 2 to 4 hr as needed
Paraldehyde		0.15 ml/kg (150 mg/kg) p.o., i.m., or rectally
Pentobarbital (Nembutal®)		2 or 3 mg/kg p.o., i.m., or rectally every 8 hr as needed
Secobarbital (Seconal®)		6 mg/kg/day p.o. in three doses
Paregoric	Narcotic withdrawal	2 to 4 drops/kg p.o. every 4 hr; increase to 20 to 40 drops/kg/day
	Sedation	0.06 ml/month (up to 12 months) every 3–4 hr p.o.
	Analgesic	0.25 to 0.5 ml/kg per dose p.o.
Steroids		
ACTH (Corticotropin)		Aqueous: 1.6 unit/kg/day i.v., i.m., or s.c. in three or four doses
		Gel: 0.8 unit/kg/day in two doses
Cortisone acetate	Physiological	30 mg/m^2/day p.o. in three doses **or** 15 mg/m^2/day i.m. in one dose

Drugs	Indications	Dosage
	Stress	Two to four times the physiological dose
Desoxycorticosterone (DOCA)		1 to 2 mg/day i.m. in oil as a single dose
Dexamethasone (Decadron®)		Initial: 0.5 to 1.0 mg/kg i.v. or i.m.
		Maintenance: 0.25 to 0.5 mg/kg/day i.v. or i.m. in four doses
Fludrocortisone (Florinef®)		0.05 to 0.2 mg/day p.o.
Hydrocortisone	Physiological	12.5 mg/m^2/day i.m. **or** 25 mg/m^2/day p.o. in three doses
	Shock (succinate)	50 mg/kg i.v. immediately, **then** 50 to 75 mg/kg/day i.v. in four doses
	Asthma	10 mg/kg/day i.v. in four doses
Prednisone		2 mg/kg/day p.o. in two to four doses
Thyroid preparations		
Levothyroxine (Synthroid)		1 to 6 months old: 12 μg/kg/day p.o.
		6 to 12 months old: 6 to 8 μg/kg/day p.o.
		1 to 5 years old: 4 to 6 μg/kg/day p.o.
		5 to 10 years old: 3 to 5 μg/kg/day p.o.
		>10 years old: 2 to 3 μg/kg/day p.o.
Potassium iodide (SSKI®)	Expectorant	2 to 4 drops in orange juice every 8 hr
	Thyrotoxicosis	0.9 ml/day (900 mg/day) p.o. in three doses
Propranolol (Inderal®)	Thyrotoxicosis	Children: 2.5 to 10 mg/kg/day p.o. in three or four doses
		Adults: 1 to 2 mg i.v. over a 10-min period
Propylthiouracil (PTU)		Initial: 5 mg/kg/day p.o. in three or four doses
		Maintenance: 75 to 200 mg/day p.o. in two or three doses
Thyroid USP		Initial: 15 mg p.o. in one dose (infants) **or** 30 mg p.o. in one dose (children)
		Maintenance: 60 to 180 mg/day p.o.
Methimazole (Tapazole®)		Initial: 0.4 mg/kg/day p.o. in three doses
		Maintenance: 0.2 mg/kg/day in three doses
Other drugs		
Allopurinol	Xanthine oxidase inhibitor	<6 years old: 150 mg/day p.o. in three doses
		6 to 10 years old: 300 mg/day p.o. in three doses (maximum dose, 800 mg/day)

Drugs Used in Pediatric Practice *(continued)*

Drugs	Indications	Dosage
Cholestyramine (Questran®)	Ion-exchange resin (bile salts)	240 mg/kg/day in three doses p.o.
Dihydrotachysterol	Antihypocalcemic	Infants: 0.05 to 0.2 mg/day p.o. Children: 0.2 to 1.0 mg/day p.o. Adjusted according to serum calcium levels
Dobutamine	Cardiotonic	2 to 10 μg/kg/min continuous i.v. (maximum dose, 40 μg/kg/min)
Edrophonium (Tensilon®)	Antidote (to curare derivatives) and diagnostic aid (myasthenia gravis); atropine should be readily available	Neonates: 0.1 mg i.v. in one dose Infants and children: 0.2 mg/kg i.v.; give 20% of dose slowly; if no response in 1 min, give 1-mg increments (maximum total dose, 5 to 10 mg)
Ergocalciferol	Vitamin	Initial: 0.125 mg/kg/day until calcium level starts to rise Maintenance: 0.05 mg/kg/day
Glucagon	Antidiabetic	0.025 to 0.1 mg/kg s.c., i.m., or i.v.; repeat every 20 min as needed (maximum total dose, 1.0 mg)
Ibuprofen	Anti-inflammatory	40 mg/kg/day p.o. in three or four doses (maximum dose, 2.4 g/day)
Iron dextran (Imferon®)	Hematinic	Total dose of iron (in mg): m^2 × 55 × 13.5 (Hgb in gm/100 ml) i.v. or i.m. (maximum i.v. dose, 2 ml/day)
Iron salts	Therapeutic	6 mg elemental iron/kg/day p.o. in three doses
	Prophylaxis	Premature infants: 2 mg/kg/day Full-term infants: 1 mg/kg/day (maximum dose, 15 mg/day)
Methenamine mandelate (Mandelamine®)	Antibacterial (urinary)	Initial: 100 mg/kg/day p.o. in three or four doses Maintenance: 50 mg/kg/day p.o. in three or four doses (maximum dose, 3 g/day)
Pancreatic enzymes (Pancrease®)	Digestant adjunct	1 or 2 capsules with meals **or** 1 capsule with snacks
Pancuronium bromide (Pavulon®)	Relaxant (skeletal muscle)	Initial: 0.02 mg/kg/dose (neonates) **or** 0.1 to 0.15 mg/kg/dose (children) Maintenance: 0.1 mg/kg/dose every 30 to 60 min i.v.
Penicillamine	Chelating agent Acute therapy	25 to 50 mg/kg/day p.o. in three doses
	Chronic therapy	Children <6 months old: 250 mg/day p.o. in one dose

Drugs	Indications	Dosage
Phenazopyridine (Pyridium®)	Analgesic (urinary tract)	Older children: 1 g/day p.o. in four doses 12 mg/kg/day p.o. in three doses
Probenecid (Benemid®)	Uricosuric	Children 2 to 14 years old: 25 mg/kg p.o. immeditely, **then** 40 mg/kg/day in four doses Adults: 250 mg 2×/day p.o. for 1 week **then** 500 mg p.o. 2×/day (maximum dose, 25 mg/day)
Scopolamine	Gonorrhea Anticholinergic	1 g 30 min before penicillin 6 µg/kg/dose p.o. or s.c.
Vasopressin (Pitressin®)	Hormone (anti-diuretic)	Aqueous: 1 to 3 ml/day s.c. in three doses Tannate in oil: 0.2 ml i.m. increase dose every 1 to 3 days as needed (maximum dose, 2 ml) Nasal drops: 1 or 2 drops in each nostril every 6 hr as needed

Drugs Used for Sedation

Drug	Neonates	Children	<1–6 months	6 months–1 year	>1 year
Premedication (for diagnostic and therapeutic procedures)					
Meperidine (Demerol®)	1.0 mg/kg	2.0 mg/kg			
Promethazine (Phenergan®)	0.5 mg/kg	1.0 mg/kg			
Chlorpromazine[a] (Thorazine®)	0.5 mg/kg	1.0 mg/kg			
Preoperative (general anesthesia)					
Atropine (maximum dose, 0.6 mg/kg)			0.01–0.02 mg/kg	0.01–0.02 mg/kg	0.01–0.02 mg/kg
Phenobarbital (maximum dose, 120 mg/kg)			—	3.0–4.0 mg/kg	3.0–4.0 mg/kg
Meperidine (maximum dose, 100 mg/kg)			—	—	1.0 mg/kg

[a]Do not use chlorpromazine in patients with hypothalamic and/or brain stem lesions; decrease the dosage by at least 50% (occasionally more) in patients being prepared for cardiac catheterization.

Gamma Globulin Prophylaxis

1. Diphtheria

   a. Diphtheria immune globulin (DIG), 20,000 to 120,000 units i.m.

   b. Immunize upon **clinical suspicion** of diphtheria, after testing for hypersensitivity to serum.

2. Hepatitis A (HAV)

   a. Immune serum globulin (ISG), 0.02 to 0.04 ml/kg i.m. (prophylactic dose) **or** 0.06 ml/kg i.m., repeated in 6 months (for continuously exposed persons).

3. Hepatitis B (HBV)

   a. Hepatitis B immune globulin (HBIG), 0.05 to 0.07 ml/kg i.m. (maximum dose, 5 ml) in adults **or** 0.5 ml i.m., repeated in 1 month, in infants.

   b. ISG, 0.12 ml/kg i.m. (maximum dose, 5 ml), repeated in 1 month, in adults **or** 2.0 ml i.m. in infants; may be used if HBIG is not available, but is not as effective.

4. Rubeola

   a. ISG, 0.25 ml/kg i.m. (prophylactic dose).

5. Tetanus

   a. Human tetanus immune globulin (HTIG), 250 to 500 units i.m. (prophylactic dose) **or** 3,000 to 6,000 units i.m. (therapeutic dose).

   b. Equine or bovine tetanus immune globulin (TIG), 3,000 to 5,000 units i.m. (prophylactic dose) **or** 50,000 to 100,000 units i.m. (therapeutic dose); may be used if HTIG is not available, after testing for hypersensitivity to the serum.

6. Varicella-zoster

   a. Zoster immune globulin: Consult with Centers for Disease Control, Atlanta, Georgia (404/329-3741).

   b. Zoster immune plasma (ZIP), 10 ml/kg i.v.

   c. ISG, 0.6 to 1.2 ml/kg i.m. (modifying dose); may be used only if ZIG or ZIP is not available.

Growth Chart: Boys

DISTRIBUTED BY MEAD JOHNSON NUTRITIONAL DIVISION

Reprinted courtesy of Mead Johnson
Nutritional Division, Evansville, Indiana

GROWTH CHARTS
WITH REFERENCE PERCENTILES
FOR BOYS
2 TO 18 YEARS OF AGE

Stature for Age
Weight for Age
Weight for Stature

NAME _____   RECORD # _____

DATE OF BIRTH _____

Date of Measurement	Age Years	Age Months	Stature	Weight		

These charts to record the growth of the individual child were constructed by the National Center for Health Statistics in collaboration with the Center for Disease Control. The charts are based on data from national probability samples representative of boys in the general U.S. population. Their use will direct attention to unusual body size which may be due to disease or poor nutrition.

Measuring: Take all measurements with the child in minimal indoor clothing and without shoes. Measure stature with the child standing. Use a beam balance to measure weight.

Recording: First take all measurements and record them on this front page. Then graph each measurement on the appropriate chart. Find the child's age on the horizontal scale; then follow a vertical line from that point to the horizontal level of the child's measurement (stature or weight). Where the two lines intersect, make a cross mark with a pencil. In graphing weight for stature, place the cross mark directly above the child's stature at the horizontal level of his weight. When the child is measured again, join the new set of cross marks to the previous set by straight lines.

Do not use the weight for stature chart for boys who have begun to develop secondary sex characteristics.

Interpreting: Many factors influence growth. Therefore, growth data cannot be used alone to diagnose disease, but they do allow you to identify some unusual children.

Each chart contains a series of curved lines numbered to show selected percentiles. These refer to the rank of a measure in a group of 100. Thus, when a cross mark is on the 95th percentile line of weight for age it means that only five children among 100 of the corresponding age and sex have weights greater than that recorded.

Inspect the set of cross marks you have just made. If any are particularly high or low (for example, above the 95th percentile or below the 5th percentile), you may want to refer the child to a physician. *Compare* the most recent set of cross marks with earlier sets for the same child. If he has changed rapidly in percentile levels, you may want to refer him to a physician. Rapid changes are less likely to be significant when they occur within the range from the 25th to the 75th percentile.

In normal teenagers, the age at onset of puberty varies. Rises occur in percentile levels if puberty is early, and these levels fall if puberty is late.

DEPARTMENT OF HEALTH, EDUCATION, AND WELFARE, PUBLIC HEALTH SERVICE
HEALTH RESOURCES ADMINISTRATION, NATIONAL CENTER FOR HEALTH STATISTICS, AND CENTER FOR DISEASE CONTROL

BOYS FROM 2 TO 18 YEARS

STATURE FOR AGE

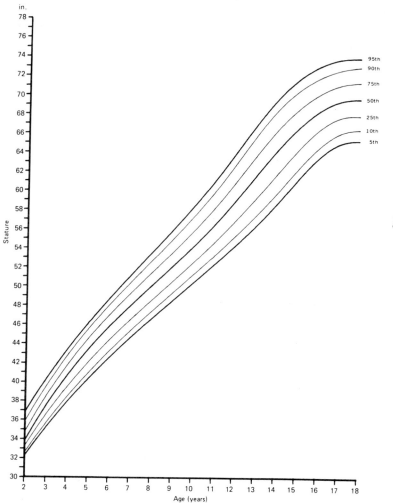

BOYS FROM 2 TO 18 YEARS
WEIGHT FOR AGE

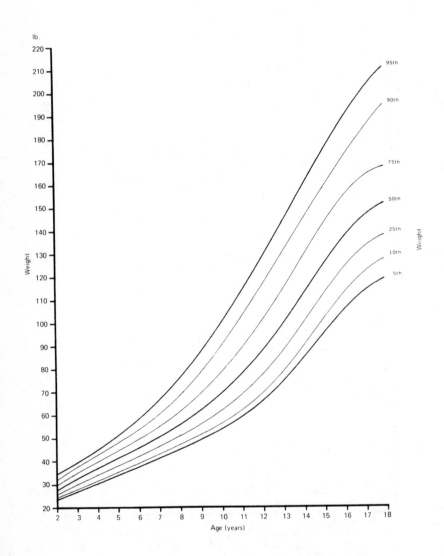

PRE-PUBERTAL BOYS FROM 2 TO 11½ YEARS

WEIGHT FOR STATURE

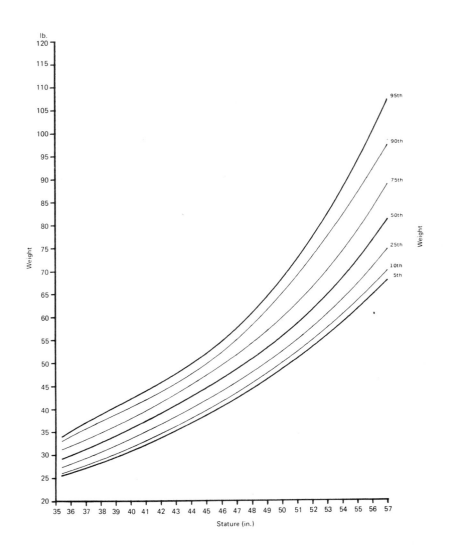

Growth Chart: Girls

DISTRIBUTED BY MEAD JOHNSON NUTRITIONAL DIVISION

Reprinted courtesy of Mead Johnson
Nutritional Division, Evansville, Indiana

GROWTH CHARTS
WITH REFERENCE PERCENTILES
FOR GIRLS
BIRTH TO 36 MONTHS OF AGE

Length for Age
Weight for Age
Head Circumference for Age
Weight for Length

NAME _____   RECORD # _____

DATE OF BIRTH _____

Date of Measurement	Age in Months	Recumbent Length	Weight	Head Circumference	

These charts to record the growth of the individual child were constructed by the National Center for Health Statistics in collaboration with the Center for Disease Control. The charts are based on data from the Fels Research Institute, Yellow Springs, Ohio. These data are appropriate for young girls in the general U.S. population. Their use will direct attention to unusual body size which may be due to disease or poor nutrition.

Measuring: Take all measurements with the child nude or with minimal clothing and without shoes. Measure length with the child lying on her back fully extended. Two people are needed to measure recumbent length properly. Use a beam balance to measure weight.

Recording: First take all measurements and record them on this front page. Then graph each measurement on the appropriate chart. Find the child's age on the horizontal scale; then follow a vertical line from that point to the horizontal level of the child's measurement (length, weight or head circumference). Where the two lines intersect, make a cross mark with a pencil. In graphing weight for length, place the cross mark directly above the child's length at

the horizontal level of her weight. When the child is measured again, join the new set of cross marks to the previous set by straight lines.

Interpreting: Many factors influence growth. Therefore, growth data cannot be used alone to diagnose disease, but they do allow you to identify some unusual children.

Each chart contains a series of curved lines numbered to show selected percentiles. These refer to the rank of a measure in a group of 100. Thus, when a cross mark is on the 95th percentile line of weight for age it means that only five children among 100 of the corresponding age and sex have weights greater that recorded.

Inspect the set of cross marks you have just made. If any are particularly high or low (for example, above the 95th percentile or below the 5th percentile), you may want to refer the child to a physician. *Compare* the most recent set of cross marks with earlier sets for the same child. If she has changed rapidly in percentile levels, you may want to refer her to a physician. Rapid changes are less likely to be significant when they occur within the range from the 25th to the 75th percentile.

DEPARTMENT OF HEALTH, EDUCATION, AND WELFARE, PUBLIC HEALTH SERVICE
HEALTH RESOURCES ADMINISTRATION, NATIONAL CENTER FOR HEALTH STATISTICS, AND CENTER FOR DISEASE CONTROL

GIRLS FROM BIRTH TO 36 MONTHS
LENGTH FOR AGE

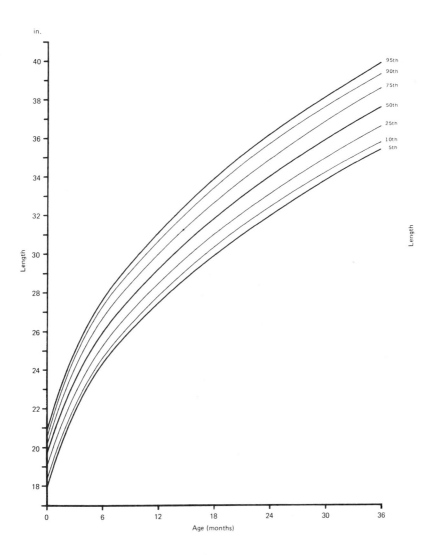

GIRLS FROM BIRTH TO 36 MONTHS
WEIGHT FOR AGE

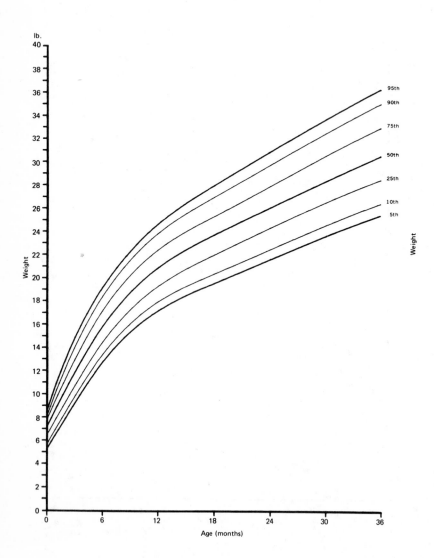

GIRLS FROM BIRTH TO 36 MONTHS

HEAD CIRCUMFERENCE FOR AGE

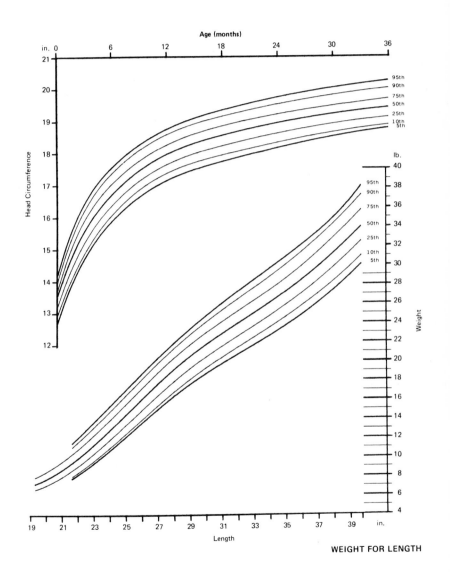

WEIGHT FOR LENGTH

Isolation Procedures

Diseases	Procedure
	Blood Precautions
Anthropod-borne viral fever Hepatitis (A, B, non-A, non-B) Malaria	Precautions are aimed at limiting the possibility of contact with blood and its products from infected patients All syringes and needles must be disposed of in such a manner that personnel will not be injured unintentionally
	Enteric Isolation
Cholera Infectious diarrhea Staphylococcal enterocolitis Hepatitis Typhoid *(Salmonella typhi)*	Separate the patient from others (private room) Gown and gloves must be worn by all persons who have direct contact with the patient or contact with articles that may be contaminated with fecal material Articles contaminated with urine or feces must be disinfected or discarded **Hands must be washed upon entering and leaving the patient's room**
	Excretion Precautions
Amebiasis Clostridial food poisoning *(C. perfringens)* Enterobiasis Giardiasis Hand, foot, and mouth disease Herpangina Infectious lymphocytosis Leptospirosis Meningitis Pleurodynia Poliomyelitis Staphylococcal food poisoning Tapeworms Enteroviral disease (other)	Dispose of excretions appropriately (adequate sewage system) **Careful handwashing after coming in contact with the patient.** The patient should also be instructed in careful handwashing after defecating
	Protective Isolation
Agranulocytosis Chemotherapy Dermatitis (especially when severe and extensive) Extensive noninfected burns Lymphomas and leukemia (in certain patients)	Separate the patient from others (private room; door must be kept closed) All persons entering the room must wear a gown, gloves, and a mask at all times **Hands must be washed upon entering and leaving the patient's room**
	Respiratory Isolation
Measles Meningococcal meningitis Meningococcemia Mumps Pertussis	Separate the patient from others (private room) A mask must be worn by all persons entering the room who are susceptible to the disease **Hands must be washed upon entering and leaving the patient's room**

Diseases	Procedure
Rubella Tuberculosis (pulmonary)	Contaminated articles must be disinfected The patient should be masked when being transported through the hospital

Secretion, Lesion

Diseases	Procedure
Actinomycosis Anthrax Brucellosis Infected burns Candidiasis (skin and mucosa) Coccidioidomycosis Conjunctivitis Gonorrhea Granuloma inguinale Herpes simplex Keratoconjunctivitis Listeriosis Lymphogranuloma venereum Nocardiosis Orf Syphilis (mucocutaneous) Trachoma (acute) Tuberculosis (draining) Tularemia (draining)	Do not touch the wound, lesion, or dressing when changing dressings or cleaning the wound or lesion **Hands must be washed before and after touching the pa- tient** Double bag soiled dressings and equipment for decontamination or disposal

Secretion, Oral

Diseases	Procedure
Herpangina Herpes oralis Infectious mononucleosis Melioidosis, pulmonary *Mycoplasma* pneumonia Pneumonia, bacterial Psittacosis Q fever Scarlet fever Streptococcal pharyngitis	Instruct the patient to cough or expectorate into a disposable tissue and dispose of the tissue in a nearby impervious bag Equipment used in respiratory management of these patients (e.g., endotracheal tubes, suction tubing, tracheostomy catheters) should be discarded in an impervious bag or bagged for disinfection

Strict Isolation

Diseases	Procedure
Anthrax Major burns Congenital rubella Diphtheria Disseminated herpes Disseminated zoster Lassa fever Marburg virus disease Pneumonic plague Pneumonia *(S. aureus* and group A *Streptococcus)* Rabies Major skin infections Smallpox Varicella Vaccinia	Separate the patient from others (private room; door must be kept closed) All persons entering the room must wear a gown, gloves, and a mask **Hands must be washed upon entering and leaving the patient's room** Articles in the room must be wrapped before being discarded or disinfected

Wound Precautions

Diseases	Procedure
Infected burns Gas gangrene	A private room is best All persons having contact with the patient must wear a gown

Isolation Procedures *(continued)*

Diseases	Procedure

Herpes zoster
Melioidosis (extrapulmonary)
Bubonic plague
Puerperal sepsis
Wound infections not covered by
  dressings
	All persons having direct contact with the lesion must also
	  wear gloves
	Instruments, dressings, and linens should be wrapped before
	  being discarded or disinfected

Modified from *Report of the Committee on Infectious Diseases*, American Academy of Pediatrics, 1982, with permission.

Normal Laboratory Values[a]

Test	Newborn	Infant	Child	Adolescent	Comments
ACTH	—	—	—	—	20–80 pg/ml at 8 a.m. (values are lower in p.m.)
Aldolase	—	1.5–18.5 units/l	2.5–13.5 units/l	1.5–12.0 units/l	Values may be higher if the patient is tested in the upright position
Aldosterone	10–35 ng/dl	30–130 ng/dl	5–50 ng/dl	5–15 ng/dl	
Ammonia	90–150 μg/dl	40–80 μg/dl	—	40–80 μg/dl	Enzymatic method (Conway method yields slightly higher values)
Amylase	—	—	—	—	45–200 dye units
α_1-Antitrypsin	113–284 mg/dl	113–284 mg/dl	113–284 mg/dl	113–284 mg/dl	
Barbiturate	0	0	0	0	Therapeutic blood level, 15–40 μg/ml
Bilirubin, direct	0–0.2 mg/dl	0–0.2 mg/dl	0–0.2 mg/dl	0–0.2 mg/dl	
Bilirubin, total	Day 1: <2 mg/dl Day 2: <8 mg/dl Day 3: <8 mg/dl Day 10: 0.2–1.0 mg/dl	0.2–1.0 mg/dl	0.2–1.0 mg/dl	0.2–1.0 mg/dl	
Calcium, total	5.9–10.7 mg/dl	9.0–11.0 mg/dl	8.5–11.0 mg/dl	8.5–10.5 mg/dl	
Carbon dioxide (P_{CO_2})	18–24 mm Hg	25–29 mm Hg	25–29 mm Hg	25–29 mm Hg	
Carbon dioxide, total	17–24 mmol/l	20–28 mmol/l	12–20 mmol/l	23–29 mmol/l	After 1 year of age, the level gradually increases to adult levels
Carbon monoxide	—	—	0–2%	0–2%	Levels for nonsmokers
Carotenoids	—	0–70 μg/dl	40–130 μg/dl	60–200 μg/dl	
Catecholamines					
Norepinephrine	—	—	—	47–69 ng/dl	
Epinephrine	—	—	—	18–26 ng/dl	
Chloride, serum	96–107 mEq/l	98–106 mEq/l	98–106 mEq/l	98–106 mEq/l	

Normal Laboratory Values[a] (continued)

Test	Newborn	Infant	Child	Adolescent	Comments
Chloride, sweat	—	0–30 mmol/l	0–30 mmol/l	0–30 mmol/l	Values > 60 mmol/l are diagnostic of cystic fibrosis
Cholesterol, total	45–150 mg/dl	70–175 mg/dl	120–200 mg/dl	120–210 mg/dl	
Human chorionic gonadotropin (HCG)	—	—	—	60,000 to 400,000 units/dl	First trimester of pregnancy
HCG (radioimmunoassay)	—	—	—	36–56 units/ml	First trimester of pregnancy
Copper	20–70 µg/dl	30–150 µg/dl	30–150 µg/dl	70–155 µg/dl	
Creatine phosphokinase (CPK)	10–300 units/l			12–65 units/l	
Creatinine	0.6–1.2 mg/dl	0.2–0.4 mg/dl	0.3–0.7 mg/dl	0.5–1.2 mg/dl	
Creatinine clearance	40–65 ml/min/ 1.73 m²		98–150 ml/min/ 1.73 m²	80–130 ml/min/ 1.73 m²	
Electrophoresis					
Total protein	4.6–7.4 g/dl	6.1–6.7 g/dl	6.0–8.0 g/dl	6.0–8.0 g/dl	
Albumin	3.6–5.4% total protein	4.4–5.3% total protein	3.5–4.7% total protein	3.5–4.7% total protein	
α1 globulin	0.1–0.3% total protein	0.2–0.4% total protein	0.2–0.3% total protein	0.2–0.3% total protein	
β globulin	0.2–0.6% total protein	0.5–0.8% total protein	0.5–1.1% total protein	0.5–1.1% total protein	
Free fatty acids	—	—	—	—	> 1 µg/ml
α-Fetoprotein	—	—	0.3–0.9 mmol/l	—	
Fibrinogen	125–300 mg/dl	150–450 mg/dl	150–450 mg/dl	150–450 mg/dl	
Follicle-stimulating hormone (FSH)	—	—	2–11 million units/ml	4–30 million units/ml	Midcycle peak, 10–90 million units/ml
Galactose	0–20 mg/dl	0–20 mg/dl	—	—	
Glucose, fasting	30–60 mg/dl	60–100 mg/dl	60–100 mg/dl	70–105 mg/dl	
Glucose 6-phosphate dehydrogenase	5.0–18.3 units/g Hb	5.0–9.7 units/g Hb	5.0–9.7 units/g Hb	5.0–9.7 units/g Hb	
Growth hormone	12–34 ng/ml	1–5 ng/ml	1–5 ng/ml	1–5 ng/ml	
Hemoglobin, serum	—	0–3 mg/dl	0–3 mg/dl	0–3 mg/dl	
Glucose insulin, fasting	<8	—	—	7–24 units/ml	
Glucose insulin, OGTT		—	—	—	0: 4–24 60: 18–276 120: 16–166 180: 4–38

Test					Comments
Iron, binding capacity	60–175 µg/dl	100–400 µg/dl	250–400 µg/dl	250–400 µg/dl	
Iron, total	100–250 µg/dl	40–100 µg/dl	50–120 µg/dl	50–150 µg/dl	
Lactic acid	—	—	—	—	Arterial whole blood: 0.35–0.75 mmol/l
Lactic dehydrogenase (LDH)	300–500 units/l	200–250 units/l	60–170 units/l	40–90 units/l	
Lead	—	—	—	—	<30 µg/dl
Magnesium	1.4–2.2 mEq/l	1.3–2.1 mEq/l	1.3–2.1 mEq/l	1.3–2.1 mEq/l	
Methemoglobin	—	—	—	—	0.0–0.3 g/dl whole blood
Osmolality	—	—	—	—	290–312 mOsm
Oxygen (P_{O_2}), arterial	65–80 mm Hg	85–110 mm Hg	85–110 mm Hg	85–110 mm Hg	Venous: 30–50 mm Hg
Oxygen saturation, arterial	40–90%	95–98%	95–98%	95–98%	Venous: 55–85%
pH	7.27–7.47	7.35–7.43	7.35–7.43	7.35–7.43	
Phenylalanine	1.2–3.4 mg/dl	0.8–1.8 mg/dl	0.8–1.8 mg/dl	0.8–1.8 mg/dl	Premature infant: 2.0–7.5 mg/dl
Phosphatase, alkaline	50–165 units/l	50–165 units/l	20–150 units/l	20–70 units/l	
Phosphorus	3.5–8.6 mg/dl	4.5–6.5 mg/dl	4.5–5.5 mg/dl	3.0–4.5 mg/dl	
Potassium	3.7–5.0 mEq/l	4.1–5.3 mEq/l	3.4–4.5 mEq/l	3.5–5.3 mEq/l	Increased with hemolysis
Salicylates	0	0	0	0	Therapeutic blood level: 15–25 mg/dl Toxic blood level: <30 mg/dl
Sodium	134–144 mEq/l	139–145 mEq/l	138–145 mEq/l	135–148 mEq/l	
T3 (resin)	27–32%	—	—	25–35%	
Thyroid-stimulating hormone (TSH)	4–15 units/ml	2–11	2–11	2–11	
Thyroxine	14–23 µg/dl	4–11 µg/dl	4–11 µg/dl	4–11 µg/dl	
Thyroxine (radioimmunoassay)	10–20.8 µg/dl	7–15 µg/dl	5–14 µg/dl	5–12 µg/dl	
Triglycerides	5–40 mg/dl	5–40 mg/dl	—	30–150 mg/dl	Diet dependent
Transaminase (SGPT)	5–28 units/l	0–54 units/l	1–30 units/l	0–19 units/l	
Transferrin	—	—	—	—	200–400 mg/dl
Urea nitrogen (BUN)	4–18 mg/dl	5–18 mg/dl	5–18 mg/dl	6–23 mg/dl	
Uric acid	5.2–9.0 mg/dl	—	2.0–5.5 mg/dl	2.6–7.2 mg/dl	
Vitamin A	35–75 µg/dl	—	60–100 µg/dl	30–65 µg/dl	
Vitamin E	—	—	—	—	5–20 µg/ml
Hematological values					
Bleeding time	1–8 min	1–6 min	1–6 min	1–6 min	
Clotting time	—	—	—	—	5–8 min
Complement, total hemolytic	25–45 units/ml	25–45 units/ml	25–45 units/ml	25–45 units/ml	

Normal Laboratory Values[a] (continued)

Test	Newborn	Infant	Child	Adolescent	Comments
Complement (C4)	—	—	20–40 mg/dl	10–40 mg/dl	
Complete blood cell count					All values are $\times 10^3$
Hemoglobin	15–22 g/dl	10–15 g/dl	11–15 g/dl	12–16 g/dl	
WBC count	6.0–30.0/mm³	6.0–17.5/mm³	4.8–10.8/mm³	4.8–10.8/mm³	
Hematocrit	50–65%	30–40%	31–45%	40–50%	
Erythrocyte sedimentation rate (ESR)	0–2 mm/hr	3–13 mm/hr	3–13 mm/hr	1–15 mm/hr	
Hemoglobin electrophoresis	—	—	—	—	A_2 and A_3 Hb: 96–98.5% A_2 Hb: 1.5–4.0%
Fetal hemoglobin	40–70%	2–20%	1–2%	1–2%	
Partial thromboplastin time (PTT)	>90 sec	25–40	25–40	25–40	Activated
Prothrombin time (PT)	<17 sec	11–14	25–40	25–40	
Reticulocyte count	1.1–4.5% of red cells	0.5–3.1% of red cells	0–2.0% of red cells	0–2.0% of red cells	

[a]Normal values differ for each laboratory; consult the hospital laboratory manual for abnormal tests.

Poisonous Plants[a]

Plant	Toxic substance	Signs and symptoms
American mistletoe	Toxic amine	Various degrees of gastroenteritis; occasionally, hypertension occurs
Autumn crocus	Source of colchicine	Burning of the mouth and throat, nausea, diarrhea, weakness, respiratory depression, and/or shock
Buttercup	Potent vesicant	Inflammation of the mouth and throat, severe gastroenteritis with occasional bloody diarrhea
Caladium	Calcium oxalate crystals (raphides)	Mucosal irritation of the oral cavity associated with pain and swelling of the mucosa
Castor bean	Phytotoxin: ricin **(extremely toxic, even in small amounts)**	Gastrointestinal hemorrhage, acute hemolysis, liver and kidney damage, burning of the mouth and throat, vomiting, and diarrhea; symptoms may be delayed for 12 to 18 hr
Christmas holly	Saponin	Causes a mild to moderate reaction with nausea, vomiting, abdominal pain, and diarrhea
Christmas rose	Glycosides	Irritation and numbing of the oral mucosa, gastrointestinal upset and, occasionally, seizures
Common nightshade	Toxic alkaloid	Muscle weakness, drowsiness, paralysis, abdominal pain, constipation, and diarrhea
Daffodil	Not isolated	Severe gastrointestinal irritation
Deadly nightshade	Belladonna alkaloids	Constipation, abdominal pain, diarrhea, muscle weakness, drowsiness, and/or paralysis
Dumbcane (*Dieffenbachia*)	Calcium oxalate crystals (raphides)	Mucosal irritation; pain and swelling of the oral mucosa
Elephant ears	Calcium oxalate crystals (raphides)	Severe mucosal irritation; pain and swelling of the oral mucosa
English ivy	Saponin	Nausea, vomiting, nervousness, respiratory difficulties and, occasionally, coma
Foxglove	Saponin, digitalis glycosides	Abdominal pain, nausea, vomiting, diarrhea, cardiac arrhythmias, confusion, and/or seizures
Fruit pits (cherry, peach, plum, apricot, nectarine, and apple)	Cyanide (typically, a large amount of the pit needs to be chewed and ingested)	Nausea, dizziness, confusion, anxiety, tremors, vocal cord paralysis, weakness, and respiratory distress

Poisonous Plants[a] *(continued)*

Plant	Toxic substance	Signs and symptoms
Hyacinth	—	Gastrointestinal irritation
Iris	—	Severe gastrointestinal irritation
Jimsonweed	Atropinelike alkaloid	Thirst, visual abnormalities, dilated pupils, excitement, delirium, hallucination, hyperthermia, and coma
Jonquil	—	Severe gastrointestinal irritation
Laurel	Andromedotoxin	Nausea, vomiting, respiratory distress, hypotension, and/or coma
Lily of the valley	Saponin, digitalislike glycosides	Abdominal pain, nausea, vomiting, diarrhea, cardiac arrhythmias, confusion, and/or seizures
Morning glory seeds	Myristicin (ingestion of more than 50 seeds is usually required for toxic effects)	Abdominal pain, hallucinations, blurred vision, and confusion
Narcissus	—	Severe gastrointestinal irritation
Nutmegs	Mystricin (the ingestion of only two seeds will cause toxic effects; the seeds must be chewed)	Abdominal pain, numbness, thirst, drowsiness, dizziness, hallucinations, delirium, and/or coma
Oleander	Saponin, digitalislike glycosides	Abdominal pain, nausea, vomiting, diarrhea, arrhythmias, confusion, seizures
Philodendron	Calcium oxalate crystals (raphides)	Mucosal irritation; pain and swelling of the oral mucosa
Poinciana	—	Severe gastrointestinal irritation, vomiting, diarrhea, and dehydration
Poinsettia	Toxic sap	Severe vomiting and diarrhea
Poison hemlock	Central nervous system stimulant	Nausea, vomiting, weakness, bradycardia, and respiratory distress
Rhododendron	Andromedotoxin	Nausea, vomiting, respiratory distress, hypotension, and/or coma
Star of Bethlehem	Saponin, digitalislike glycosides	Abdominal pain, nausea, vomiting, diarrhea, cardiac arrhythmias, confusion, and/or seizures
Wild parsnip	Cicutoxin **(extremely toxic, even in small amounts)**; one of the most toxic plants affecting humans; it is also called water hemlock	Abdominal pain, mental excitement, seizures, and death
Yew	Taxine **(extremely toxic, even in small amounts)**	Gastrointestinal distress, pupillary dilatation, weakness, seizures, respiratory depression, and cardiac depression

[a]Most plants are nontoxic and those that are usually require ingestion of rather large amounts before symptoms of toxicity appear. Several plants, however, are extremely poisonous, even in small amounts. Treatment for ingestion of poisonous plants is similar to that of ingestion of other toxic substances and the usual protocol should be followed; other measures are generally supportive and symptomatic.

Pupil Reactions

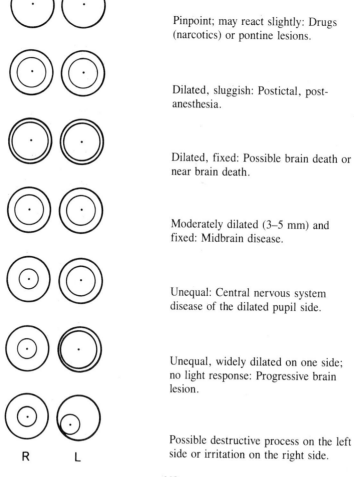

Pinpoint; may react slightly: Drugs (narcotics) or pontine lesions.

Dilated, sluggish: Postictal, post-anesthesia.

Dilated, fixed: Possible brain death or near brain death.

Moderately dilated (3–5 mm) and fixed: Midbrain disease.

Unequal: Central nervous system disease of the dilated pupil side.

Unequal, widely dilated on one side; no light response: Progressive brain lesion.

Possible destructive process on the left side or irritation on the right side.

R   L

643

Scoring Systems

Apgar score

Sign	0	1	2
Color	Blue	Acrocyanosis	Pink
Heart rate	0	100	100
Reflex irritability	No response	Grimace	Cry
Muscle tone	Flaccid	Flexion of extremities	Active
Respiratory effort	Absent	Slow, irregular	Strong, crying

Apgar score 0–3: Full resuscitation.
Apgar score 4–6: Suction and temperature support.
Apgar score 7–10: Best possible condition; transfer to newborn nursery.

Asthma score

Signs and symptoms	0	1	2
Cyanosis	None	Present on room air	Present in 40% oxygen
Wheezing	None	With stethoscope	Audible without stethoscope
Distress	None	Intercostal retractions	All accessory muscles used
Breath sounds	Normal	Asymmetrical	Decreased to absent
Cerebral function	Normal	Depressed or agitated	Comatose

Score ≥5 indicates impending respiratory failure: Monitor arterial blood gases, initiate intravenous fluids and bronchodilator therapy, administer oxygen, and be prepared to intubate the patient (notify the anesthesiologist).

Score ≥7 indicates respiratory failure: Intubate the patient, monitor arterial blood gases, initiate intravenous fluids and bronchodilator therapy, provide cardiovascular support, if necessary, and mechanically ventilate the patient.

Modified from Wood and Downes, 1972, with permission.

Newborn Maturity Rating and Classification

ESTIMATION OF GESTATIONAL AGE BY MATURITY RATING

Symbols: × - 1st Exam   ○ - 2nd Exam

Gestation by Dates _____ wks

Birth Date _____ Hour _____ am / pm

APGAR _____ 1 min _____ 5 min

MATURITY RATING

Score	Wks
5	26
10	28
15	30
20	32
25	34
30	36
35	38
40	40
45	42
50	44

NEUROMUSCULAR MATURITY

	0	1	2	3	4	5
Posture						
Square Window (Wrist)	90°	60°	45°	30°	0°	
Arm Recoil	180°		100°-180°	90°-100°	<90°	
Popliteal Angle	180°	160°	130°	110°	90°	<90°
Scarf Sign						
Heel to Ear						

PHYSICAL MATURITY

	0	1	2	3	4	5
SKIN	gelatinous red, transparent	smooth pink, visible veins	superficial peeling &/or rash, few veins	cracking pale area, rare veins	parchment, deep cracking, no vessels	leathery, cracked, wrinkled
LANUGO	none	abundant	thinning	bald areas	mostly bald	
PLANTAR CREASES	no crease	faint red marks	anterior transverse crease only	creases ant. 2/3	creases cover entire sole	
BREAST	barely percept.	flat areola, no bud	stippled areola, 1–2 mm bud	raised areola, 3–4 mm bud	full areola, 5–10 mm bud	
EAR	pinna flat, stays folded	sl. curved pinna, soft with slow recoil	well-curv. pinna, soft but ready recoil	formed & firm with instant recoil	thick cartilage, ear stiff	
GENITALS Male	scrotum empty, no rugae		testes descending, few rugae	testes down, good rugae	testes pendulous, deep rugae	
GENITALS Female	prominent clitoris & labia minora		majora & minora equally prominent	majora large, minora small	clitoris & minora completely covered	

SCORING SECTION

	1st Exam=X	2nd Exam=O
Estimating Gest Age by Maturity Rating	_____ Weeks	_____ Weeks
Time of Exam	Date _____ am pm Hour _____	Date _____ am pm Hour _____
Age at Exam	_____ Hours	_____ Hours
Signature of Examiner	_____ M.D.	_____ M.D.

Scoring System from J. L. Ballard, et al. 1977. Figures adapted from A. Y. Sweet, 1977.

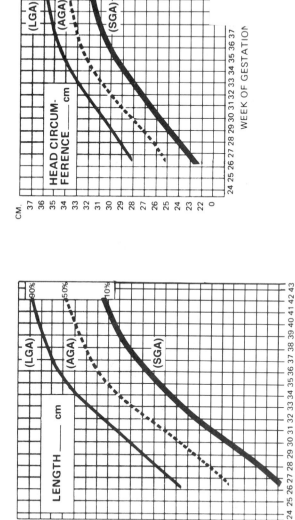

CLASSIFICATION OF NEWBORNS—
BASED ON MATURITY AND INTRAUTERINE GROWTH
Symbols: × - 1st Exam   ○ - 2nd Exam

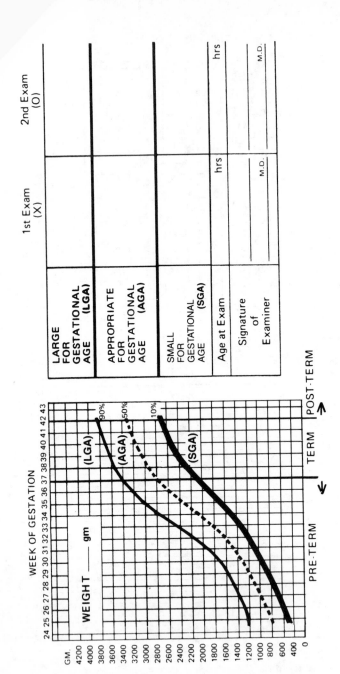

Adapted from L. C. Lubchenco, *et al.* (1966) and F. C. Battaglia and L. C. Lubchenco (1967).

Vitamin Deficiencies and Excesses

Diagnosis	Treatment

Vitamin A Deficiency

Clinical manifestations
  Insidious onset
  Impairment of dark adaptation (night blindness)
  Drying of conjunctiva and cornea
  Bitot spots (gray plaques on the bulbar conjunctiva)
  Mental and growth retardation
  Anemia
  Apathy
  Increased intracranial pressure
Laboratory and clinical tests
  Dark adaptation test
  Serum carotine level (decreased absorption of vitamin A in malabsorptive states)
  Vitamin A absorption test

Night blindness and conjunctival disease:
  Vitamin A, 5,000 to 10,000 units/day for 10 days **or** 200,000 units i.m. once
Corneal lesions: Vitamin A,
  100,000 units i.m. once, **then**
  200,000 units p.o. once 7 days after the first dose. Antibiotic ophthalmic ointment may be required
Provide adequate nutrition
Water-soluble vitamin A preparation (2,000 units/day) should be provided to patients with chronic fat malabsorption

Vitamin A Excess (Hypervitaminosis A)

Clinical manifestations
  Vomiting and drowsiness
  Pseudotumor cerebri (vomiting, papilledema, bulging of the anterior fontanelle, and increased intracranial pressure)
  Chronic ingestion may lead to failure to thrive, anorexia, irritability, chelosis, alopecia, seborrheic lesions, plantar desquamation of the skin, and hepatomegaly
  Tender swelling of the bones may occur
Laboratory and clinical tests
  Vitamin A level is increased
  Radiographs of the long bones show midshaft hyperostosis
  Hypercalcemia may occur

Discontinue intake of vitamin A
Give supportive and symptomatic treatment
Restrict intake of calcium if hypercalcemia is present
If hypercalcemia is severe:
  Hydrate with half-normal saline and assure a good urine output
  Furosemide, 0.5 to 1.0 mg/kg every 6 to 12 hr, is given until the calcium level falls
  Steroids (prednisone, 2 mg/kg/day) is given initially, then tapered

Vitamin D Deficiency

Clinical manifestations
  Craniotabes
  Palpable and visable enlargement of the costochondral junctions (rachitic rosary)
  Cranial asymmetry and bossing
  Abnormal eruption and calcification of teeth and extensive dental caries
  Scoliosis and thoracolumbar kyphosis
  Epiphyseal enlargement of the wrists and ankles

Nutritional deficiency
  Vitamin D_2 (ergocalciferol), 5,000 to 10,000 units/day p.o. until the biochemical abnormalities resolve and healing is complete; **then,** 400 IU/day, **or** Vitamin D_2, 600,000 IU in a single dose (this is not mentioned in the manufacturer's directions for use)
Chronic renal disease
  Normalize hyperphosphatemia by

Vitamin Deficiencies and Excesses *(continued)*

Diagnosis	Treatment

Bending of the shafts of the long bones causing genu varum or genu valgum
Short stature
Lax ligaments
Poorly developed musculature and decreased muscle tone
Laboratory and clinical tests
  Calcium level is normal or low
  Phosphorus level is low
  Alkaline phosphatase level is high
  Urine cyclic AMP level is elevated
  1,25-dihydroxycholecalciferol (1,25-DHCC) level is low
  Radiographs show cupping and fraying of the distal radius and ulna, decreased bone density, and, during healing, a line of preparatory calcification
	dietary restriction and phosphate-binding agents
	1,25-DHCC and vitamin D_3, 0.25 to 0.50 μg/day p.o.; calcium levels must be closely followed since hypercalcemia can occur.
	Vitamin D-dependent rickets (autosomal recessive)
	  Vitamin D_2 40,000 to 50,000 IU/day **or** vitamin D_3, 1 to 2 μg/day

Vitamin D Excess

Clinical manifestations
  Hypercalcemia and hypercalciuria
  Generalized osteoporosis
  Metastatic calcifications
  Dehydration
  Hypotonia, irritability, constipation, and anorexia
  Hypertension, aortic stenosis, and retinopathy
	Discontinue vitamin D
	Decrease calcium intake
	Assure adequate hydration and urine output
	If hypercalcemia is severe, steroids, EDTA, and/or aluminum hydroxide orally may be required (see treatment of Vitamin A excess for recommendations for treatment of hypercalcemia)

Vitamin E Deficiency

Clinical manifestations (variable and questionable)
  Muscle weakness and focal necrosis of striated muscle
  Creatinuria
  Anemia (hemolytic and nonhemolytic)
Laboratory and clinical tests
  Vitamin E level
  Peroxice hemolysis test on the patient's red blood cells
	Provide an adequate diet (the exact requirement is not known)
	Provide vitamin E supplementation to patients with conditions that cause fat malabsorption
	Provide vitamin E supplementation to premature infants (15 to 25 IU/day)

Vitamin K Deficiency

Clinical manifestations
  Hypoprothrombinemia
  Hemorrhagic diseases
Laboratory and clinical tests
  Prolonged prothrombin time (PT) and partial thromboplastin time (PTT)
	Mild deficiencies: Vitamin K_1, 1 to 2 mg/day p.o.
	Severe deficiencies: Vitamin K_1, 5 mg/day i.m. or i.v.
	Salicylate intoxication: Vitamin K_1, 1 to 2 mg i.m. or i.v.
	Severe liver disease
	  Frequently does not respond to vitamin K administration; whole blood transfusion is usually required

Vitamin B₁ Deficiency (Beriberi)

Clinical manifestations
  Classical triad: Peripheral neuritis, congestive heart failure, and psychiatric disturbances
  Dry beriberi: Patients are pale, listless, and apathetic; dyspnea is usually present; ankle
	Thiamin HCl,
	  5 to 25 mg i.m. or i.v. initially, **then** 5 to 10 mg/day for 1 month
	  Diet should contain a minimum of 1.5 g of protein/kg of body weight/day

Diagnosis	Treatment

and knee jerks are absent
Wet beriberi: Signs of congestive heart failure
    predominate; patients appear pale,
    malnourished, and edematous; dyspnea,
    tachycardia, vomiting, and absent ankle
    jerks occur
Hoarseness is characteristic
Increased intracranial pressure and coma
    may predominate the clinical picture.
Laboratory and clinical tests
    Clinical response after the administration of
        thiamin is the best test for deficiency
    Monitor blood lactic acid and pyrivic acid level

Vitamin B$_2$ (Riboflavin) Deficiency

Clinical manifestations
    Chelosis (perlèche)
    Inflammation of the tongue, resulting in loss
        of papillary structures (smooth appearing)
    Conjunctivitis, keratitis, and photophobia
    Seborrheic dermatitis
Laboratory and clinical tests
    Urinary excretion of vitamin B$_2$ is <30 µg/day

Provide a diet adequate in riboflavin
Riboflavin, 6 to 20 mg/day p.o.
Severe deficiency; Vitamin B$_2$, 25 mg initially,
    then 6 to 20 mg/day p.o.
Recovery from symptoms is usually rapid if
    treatment is adequate

Niacin Deficiency (Pellegra)

Clinical manifestations
    Dermatitis, diarrhea, dementia
    Glossitis
    Characteristic skin manifestations:
        symmetrical sharply demarcated sunburn-
        like rash; exacerbated by light causing a
        "pellagrous glove" (hand involvement),
        "pellagrous boot" (foot involvement), and/or
        "Casal's necklace" (neck involvement)
Laboratory and clinical tests
    There is a rapid response to the
        administration of niacin
    Urine levels of n-methylnicotinamide are low

Provide a diet adequate in tryptophane
Nicotinamide, 50 mg s.c. three times a day
    until there is significant clinical
    improvement
After improvement, supplement the diet with
    10 to 20 mg/day p.o.

Vitamin B$_6$ (Pyridoxine) Deficiency

Clinical manifestations
    Seizures (infants and older children)
    Peripheral neuritis
    Microcytic hypochromic anemia
    Chelosis, glossitis, seborrhea
Laboratory and clinical tests
    After other causes of neonatal seizures are
        ruled out, inject 100 mg of pyridoxine;
        seizure cessation is diagnostic
    In older children, improvement of EEG tracing
        with injection of pyridoxine is diagnostic

Infants: Pyridoxine, 10 to 20 mg p.o. for 3
    weeks, **then** 2 to 5 mg/day for 3 weeks
Older children on isoniazid: 10 mg pyridoxine/
    100 mg isoniazid/day

Folic Acid Deficiency

Clinical manifestations and laboratory tests
    Decrease in serum folate level
    Hypersegmented neutrophils in the peripheral
        smear (3.42 segments/cell/100 cells)
    Megaloblastic changes in the blood and
        marrow

Folic acid, 5 mg/day p.o. for 2 or 3 weeks
Adequate folic acid in the diet:
    Infants require 50 µg/day,
    children require 100 to 300 µg/day, and
    children >10 years old require 400 µg/day

Vitamin Deficiencies and Excesses *(continued)*

Diagnosis	Treatment

Anemia
Sleeplessness and irritability
Vitamin B_{12} level is normal (or low if a
  combined deficiency is present); folate
  administration to patients with vitamin B_{12}
  deficiencies will correct the hematological
  abnormality, but will not affect the CNS
  manifestations

Vitamin B_{12} Deficiency

Clinical manifestations
  Pernicious anemia (megaloblastic)
  Neurological changes resulting from posterior
    and lateral column demyelinization
    (paresthesias, sensory deficits, decreased
    or absent deep tendon reflexes, confusion,
    and abnormalities of memory)
Laboratory and clinical tests
  Hypersegmentation of the neutrophils
  Megalocytes on the peripheral smear
  Vitamin B_{12} level is <100 μg/ml
  Shilling test: Cobalt-labeled vitamin B_{12}, 0.5
    μg given orally, followed in 2 hr by 1,000 μg
    parenterally; urine is collected; less than 7%
    of labeled vitamin B_{12} in 24 hr in the urine
    indicates a lack of intrinsic factor
  Occasionally, gastric mucosal biopsy is
    required for diagnosis
  Urine level of methylmalonic acid is increased

Uncomplicated deficiency
  Cyanocobalamine, 1 μg/day i.m. for 10 days,
  then 1 to 2 μg/month i.m.
Complicated deficiency
  Cyanocobalamin, 15 to 50 μg every other day
  for 2 to 4 weeks, *then* 30 to 100 μg/month
  i.m.
In most cases, treatment must continue for life

Vitamin C Deficiency (Scurvy)

Clinical manifestations
  Early symptoms are vague; irritability,
    vomiting, diarrhea, and anorexia may occur
  Irritability increases and the child resists
    being moved because of tenderness of the
    legs
  Pseudoparalysis occurs from pain and the
    child lies in a frog position
  Swelling along the long bone shafts;
    subperiosteal hemorrhage can be palpated
  Apprehensive facial expression
  Bluish-purple spongy swelling of the gums
    (especially in the region of the upper
    incisors) and other areas of the mucous
    membranes
  Delayed wound healing
  Anemia, petechiae, fever, and joint swelling
Laboratory and clinical tests
  The diagnosis is made by identifying the
    clinical syndrome and characteristic
    radiographic findings
    Changes are greatest around the knees
    Bones have a ground-glass appearance

Provide an adequate diet
Ascorbic acid,
  100 to 200 mg/day p.o., i.m. or i.v. for 1 or 2
  weeks

Diagnosis	Treatment
The cortex is thin	
There is a sharp outline of the epiphysis	
"White line of Fränkel" occurs at the metaphysis	
Zone of rarefaction beneath the white line is present	
Elevated and calcified periosteum is present; subperiosteal hemorrhage is seen during healing	

References and Bibliography

Alexander, J. W., and Good, R. A. (1970): *Immunobiology for Surgeons.* Saunders, Philadelphia.

American Academy of Pediatrics (1982): Report of the Committee on Infectious Diseases.

Apley, J. (1974): The child with abdominal pain. *Ped. Clin. North Am.,* 21:991.

Aranda, J. V., Grondin, D., and Sasyniuk, B. I. (1981): Pharmacologic considerations in the therapy of neonatal apnea. *Ped. Clin. North Am.,* 28:113.

Arena, J. M. (1974): *Poisoning: Toxicology—Symptoms—Treatments.* Charles C Thomas, Springfield, Illinois.

Artman, M., and Graham, T. P., Jr. (1982): Congestive heart failure in infancy: Recognition and management. *Am. Heart J.,* 103:1040–1055.

Anderson, B. J., McDonald, F. J., et al. (1976): Clinical disorders of water metabolism. *Kid. Int.,* 10:117.

Avery, G. B., ed. (1975): *Neonatology, Pathophysiology and Management of the Newborn.* J. B. Lippincott, Philadelphia.

Aynsley-Green, A. (1982): Hypoglycemia in infants and children. *Clin. Endocrinol. Metab.,* 11:159–194.

Ballard, J. L., et al. (1977): A simplified assessment of gestational age. *Pediatr. Res.,* 11:374.

Barrows, H. S., and Tamblyn, R. M. (1980): *Problem-Based Learning: An Approach to Medical Education,* p. 206. Springer, New York.

Battaglia, F. C., and Lubchenco, L. C. (1967): Classification of newborns based on maternity and intrauterine growth. *J. Pediatr.,* 71:159.

Beaudet, A. L. (1978): Genetic diagnostic studies for mental retardation. In: *Current Problems in Pediatrics,* Vol. 8, No. 5. Year Book, Chicago.

Beckwith, J. B. (1973): The sudden infant death syndrome. In: *Current Problems in Pediatrics,* Vol. 3, No. 8. Year Book, Chicago.

Beckwith, J. B., and Palmer, N. F. (1978): Histopathology and prognosis of Wilm's tumor. *Cancer,* 41:1937.

Bell, W. E. (1978): Increased intracranial pressure—Diagnosis and management. In: *Current Problems in Pediatrics,* Vol. 8, No. 4. Year Book, Chicago.

Berquest, W. E., et al. (1981): Gastroesophageal reflux—Associated recurrent pneumonia and chronic asthma in children. *Pediatrics,* 68:29–35.

Berritz, W. E., and Talro, D. S. (1981): *The Pediatric Drug Handbook,* p. 475. Year Book, Chicago.

Biller, J. A., and Yeager, A. M., eds. (1981): *The Harriet Lane Handbook,* 9th ed. Year Book, Chicago.

Blanksma, L. A., et al. (1969): Incidence of high blood lead levels in Chicago children. *Pediatrics,* 44:661.

Bond, J. V. (1976): Neuroblasoma metastatic to the liver in infants. *Arch. Dis. Child,* 51:879.

Breslow, N. W., et al. (1978) Wilm's tumor: Prognostic factors for patients without metastasis at diagnosis. *Cancer,* 41:1577.

Brooks, J. G. (1981): The child who nearly drowns. *Am. J. Dis. Child,* 135:999.

Brooks, J. G. (1982): Apnea of infancy and sudden infant death syndrome. *Am. J. Dis. Child,* 136:1012–1023.

Brooks, L. J., and Cropp, G. J. A. (1981): Theophylline therapy in bronchiolitis. *Am. J. Dis. Child,* 135:934.

Carter, S., and Gold, A. P. (1974): Limp infant syndrome. In: *Neurology of Infancy and Childhood*, p. 216. Appleton-Century-Crofts, Norwalk, Connecticut.

Chamberlin, R. W. (1982): Prevention of behavioral problems in young children. *Ped. Clin. North Am.*, 29:239.

Chisolm, J. J. (1968): The use of chelating agents in the treatment of acute and chronic lead intoxication in childhood. *J. Pediatr.*, 73:1.

Chisolm, J. J., and Kaplan, E. (1968): Lead poisoning in childhood—Comprehensive management and prevention. *J. Pediatr.*, 73:492.

Clyman, R. I., and Hegmann, M. A. (1981): Pharmacology of the ductus arteriosus. *Ped. Clin. North Am.*, 28:77.

Committee on Accident and Poison Prevention. (1981): First aid for the choking child. *Pediatrics*, 67:744.

Committee on Accident and Poison Prevention (1981): Trampolines II. *Pediatrics*, 67:438.

Crone, R. K. (1980): Acute circulatory failure in children. *Ped. Clin. North Am.*, 27:525.

Cupoli, J. M., et al. (1980): Failure to thrive. In: *Current Problems in Pediatrics*, Vol. 10, No. 11. Year Book, Chicago.

Dean, J. M., and McComb, J. G. (1981): Intracranial pressure monitoring in severe near-drowning. *Neurosurgery*, 9:627.

DeLemarens, S. A. (1978): Management of Wilm's tumor. *Ped. Ann.*, 7(8):52.

Dodge, W. F. (1969): Detection of bacteriuria in children. *J. Pediatr.*, 74:107–110.

Donegan, J. H. (1981): New concepts in cardiopulmonary resuscitation. *Anesth. Anal.* 60:100–108.

DuBrow, I. W., Fisher, E. A., Amat-Y-Leon, F., Denes, P., Wu, D., Rosen, K., and Hastreiter, A. R. (1975): Comparison of cardiac refractory periods in children and adults. *Circulation*, 51:485.

Duchett, J. W., and Koop, C. E. (1977): Neuroblastoma. *Urol. Clin. North Am.* 4:258.

Ellis, M., Robertson, W. O., and Rumack, B. (1979): Plant-ingestion poisoning from A to Z. *Patient Care*, 13:86–140.

Fine, P. R., et al. (1972): Pediatric blood levels: A study in 14 Illinois cities of intermediate population. *JAMA*, 221:13.

Francis, D. E. M., ed. (1974): *Diets for Sick Children*, 3rd ed. Blackell, London.

Frates, R. C. (1981): Analysis of predictive factors in the assessment of warm water near drowning in children. *Am. J. Dis. Child*, 135:1006.

Fritz, G. K., and Armbrust, J. (1982): Enuresis and encopresis. *Psychiatr. Clin. North Am.*, 5:283–296.

Galler, J. R., Neustein, S., and Walker, W. A. (1980): Clinical aspects of recurrent abdominal pain in children. *Adv. Ped.* 27:31–53.

Gardner, L. I., ed. (1969): *Endocrine and Genetic Diseases of Childhood and Adolescence*, 2nd ed. Saunders, Philadelphia.

Gersony, W. M., and Hordof, A. J. (1978): Infective enocarditis and diseases of the pericardium. *Ped. Clin. North Am.*, 25:831.

Goodman, R. M., and Gorlin, R. J. (1977): *Genetic Disorders*, 2nd ed. Mosby, St. Louis.

Gorman, R. J., Saxon, S., and Snead, O. C. (1981): Neurologic sequelae of Rocky Mountain spotted fever. *Pediatrics*, 67:354.

Gosselin, R. E., et al. *Clinical Toxicology of Commercial Products*. Williams and Wilkins, Baltimore, Maryland.

Gould, J. B. (1979): Management of the near-miss infant: A personal perspective. *Ped. Clin. North Am.*, 26:857.

Guntheroth, W. G. (1978): Disorders of heart rate and rhythm. *Ped. Clin. North Am.* 25:869.

Hahn, J. F. (1980): Cerebral edema and neurointensive care. *Ped. Clin. North Am.* 27:587.

Handsfield, H. H. (1982): Sexually transmitted diseases. *Hosp. Pract.*, 18:99–116.

Hanson, P. A. (1977): Floppy baby. Oppenheim's disease, amyotonic congenita. *Ped. Ann.*, 6:194–202.

Harmitz, P. R., and Walker, W. A. (1980): Nausea and vomiting. In: *Current Pediatric Therapy*. Vol. 9, p. 168. Saunders, Philadelphia.

Harrison, H. E., and Harrison, H. C. (1979): Disorders of calcium and phosphate metabolism in childhood and adolescence. In: *Major Problems in Clinical Pediatrics*, Vol. 20, Saunders, Philadelphia.

Hart, N. J.: Therapeutic considerations in the treatment of common cardiac arrhythmias. In: *Cardiovascular Therapy*, edited by D. G. Vidt. F. A. Davis, Philadelphia.

Hauger, S. V. (1981): Facial cellulitis: An early indicator of group B streptococcal bacteremia. *Pediatrics*, 67:376.

Helefant, R. H. (1980): *Bellet's Essentials of Cardiac Arrhythmias*. Saunders, Philadelphia.

Hellerstein, H. K., and Turell, D. J. (1964): Mode of death in coronary artery disease: Electrocardiographic and clinicopathological correlation. In: *Sudden Cardiac Death*, edited by B. Surawicz and E. D. Pellegrino, p. 17. Grune and Stratton, New York.

Herbst, J. J. (1981): Gastroesophageal reflux. *J. Pediatr.*, 98:859–870.

Hoekelman, R. A., ed. (1978): *Principles of Pediatrics: Health Care of the Young*. McGraw-Hill, New York.

Holmes, L. B. (1972): Mental retardation. In: *Atlas of Diseases with Associated Physical Abnormalities*. Macmillan, New York.

Hughes, I. A. (1982): Congenital and acquired disorders of the adrenal cortex. *Clin. Endocrinol. Metab.*, 11:89–125.

Jolley, H. (1981): *Diseases of Children*. Blackwell, London.

Jones, K.L. (1978): Dysmorphology: An approach to a child with structural defects. In: *Current Problems in Pediatrics*, Vol. 8, No. 3. Year Book, Chicago.

Illinois Association for Retarded Citizens and C. D. C. (1977): *Medical Treatment Guide for Pediatric Lead Poisoning*. Atlanta.

Kanarek, K. S., Williams, P. R., and Curran, J. S. (1982): Total parenteral nutrition in infants and children. *Adv. Ped.*, 29:151.

Kaplan, E. I. (1978): Acute rheumatic fever. *Ped. Clin. North Am.*, 25:817.

Kaplan, S. A. (1979): Disorders of the adrenal cortex, I and II. *Ped. Clin. North Am.*, 26:65.

Kelalis, P. P., and King, L. R. (1976): *Clinical Pediatric Urology*. Vols. I and II. Saunders, Philadelphia.

Kelly, D. H., and Nelson, N. M. (1981): Should infants at risk for sudden infant death syndrome be monitored? In: *Controversies in Child Health and Pediatric Practice*, pp. 59–88. McGraw-Hill, New York.

Kempe, C. H., Silver, H. K., and Brien, D., eds. (1982): *Current Pediatric Diagnosis and Therapy*, 7th ed. Lange Medical Publishers, Los Altos, California.

Knobloch, H., and Pacamanick, B., eds. (1974): *Gesel and Amatruda's Developmental Diagnosis*, 3rd ed. Harper and Row, Hagerstown, Maryland.

Landtman, B. (1947): Heart arrhythmias in children. *Acta Pediatr.* 34:(Suppl. I).

LanFranchi, S. H. (1979): Hypothyroidism. *Ped. Clin. North Am.*, 26:33.

Lansky, L. L. (1975): *Pediatric Neurology: A Practitioner's Guide*, p. 275. Medical Examination Publishing, New York.

Lanzkowsky, P. (1980): *Pediatric Hematology–Oncology: A Treatise for the Clinician*. McGraw-Hill, New York.

Leap, L. L., Breslow, N. E., and Bishop, H. C. (1978): The surgical treatment of Wilm's tumor: Results of the national Wilm's tumor study. *Ann. Surg.*, 187:351.

Leff, A. (1982): Pathogenesis of asthma. *Chest*, 81:224–229.

Leffert, F. (1980): The management of chronic asthma. *J. Pediatr.*, 97:875–885.

Levine, M. D. (1982): Encopresis—Its potentiation, evaluation and alleviation. *Ped. Clin. North Am.*, 29:315.

Levine, M. D. (1982): The high prevalence—low severity developmental disorders. *Adv. Ped.*, 29:529.

Levison, H., Tabachnik, E. and Newth, C. J. L. (1982): Wheezing in infancy, croup and epiglottis. In: *Current Problems in Pediatrics*, Vol. 12. Year Book, Chicago.

Levy, J. S., Winters, R. W., and Heird, W. C. (1980): Total parenteral nutrition in pediatric patients. *Pediatr. Rev.*, 2:99–106.

Lieberman, E. (1980): Blood pressure and primary hypertension in childhood and adolescence.

In: *Current Problems in Pediatrics*, Vol. 10. No. 4. Year Book, Chicago.

Lubchenco, L. O. (1976): *The High Risk Infant—Major Problems in Clinical Pediatrics*, Vol. 14. Saunders, Philadelphia.

Malinowski, S. W., et al. (1979): Management of human bite injuries of the hand. *J. Trauma*, 19:655.

March, J. L. (1980): Comprehensive care for craniofacial anomalies. In: *Current Problems in Pediatrics*, Vol. 10, No. 9. Year Book, Chicago.

McCarthy, P. L., et al. (1980): Evaluation of arthritis and arthralgia in the pediatric patient. *Clin. Pediatr.*, 19:183.

McMillan, J. A., Nieburg, P. I., and Oski, F. A. (1977): *The Whole Pediatrician's Catalog*, Saunders, Philadelphia.

McMillan, J. A., Stockman, J A., III, and Oski, F. A. (1979): *The Whole Pediatrician's Catalog*, Vol. 2. Saunders, Philadelphia.

Moodie, D. S. (1982): Medical management of infants and children with congenital heart disease. In: *Cardiovascular Therapy*, edited by D. G. Vidt. F. A. Davis, Philadelphia.

Muldoon, R. L., Jaecker, D. L., and Kiefer, H. K. (1981): Legionnaire's disease in children. *Pediatrics*, 67:329.

New, M. I., and Levine, L. S. (1981): Congenital adrenal hyperplasia. *Clin. Biochem.*, 14:258–272.

Orlowski, J. P. (1980): Cardiopulmonary resuscitation in children. *Ped. Clin. North Am.*, 27:495.

Paul-Lee, W. N. (1979): Thyroiditis, hyperthyroidism and tumors. *Ped. Clin. North Am.*, 26:53.

Pearn, J. H., et al. (1970) Bathtub drownings: Report of seven cases. *Pediatrics*, 64:68.

Perkin, R. M., and Levin, D. L. (1982): Shock in the pediatric patient. Parts I and II. *J. Pediatr.*, 101:163–169.

Piomelli, S. et al. (1973): The FEP (free erythrocyte prophyrins) test: A screening micromethod for lead poisoning. *Pediatrics*, 51:254.

Pizzo, P. A., Lovejoy, F. H., and Smith, D. H. (1975): Prolonged fever in children: Review of 100 cases. *Pediatrics*, 55:468.

Plotkin, S. A. (1981): New rabies vaccine. *Pediatrics*, 68:131.

Powers, D. R. (1974): Wilm's tumor: Recent advances and unsolved problems. *Ped. Ann.*, I:55–70.

Press, E. (1956): *Accidental Poisoning in Childhood*. American Academy of Pediatrics, Evanston, Illinois.

Rabe, E. F. (1964): The hypnotic infant. *J. Pediatr.*, 64:422.

Reimer, S. L., Michener, W. M., and Steiger, E. (1980): Nutritional support of the critically ill child. *Ped. Clin. North Am.*, 27:647.

Reiter, E. O., Roof, A. W., Rettig, K., and Vargas, A. (1981): Childhood thyromegaly: Recent developments. *J. Pediatr.*, 99:507–518.

Ried, D. H. S. (1970): Treatment of the poisoned child. *Arch. Dis. Child*, 45:428.

Riley, H. D. (1975): Management of urinary tract infections in children. *Urol. Clin. North Am.*, 2(3):537–556.

Robert, N. K. (1975): *The Cardiac Conducting System and the His' Bundle Electrogram*. Appleton-Century-Crofts, Norwalk, Connecticut.

Roberts K. B. (1979): *Manual of Clinical Problems in Pediatrics*, p. 459. Little Brown, Boston.

Root, A. W., et al. (1979): The thyroid—Recent advances in normal and abnormal physiology. *Adv. Ped.*, 26:441–534.

Rosen, M. R., Hoffman, B. F., and Wit, A. L. (1975): Electrophysiology and pharmacology of cardiac arrhythmias. III. The causes and treatment of cardiac arrhythmias. *Am Heart J.*, 89:115.

Rosen, M. R., Wit, A. L., and Hoffman, B. F. (1974): Electrophysiology and pharmacology of cardiac arrhythmias. I. Cellular electrophysiology of the mammalian heart. *Am. Heart J.*, 88:380.

Rosenfield, R. L., et al. (1980): The diagnosis and management of intersex. In: *Current Problems in Pediatrics*, Vol. 10, No. 7. Year Book, Chicago.

Rothner, A. D. (1979): Headaches in children—A review. *Headache*, 19:156.

Roy, C. C., Silverman, A., and Cozetto, F. J. (1975): *Pediatric Clinical Gastroenterology.* Mosby, St. Louis.

Rubin, P. (1968): Cancer of the myogenital tract: Wilm's tumor and neuroblastoma. *JAMA,* 204:123.

Rudolph, A. M., ed. (1982): *Pediatrics.* Appleton-Century-Crofts, Norwalk, Connecticut.

Rumack, B. H., and Matthew, H. (1975): Acetaminophen poisoning and toxicity. *Pediatrics,* 55:873.

Schwartz, A. D., et al. (1974): Spontaneous regression of disseminated neuroblastoma. *J. Pediatr.,* 85:760.

Senior, B., and Wolfsdorf, J. I. (1979): Hypoglycemia in children. *Ped. Clin. North Am.,* 26:171.

Sheldon, S. H. (1979): *Pediatric Differential Diagnosis: A Problem Oriented Approach,* p. 147. Raven Press, New York.

Sheldon, S. H. (1981): *Manual of Practical Pediatrics,* p. 289. Raven Press, New York.

Shepard, T. H. (1976): *A Catalog of Teratogenic Agents,* 2nd ed. Johns Hopkins University Press, Baltimore.

Shinnar, S., and D'Souza, B. J. (1982): The diagnosis and management of headaches in childhood. *Ped. Clin. North Am.,* 29:74–79.

Shnaps, Y., et al. (1981): The chemically abused child. *Pediatrics,* 68:119

Shwachman, H. (1978): Cystic fibrosis. In: *Current Problems in Pediatrics,* Vol. 10, No. 7. Year Book, Chicago.

Sims, D. G. (1977): Histiocytosis X. *Arch. Dis. Child,* 52:433.

Smith, D. W. (1976): *Recognizable Patterns of Human Malformation,* 2nd ed. Saunders, Philadelphia.

Smith, D. W. (1977): Growth and its disorders. In: *Major Problems in Clinical Pediatrics,* Vol. 15. Saunders, Philadelphia.

Spiro, A. T. (1977): Approach to diagnosis in the child with muscle weakness. *Pediatr. Ann.,* 6(3):149–161.

Stewart, A. L., Reynolds, E. O., and Lipscomb, A. P. (1981): Outcome for infants of very low birthweight—Survey of world literature. *Lancet,* 1:1034–1040.

Stollerman, G. H. (1975): *Rheumatic Fever and Streptococcal Infections.* Grune and Stratton, New York.

Strassburg, M.A., et al. (1981): Animal bites: Patterns of treatment. *Ann. Emerg. Med.,* 10:193.

Sulayman, R. F., and Thilenius, O. G. (1981): Complication of heart disease in children. *Pediatrician,* 10:99.

Summitt, R. L., and Etteldorf, J. N. (1964): Salicylate intoxication in children—Experience with peritoneal dialysis and alkalinization of the urine. *J. Pediatr.,* 64:803.

Thompson, A. J. (1980): Diagnosis and treatment of headaches in the pediatric patient. *Curr. Probl. Pediatr.,* 10:5–52.

Thompson, C. E. (1981): Diagnosis of proximal muscle weakness in childhood. *Pediatric Basics,* 31:4–7.

Truex, R. C. (1973): Anatomy of the specialized tissues of the heart. In: *Cardiac Arrhythmias,* edited by L. S. Dreifus and W. Likoff, pp. 1–12. Grune and Stratton, New York.

Vaughan, V. C., McCay, R. J., and Behrman, R. E., eds. (1979): *Nelson Textbook of Pediatrics,* 11th ed. Saunders, Philadelphia.

Voorhess, M. L. (1979): Disorders of the adrenal medulla and multiple endocrine adenomatosus. *Ped. Clin. North Am.,* 26:2ᴜ9.

Walsh, J. K. (1981): Gastroesophageal reflux in infants. *J. Pediatr.,* 99:197–201.

Wasserman, E., and Gzomisch, D. S. (1976): *Pediatrics: A Problem Oriented Approach.* Medical Examination Publishers, New York.

Watanabe, Y., and Dreifus, L. S. (1973): Arrhythmias: Mechanisms and pathogenesis. In: *Cardiac Arrhythmias,* edited by L. S. Dreifus and W. Likoff, pp. 35–54. Grune and Stratton, New York.

Weinberger M., Hendeles, L., and Ahrens, R. (1981): Clinical pharmacology of drugs used in asthma. *Ped. Clin. North Am.,* 28:47.

White, C. B., et al. (1981): Soft tissue infections associated with *Hemophilis aphrophilus*. *Pediatrics*, 67:434.

Wilkinson, J. D., Dudgeon, L., and Sondheimer, J. M. (1981): A comparison of medical and surgical treatment of gastroesophageal reflux in severely retarded children. *J. Pediatr.*, 99:202–205.

Wit, A. L., Rosen, M. R., and Hoffman, B. F. (1974): Electrophysiology and pharmacology of cardiac arrhythmias. II. Relationship of normal and abnormal activity of cardiac fibers to the genesis of arrhythmias. *Am. Heart J.*, 88:515,664,798.

Wood, W., Downes, J., and Lecks, H. (1972): A clinical scoring system for the diagnosis of respiratory failure: A preliminary report. *Am. J. Dis. Child*, 123:227.

Yunginger, J. W. (1981): Advances in the diagnosis and treatment of stinging insect allergy. *Pediatrics*, 67:325.

Subject Index

Notes

Notes

Notes

Notes

Notes

Notes

Notes